Coronary Magnetic
Resonance Angiography

Springer
New York
Berlin
Heidelberg
Barcelona
Hong Kong
London
Milan
Paris
Singapore
Tokyo

André J. Duerinckx, MD, PhD

Chief of Radiology Service, VA North Texas
Healthcare System, and Professor of Radiology and
Medicine, The University of Texas Southwestern
Medical Center, Dallas, Texas

Editor

Coronary Magnetic Resonance Angiography

With 417 Figures

With a Foreword by Arthur E. Stillman

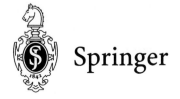 Springer

André J. Duerinckx, MD, PhD
Chief of Radiology Service
VA North Texas Healthcare System
Dallas, TX 75216, USA
and
Professor of Radiology and Medicine
University of Texas Southwestern Medical Center
Dallas, TX 75235, USA
e-mail: andréjd@earthlink.net

Cover illustration: Chapter 9, Figures 3c and 3e. Reprinted from Duerinckx AJ, Shaaban A, Lewis A, Perloff J, Laks H. 3D MR imaging of coronary arteriovenous fistulas. European Radiology 2000;10(9): 1459–1963.

Library of Congress Cataloging-in-Publication Data
Coronary magnetic resonance angiography / editor, André J. Duerinckx.
   p. cm.
   Includes bibliographical references and index.
   ISBN 0-387-94959-3 (hardcover : alk. paper).
   1. Coronary magnetic resonance angiography.   2. Angiocardiography.
I. Duerinckx, André J.
RC683.5.M35 C67 2000
616.1'207548—dc21   99-053567

Printed on acid-free paper.

Production coordinated by Chernow Editorial Services, Inc., and managed by Lesley Poliner; manufacturing supervised by Jerome Basma.
Typeset by Matrix Publishing Services, York, PA.
Printed and bound by Maple-Vail Book Manufacturing Group, York, PA.
Printed in the United States of America.

9 8 7 6 5 4 3 2 1

ISBN 0-387-94959-3   SPIN 10553128

Springer-Verlag   New York Berlin Heidelberg
A member of BertelsmannSpringer Science+Business Media GmbH

To
My parents and family in Belgium
To
David, Lucy, Cleo, and Ricky

Foreword

This is an extraordinary time for cardiac imaging. Coronary magnetic resonance angiography (MRA) was first described in 1991. After years of steady, albeit slow, progress, pioneers in coronary imaging are on the verge of seeing the fruits of their hard work. Manufacturers are investing their technical know-how in incorporating essential cardiac capabilities into their scanners and marketing dedicated cardiac magnetic resonance imaging (MRI) scanners. Coronary MRA has become a useful noninvasive clinical test. While large series patient studies have not yet been reported, it appears that the latest coronary MRA techniques may be used for screening at least select patient populations. In 1999, multidetector computed tomography (CT) has emerged as another important noninvasive coronary imaging modality. The winners of this competition are cardiac imagers and the patients they serve as each modality spurs the other on to greater capabilities.

This book by experts in their fields is an excellent resource for those already involved in cardiac imaging, as well as for the novice. Together with attending categorical courses, such as those offered by the North American Society for Cardiac Imaging and the Society for Cardiovascular Magnetic Resonance, hands-on workshops, and minifellowships, this book should aid those who wish to share in the excitement. It does no good to build demand for services that cannot be delivered. For this reason, greater involvement is strongly encouraged.

Arthur E. Stillman, MD, PhD
Cleveland Clinic Foundation
Cleveland, Ohio

Preface

Magnetic resonance angiography (MRA) of the coronary arteries has become a new clinical tool based on ultrafast magnetic resonance imaging (MRI) sequences first described in 1991. Coronary arteries are small, tortuous vessels subjected to significant physiological motions (respiration and cardiac contractions) and thus present a special challenge for MRA, unlike other vascular structures. Coronary MRA can play a clinical role in the noninvasive evaluation of congenital coronary artery anomalies, in the follow-up of coronary lesions after angioplasty, and in the evaluation of the patency of bypass grafts and coronary stents. Its clinical utility for detecting coronary lesions is still being defined. Even in this early stage of development, there are several advantages to using coronary MRA as a screening tool for proximal coronary disease in patients with ischemic heart disease. MRA is a noninvasive procedure, does not expose the patient or physician to X-ray radiation or iodinated contrast media, and may be combined with MR perfusion and functional studies. As such, even with the great potential of multislice computed tomography (CT), the use of MRA for the evaluation of coronary artery disease remains important.

We were motivated to write this book because of the increasing interest in the already-proven clinical applications of coronary MRA techniques and the fact that many commercial implementations of coronary MRA pulse sequences have become available. The interest in cardiac MRI at international meetings has dramatically increased because of all this scientific progress. It has now become obvious that cardiac MRI together with cardiac CT are important and essential noninvasive imaging and clinincal tools. Coronary MR angiographic techniques will also impact our approach to MRA of the thorax and abdomen.

This book is a review of established and most likely to succeed coronary MR angiographic techniques, with special attention to the clinical practitioner who would like to be part of this exciting activity. We also want to help the many scientists involved in this field, who may feel intimidated by the complexity of the coronary and cardiac anatomy.

Although coronary MRA may be relatively easy to perform for a cardiac-trained imager, it represents a challenge to others with less exposure to this new clinical application. The understanding of advanced MR pulse sequences and strategies may be overwhelming to some. This book on Coronary MRA attempts to demystify the art of coronary MRA by providing several "how do I do it" chapters in nontechnical language (both to the physicist and the clinician), with clearly illustrated imaging steps and protocols. The book provides a comprehensive overview of coronary MRA for those scientists and physicians planning to incorporate coronary MRA into their research or clinical practice. At the same time, it also offers a glimpse into the future.

Coronary MRA is a relatively young field that is still developing. The coronary MR angiographic techniques are in continuous flux and continue to evolve. We hope that this book will encourage more clinicians to use these new applications of magnetic resonance imaging (MRI) and MRA. We also hope that it will provide an interface among MR physicists, clinicians, and industry people to impact the diagnosis and treatment of patients with cardiovascular disease.

I want to thank my many colleagues who have contributed to this book, and who have been so patient with the many revisions. We have made an effort to keep this book as up to date as possible. I also want to thank the people at Springer-Verlag and Chernow Editorial Services, Inc. for working with me on this project. Specifically, I wish to thank Kathy Jackson and Barbara Chernow of Chernow Editorial Services and Robert Albano at Springer-Verlag for guidance and help.

André J. Duerinckx, MD, PhD
Dallas, Texas
February 2001

Contents

Contributors

Stephan Achenbach, MD
Medizinische Klinik II (Kardiologie) mit Poliklinik, University of Erlangen-Nuremberg, 91054 Erlangen, Germany

Dennis Atkinson, Msc
Academic Research Manager, General Electric Medical Systems, Irvine, CA 92612, USA

Kostaki G. Bis, MD
Department of Radiology, William Beaumont Hospital, Royal Oak, MI 48073, USA

Jan Bogaert, MD, PhD
Universitaire Ziekenhuizen Leuven-KUL, U.Z. Gasthuisberg, Leuven 3000, Belgium

Hugo G. Bogren, MD, PhD
University of California, Davis, Medical Center, Sacramento, CA 95825, USA

Michael H. Buonocore, MD, PhD
University of California, Davis, Imaging Center, Sacramento, CA 95817, USA

Daniel M. Chernoff, MD, PhD
Department of Radiology, University of California, San Francisco, Medical Center, San Francisco, CA 94143, USA

Peter G. Danias, MD, PhD, FACC
Assistant Professor of Medicine, Director, Nuclear Cardiology, Beth Israel Deaconess Medical Center and Harvard Medical School, Boston, MA 02215, USA

André J. Duerinckx, MD, PhD
Radiology Service, VA North Texas Healthcare System, Dallas, TX 75216, and Department of Radiology and Medicine, The University of Texas Southwestern Medical Center, Dallas, TX 75235, USA

Steven Dymarkowski, MD
Universitaire Ziekenhuizen Leuven-KUL, U.Z. Gasthuisberg, Leuven 3000, Belgium

Peter J. Fitzgerald, MD
Stanford University Medical Center, Stanford, CA 94305-5105, USA

E. Mark Haacke, PhD
MRI Institute for Biomedical Research, Brentwood, MI 63144, USA

Christopher J. Hardy, PhD
GE Corporate Research and Development, Schenectady, NY 12309, USA

Ali Hassan, MD
Stanford University Medical Center, Stanford, CA 94305-5105, USA

Mark B.M. Hofman, PhD
Academisch Ziekenhuis V.U., Amsterdam 1007 MB, The Netherlands

Michael Jerosch-Herold, PhD
Department of Radiology, University of Minnesota Medical Center, Minneapolis, MN 55455, USA

Hillel Laks, MD
Division of Cardiothoracic Surgery, University of California, Los Angeles, Center for Health Sciences, Los Angeles, CA 90095, USA

Anthony Lewis, MD
29002 Old Carriage Court, Agoura Hills, CA 91301, USA

Debiao Li, PhD
Northwestern University Medical School, Chicago, IL 60611, USA

Christine H. Lorenz, PhD
Royal Brompton Hospital, London SW3 6NP, UK

Warren J. Manning, MD
Associate Professor of Medicine and Radiology, Section Chief, Non-invasive Cardiac Imaging, Beth Israel Deaconess Medical Center and Harvard Medical School, Boston, MA 02215, USA

Werner Moshage, MD
University of Erlangen-Nuremberg, 91054 Erlangen, Germany

Antonino Nicosia, MD
Institute of Cardiology, Ferrarotto Hospital, University of Catania, 95124 Catania, Italy

Dudley Pennell, MD, FRCP, FACC, FESC
Director Cardiovascular MR Unit, Royal Brompton Hospital, London SW3 6NP, UK

Joseph Perloff, MD
Adult Congenital Heart Disease Center, University of California, Los Angeles, Center for Health Sciences, Los Angeles, CA 90095, USA

Johannes C. Post, PhD
Department of Cardiology, VU Medical Center, 1081 HV, Amsterdam, The Netherlands

M.B. Scheidegger
Institute of Biomedical Engineering, University and ETH Zürich, MR-Center USZ, CH-8091 Zürich, Switzerland

Akram Shaaban, MD
Department of Radiology, University of Utah Health Science Center, Salt Lake City, UT 84132, USA

Orlando Simonetti, PhD
Cardiac R&D Group, Siemens Medical Systems, Inc., Chicago, IL 60611, USA

Arthur E. Stillman, MD, PhD
Cleveland Clinic Foundation, Cleveland, OH 44195, USA

Albert C. van Rossum, MD, PhD
Professor of Cardiology, Department of Cardiology, VU Medical Center, 1081 HV, Amsterdam, The Netherlands

Thomas G. Vrachliotis, MD
Department of Cardiovascular/Interventional Radiology, Beth Israel and Deaconess Medical Center and Harvard Medical School, Boston, MA 02215, USA

Yi Wang, PhD
Radiology Service, Cornell University Medical College, New York, NY 10021, USA

Norbert Wilke, MD, PhD
Center for MR Research, University of Minnesota Medical Center, Minneapolis, MN 55455, USA

Bernd J. Wintersperger, MD
Department of Clinical Radiology, University of Munich—Grosshadern Campus, 81377 Munich, Germany

Pamela K. Woodard, MD
Washington University Medical Center, St. Louis, MO 61310, USA

1
Coronary MRA: What It Is, and Why We Should Be Interested

André J. Duerinckx

Magnetic resonance angiography (MRA) of the coronary arteries became possible in 1991 with the development of a new group of fast magnetic resonance imaging (MRI) sequences. Coronary MR angiography has since been used with great success in key clinical applications, such as the detection of coronary artery variants, and the imaging of coronary stents and bypass grafts. The new MRI techniques also allow quantification of velocity and flow in coronary arteries. The most promising aspect is the potential role of coronary MR angiography in screening for coronary artery lesions, which is actively being investigated.

Coronary artery disease remains the leading cause of death in the United States, and is responsible for an estimated 900,000 deaths per year. The estimated cost of these deaths and the additional 1.5 million heart attacks annually exceeds $60 billion in the United States alone (1). X-ray contrast angiography is widely accepted as the definitive method to define coronary anatomy; however, given that currently more than 1 million diagnostic cardiac catheterizations are performed annually in the United States (2), and the relative high procedural cost of $3000–$5000, any less-expensive noninvasive alternate test would be welcome. Coronary MRA offers the potential to replace diagnostic and screening X-ray coronary angiography in the near future in selected population groups. The impact of cardiac MRI on the global cost of healthcare and the use of diagnostic tests for myocardial ischemia will be enormous. This book will introduce the novice to these new cardiac MRI technologies and their proven and future applications. The more advanced readers will find extensive discussions of the research and preclinical work done by many investigators since 1991.

What Is Coronary MRA?

Unlike other blood vessels, coronary arteries are small tortuous vessels subjected to significant physiological motion, both cardiac and respiratory, which present a tremendous challenge to conventional MRI and MRA techniques (see Chap. 2). With the development in 1991 of a new group of fast MRI pulse sequences "reliable and reproducible" MRA of the coronary arteries has become possible and was described in the first preclinical studies published in 1993 and 1994 (3–5) (see also review in Chap. 3, and more details in Chap. 15). The term *reliable* means simply that images of good quality can routinely and reproducibly be obtained in the majority of patients. Prior to the development of these newer techniques coronary artery MRI was possible, but it was much less reliable and not considered a clinical application of cardiac MRI (see Chap. 4).

Several generations of coronary MRA techniques have since been described. All techniques use electrocardiogram (EKG) triggering. First-generation breath-hold techniques, as described in 1991, acquire one two-dimensional (2-D) image per breathhold and are commercially available on almost all new MRI scanners. They are robust and have successfully been used for specific clinical applications (see Chaps. 7–11). All imagers should become familiar with their use. The second-generation techniques use navigator pulses for respiratory gating or triggering and are referred to as "non-breathholding" or "free-breathing" techniques because they do not require breathholding. Although the initial implementations were somewhat unreliable, dramatic improvements have since been made. Third-generation techniques allow three-dimensional (3-D) volume acquisitions (multiple 2-D images) in a single breathhold, which in combination with real-time interactive slice positioning appears very promising. MR contrast agents, real-time slice positioning, and higher-resolution acquisition schemes (e.g., spiral MRA) can further improve and facilitate the use of these coronary MRA techniques.

Technical progress and changes in this subfield of cardiac MRI have been so fast that large-scale preclinical trials have not been (and probably never will be) conducted with the majority of the first- and second-generation coronary MRA pulse sequences as known today. In this chapter we will provide an overview of the book and review the development of these new cardiac MRI techniques and the initial successes with clinical applications using commercial MR scanners.

Clinical Indications for Coronary MRA

Coronary MRA is a cardiac MRI technique used to visualize the proximal and middle portion of most coronary arteries and some coronary artery branches. The techniques and practice of coronary MRA can easily be learned (see Chaps. 5 and 6). Even though it is not equivalent to conventional X-ray based coronary angiography, coronary MRA can and should be used for noninvasive imaging in a variety of clinical situations (Chap. 7). We will discuss in detail the evaluation of congenital coronary artery anomalies (Chaps. 8 and 9), and the noninvasive determination of the patency of bypass grafts (Chaps. 10 and 11) and coronary stents (Chap. 17). Coronary MRA can also be used in the follow up of known proximal coronary lesions (e.g., after angioplasty). The use of coronary MRA for blind prospective detection of unknown coronary lesions, however, is still being evaluated (Chap. 12). Coronary MRA techniques may become an integral part of the clinical evaluation and screening of patients with ischemic heart disease. Coronary MRI techniques appear to be very promising in the quantification of coronary flow and flow reserve (Chaps. 13 and 14).

Why Are Traditional Cardiac-Gated MRI and MRA Inadequate to Visualize Coronary Vessels?

Conventional cardiac-triggered MRI has provided reliable, clinically useful, and diagnostic images of cardiac structures and large vessels within the thorax for many years (6–10). With conventional cardiac MRI it has been possible to visualize coronary bypass grafts, evaluate bypass graft patency, and quantitate flow in bypass grafts (Chaps. 10 and 11). Bypass grafts are generally easier to image than are native coronary vessels because they are larger in size and because they are usually located further away from the heart and therefore undergo less cardiac motion. It is well known that traditional cardiac-triggered spin-echo (SE) and gradient-recalled-echo (GRE) images can occasionally show small portions of the native coronary artery tree (11–13), and they have been used to visualize congenital coronary artery variants (14,15). These techniques, however, have significant limitations: Motion artifacts and pulsatile flow artifacts preclude visualization of all except the very proximal or

abnormally dilated vessel anatomy; it is difficult to distinguish between coronary arteries and veins; and the pericardial space can easily be mistaken for portions of a vessel or bypass graft. In contrast to this, the new coronary MRA techniques allow much more reliable and consistent visualization of the proximal native coronary tree (16–22).

Conventional MRA techniques depict and characterize blood vessels and blood flow, and they are relatively well established in clinical practice (23–28). The term *MRA* refers to a broad array of approaches based on various physical properties of blood and blood flow. MRA techniques for body MRA have also undergone tremendous changes since the advent of dynamic contrast-enhanced (CE) breathhold 3-D MRA techniques (28). The more traditional older MRA techniques, which are still used for neuroimaging and a few other applications, rely on either time of flight (TOF) or phase contrast (PC) approaches. Modifications, such as bolus tagging and multiple velocity-encoded phase contrast acquisitions, permit quantification of velocity and flow. Even for flow within large vessels traditional TOF techniques have known limitations due to the fact that they are not cardiac triggered. Cardiac triggering improves TOF MRA for vessels with significant pulsatile flow (29,30). PC MRA techniques routinely use cardiac gating. With the use of respiratory gating or multiple respiratory averages, both cardiac triggered TOF and PC MRA perform adequately when imaging flow in large vessels even in the presence of significant pulsatile flow and moderate respiratory motion. When it comes to imaging small tortuous vessels in the chest or abdomen, however, or even any large vessel in the thorax, none of these traditional MRA techniques have been able to perform consistently or adequately. The newer CE 3-D MRA techniques now provide reliable techniques in both the abdomen and periphery as well as in the chest. MRA of pulmonary arteries, the aortic arch, and even coronary bypass grafts (see Chaps. 10 and 11) using these new CE 3-D MRA techniques is used in daily clinical practice at many centers. These newest MRA techniques, however, are not routinely cardiac-gated and are thus inadequate for imaging of native coronary vessels or the distant anastomoses of coronary bypass grafts.

Coronary MRA Pulse Sequences

Advances in MR pulse sequence design (with the first described cardiac applications in 1991) have resulted in a significant reduction of both respiratory motion artifacts (i.e., by eliminating, correcting, or compensating for respiratory motion) and pulsatile flow artifacts (i.e., by always using cardiac triggering and middiastolic acquisitions), while maintaining a reasonable short-image acquisition time (i.e., by segmenting the data acquisition in *k*-space) (31–33). Coronary MRA does significantly differ from conventional MRA in that it incorporates mechanisms to compensate for both cardiac and respiratory motion. We will always refer to these MR techniques as "coronary MRA" even though some of the techniques are variants of 2-D MRI sequences, and not really MRA techniques. Because they are used to visualize coronary vessels, however, the terminology *MRA* will be used. Most of the new coronary MRA techniques can also be applied to image larger thoracic vessels (34,35) and improved cardiac imaging in general (10,36,37). Knowledge of coronary MR imaging is relevant to any imager (radiologist, cardiologist or other physicians) interested in improving the quality of vascular imaging using MRI or MRA.

The new MRI sequences that allow reliable and reproducible MRA of the coronary arteries can be classified in many ways. In this book we opted for a classification based partially on historical developments as well as on the amount of information obtained (single 2-D images vs. 3-D slabs) for a given level of patient comfort (breathholding vs. non-breathholding) and the total duration of the data acquisition. A first generation of coronary MRA techniques was first described in 1991 and is now commercially available on most clinical MRI scanners. These techniques rely upon a combination of segmental acquisition in *k*-space of the data to minimize cardiac motion and the use of a single breathhold to minimize respiratory motion artifacts. They require sequential single breathholds, with a total examination time from 30 to 60 minutes. The typical coronary MRI quality obtained is illustrated in Figures 1.1 and 1.2. These first-generation techniques are described in Chapters 5, 14, and 15. A second generation of techniques de-

scribed in 1993–1994 allows image acquisition during repeated breathholding or during "free breathing," and opens the way for higher resolution coronary MRA with increased patient comfort. These techniques are referred to as the "navigator" techniques and are based on concepts developed for abdominal imaging many years ago. They are still undergoing extensive fine tuning. They typically require 5–12 minutes per 3-D slab acquisition, with three slabs being adequate to cover most of the heart. The coronary MRI quality that can be obtained is illustrated in Figure 1.3. These second-generation techniques are described in Chapters 6 and 16–19. Improvements to these techniques have made them into very robust and clinically useful techniques

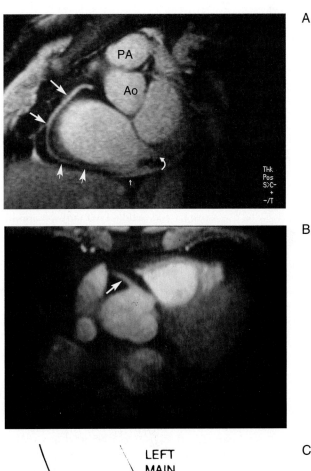

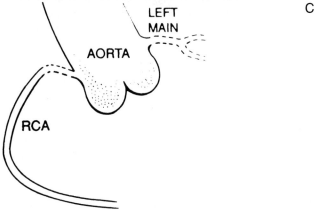

Figure 1.1. The right coronary artery (RCA) imaged with a first-generation coronary MRA technique. Each image was obtained within a breathhold. The RCA lies in the anterior atrioventricular groove. A large portion of the RCA (arrows) can usually be visualized with a single imaging plane through the anterior atrioventricular groove (A). One additional transaxial plane is often needed to show the ostium of the RCA clearly (B). A schematic drawing of the typical appearance of the RCA on coronary MR angiograms is shown (C). (A) The proximal and middle RCA are shown (long white arrow); the distal RCA (short white arrows) is slightly out-of-plane and better seen in an image obtained in a parallel imaging plane. The origin of the RCA is out-of-plane. (B) Origin of the RCA best seen on oblique transaxial plane. (C) Schematic drawing of a typical appearance of the proximal and mid-RCA on coronary angiograms. The origin is shown in dashed (thin) lines to emphasize the point that the origin is often better seen in an additional plane. Also shown are: the pericardial sac (thin arrows); Ao = ascending aorta; PA = main pulmonary artery; coronary sinus (curved arrow). (Figures 1A and 1C: reprinted with permission from Duerinckx (18). Figure 1B: reprinted with permission from Duerinckx (19).)

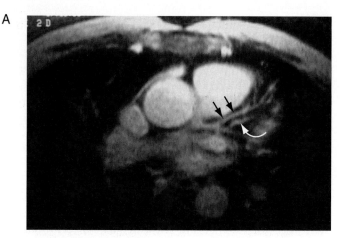

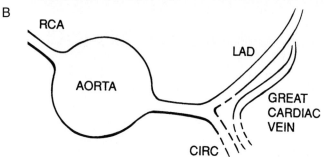

Figure 1.2. Left coronary artery system imaged with a first-generation coronary MRA technique. The left coronary artery system is relatively complex and requires multiple imaging planes to visualize its proximal course. (A) Oblique transaxial plane showing the proximal and middle LAD (arrows) and the great cardiac vein (curved arrows). (B) Schematic drawing of a typical appearance of the left main, LAD, proximal circumflex, and great cardiac vein on oblique transaxial planes. The origin of the LAD and circumflex are shown in dashed (thin) lines to emphasize the point that often these origins are better seen in another plane. Also shown are: the pericardial sac (thin arrows); Ao = ascending aorta; RV = right ventricle; LV = left ventricle; LA = left atrium; DA = descending aorta; S = superior vena cava. (Reprinted with permission from Duercinkx (19).)

results in animals (40–43). The use of new MR blood pool contrast agents may open up a whole new world for coronary MRA similar to what happened after Martin Prince introduced the concept of CE 3-D MRA for body, peripheral, and chest MRA applications.

Because only the first- and second-generation coronary MRA techniques are now universally available on most commercial MRI, the bulk of the published preclinical literature on this topic has been limited to these techniques. One of the purposes of this book is to pro-

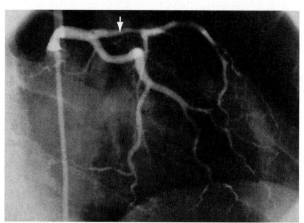

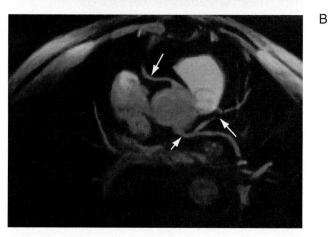

Figure 1.3. Proximal right and left coronary arteries imaged with an early version of a second-generation coronary MRA technique and intensive postprocessing of the data, and a maximum intensity projection (MIP) of a 3-D coronary MR angiogram acquired in a patient without breatholding but with retrospective respiratory gating. (A) Conventional angiogram, right anterior oblique view: A 50–70% stenosis of the proximal LAD is present (arrow). The distal LAD can not be distinguished from overlapping diagonal branches. (B) A maximum intensity projection (MIP) image derived from a 3-D MRA data set with 16 partitions, 1.2 × 2 × 2 mm³ resolution, and five averages. Overlapping blood pool signal was removed prior to the MIP reconstruction. An edge-preserving filter was applied to improve signal-to-noise. Note the excellent delineation of the RCA (small arrow), circumflex (arrowhead), and a 50–75% stenosis of the proximal LAD (thin arrow). (Reprinted with permission from Li D, et al. (41).)

that are now available on several commercial scanners (38,39). Exciting and promising third-generation techniques have been described since 1995 and are still in full development. The combination of second- and third-generation techniques provides the ultimate compromise between user friendliness, high spatial resolution and acquisition speeds. The best approach may indeed be to use both techniques at all times, as needed. They require one or several breatholds for a full survey of the heart and coronary vessels. The coronary MRI quality that can be obtained is illustrated in Figure 1.4. These third-generation techniques are described in Chapters 20 and 21. The combination of MR contrast agents (and, in the near future, MR blood pool agents) with any of these coronary MRA techniques seems very promising, as illustrated in Figure 1.5 based on initial

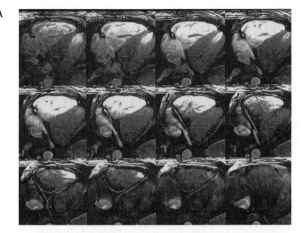

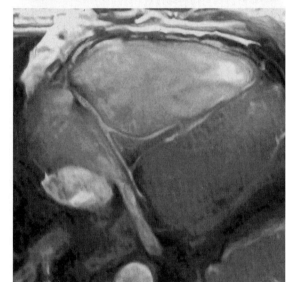

Figure 1.4. Distal RCA and posterior descending artery (PDA) imaged with a third-generation technique. (A) The center nine sections (from the 16 reconstructed for VCATS) are displayed. (B) Volume rendering integrates the entire course of the distal RCA. Acquisition parameters are: Sixteen 1.5-mm-thick sections were reconstructed for VCATS by using 21 heartbeats, a 126 × 256 matrix with partial Fourier encoding, and an FOV of 240 × 320 mm. (Reprinted with permission from Wielopolski PA, et al. Breathhold coronary MR angiography with volume targeted imaging. *Radiology* 1998;209:209–19.)

vide an understanding of these techniques, and to discuss their use for MRI of normal coronary anatomy. We refer the reader to other detailed reviews of these coronary MRA techniques (16–22, 44–46).

Other Techniques for Noninvasive Imaging of the Coronary Arteries

Many imaging tools exist to evaluate the coronary artery anatomy directly: electron-beam computed tomography (EB-CT) (Chaps. 27 and 28), coronary MRA, echocardiography (both transthoracic and transesophageal), in-travascular ultrasound (Chap. 29), and invasive X-ray coronary angiography, which is today's gold standard. EB-CT and MRI appear very close competitors for the same market. Unlike EB-CT, however, coronary MRA does not require iodinated contrast agents or X-ray radiation, and it has the potential to become a more widespread and easy-to-use cardiac screening tool.

Why Should We Care About Coronary MRA in 2001 and Later?

Atherosclerosis, specifically coronary artery disease, is the most common cause of adult mortality in the western hemisphere. Cardiac imaging represents an enormous percentage of all diagnostic imaging procedures. In 1993 an estimated $1.67 billion (or 32% of all costs for imaging) was spent in the United States by Medicare (Part B) for reimbursement of the 10 most common imaging procedures that are all primarily cardiovascular in nature (51). Atherosclerosis remains an elusive, progressive, and devastating disease, despite the enormous investment of research dollars by government and industry. Invasive selective coronary angiography has long been and is still the gold standard for defining the site and severity of stenotic lesions in the coronary arteries. The functional significance of lesions can be determined with myocardial perfusion tests with and without stress using nuclear cardiology, echocardiography, or, most recently, MRI. In the more recent literature, the importance of the mechanisms involved in plaque formation and rupture as well as thrombus formation has been emphasized. Plaque histology and plaque stability are and should be critical factors in predicting the importance of a small plaque or a coronary lesion for future events. Nevertheless, in the day-to-day practice of cardiology, the traditional criteria of lesion stenosis and physiological significance of lesion severity (coronary flow reserve) are still routinely used.

Thus, for the day-to-day clinical practice of cardiology, the need to image the coronary vessel's lumen and to exclude the presence of significant coronary lesions remain. Conventional X-ray coronary angiography is now used almost exclusively for the direct visualization of the coronary lumen. Intravascular ultrasound has provided an alternative, but it is still very invasive (see Chap. 29). Noninvasive alternatives, such as echocardiography (for infants and some pediatric patients), EB-CT angiography, and MRA, have all been evaluated. Electron-beam CT angiography offers a good solution, although it requires the use of X-ray radiation and the injection of a potentially harmful iodinated contrast agent (47–51). Cardiac-triggered multislice helical CT has also been shown to offer great promise for coronary artery imaging. Coronary MRA is less invasive and can be used in a wider patient population (e.g., those with

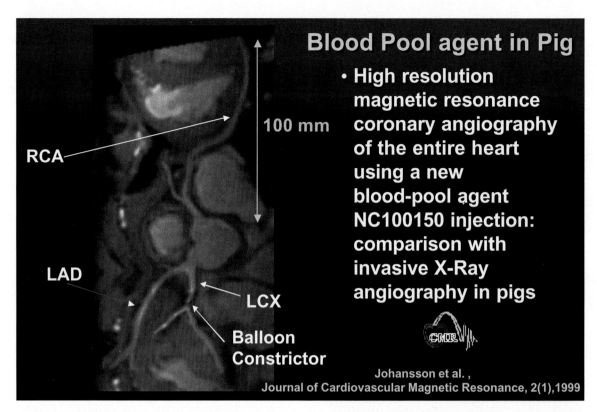

Figure 1.5. Coronary MR angiogram (curved reformat) in a pig with an externally placed balloon constrictor on the left circumflex artery. Images were obtained with NC100150 Injection, 5 mg Fe/kg body weight (Nycomed Amersham Imaging) using a 3-D spoiled gradient echo sequence with fat suppression and a flip angle sweep optimized to maintain constant maximum signal in the blood (TR/TE 6.7/2.3 ms). A 2-D RF selective navigator placed on the diaphragm was used for motion compensation. Images were obtained on a 1.5 T Gyroscan NT, PT 6000 (Philips Medical Systems, the Netherlands). Resolution was $0.9 \times 0.9 \times 0.9$ mm^3, and the acquisition window per cardiac cycle was 55 ms. (Images courtesy of Lars Johansson, Nycomed, Olso, Norway, and Christine Lorenz, Siemens Medical Center, London, UK; images acquired while both were working at the Center for Cardiovascular MR, Barnes-Jewish Hospital at Washington University Medical Center, St. Louis, MO.)

renal failure), but it is excluded in others (e.g., patients with pacemakers, etc.). Efforts are being made to teach the performance of coronary MRA to the point where it can be used in many clinical settings with existing commercial MR scanners and pulse sequences (52) (see also Chaps. 4 and 5). The use of cardiac MRI in general is receiving a lot of attention, and several medical societies [e.g., the North American Society for Cardiac Imaging (53) and the Society for Cardiovascular Magnetic Resonance] now organize yearly educational symposia to increase the numbers of users who can perform these studies (53–55). Dramatic improvements in the technology (i.e., newer and better cardiac MRI pulse sequences) and a trend to teach the performance of coronary MRA to more end-users (e.g., radiologists and cardiologists) are both important. This book hopes to reflect on these trends in this subfield of cardiac MRI.

The future role of coronary MRA as a screening tool for coronary lesion detection has been debated by many authors (56–61). Both Higgins and Duerinckx have postulated that the availability of coronary MRA technique is an essential prerequisite before the widespread routine use of cardiac MRI in the evaluation of patients with ischemic heart disease will take off (62,63). One such discussion was held during a meeting on October 28–29, 1996, of a working group sponsored by the National Heart, Lung and Blood Institute (NHLBI) in Bethesda, MD (55). This working group recommended future work on coronary artery visualization and flow quantification as the number one high-risk–high-benefit activity for academic researchers and as a special area of emphasis for the NIH. Lee Rogers, editor-in-chief of the *American Journal of Radiology*, presented a similar discussion in the *American Journal of Roentgenology*, in the April 1998 issue (58). Dr. Rogers pointed out that coronary artery imaging is still difficult and technically demanding, but not impossible. Neither MR imaging nor EB-CT have sufficiently solved their inherent problems to make noninvasive coronary artery imaging a clinical reality. Whenever a noninvasive procedure (even if not perfect) replaces an invasive one, however, the number of examinations has the potential of increasing dramatically. There is thus an enormous potential market for noninvasive coronary MRA. The manufacturers and users will be extremely interested in this market. Potential turf battles between radiologists and cardiologists may erupt given the potential for new revenues.

One should also not forget that in the work up of patients with coronary artery disease the total atherosclerotic burden in the aorta, carotid, and femoral arteries are good predictors of coronary artery disease. A good correlation has been shown between the severity of atherosclerotic disease in one arterial bed and involvement of other vessels (64). This also opens the potential for more involvement by imagers in noninvasive screening for ischemic heart disease, beyond the already established involvement in coronary calcium screening. Measuring the intimal–medial wall thickness in the carotid arteries and the femoral arteries can be easily performed by most radiology practices using ultrasound and could also become an important parameter, in addition to the more traditional screening factors, for the early prediction of coronary artery disease.

It is extremely important that all cardiac imagers (i.e., radiologists, cardiologists, and others) keep up with the latest advances in this subfield of cardiac MRI so that we can offer these new cardiac MRI studies to our patients. In order to do this, however, we need to be knowledgeable about the coronary MRA sequences available today on commercial MRI scanners. Radiologists need to be prepared to work with cardiologists when using these new cardiac MRI applications, and vice versa. Both groups need each other to fully utilize the potential of cardiac MRI and make this available to patients. In this book, we will describe the coronary MRA techniques that have been developed and tested in preclinical trials. We will direct the imager who is not yet a specialist in cardiac MRI and coronary MRA to those MR techniques that in our view seem the most likely to provide good results in the hands of the majority of users. Very promising future developments, such as a combination of second- and third-generation approaches to coronary MRA and the use of MR blood pool contrast agents, will also be described. We refer the readers to the specialized literature and conference proceedings for further information on these topics beyond May 2000.

There are differences from country to country and from continent to continent as to what are realistic clinical applications of and expectations for coronary MRA. In the November 1999 special issue on Cardiovascular MRI of the *Journal of Magnetic Resonance Imaging*, the clinical experiences with coronary MRA in Japan, the United States, and Europe were described (65–67). In general the future of coronary MRA appears very promising (68–72).

We refer the readers to the specialized literature, conference proceedings and web sites for further information on these topics beyond May 2000. Specifically, the program and proceedings of the First International Workshop on Coronary MR & CT angiography, held October 1–3, 2000, in Lyon, France, and organized by the North American Society for Cardiac Imaging (NASCI) provides added information ⟨www.nasci.org⟩ (73). Other good sources of added information are the Society for Cardiovascular Magnetic Resonance ⟨www.scmr.org⟩ and the International Society for Magnetic Resonance in Medicine ⟨www.ismrm.org⟩. Other web sites provide direct links to information on cardiac MRI in general ⟨www.cardiac-mri.com⟩ and coronary MRA specifically (for example, ⟨www.bidmc.harvard.edu/cmr/cmr-network.html⟩ and ⟨www.nasci.org⟩). Results of multicenter, industry-sponsored trials to test new coronary MRA techniques and contrast agents are under way and will undoubtedly further increase our confidence in coronary MRA.

References

1. Heart and stroke facts: 1996 statistical supplement. Dallas: American Heart Association.
2. Johnson LW, Lozner EC, Johnson S, et al. Coronary arteriography 1984–1987: A report of the registry of the society for cardiac angiography and interventions. Cathet Cardiovasc Diagn 1989;17:5–10.
3. Manning WJ, Li W, Edelman RR. A preliminary report comparing magnetic resonance coronary angiography with conventional angiography. N Engl J Med 1993;328:828–32.
4. Manning WJ, Li W, Boyle NG, Edelman RE. Fat-suppressed breath-hold magnetic resonance coronary angiography. Circulation 1993;87:94–104.
5. Duerinckx AJ, Urman M. Two-dimensional coronary MR angiography: analysis of initial clinical results. Radiology 1994;193:731–38.
6. Higgins CB, Silverman NH, Kersting-Sommerhoff VA, Schmidt K. Congenital heart disease: echocardiography and magnetic resonance imaging. New York: Raven Press, 1990.
7. Higgins CB. Essentials of cardiac radiology and imaging. Philadelphia: J.B. Lippincott Company, 1992.
8. Blackwell GG, Cranney GB, Pohost GM. MRI: cardiovascular system. New York: Gower Medical Publishing, 1992.
9. Duerinckx A, Higgins C, Pettigrew R. MRI of the cardiovascular system (The Raven Press MRI Teaching File). New York: Raven Press, 1994.
10. Bogaert J, Duerinckx AJ, Rademakers FE. Magnetic resonance of the heart and great vessels: clinical applications. Springer-Verlag, 1999.
11. Lieberman LM, Botti RE, Nelson AD. Magnetic resonance of the heart. Radiol Clin North Am 1984;22:847–58.
12. Paulin S, vonSchulthess GK, Fossel E, Krayenbuehl HP. MR imaging of the aortic root and proximal coronary arteries. Am J Roentgenol 1987;148:665–70.
13. Cassidy M, Schiller N, Botvinick E, et al. Assessment of coronary artery imaging by gated magnetic resonance: an evaluation of the utility and potential of the currently available imaging methods. Am J Card Imag 1989;3:100–7.
14. Bisset GS, Strife JL, McCloskey J. MR imaging of coronary artery aneurysms in a child with Kawasaki disease. Am J Roentgenol 1989;152:805–7.

15. Doorey AJ, Wills JS, Blasetto J, Goldenberg EM. Usefulness of magnetic resonance imaging for diagnosing an anomalous coronary artery coursing between aorta and pulmonary trunk. Am J Cardiol 1994;74:198–99.

16. Manning W, Edelman R. Magnetic resonance coronary angiography. Magn Reson Q 1993;9(3):131–51.

17. Pennell DJ, Keegan J, Firmin DN, Gatehouse PD, Underwood SR, Longmore DB. Magnetic resonance imaging of coronary arteries: technique and preliminary results. Br Heart J 1993;70(4):315–26.

18. Duerinckx AJ. Review: MR angiography of the coronary arteries. Top Magn Reson Imag 1995;7(4):267–85.

19. Bogaert J, Duerinckx AJ, Baert AL. Coronary MR angiography: a review. J Belge de Radiologie / Belgisch Tijdschrift voor Radiologie. 1994;77:255–61.

20. Duerinckx AJ. Coronary MR angiography. In: Cardiac MR imaging. Boxt LM, ed. MRI Clin North Am 1996;4(2): 361–418.

21. Wielopolski PA, van Geuns RJ, de Feyter PJ, Oudkerk M. Coronary arteries. Eur Radiol 1998;8(6):873–85.

22. Duerinckx AJ. Coronary MR Angiography (invited article). In: Cardiac Radiology. Boxt LM, ed. Radiol Clin North Am 1999;37(2):273–318.

23. Arlart IP, Bongartz GM, Marchall G. Magnetic resonance angiography. New York: Springer-Verlag, 1996.

24. Anderson CM, Edelman RR, Turski PA. Clinical magnetic resonance angiography. New York: Raven Press, 1993.

25. Potchen EJ, Haacke EM, Siebert JE, Gottschalk A. Magnetic resonance angiography: concepts & applications. St Louis: Mosby, 1993.

26. Atkinson D, Teresi L. Magnetic resonance angiography (review article). Magn Reson Q 1995;10(3):149–72.

27. Brant-Zawadzki M, Boyko OB, Jensen MC, Gillan GD. MR angiography: a teaching file. New York: Raven Press, 1993.

28. Prince MR, Grist TM, Debatin JF. 3D contrast MR angiography, 2nd ed. Berlin: Springer-Verlag, 1999.

29. Saloner D, Selby K, Anderson CM. Diastolic acquisition of arterial stenosis: improvements by diastolic acquisition. Magn Reson Imag 1994;31:196–203.

30. Franck A, Selby K, vanTyen R, Nordell B, Saloner D. Cardiac-gated MR angiography of pulsatile flow: k-space strategies. JMRI 1995;5:297–307.

31. Pearlman JD, Edelman RE. Ultrafast magnetic resonance imaging: segmented TurboFLASH, echo-planar, and real-time nuclear magnetic resonance. Radiol Clin North Am 1994;32(3):593–612.

32. Lauzon ML, Rutt BK. Generalized k-space analysis and correction of motion effects in MR imaging. Magn Reson Med 1993;30:438–46.

33. Mezrich R. A perspective on k-space. Radiology 1995; 195:297–315.

34. Hartnell GG, Finn JP, Zenni M, et al. MR imaging of the thoracic aorta: comparison of spin-echo, angiographic and breath-hold techniques. Radiology 1994;191(3):697–704.

35. Hernandez RJ, Aisen AM, Foo TKF, Beekman RH. Thoracic cardiovascular anomalies in children: evaluation with a fast gradient-recalled-echo sequence with cardiac-triggered segmented acquisition. Radiology 1993;188: 775–80.

36. Bluemke DA, Boxerman JL, Mosher T, Lima JA. Segmented K-space cine breath-hold cardiovascular MR imaging: part 2. Evaluation of aortic vasculopathy. Am J Roentgenol 1997;169(2):401–7.

37. Bluemke DA, Boxerman JL, Atalar E, McVeigh ER. Segmented K-space cine breath-hold cardiovascular MR imaging: part 1. Principles and technique. Am J Roentgenol 1997;169(2):395–400.

38. Stuber M, Botnar RM, Danias PG, et al. Double-oblique free-breathing high resolution three-dimensional coronary magnetic resonance angiography. J Am Coll Cardiol 1999;34(2):524–31.

39. Stuber M, Botnar RM, Danias PG, Kissinger KV, Manning WJ. Submillimeter three-dimensional coronary MR angiography with real-time navigator correction: comparison of navigator locations. Radiology 1999;212(2):579–87.

40. Johansson LO, Nolan NM, Taniuchi M, Fischer SE, Wickline SA, Lorenz CH. High resolution magnetic resonance coronary angiography of the entire heart using a new blood-pool agent, NC100150 injection: comparison with invasive x-ray angiography in pigs. J Cardiovasc Magn Reson 1999;2(1):139–44.

41. Li D, Kaushikkar S, Haacke EM, et al. Coronary arteries: three-dimensional MR imaging with retrospective respiratory gating. Radiology 1996;201(3):857–63.

42. Sakuma H, Goto M, Nomura Y, Kato N, Takeda K, Higgins CB. Three-dimensional coronary magnetic resonance angiography with injection of extracellular contrast medium [in process citation]. Invest Radiol 1999;34(8): 503–8.

43. Taylor AM, Panting JR, Keegan J, et al. Safety and preliminary findings with the intravascular contrast agent NC100150 injection for MR coronary angiography. J Magn Reson Imag 1999;9(2):220–27.

44. Duerinckx AJ. MRI of coronary arteries. Int J Card Imag 1997;13(3):191–97.

45. Duerinckx AJ, Lipton MJ. Noninvasive coronary artery imaging using CT and MR imaging [comment] [see comments]. Am J Roentgenol 1998;170(4):900–2.

46. Danias PG, Edelman RR, Manning WJ. Coronary MR angiography. Cardiol Clin 1998;16(2):207–25.

47. Moshage WEL, Achenbach S, Seese B, Bachman K, Kirchgeorg M. Coronary artery stenosis: three-dimensional imaging with electrocardiographically triggered, contrast agent-enhanced, electron-beam CT. Radiology 1995; 196(3):707–14.

48. Chernoff DM, Ritchie CJ, Higgins CB. Evaluation of electron beam CT coronary angiography in healthy subjects. Am J Roentgenol 1997;169(1):93–99.

49. Achenbach S, Moshage W, Ropers D, Nossen J, Daniel WG. Value of electron-beam computed tomography for the noninvasive detection of high-grade coronary artery stenoses and occlusions. N Engl J Med 1998;339(27): 1964–71.

50. Achenbach S, Moshage W, Bachmann K. Detection of high-grade stenosis after PTCA using contrast-enhanced electron beam CT. Circulation 1997;96(9):2785–88.

51. Schmermund A, Rensing BJ, Sheedy PF, Bell MR, Rumberger JA. Intravenous electron-beam computed tomographic coronary angiography for segmental analysis of coronary artery stenoses. J Am Coll Cardiol 1998;31(7): 1547–54.

52. Duerinckx AJ. Coronary arteries: How do I image them?

In: Bogaert J, Duerinckx AJ, Rademakers F, eds. Magnetic resonance of the heart and great vessels: clinical applications. Berlin: Springer-Verlag, 1999:223–43.

53. Boxt LM, Lipton MJ. Future direction of cardiovascular research. The North American Society of Cardiac Imaging. Radiology 1998;208(2):283–84.

54. Reiber JHC, vanderWall EE. What's new in cardiovascular imaging? Dordrecht: Kluwer Academic Publishers, 1998.

55. Budinger TF, Berson A, McVeigh ER, et al. Cardiac MR imaging: report of a working group sponsored by the National Heart, Lung, and Blood Institute. Radiology 1998; 208(3):573–76.

56. Caputo GC. Coronary arteries: potential for MR imaging (editorial). Radiology 1991;181(3):629–30.

57. Caputo GC. Coronary MR angiography: a clinical perspective (editorial). Radiology 1994;193(3):596–98.

58. Rogers LF. The heart of the matter: noninvasive coronary artery imaging (editorial). Am J Roentgenol 1998;170:841.

59. Josefson D. MRI found suitable for detecting coronary heart disease. Br Med J 1999;319(7217):1092A.

60. Kates AM, Vedala G, Woodard PK, Davila-Roman VG, Gropler RJ. Noninvasive coronary artery imaging in the diagnosis and management of patients with ischemic heart disease. Curr Opin Cardiol 1999;14(4):314–20.

61. Marano P. The emerging role of MRI in coronary artery disease. Rays 1999;24(1):1–3.

62. Higgins CB. Prediction of myocardial viability by MRI [editorial]. Circulation 1999;99:727–29.

63. Duerinckx A. Myocardial viability by MRI: is it ready for clinical use? Am J Roentgenol 2000;174:1741–1743.

64. Khoury Z, Schwartz R, Gottlieb S, Chenzbraun A, Stern S, Keren A. Relation of coronary artery disease to atherosclerotic disease in the aorta, carotid, and femoral arteries evaluated by ultrasound. Am J Cardiol 1997;80:1429–33.

65. Nitatori T, Yoshino H, Yokoyama K, Hachiya J, Ishikawa K. Coronary MR angiography–a clinical experience in Japan. J Magn Reson Imag 1999;10(5):709–12.

66. Danias PG, Stuber M, Edelman RR, Manning WJ. Coronary MRA–a clinical experience in the United States. J Magn Reson Imag 1999;10(5):713–20.

67. Bunce NH, Pennell DJ. Coronary MRA–a clinical experience in Europe. J Magn Reson Imag 1999;10(5):721–27.

68. Duerinckx AJ. Coronary MR angiography. Radiol Clin North Am 1999;37(2):273–318.

69. Wielopolski PA, van Geuns RJ, de Feyter PJ, Oudkerk M. Coronary arteries. Eur Radiol 2000;10(1):12–35.

70. Polak JF. MR coronary angiography: are we there yet? [editorial; comment]. Radiology 2000;214(3):649–50.

71. Hardy CJ, Saranathan M, Zhu Y, Darrow RD. Coronary angiography by real-time MRI with adaptive averaging. Magn Reson Med 2000;44(6):940–46.

72. Serfaty JM, Yang X, Aksit P, Quick HH, Solaiyappan M, Atalar E. Toward MRI-guided coronary catheterization: visualization of guiding catheters, guidewires, and anatomy in real time. J Magn Reson Imag 2000;12(4):590–94.

73. Proceedings and Abstracts of the First International Workshop on Coronary MR & CT Angiography, Oct 1–3, 2000, Lyon, France, organized by the North American Society for Cardiac Imaging. In: Duerinckx AJ, ed. Int J Card Imag 2000;16(3).

2
Anatomy and Physiology of Coronary Arteries

André J. Duerinckx

The anatomy and physiology of coronary vessels are so significantly different from those of other larger vessels in the body that a brief description is needed to understand better some of the design considerations for coronary magnetic resonance angiography (MRA) pulse sequences. Coronary arteries are small, tortuous vessels that are subjected to significant physiological motion, including cardiac motion, respiratory motion, and vascular pulsations. Knowledge of coronary artery motion, coronary artery wall contractions, and coronary flow variability throughout a cardiac cycle is also needed to design coronary MRA pulse sequences and imaging strategies better.

Coronary Vessel Anatomy and Size

Detailed information about the general appearance, distribution, and normal variants of coronary vessels can be found in multiple cardiology textbooks and will not be repeated here (1,2). Studies of normal coronary anatomy based on MR images are also available (3). The fact that both arteries and veins are visible on MR images requires a detailed knowledge of both the arterial and venous coronary artery anatomy (4).

We will only briefly review the morphology of the coronary arteries, using a graphical representation from a textbook by Soto et al. (5). The right and left coronary arteries usually originate from the aorta as separate channels (rarely, from a single trunk—see Chap. 8). The right coronary artery (RCA) arises from the anterior (right) coronary cusp; the left coronary artery arises from the posterior (left) coronary cusp. The course of the major coronary arteries is shown schematically in Figure 2.1A. The RCA is a large vessel that runs within the right atrioventricular groove (separating the right atrium and ventricle) to the inferior wall of the heart. It bifurcates there into the posterior descending artery (PDA) and the posterolateral branches. The PDA runs in the posterior interventricular sulcus toward the cardiac apex. The left

coronary artery is a much shorter vessel (10–15 mm in length) that runs just posterior to the pulmonary trunk. It then bifurcates into two large branches: the left anterior descending (LAD) artery and the circumflex artery. The LAD runs from the base of the heart to the apex along the anterior interventricular groove. The circumflex artery runs along the left (posterior) atrioventricular groove. For the purposes of coronary MRA there is no need to know more about coronary anatomy (e.g., side-branches and their nomenclature) because the spatial resolution of today's techniques does not yet allow routine visualization of these branches.

It is important for the cardiac imager to be able to select appropriate imaging planes quickly along the course of the main coronary vessel. This will be dealt with in detail in a later chapter (Chap. 5). A simplified diagram of the coronary vessels is shown in Figure 2.1b. The RCA and circumflex arteries form a circle within the atrioventricular groove. The LAD and PDA branch of the RCA form a loop within the anterior and posterior interventricular sulci.

Variations of the coronary arterial pattern are common and occur in about 10% of the population. The most common variant is a nondominant (hypoplastic) RCA. In such cases the circumflex artery is dominant and provides circulation to the posterior septum and to the left inferior ventricular wall.

We will now discuss the size of coronary vessels because it is relevant to the design of coronary MRA techniques. First, coronary MRA show both arteries and veins, unlike X-ray contrast angiograms. Coronary veins usually appear larger than the arteries, which helps in distinguishing them. Following the course of the vessels is another good way to distinguish between the two.

Detailed studies on the size of typical coronary arteries are available and will be reviewed. The luminal diameter of normal coronary arteries has been well studied (6,7). In a group of 20 right-dominant men, the left main (LM) coronary artery measured 4.5 ± 0.5 mm, the

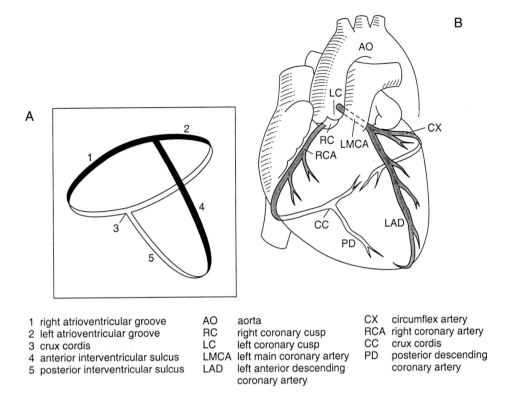

1	right atrioventricular groove	AO	aorta	CX	circumflex artery
2	left atrioventricular groove	RC	right coronary cusp	RCA	right coronary artery
3	crux cordis	LC	left coronary cusp	CC	crux cordis
4	anterior interventricular sulcus	LMCA	left main coronary artery	PD	posterior descending
5	posterior interventricular sulcus	LAD	left anterior descending		coronary artery
			coronary artery		

Figure 2.1. Course of the coronary arteries around the heart. (A) The course of the coronary arteries and their major branches is shown schematically (see text for abbreviations). (B) In this schematic representation, the cardiac apex is oriented anteriorly, inferiorly, and to the left, following the usual anatomic arrangement of the heart. The atrioventricular groove is represented by a circle, and the anterior and posterior interventricular sulci by a loop (the right ventricle is on the right and the left ventricle is on the left). The right part of the circle represents the right atrioventricular groove and marks the course of the RCA. The left part of the circle represents the left atrioventricular groove and marks the course of the circumflex artery. The anterior (superior) part of the loop marks the course of the LAD. The inferior part of the loop marks the course of the PDA in the 90% of patients with right dominant coronary system. (Reprinted with permission from Soto et al. (5).)

proximal LAD coronary artery measured 3.7 ± 0.4 mm, and the distal LAD 1.9 ± 0.4 mm. Variations with anatomic dominance (right vs. left) were seen in the RCA and left circumflex (LCx). For the RCA proximal diameter varied between 3.9 ± 0.6 and 2.8 ± 0.5 mm (right vs. left dominance) and for the LCx between 3.4 ± 0.5 and 4.2 ± 0.6 mm ($p < 0.01$ significance). Women had a smaller epicardial arterial diameter than men, even after normalization for body surface area. Side branches (e.g., marginals and diagonals) were smaller.

Similar studies on the size of coronary veins are not as readily available. Based on a large number of MRI studies, however, and except for the coronary sinus, veins appear to have a similar size and MR appearance to the adjacent arteries.

Frequency and Distribution of Coronary Artery Lesions

The need for a noninvasive screening test for coronary artery disease (CAD) increases when the "gold standard," which is invasive contrast angiography, demonstrates no evidence of CAD in large groups of patients. To judge the potential impact of a noninvasive screening test better, we will first review published literature on the frequency of normal coronary angiograms in symptomatic population groups.

The frequency of normal coronary angiograms in patients presenting with chest pain, angina pectoris, or prior myocardial infarct has been reported in several studies. Bergstrand et al. (8) studied 216 men evaluated for angina pectoris, including 127 men with prior myocardial infarct. In 7.8% of these patients, no atherosclerotic changes were found in the coronary vessels; in addition, 16.7% had lesions considered to be without hemodynamic implications. Another similar study found no evidence of atherosclerotic changes in the coronary arteries in 8% of a group of 71 males suffering from severe angina pectoris (9). Another study by Freedman et al. (10) describing the distribution of coronary atherosclerosis in 4722 men, found no such changes in 7.8% of men. A more recent study by Perez et al. (11) obtained more than 30% of normal angiograms in 101 men with chest pain. As patients are being more aggressively evaluated and referred for coronary angiography with less advanced coronary disease, these numbers will probably increase.

In order to evaluate the clinical impact of a new noninvasive diagnostic test, it is also important to know the a priori probability for disease distribution in a given population (12). To be specific, if a diagnostic screening test has limitations (e.g., a low sensitivity in picking up lesions in specific locations), knowing how often such lesions occur is important to evaluate the clinical utility of the test. This is very relevant for coronary MRA, where the early 2-D techniques had great difficulty in visualizing the LCx (see Table 2.4) and thus could not detect most LCx lesions (see later discussion). We will thus review data from published studies describing the distribution of CAD in patient groups with known angina pectoris and/or prior myocardial infarcts, and studies on the frequency of disease within each vessel.

In the study by Bergstrand et al. (8) involving 216 men with angina pectoris, the proximal RCA was the most frequent site of coronary atherosclerosis. The proximal RCA was affected by atherosclerosis in 57.5% with 30.1% having an occlusion between the first ventricular branch and the marginal branch. In the same group of patients, 29% had significant stenosis or occlusion of the LAD between the first and second diagonal branches. The left circumflex coronary artery was free of any disease in its proximal portion (ostium to first obtuse marginal branches) in 67% of patients, free of disease in its middle portion (between the first and second obtuse marginal branches) in 71% of patients and free of disease in its distal course (the third obtuse marginal branch or the posterior descending artery when derived from the left coronary artery) in 79.5% of patients. If one includes hemodynamically nonsignificant lesions (diameter narrowing < 50%), there was no significant disease in the proximal LCx in 78.7%, in the middle LCx in 74%, and in the distal LCx in 79.5% of patients. There was similarly no disease in 86% of left main arteries. Several other studies have suggested that atherosclerotic CAD occurs relatively infrequently in the LCx artery. Hillis et al. (13) reviewed selective coronary angiograms performed in a group of 1436 patients evaluated for chest pain. Of these, 17% had no significant CAD and 27% had single-vessel CAD. The distribution of coronary stenosis in the patients with single-vessel CAD was: The LAD was narrowed in 51%, the RCA in 35%, and LCx in 14%. Even in the subgroup of 217 patients with two-vessel coronary disease, the frequency of disease in the LCx was also less than it was in the other vessels (i.e., the LAD–RCA combination occurred more frequently than did the LAD–LCx and LCx-RCA combinations). Hillis et al. discuss several other studies that showed frequencies of LCx disease in patients with single coronary artery disease varying from 3% to 13%. These include a study by Feit et al. (14) of 402 consecutive abnormal coronary angiograms, including 54 patients with single-vessel disease. Only 7 (13%) of 54 patients among this group had LCx disease. There are several possible reasons for the relative infrequency of LCx involvement. This may possibly reflect some degree of LCx protection, due to differences in coronary artery anatomy and the resultant flow patterns and turbulence. Another study (15) reviewed patients who died from CAD and found the following distribution: The LAD was the most frequently diseased coronary vessel (58%), followed by the RCA (33%), the LCx (25%), and the left main (LM) (16%).

This relative low-frequency of LCx artery disease (from 7% to 25%) is significant when evaluating the clinical utility of early coronary MRA technique.

Motion of Coronary Arteries Due to Cardiac Motion

The primary challenge for coronary angiography is to overcome the effects of motion of the coronary arteries due to respiration and cardiac contraction. Most of the initial efforts to reduce motion artifacts have centered on respiratory motion as discussed in the next section. Many coronary MRA studies can be acquired in a 100–160-msec window during mid- to late diastole, when cardiac motion is minimal; however, this rest period of the cardiac cycle for coronary artery imaging varies substantially from patient to patient, as described by Wang et al. (16). This may explain why even with short acquisition times within each heartbeat, and even when no arrhythmias are present, the quality and accuracy of coronary MRA may remain variable. This variability in the cardiac rest period will also affect the image quality obtained with electron-beam and multislice helical computed tomography (CT). We will first review the indirect evidence and data on the effect of cardiac motion on coronary artery motion.

Motion of the coronary arteries follows the motion of the ventricular chambers. Karwatowski et al. (17,18) have quantitated the left ventricular long-axis motion with MR velocity mapping perpendicular to a basal short-axis plane in healthy subjects and in patients with ischemic heart disease. They found a maximum early diastolic long-axis velocity of 125 ± 33 mm/sec, with a mean peak early diastolic velocity of 82 ± 22 m/sec in a group of 19 controls (age 35–76). Velocities were less in patients with ischemic heart disease. In another study (19) cardiac wall contraction during middiastole was about 10 mm/sec, which is much less. This motion has been well described in the cardiac literature, and will not be discussed further. Cardiac triggering will compensate for most of this motion. Most coronary MRA are acquired in middiastole over a 70–300-msec period, with a 0.7–3.0-mm displacement due to cardiac motion, which is much less than the displacement due to respiratory variations, which will be discussed next.

Hofman et al. have also measured the in-plane coronary motion of the coronary artery by using respiratory-triggered cine MRI (20). Motion depicted in cine MRI is not in real-time; rather, it is averaged over many heartbeats. These measurements were performed in a fixed plane, so the "motion" observed was not the motion of a fixed point on the coronary artery, but was instead the appearance of different points along the coronary artery as the vessel moved through the fixed plane. Furthermore, cine MRI still lacks adequate spatial resolution and image quality for precise measurements of coronary motion.

Wang et al. (16) measured the motion of coronary arteries in 13 patients by using breathhold, biplane, conventional angiography, with frontal and lateral projections of the left and right coronary arteries acquired at 30 frames/sec. The time courses of the coordinates of bifurcations of proximal parts of the coronary arteries were measured, from which the rest period (motion <1 mm in orthogonal axes), velocity, displacement range, motion correlation, and reproducibility from heartbeat to heartbeat were estimated. Both the motion and the amplitude varied substantially from patient to patient. The rest period varied from 66 to 333 msec (mean, 161 sec) for the left coronary artery and from 66 to 200 msec (mean, 120 msec) for the right coronary artery.

Motion of Coronary Arteries Due to Respiratory Motion

Many coronary MRA techniques, and most recent cardiac magnetic resonance imaging (MRI), is performed during a breathhold. This more or less eliminates all motion due to respiration. Holland et al. (21) investigated and quantified the motion of the diaphragm and heart during suspended breathing at end inspiration and end expiration. In 10 healthy adult volunteers, line scanning was performed to monitor the position of the diaphragm during a breathhold at end inspiration and end expiration, with a spatial and temporal resolution of 0.25 mm and 200 msec, respectively. Electrocardiographically gated, turbo fast low-angle shot (FLASH) MRI was performed to monitor movement of the diaphragm and heart. Holland et al. (21) found that the diaphragm moved upward during a breathhold. At end expiration, the velocity of the diaphragm during suspended breathing was constant (mean, 0.15 mm/sec). At end inspiration, motion of the diaphragm during suspended breathing was more complex (range, 0.1–7.9 mm/sec). During a 20-second breathhold, mean displacement of the diaphragm was 25% of that during normal breathing. FLASH MRI revealed variations in the position of the heart during a breathhold. During suspended respiration, the heart did not return to the same position on consecutive heartbeats; consequently, the margins of the heart typically moved inward. Holland et al. (21) concluded that breathholding does not eliminate motion of the diaphragm. Changes in the motion of the diaphragm and transthoracic pressure during a breathhold result in complex movement of the heart and may cause blurring during breathhold MRI.

Adaptive real-time or retrospective correction of motion due to respiration during free-breathing coronary MRA (the second-generation technique) is a very important improvement of the early implementations of the technique, as will be discussed elsewhere in this book. Many investigators have studied the relationship between coronary artery motion and respiratory motion.

Studies initially quantitated the extent of additional motion due to respiration for MRI applications in the abdomen and thorax (22–25). Wang et al. (23) studied the effects of respiration on the cardiac position quantitatively by imaging the heart during diastole at various positions of tidal respiration. This was done in 10 healthy subjects (age: 23–37; three females, seven males) using a 2-D breathhold technique for coronary MRA, as described later in this chapter. Coronary MRA was performed in left anterior oblique (LAO) and right anterior oblique (RAO) equivalent planes. Each measurement was repeated seven times. Averaged results are shown in Table 2.1.

These figures have a practical importance when comparing different data acquisitions schemes. For example, when comparing a 2-D breathhold and 3-D nonbreathhold technique the 3-D acquisition time per heartbeat can be 40 ms longer than the typical 2-D acquisition (22). The coronary displacement caused by the cardiac motion during the extra 40 ms is negligible (0.4 mm), whereas the added respiratory motion can be up to 10.5 mm for the RCA root. It should also be mentioned that the total acquisition times are continually decreasing, as they do with the newer 3-D implementations that have acquisition times as short as 120 ms for 16 slices (26).

Table 2.1. Displacements of key anatomical landmarks during tidal respiration in normal volunteers.

Anatomical landmarks	Range (mm)	Direction
Heart (inf. margin)	18.1 ± 9.1 mm	SI
Heart (ant. margin)	2.4 ± 1.5 mm	AP
Apex	16.0 ± 7.1 mm	SI
RCA root	10.5 ± 4.8 mm	SI
	2.3 ± 1.4 mm	AP
LAD prox	13.1 ± 4.1 mm	SI

SI = Superior-inferior; AP = Anterior–Posterior; mean ± standard deviation over 10 subjects
Source: Modified from Table 1 in Ref. (23).

Diaphragmatic navigators are frequently used in free-breathing coronary MRA, either to gate or prospectively correct slice position, or both. For such approaches, a constant relationship between coronary and diaphragmatic displacement throughout the respiratory cycle is assumed. Two studies have shown significant interpatient variability in this relation. Taylor et al. (27,28) have calculated a subject-specific motion-correction factor for free-breathing coronary MRA. The motion-correction factor refers to the ratio of the diaphragm displacement against coronary displacement for a single subject. This is usually measured in the superior/inferior (SI) direction, although it can and has been extended in all three dimensions. Taylor et al. have measured the SI correction factor in 25 subjects and found a wide variation of correction factors between subjects: proximal RCA, mean 0.49 ± 0.15, range 0.20–0.70; proximal left coronary artery, mean 0.59 ± 0.15, range 0.20–0.85. The subject-specific correction factor was accurately calculated from motion of the aortic root in the coronal plane between expiratory and inspiratory breathhold. Danias et al. (29) also studied the relationship between motion of coronary arteries and diaphragm during free breathing. They evaluated the relationship between diaphragmatic and coronary artery motion during free breathing. A real-time echoplanar MRI sequence was used in 12 healthy volunteers to obtain 30 successive images each (one per cardiac cycle) that included the left main coronary artery and the domes of both hemidiaphragms. The coronary artery and diaphragm positions (relative to isocenter) were determined and analyzed for effective diaphragmatic gating windows of 3, 5, and 7 mm (i.e., diaphragmatic excursions of 0–3, 0–5, and 0–7 mm from the end-expiratory position, respectively). Danias et al. (29) found that although the mean slope correlating the displacement of the right diaphragm and the left main coronary artery was approximately 0.6 for all diaphragmatic gating windows, they also found great variability among individual volunteers. Linear regression slopes varied from 0.17 to 0.93, and $r2$ values varied from 0.04 to 0.87. They conclude that individual variability exists in the relationship between coronary and diaphragmatic respiratory motion during free breathing. Coronary MRA approaches that use diaphragmatic navigator position for prospective slice correction may therefore benefit from patient-specific correction factors. On the other hand coronary MRA may benefit from a more direct assessment of the respiratory displacement of the heart and coronary arteries using left ventricular navigators.

In a study based on 17 normal subjects and 15 patients Taylor et al. (30) also showed that there is great variability in the capability of patients to hold their breath when compared to normal volunteers. This is not surprising but very important when evaluating and comparing coronary MRA techniques; however, this is just one study that may exaggerate the problems encountered with breathhold imaging in real patients. Being able to perform breathholding (required for first- and third-generation techniques) is not the same as being able to perform breathholding with the diaphragm at the same position (as required for many implementations of second-generation techniques). This last criterion is too restrictive when all one cares about is image quality. Multiple preclinical studies (as discussed later in the book), including the first one by Manning et al. in the *New England Journal of Medicine* in 1993 (31), have clearly shown that good-quality breathhold coronary MRA can be performed in patients.

Duerinckx et al. (4) have also documented variability of diaphragm position in patients and in normal volunteers during sequential breathhold maneuvers. In the early days of coronary MRA (first-generation techniques), investigators were forced to use prone positioning because in the very early days of coronary MRA, phased array thoracic coils were not yet available. With the advent of phased-array thoracic coils, supine positioning during coronary MRA became possible. This was viewed as a major advance because of increased patient comfort. Since then, the use of prone imaging (as opposed to the routine supine imaging) has been reconsidered for free-breathing real-time navigator corrected 3-D coronary MRA techniques (work-in-progress). Chest-wall motion and diaphragmatic motion are not always synchronized, which is a fact known from prior physiology literature. This is an important additional complicating factor in the evaluation of navigator based free breathing 3-D coronary MRA techniques. Even though prone positioning may indeed help further improve the image quality, many studies have shown acceptable images obtained with 3-D coronary MRI MRA using supine positioning. This is an open debate at the present time.

Coronary Blood Velocity

The flow pattern in coronary vessels and grafts is biphasic, consisting of systolic and diastolic phases with higher velocity in diastole than systole (32). This is illustrated in Figure 2.2 for flow in a normal bypass graft. Flow in the coronary sinus is characterized by biphasic systolic–diastolic flow and a short period of end-diastolic retrograde flow (33). Thus, flow within the coronary arteries is pulsatile and highly variable during the cardiac cycle with additional differences between the left coronary artery (LCA) and right coronary artery (RCA) circulation.

The range of velocities in native coronary arteries (32,34), in coronary artery bypass graft (CABG) (35,37), and in the coronary sinus (38) have been well studied (Table 2.2). Flow in the left coronary system is maximal during early diastole, and during late systole in the right coronary artery system (32,39,40). The ratio of peak ve-

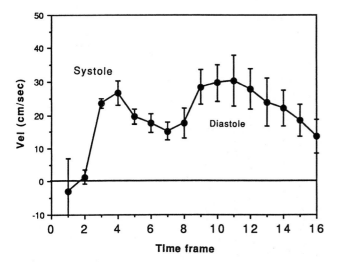

Figure 2.2. (Reprinted with permission from Duerinckx AJ. Coronary MR Angiography. MRI Clin N Am 1996;4(2):361–418.)

locity in early diastole to peak velocity in systole is greater than 2 for the left coronary system, whereas it is equal to or less than 1.5 for the RCA (see Table 2.2). Somewhat more than half the RCA flow is supplied during systole. This variability in the intensity of flow throughout the cardiac cycle will affect the selection of optimal timing of image data acquisition within the cardiac cycle.

Based on a noninvasive study (35) using combined 2-D and pulsed Doppler echocardiography, a significant difference in the velocity profiles in internal mammary artery (IMA) and saphenous vein (SV) grafts has been demonstrated (see Table 2.2). In patients with internal mammary artery grafts, the blood velocity in the recip-

ient artery was not as high as that in patients with an SV graft. In the recipient coronary artery in patients with SV grafts there was high velocity and very large variations in velocity during diastole. Other studies have confirmed these findings (33,43,44).

An update on MR-based studies of coronary flow is provided later (see Chaps. 13 and 14).

Coronary Wall Motion

The cross-sectional area of normal coronary vessels changes by as much as 10% throughout the cardiac cycle (45,46). Previous studies have demonstrated the mean variation in coronary vessel size of 3% from beat to beat, and of 6% from systole to diastole, suggesting that beat to beat and phasic changes in coronary arterial diameter would probably not be well detected at the MRI spatial resolutions used today (45). These changes in cross-sectional size of the vessel will have minimal effect on coronary MRA imaging techniques, but they might have a significant effect when estimating coronary artery flow or flow reserve (47).

Coronary Flow Reserve

Coronary flow reserve refers to the increment in coronary flow above the resting level during a stimulus that produces coronary vasodilatation. It gives information about the coronary vascular bed, but it is easy to misinterpret (48). Factors such as heart rate, contractility, end-diastolic pressure, and blood viscosity can all interfere with measuring maximal flow reserve. Peak di-

Table 2.2. Typical values for peak velocity of blood flow in native coronary arteries, bypass grafts, and coronary sinus based on Doppler and early MR measurements (normal vessels, no lesions).

Vessel type	Number normals	Peak-diastolic velocity (cm)	Peak-systolic velocity (cm)	Ratio of peak diastolic/systolic velocities	Ref.
Native coronary vessel (LAD)	9	35 ± 11	24 ± 7	n/a	(34)
Native vessel (LAD and RCA) (peak)	9	35 ± 2.1	16 ± 1.4	2.2	(41)
Native vessel (mean)	9	26 ± 1.9	11 ± 0.8	2.4	(41)
RCA				1.5 ± 0.5	(42)
LAD				2.0 ± 0.5	(42)
Coronary sinus (MR)		22.6 ± 5.9			(38)
Coronary sinus (US)*	8	26 ± 4	34 ± 21	0.8	(33)
IMA Graft (IMAG)	11	57.7 ± 9.9	30.9 ± 5.6	1.9	(35)
SV Graft (SVG)	20	28.0 ± 8.9	15.0 ± 4.9	1.9	(35)
Recipient vessel (IMAG)	10	55.1 ± 7.2	29.0 ± 5.0	1.9	(35)
Recipient vessel (SVG)**	17	93.5 ± 14.7	50.2 ± 10.8	1.9	(35)

From: Duerinckx AJ. Coronary MRA. MRI Clin N Am 1996;4(2):361–418; with permission.
RCA = right coronary artery; LAD = left anterior descending coronary artery; IMA = internal mammary artery; SV = saphenous vein.
* Also contains an end-diastolic retrograde flow peak of 20 ± 6 cm/s.
** Very large variations in velocity during diastole, with an abrupt fall from high to fairly low.

Table 2.3. Typical values for changes in blood velocity ranges in native coronary arteries before and after pharmaceutical stress (34).

Vessel type	Normal LAD	Diseased LAD (75% stenosis)
Number of patients	9	6
Peak diastolic velocity (at rest)	35 ± 11 cm/s	54 ± 14 cm/s
Peak systolic velocity (at rest)	24 ± 7 cm/s	29 ± 10 cm/s
Peak diastolic velocity (stress)	104 ± 21 cm/s	76 ± 20 cm/s
Peak systolic velocity (stress)	48 ± 7 cm/s	40 ± 19 cm/s
Stress/rest diastolic velocity ratio	3.22 + 0.96	1.46 ± 0.45

From: Duerinckx AJ. Coronary MR angiography. MRI Clin N Am 1996;4(2):361–418; with permission.

astolic velocity in normal coronary vessels increases three- to fourfold during stress (34).

Typical changes in coronary blood velocity from baseline to stress (dipyridamole-induced coronary vasodilatation) based on a transesophageal echo (TEE) study (34) are summarized in Table 2.3.

Coronary Vessel Background

Coronary arteries are usually embedded in epicardial fat most of their course. Therefore some form of fat-suppression scheme to separate the signal from the coronary artery lumen from the surrounding perivascular fat is needed (at least for the "bright-blood" sequences). Occasionally, coronary arteries course through the myocardium and are surrounded by myocardial tissue. To improve the contrast between blood and myocardium a magnetization scheme prior to data collection can enhance the contrast. Both magnetization transfer (49,50) and T2-weighted preparation (51,52) have been described. The T2-weighted preparation takes advantage of the T2 differences between myocardium, oxygenated blood in coronary arteries (233 msec), and the saturated venous blood (35 msec for 20% O_2 saturation).

After surgical intervention or stent, placement metal, such as surgical clips or stents, may surround portions of the vessel. In order to enhance the vessel-to-surrounding tissue ratio, one has to take into account the surroundings of the coronary vessels when optimizing pulse sequences.

Coronary Wall and Plaque

Coronary MRA can be performed using bright blood or black blood sequences (see Chap. 3). With some of the bright blood sequences, the wall and arterial blood inside the vessel wall may have very similar signal characteristics. The use of black blood imaging or MR contrast agents may be needed to distinguish between wall and blood content. T2-weighted preparation may also improve the distinction between coronary vessel wall and blood content.

Imaging of the coronary wall and plaque inside the wall has been described by several groups (Meyer, unpublished; 53–57). This is an extension to coronary MRA of very exciting work on the use of MRI for atherosclerotic plaque characterization (58–73).

References

1. Higgins CB. Essentials of cardiac radiology and imaging. Philadelphia: J.B. Lippincott Company, 1992.
2. Grossman W. Cardiac catheterization and angiography, 3rd ed. Philadelphia: Lea and Febiger, 1986:31.
3. van Rossum AC, Bedaux WL, Hofman MB. Morphologic and functional evaluation of coronary artery bypass conduits. J Magn Reson Imag 1999;10(5):734–40.
4. Duerinckx AJ, Atkinson DP, Mintorovitch J, Simonetti OP, Urman MK. Two-dimensional coronary MR angiography: limitations and artifacts. Eur Radiology 1996;6(3):312–25.
5. Soto B, Kassner EG, Baxley WA. Imaging of cardiac disorders. Volume 2: acquired diseases. Philadelphia: J.B. Lippincott/Gower Medical Publishing, 1992.
6. Dodge JT Jr, Brown BG, Bolson EL, Dodge HT. Lumen diameter of normal human coronary arteries. Influence of age, sex, anatomic variation, and left ventricular hypertrophy and dilatation. Circulation 1992;86:232–46.
7. MacAlpin RN, Abbassi AS, Grollman JH, Eber L. Human coronary artery size during life. A cinearteriographic study. Radiology 1973;108:567–576.
8. Bergstrand L, Bylund H, Erikson U, et al. Distribution of coronary atherosclerosis and its correlation to metabolic risk factors and femoral atherosclerosis. Acta Radiol 1994;33:481–86.
9. Aro A, Soimakallio S, Voutilainen E, Ehnholm C, Wiljasalo M. Serum lipoprotein and apoprotein levels as indicators of the severity of angiographically assessed coronary artery disease. Atherosclerosis 1986;62:219–25.
10. Freedman DS, Gruchow HW, Jacobsen SJ, Anderson AJ, King JF, Barboriak JJ. Risk factors and the anatomic distribution of coronary artery disease. Atherosclerosis 1989; 75:227–36.
11. Perez GO, Mendez AJ, Goldberg RB, et al. Correlates of atherosclerosis in coronary arteries of patients undergoing angiographic evaluation. Angiology 1990;41:525–32.
12. Chang PJ, Bayesian analysis revisited: a radiologist's survival guide. Am J Roentgenol 1989;152:721–27.
13. Hillis LD, Winniford MD. Frequency of severe (70% or more) narrowing of the right, left anterior descending, and left circumflex coronary arteries in right dominant circulations with coronary artery disease. Am J Cardiol 1987;59:358–59.
14. Feit A, Khan R, Sheriff NE, Reddy CVR. Nonrandom occurrence of single-vessel coronary artery disease. Am J Med 1984;77:683–84.
15. Waller B. Anatomy, histology, and pathology of the major epicardial coronary arteries relevant to echocardiographic imaging techniques. J Am Soc Echocardiogr 1989;2(4):232–52.

16. Wang Y, Vidan E, Bergman GW. Cardiac motion of coronary arteries: variability in the rest period and implications for coronary MR angiography. Radiology 1999; 213(3):751–58.

17. Karwatowski SP, Mohiaddin RH, Yang GZ, Firmin DN, St John Sutton M, Underwood SR. Regional myocardial velocity image by magnetic resonance in patients with ischaemic heart disease. Br Heart J 1994;72(4):332–38.

18. Karwatowski SP, Mohiaddin R, Yang GZ, et al. Assessment of regional left ventricular long-axis motion with MR velocity mapping in healthy subjects. J Magn Reson Imag 1994;4(2):151–55.

19. Kong Y, Morris JJ, McIntosh HD. Assessment of regional myocardial performance from biplane coronary cineangiograms. Am J Cardiol 1971;27:529–37.

20. Hofman MB, Wickline SA, Lorenz CH. Quantification of in-plane motion of the coronary arteries during the cardiac cycle: implications for acquisition window duration for MR flow quantification. J Magn Reson Imag 1998; 8(3):568–76.

21. Holland AE, Goldfarb JW, Edelman RR. Diaphragmatic and cardiac motion during suspended breathing: preliminary experience and implications for breath-hold MR imaging. Radiology 1998;209(2):483–89.

22. Wang Y, Grist TM, Korosec FR, et al. Respiratory blur in 3D coronary MR imaging. Magn Reson Med 1995;33(4): 541–48.

23. Wang Y, Riederer SJ, Ehman RL. Respiratory motion of the heart: kinematics and implications for the spatial resolution in coronary imaging. Magn Reson Med 1995;33(5): 713–19.

24. Sachs TS, Meyer CH, Hu BS, Kohli J, Nishimura DG, Macovski A. Real-time motion detection in spiral MRI using navigators. Magn Reson Med 1994;32(5):639–45.

25. Fu Z, Wang Y, Grimm RC, et al. Orbital navigator echoes for motion measurement in magnetic resonance imaging. Magn Reson Med 1995;34(5):746–53.

26. Li D, Kaushikkar S, Woodard P, Dhawale P, Haacke EM. Three-dimensional MRI of coronary arteries (abstr). In: Book of abstracts of VII International Workshop on Magnetic Resonance Angiography. Matsuyama, Japan: October 12–14, 1995.

27. Taylor AM, Jhooti P, Firmin DN, Pennell DJ. Automated monitoring of diaphragm end-expiratory position for real-time navigator echo MR coronary angiography. J Magn Reson Imag 1999;9(3):395–401.

28. Taylor AM, Keegan J, Jhooti P, Firmin DN, Pennell DJ. Calculation of a subject-specific adaptive motion-correction factor for improved real-time navigator echo-gated magnetic resonance coronary angiography. J Cardiovasc Magn Reson 1999;1(2):131–38.

29. Danias PG, Stuber M, Botnar RM, Kissinger KV, Edelman RR, Manning WJ. Relationship between motion of coronary arteries and diaphragm during free breathing: lessons from real-time MR imaging. Am J Roentgenol 1999;172(4):1061–65.

30. Taylor AM, Keegan J, Jhooti P, Gatehouse PD, Firmin DN, Pennell DJ. Differences between normal subjects and patients with coronary artery disease for three different MR coronary angiography respiratory suppression techniques. J Magn Reson Imag 1999;9(6):786–93.

31. Manning WJ, Li W, Edelman RR. A preliminary report comparing magnetic resonance coronary angiography with conventional angiography. N Engl J Med 1993;328: 828–32.

32. Iliceto S, Memmola C, Marangelli V, Caiato C, Rizzon P. Evaluation of coronary artery anatomy and physiology with the use of transesophageal echocardiography. Cor Art Dis 1992;3:357–63.

33. Siostrzonek P, Kranz A, Heinz G, et al. Noninvasive estimation of coronary flow reserve by transesophageal Doppler measurements of coronary sinus flow. Am J Cardiol 1993;72:1334–37.

34. Iliceto S, Marangelli V, Memmola C, Rizzon P. Transesophageal Doppler echocardiography evaluation of coronary blood flow velocity in baseline conditions and during dipyridamole-induced coronary vasodilation. Circulation 1991;83:61–69.

35. Fusejima K, Takahara Y, Sudo Y, Murayama H, Masuda Y, Inagaki Y. Comparison of coronary hemodynamics in patients with internal mammary artery and saphenous vein coronary artery bypass grafts: a noninvasive approach using combined two-dimensional and Doppler echocardiography. J Am Coll Card 1990;15(1):131–39.

36. Bandyk D, Galbraith T, Haasler G, Almassi H. Blood flow velocity of internal mammary artery and saphenous vein grafts to the coronary arteries. J Surg Res 1988;44:342–51.

37. Fujiwara T, Kajiya F, Kanazawa S, et al. Comparison of blood-flow velocity waveforms in different coronary artery bypass grafts: sequential saphenous vein grafts and internal mammary artery grafts. Circulation 1988;78:1210–17.

38. vanRossum AC, Visser FC, Hofman MBM, Galjee MA, Westerhof N, Valk J. Global left ventricular perfusion: noninvasive measurement with cine MR imaging and phase velocity mapping of coronary venous outflow. Radiology 1992;182:685–91.

39. Paschal C, Haacke E, Adler L, Finelli DA. Magnetic resonance coronary artery imaging. Cardiovasc Intervent Radiol 1992;15:23–31.

40. Mukundan S, Oshinski JN, Pettigrew RI. Breath-hold turbo cine MRI for 4D localization of coronary arteries (abstr.). In: Printed program of the first meeting of the Society of Magnetic Resonance (SMR). Dallas, Texas, March 5–9, 1994; J Magn Reson Imag 1994;4(P):80.

41. Kenny A, Shapiro LM. Identification of coronary artery stenosis and poststenotic blood flow patterns using a miniature high-frequency epicardial transducer. Circulation 1994;89:731–39.

42. Ofili EO, Labovitz AJ, Kern MJ. Coronary flow velocity dynamics in normal and diseased arteries. Am J Cardiol 1993;71:30D–39D.

43. DeBono DP, Samani NJ, Spyt TJ, Hartshorne T, Thrush AJ, Evans DH. Transcutaneous ultrasound measurements of blood-flow in internal mammary artery to coronary artery grafts. Lancet 1992;339:379–81.

44. Canver CC, Dame NA. Ultrasonic assessment of internal thoracic artery graft flow in the revascularized heart. Ann Thorac Surg 1994;58:135–38.

45. Ge J, Erbel R, Gerber T, et al. Intravascular ultrasound imaging of angiographically normal coronary arteries: a prospective study in vivo. Br Heart J 1994;71:572–78.

46. Tomoike H, Ootsubo H, Sakai K, Kikuchi Y, Nakamura

M. Continuous measurements of coronary artery diameter in situ. Am J Physiol 1981;240:H73–H79.

47. Clarke GD, Eckels R, Chaney C, et al. Measurement of absolute epicardial coronary artery flow and flow reserve with breathhold cine phase-contrast magnetic resonance imaging. Circulation 1995;91(10):2627–34.

48. Hoffman JIE. Maximal coronary flow and the concept of coronary vascular reserve. Circulation 1984;70:153–59.

49. Li D, Paschal CB, Haacke EM, Adler LP. Coronary arteries: three-dimensional MR imaging with fat saturation and magnetization transfer contrast. Radiology 1993;187:401–6.

50. Wielopolski P, van Geuns RJ, de Feyter PJ, Oudkerk M. Breath-hold coronary MR angiography with volume targeted imaging. Radiology 1998;209:209–20.

51. Brittain JH, Hu BS, Wright GA, Meyer CH, Macovski A, Nishimura DG. Coronary angiography with magnetization-prepared T2 contrast. Magn Reson Med 1995;33(5): 689–96.

52. Botnar RM, Stuber M, Danias PG, Kissinger KV, Manning WJ. Improved coronary artery definition with T2-weighted, free-breathing, three-dimensional coronary MRA. Circulation 1999;99(24):3139–48.

53. Worthley SG, Helft G, Fayad Z, et al. MR imaging documents coronary artery atherosclerotic severity and composition: Ex vivo and in vivo studies in a porcine model (abstr.). In: Cardiovascular Imaging 1999. The 27th Annual Meeting of the North American Society for Cardiac Imaging (NASCI), Nov 6, 1999, Atlanta, GA: 1999.

54. Botnar RM, Stuber M, Kissinger KV, Manning WJ. Real-time navigator gated and corrected coronary vessel wall imaging (abstr.). In: Cardiovascular Imaging 1999. The 27th Annual Meeting of the North American Society for Cardiac Imaging (NASCI), Nov 6, 1999, Atlanta, GA: 1999.

55. Botnar RM, Stuber M, Kissinger KV, Manning WJ. In vivo imaging of coronary artery wall in humans using navigator and free-breathing (abstr.). In: Book of Abstracts and Proceedings of the 8th Meeting of the International Society of Magnetic Resonance in Medicine (ISMRM 2000 Proceedings Available on CD-ROM). Denver, CO April 1–7, 2000.

56. Fayad ZA, Fuster V, Fallon JT, et al. Noninvasive in vivo human coronary artery lumen and wall imaging using black blood MR (abstr.). In: Book of Abstracts and Proceedings of the 8th Meeting of the International Society of Magnetic Resonance in Medicine (ISMRM 2000 Proceedings Available on CD-ROM). Denver, CO April 1–7, 2000.

57. Zheng J, Li D, Finn JP, Simonetti O, Cavagna FM. Coronary vessel wall MR imaging: Initial experience. (abstr.). In: Book of Abstracts and Proceedings of the 8th Meeting of the International Society of Magnetic Resonance in Medicine (ISMRM 2000 Proceedings Available on CD-ROM). Denver, CO April 1–7, 2000.

58. Yuan C, Petty C, O'Brien KD, Hatsukami TS, Eary JF, Brown BG. In vitro and in situ magnetic resonance imaging signal features of atherosclerotic plaque-associated lipids. Thrombosis, . . . , Arteriosclerosis 1997;17(8):1496–1503.

59. Trouard TP, Altbach MI, Hunter GC, Eskelson CD, Gmitro AF. MRI and NMR spectroscopy of the lipids of atherosclerotic plaque in rabbits and humans. Magn Reson Med 1997;38(1):19–26.

60. Toussaint JF, Southern JF, Kantor HL, Jang IK, Fuster V. Behavior of atherosclerotic plaque components after in vitro angioplasty and atherectomy studied by high field MR imaging. Magn Reson Imag 1998;16(2):175–83.

61. Hatsukami TS, Ferguson MS, Beach KW, et al. Carotid plaque morphology and clinical events. Stroke 1997;28(1): 95–100.

62. Bonn D. Plaque detection: the key to tackling atherosclerosis? [news]. Lancet 1999;354(9179):656.

63. Luk-Pat GT, Gold GE, Olcott EW, Hu BS, Nishimura DG. High-resolution three-dimensional in vivo imaging of atherosclerotic plaque. Magn Reson Med 1999;42(4):762–71.

64. Shinnar M, Fallon JT, Wehrli S, et al. The diagnostic accuracy of ex vivo MRI for human atherosclerotic plaque characterization. Arterioscler Thromb Vasc Biol 1999;19(11): 2756–61.

65. Zimmermann-Paul GG, Quick HH, Vogt P, von Schulthess GK, Kling D, Debatin JF. High-resolution intravascular magnetic resonance imaging: monitoring of plaque formation in heritable hyperlipidemic rabbits. Circulation 1999;99(8):1054–61.

66. Fayad ZA, Fuster V, Fallon JT, et al. Noninvasive in vivo human coronary artery lumen and wall imaging using black-blood magnetic resonance imaging. Circulation 2000;102(5):506–10.

67. Fayad ZA, Fuster V. Characterization of atherosclerotic plaques by magnetic resonance imaging. Ann NY Acad Sci 2000;902:173–86.

68. Fischer A, Gutstein DE, Fayad, ZA, Fuster V. Predicting plaque rupture: enhancing diagnosis and clinical decision-making in coronary artery disease. Vasc Med 2000;5(3): 163–72.

69. Rogers WJ, Prichard JW, Hu YL, et al. Characterization of signal properties in atherosclerotic plaque components by intravascular MRI. Arterioscler Thromb Vasc Biol 2000; 20(7):1824–30.

70. Worthley SG, Helft G, Fuster V, et al. Serial in vivo MRI documents arterial remodeling in experimental atherosclerosis. Circulation 2000;101(6):586–89.

71. Worthley SG, Helft G, Fuster V, et al. Noninvasive in vivo magnetic resonance imaging of experimental coronary artery lesions in a porcine model. Circulation 2000;101(25): 2956–61.

72. Worthley SG, Helft G, Fuster V, et al. High resolution ex vivo magnetic resonance imaging of in situ coronary and aortic atherosclerotic plaque in a porcine model. Atherosclerosis 2000;150(2):321–29.

73. Worthley SG, Helft G, Fayad ZA, et al. Images in cardiovascular medicine. Magnetic resonance imaging and asymptomatic aortic dissection. Circulation 2000;101(23):2771.

3
Coronary MR Angiographic Techniques

Dennis Atkinson, Orlando Simonetti, and André J. Duerinckx

Introduction

Coronary magnetic resonance imaging (MRI) is not the same as conventional X-ray angiography (XRA). The two techniques differ in many and profound ways. They differ in how they acquire and produce images, how their systems are operated, and, eventually, how the methods are used clinically. XRA is a high-resolution projection method that is capable of delineating very fine structures of the beating heart. Magnetic resonance angiography (MRA) of the coronaries is a medium-resolution method that can produce thin section views along any arbitrary projection. It typically requires synchronization of multiple heartbeats to elicit an image reliably. XRA of the coronary tree is a widely used and accepted means for assessing the caliber of the cardiac vessels. Generations of radiologists and cardiologists have studied coronary images. MR is still in a state of relative infancy.

Given the current success of conventional angiography, why is there any interest in MRI of the coronaries? First, conventional X-ray angiography is not without its disadvantages. It is an invasive technique with some patient risk. It is also a projection method lacking three-dimensional information. Furthermore, it is restricted to specific view angles by instrumentation and patient location. It is expensive. It lacks the facility to acquire additional cardiac physiologic data in the same setting (e.g., wall motion, perfusion, or characterization of infarcted regions and/or ischemic risk). It requires a team of well-trained experts to perform, and it exposes them and the patient to ionizing radiation.

MRA does not offer an advantage compared to XRA in each of these issues. Rather, MRA has some unique capabilities that may define a complementary role for the technique in the clinical setting. MRA has gained clinical acceptance in other areas of the body and may offer a noninvasive means for assessing the health of coronary vessels. This chapter is intended to be a brief technical introduction into the process of MRI and MRA. Subsequent chapters will detail the methods and describe clinical experience to date.

MRI and Conventional X-ray Imaging

MR imaging and conventional X-ray imaging use completely different acquisition methods with different equipment. In conventional angiography, radiation floods the entire imaging field-of-view (FOV), through the patient and onto a detector apparatus. Radiation is attenuated as it passes through the body, resulting in dark, low signal areas where the projection passes through areas of high electron density. The overall image contrast is adjusted by varying the number (via mA) and energy (keV) of the photons used in imaging. Intravascular contrast is achieved in two steps. A fine-tipped catheter is typically inserted into the femoral artery and passed retrograde through the aorta to the artery of interest. This is performed using X-ray fluoroscopy to monitor the progression of the tip to the proper vessels. Once in place, high-density iodinated contrast agent is released into the vessels opacifying the lumen. Conventional angiography is a very rapid technique that can generate up to 30 frames per second. It is also a high-resolution method that can accurately depict features as low as 0.1 mm. Used properly in the hands of trained experts, XRA has been a technique widely recognized as the gold standard for the detection of coronary arterial stenoses.

MRI

MRA uses a completely different manner for making images. No ionizing radiation is used. The MRI signal comes instead from hydrogen protons within the body. Scientists have known since the 1920s that nuclei precess when in the presence of a strong, externally applied magnetic field. [In fact, MRI was called nuclear magnetic resonance (NMR) in early clinical use.] The rate precession or frequency is characteristic of both the strength of the magnetic field and the type of nuclei. Typical clinical MR scanners today operate at 1.5 Tesla with a precessional frequency of about 63 MHz, although routine clinical imaging is performed at field strengths between 0.2 and 2.0 Tesla. In general, the signal–noise improves linearly with field strength (or frequency), with most coronary studies to date being done at 1.0 Tesla or higher.

Precession alone is not sufficient to produce an image. Knowing the precessional frequency gives only the bulk resonance of all tissues within the magnetic field. In order to produce images, the magnetic resonance technique needs to modify the precession rate in the magnet to localize tissues within the body. Localization of tissues is accomplished by applying specific local changes to the magnetic field within the main field of the magnet. These field gradients are small, typically 0.001–0.01% of the main field, but sufficient uniquely to identify locations within the body. Local field changes are done via three separate coils within the main field and can be heard during the operation of the MR scanner as they turn on and off with rapidity. The coils, or gradients, are typically linear and define an imaging plane or volume with rectangular or square pixels. Because the three gradients may be turned on or off together, it is possible to define imaging planes that are as thin as 0.5 mm or thick as 200 mm and oriented along any oblique axis. Indeed, this is one of the unique features of MRI: It can arbitrarily change imaging orientation and slice thicknesses without any modification to the equipment.

In conventional X-ray imaging, an incident beam of high-energy photons passes through the body and an image is then produced from those remaining. This is the process for a simple wrist X-ray, a coronary angiogram, or computed tomography (CT) image. MR is different. In MRI, an incident radiation of radiofrequency (RF) energy is not transmitted through the body onto a detecting device. RF energy is instead broadcast uniformly and throughout the area of interest from almost all sides. After this brief burst of energy, there is a short waiting period, then time to "listen" and sample the returning energy. If the RF frequency is chosen along with the applied field gradients, the sampling volume can be well localized to resonate only in one area of the body. Most MR protocols operate by forcing the protons to re-emit their energy in concert to create an echo of the initial RF pulse, an echo well localized by the application of the field gradients during the brief wait. The returning energy is greatly diminished (on the order of microwatts), so small receivers, also called surface coils, are placed as close as possible to the area of

interest to minimize signal loss. (Because the MRI operating frequency is close to standard radio and television frequencies, and the receivers have such a high sensitivity, most MRI facilities enclose the imaging area with conductive material that screens outside interference.)

This process of broadcasting, forming an echo, and sampling the returning echo forms the heart of all MR imaging. Almost all MR protocols use this concept to create images of different size and location. This process alone, however, does not create image contrast. If all we did was broadcast, form an echo, and sample that echo, the result would be an image whose signal would be dependent upon the number of hydrogen protons in the volume of interest. Water, fat, muscle, and blood would all have a high density of protons and, thus, a high signal. Low-density material (e.g., air and lung pa-renchyma) would have a low signal. Cortical bone also has low signal because it is largely calcium that resonates at a different frequency than hydrogen.

Unlike many other radiologic methods, MR provides other contrast mechanisms that use inherent tissue differences. One such mechanism can create contrast between muscle and fat, flowing and nonflowing blood, and normal and pathologic tissues.

Precessing nuclei can be deflected away from the magnetic axis, much like a gyroscope spinning on a stand. Like a gyroscope, they will also return in alignment in time. MRI is based on our ability to move these spin axes away from alignment using a strong magnetic field and our ability to observe their recovery. This recovery process is an exponential one (see Fig. 3.1). By definition, recovery to 63% of the initial, or complete, longitudinal magnetization is called the T1 time. Over two times the T1 period recovery is to 85%, with essentially full recovery after four to five times the T1 times. Myocardial tissue has a T1 of approximately 650 msec, circulating blood has a T1 of about 1300 msec, and typical body fat has a brief T1 of 150 msec. These T1 recovery time differences provide a basis for creating image contrast. Repeating the RF pulse before there is complete T1 recovery of the longitudinal magnetization results in a reduced longitudinal vector for the next data acquisition. This repetition time, or TR, is one of the variables frequently adjusted in MR protocol to accentuate or diminish differences in tissues. Extremely rapid TRs (typically less than 50 msec) substantially reduce T1 recovery to suppress or saturate unwanted tissues effectively. As seen later in this chapter and throughout the book, suppression of unwanted signals is a significant part of the success of MRA techniques.

Finally, one significant difference between conventional X-ray based angiography and MRA is that the MRI process is much longer. Even though each sampling period is brief (< 10 msec), hundreds, maybe even

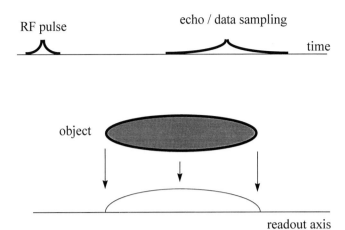

Figure 3.1. Schematic representation of the MRI process for projection imaging. A simple gradient echo is formed from a single RF excitation pulse by reversal of gradients (not shown). Absent any additional encoding steps, the signal from the object is merely projected onto a readout axis. Encoding spatial information along the readout axis is accomplished with a readout gradient applied during the echo. The result is that the Fourier transform of the returning signal gives an indication of the amount of the object within each vertical column (down arrows). This process gives no indication of spatial position within the column and may be considered as a $1 \times N$ matrix, where N is the number of data columns defined along the readout direction.

thousands, of MR samples are required to create a viable image. Because the heart beats during this acquisition, cardiac motion is a serious problem. Left uncorrected, it results in smearing of features and substantial ghosting. Scan times over 20–30 seconds will have further artifact if respiratory motion is compensated. To overcome cardiac motion problems, one simple and commonly used strategy is to trigger the acquisition to begin only when the heart is at a consistent point within the cardiac cycle. Similar to a strobe light, acquisitions at a consistent time delay make the heart appear to be at a constant location. The time delay is frequently set to be later in the cardiac cycle to make use of the longer quiescent diastolic period. This strategy is also called *prospective gating* because the delay from the R-wave is known prior to the acquisition. An alternative strategy is to acquire data repetitively and merely note the R-wave delay for each piece of data. Then, during the reconstruction process, data is re-sorted into similar delay times, or bins, where the heart would appear to be in a constant position. This method is called *retrospective gating*. Similar strategies can also be used to address the problem of respiratory motion.

This chapter is developed in a series of stages. The first is a review of the MRA imaging process that makes noninvasive visualization of arteries possible. Next is a survey of basic cardiac imaging methods and their applications for the coronaries. This is followed by results

of coronary imaging research that has shown promise in improving the spatial resolution and clinical applicability of coronary MRI. Finally, the latter part of the chapter is to introduce other techniques that make use of MR's ability to assess flow and motion of the heart.

Visualizing Flow: MRA Basics

For most routine MRI signals from moving objects are suppressed to avoid artifact and improve the overall image quality. For example, imaging of the abdomen is hindered by motion of the anterior subcutaneous fat during the study, resulting in ghosting and smearing of the fat over the FOV. In contrast, MRA seeks to accentuate those signals from moving objects while suppressing signals from stationary background areas. Indeed, it is good flow-to-background contrast that provides the basis for vessel definition and flow characterization in MRA. The development of MRA methods initially focused on the relatively simpler problem of noninvasive visualization of the carotid and intracranial vessels because these were nonmoving structures. Although the same principles and techniques were available, visualization at that time of the coronary tree with the beating heart and chest motion seemed a daunting task.

Hundreds of MRA pulsing schemes may exist, each with a slight variation in the acquisition or data manipulation (1). In general, they may be categorized into groups based on their ability to manipulate the longitudinal magnetization (Mz) or transverse magnetization (Mxy) vectors. These groupings are designated amplitude-based (Mz), phase-based (Mxy), or a combination of both amplitude- and phase-based (Mz and Mxy) techniques. The amplitude-based techniques work by producing significantly different Mz vectors for moving spins than for stationary tissues. The phase methods are based on advancement or retardation of moving spins in the presence of a spatial magnetic field gradient. Both amplitude and phase-based methods may be combined synergistically in a third category of imaging, potentially further improving flow-to-background contrast.

Amplitude-Based Methods

To provide a good illustration of the interplay between various physical parameters, let us look at a very simple amplitude-based MRI method that is most often used for 2-D coronary imaging. This most basic MRA sequence is a thin-slice, 2-D gradient-echo sequence, with a short repetition time, a high RF flip angle, and gradient pulses calibrated to reduce phase dispersal from moving spins.

After the repetition of a few RF pulses, the stationary spins within the slice become saturated due to the short repetition time (TR) and the high flip angle, and the background signal drops. On the other hand, the moving protons of the coronary arteries entering into the plane have their full magnetization because they are not yet saturated and produce a high MR signal. A constant stream of new blood protons provides a steady replenishment of new magnetization and signal. These so-called bright blood techniques are influenced by the RF flip angle, slice thickness, and the rapidity of moving spins entering the plane (e.g., a thick slice or slow flow would allow the vessel signal to saturate and appear no brighter than background). They are also called time-of-flight (TOF) methods because this technique depends on the speed of the inflow to produce enhanced blood signal.

This simple technique illustrates two essential and interdependent principles used for all MR TOF methods: (1) background signal suppression with (2) enhancement of blood signal. The clinical practice further influences these compromises of MRA with limitations imposed by the patient, the operator, and/or the MRI instrumentation.

Background Signal Suppression
If the background signal is not adequately suppressed, there is very little contrast between the vessel and pericardial fat or myocardium. The use of rapid repetition times and relatively high RF power levels (i.e., flip angles) work well to suppress some of these stationary background signals, but they can also reduce the signal from flowing protons. This process works well only when the inflow into the plane of section is sufficiently rapid to replenish already saturated spins within the vessel. Coronary blood flow (during the nonquiescent phase) is fortunately more than sufficient (up to 1 m/sec) to avoid this problem.

To suppress fat signal better, additional RF pulses are also used. A major component of flowing blood is the plasma bulk water. Within a homogeneous magnetic field, the protons in bulk water and those in aliphatic lipids resonate at a difference in frequency of about 3.4 ppm. This difference translates into 217 Hz separation at 1.5 Tesla, or 145 Hz at 1.0 Tesla. It is possible to reduce lipid signal selectively with little effect on that from the blood pool by applying a second RF pulse offset by this frequency difference (2). This frequency offset chemical-shift-selective (CHESS) (3) suppression mechanism is very helpful when examining flow in the fat-containing areas of the body (e.g., coronary and abdominal vessels). Magnetic field inhomogeneity is present whenever a patient is introduced into an otherwise very homogeneous field (i.e., the local magnetic field will vary due to their air–tissue boundaries and intrinsic diamagnetic characteristics of the tissues). If the magnetic field varies more than a few parts per million, the lipid suppression is ineffective and/or the blood signal may be eliminated because the RF energy is no longer applied to the lipid resonating frequency. To limit this

effect, the magnetic field may be re-adjusted (or shimmed) for each patient via a tuning process that changes or distorts the magnetic field. These fat-suppression, or "fat-sat," methods were key to the early success of coronary MRA and are a staple for most protocols today.

These frequency differences influence coronary protocols in a second way. After the RF pulse has been applied, the water–lipid vectors rotate around the x–y plane and cycle in phase and out of phase with respect to one another over time. The out-of-phase images are useful for coronary imaging because voxels may contain both water and pericardial lipid. With lipid and water vectors in opposition, there is intravoxel cancellation and loss of signal along the borders of the vessels. This marked local signal loss aids in better defining small vessels or depicting local stenoses. At 1.5 Tesla, gradient echo images are out of phase at 2.2, 6.6, and 11.0 msec, and in phase at 4.4, 8.8, and 13.2 msec. At lower field strengths, the fat and water vectors rotate proportionately slower. Thus, for example, at 1.0 Tesla vectors are out of phase at echo times of 3.3, 9.9, and 16.5 msec.

It is also possible via a process called *magnetization transfer* (MT) (4) to reduce nonlipid background signals (e.g., myocardial muscle using a second RF pulse tuned to a slightly different frequency). Protons in proteins and other macromolecules differ in their magnetic environment from those found in free, or bulk, water. In bulk water, there is an unfettered mobility of molecules. That is, each hydrogen proton in the water molecule "sees" the same environment nearby and with it resonates at about the same frequency. A very long T2 value and a single sharp resonance are indicators of this. Proton in water molecules that are immobile ("bound") have relatively fixed neighbors and local magnetic environments. Because of this, they each experience a differing local magnetic environment and resonate over a broader range of frequencies than unbound water. By irradiating these protons with an off-resonance RF pulse, they become saturated, whereas the bulk water (e.g., blood) signal remains largely unaffected. Through the ongoing exchange of water between the different layers, transference of saturation takes place from the immobile protons to water in a nearby hydration layer. This magnetization transference enables a larger number of bound protons to be saturated with minimal effect on the more distal, bulk water protons. This unique contrast mechanism, called either *magnetization transfer contrast* (MTC) (5) or *saturation transfer contrast* (STC) (6), has been used for applications to define tissue characteristics.

For MRA applications, the specific contrast produced via magnetization transfer is not as critical; rather, its ability to further suppress background signal is important. In this context, this application of MT presaturation has sometimes been referred to as *magnetization transfer suppression* (7) (MTS) because it can aid in suppressing background tissues with little influence on the blood and vascular signal.

Various RF pulse types and pulsing sequences have been proposed to incorporate MT presaturation into an angiographic sequence (8). Edelman et al. (9) reported an MTS experiment where a conventional gradient echo sequence was combined with a Gaussian-shaped off-resonance RF pulse set at 1.5 kHz away from the water signal. The net effect was a significantly reduced background signal and a qualitative improvement in conspicuity in 71% of the vessels in the brain.

The MT effect becomes more pronounced as the irradiation frequency approaches that of the bulk water resonance (10). In theory, on-resonance excitation should also reduce the water signal; however, there are orders of magnitude difference in T2 times between the immobile, restricted protons (Hr) and those in the free water pool (Hf) is (< 200 msec vs. > 10 msec). Selective excitation of the Hr magnetization pool can be achieved via a short duration 121 binomial pulse that reduces the Mz for short T2 tissues (Hr), whereas the Mz of longer T2 tissues (Hf) is unaffected (11). Using this sequence, Pike reported that background signal could be reduced by 39% versus a blood signal reduction of only 17%. One potential problem with the application of these off-resonance MT pulses is that of inadvertent saturation of distal blood. Introducing a patient into the magnet causes local field changes due to the air–tissue interfaces. These changes are minor and within the ability of the system to produce good image quality. Distal to the imaging area, however, what may happen is that the field (and resonant frequency) may vary such that the RF pulse that is off-resonance in one region may be on-resonance in another. This is not a problem for non-moving spins, but for flowing blood the result may be saturation of the incoming blood with attendant loss of signal. To minimize saturation of the blood pool, Kojima et al. introduced a slice-selection gradient to irradiate only the plane of section. This limited any flow saturation effect to only the slice location and avoided potential diminution of the inflowing blood signal as it passed through magnetic field inhomogeneities. The result was that blood–background ratio improved from 1.25:1 to 1.53:1 when compared with a nonselective 121 binomial method (12).

There has been limited use to date of MT effects to improve visualization of the coronary arteries.

Inversion Recovery Methods

As seen earlier, reduction of stationary spin longitudinal magnetization (Mz) can be accomplished via strategy of rapid RF excitations and the introduction of off-resonance RF presaturation. In either case, some reduction in flowing spin magnetization cannot be avoided. An alternative background method exists that uses long delays between suppression of background and the measuring of flow information. Inversion recovery (IR) is a widely accepted MRI method that uses a single pulse to tip protons upside down, then a delay before reading out the remaining signal. IR offers some unique strategies for MRA and has been used in coronary imaging (13,14). Edelman et al. implemented a version of IR where a slice-selective 180-degree pulse was followed by a variable delay (TI), then by a series of short TR (7–8 msec) gradient echo sequences to read out the data (15). By varying the TI, background tissues could be selectively nulled. Unlike the off-resonance saturation, this method does not suffer in the presence of local magnetic field inhomogeneities. When used in a single-shot mode, where the imaging data is read out for 600–1000 msec, T1 relaxation during the sampling compromised the ability to null tissues. To improve tissue nulling, the process was broken up, or segmented, into 2, 4, 8, or 16 passes. With this method, an improvement in blood–tissue signal difference-to-noise was demonstrated of 73% (49.5 vs. 28.6). This technique unfortunately suffers in the imaging of the coronary arteries as the heart moves substantially between the tag and read events, resulting in a mismatch between inverted and noninverted regions.

A simple IR technique is most effective when a homogeneous background tissue (with a single T1 recovery time) is to be suppressed. With coronary imaging this is not the case. Overlying pericardial fat and underlying myocardium both surround the vessel interfere with the vascular signal. Li expanded the IR technique into 3 dimensions and added fat saturation to improve background suppression (16). In their method [selective inversion recovery rapid acquisition with gradient echo (SIR-RAGE)], a selective inversion pulse is applied to the imaging plane shortly after the R-wave. During the TI time, fresh noninverted blood flows into the slab, replacing the blood pool in the imaging plane, producing bright blood signal against a diminished background. Given the short T1 of fat and the long TI needed to allow inflow, lipid signals could potentially limit blood–background contrast. To improve this contrast, an additional chemically selective presaturation pulse was inserted immediately prior to the 3-D acquisition; that is, the sequence became:

$$(180° - TI - fat\ saturation - (GRE\ 3D\ acquisition)NzNy$$

where Nz is the number of partitions along the slice-selection direction, and Ny the number of phase encoding lines within the imaging plane. Fat suppression without chemically selective pulses was accomplished by Richardson et al. by inserting a second inversion pulse prior to the acquisition (17). In their report, they further improved the method by employing the long TI delay time prior to acquisition to insert a series of saturation pulses to preferentially eliminate upstream venous signal.

Improved background suppression can be accomplished by using two sets of registered images: one flow encoded; the other as a mask to subtract out nonflowing signals. By using the signal differentials rather than an imperfect tissue-specific prepulse, nonmoving structures can be eliminated regardless of their T1 values, local inhomogeneities, or chemical shift. Edelman introduced this method [Signal Targeting with Alternating Radiofrequency (STAR)] as a simple pair of acquisitions. One pass tags the upstream spins with an inversion pulse, on the next, there is no inversion:

Pass (1) (Invert–delay–read)
Pass (2) (no invert–delay–read)

The result is that only the longitudinal magnetization (Mz) of the inflowing spins is affected. By subtracting one image from the other the extent and direction of flow is demonstrated by this difference of passes (1) and (2) (18). Visualizing fast flowing blood, such as the coronary arteries, uses a rather short time between the tag and read events (19), slower flow may be visualized by using longer delay times. The initial application of this black blood strategy has been to use a rapid series of gradient echos to read out the residual signal after the preparation pulses.

Others have taken advantage of some of the benefits of spin echo imaging, such as improved signal-to-noise (S/N), reduced artifact from field inhomogeneity (i.e., with postsurgical clips/wires), and in-flow. Because spin echos require tissues to be present for both the initial 90-degree excitation and the 180-degree refocusing pulse, they are very effective for black blood imaging. Moving blood courses through the vessel and is quickly replaced by nonexcited (i.e., nonsignal producing) blood, a process enhanced by the delayed and multiply refocused echos with fast, or turbo, spin-echo imaging (20).

Blood Signal Enhancement
Imaging of moving blood is complicated by the many and varied physiologic processes in the body. Traveling at velocities that range from near zero up to 1 m/second, blood moves through the heart, the coronary branches, the great vessels, and into the body. Throughout the cardiac cycle, blood presses forward, slows down, and may even reverse direction. Blood may pass through tortuous vessels and focal constrictions that reduce the cross-section by 95% or more. Surface irregularities, such as ulcerations and atherosclerotic plaque, further complicate the intravascular flow by disturbing the smooth laminar flow through the vessel. The coronaries lay upon a beating heart that contracts, twists, and is pulled to its base throughout the cardiac cycle

while also moving with each breath. It is not suprising that imaging of the coronary arteries has been one of the most difficult challenges for MRI.

Together these physiologic effects present significant technical challenges for MRA. To be clinically useful, the MRA protocol must produce high-flow/stationary contrast, proper spatial registration of both moving and stationary spins, and minimal artifact even in the presence of wide physiological and pathological variants. This protocol ideally must work in a broad population, typically including patients with severely compromised health, for it to be clinically useful.

Vascular signal enhancement in MRA comes from our ability to produce high signal from flowing blood and the proper capture of that signal during the MRI process.

Echo Times and Gradients

The duration from the initial excitation of the spins to the readout of the signal echo is called the *echo time* (TE) (see Figs. 3.1 and 3.2). This duration is typically from the peak of the RF pulse amplitude to the highest amplitude of the received signal envelope at the center of the sampling period. The field echo (FE) is defined slightly differently. The duration of the FE time is similar to that for the TE, except that its starting point begins at the first onset of dephasing gradient and goes to the peak of the echo signal. Because dephasing gradients are applied after the RF pulse FE times are shorter

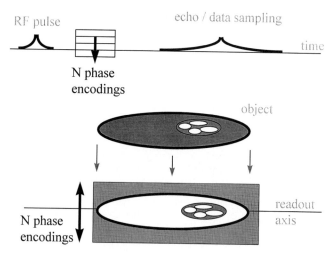

Figure 3.2. Schematic representation of the phase encoding process for a transverse image through the chest. Like Figure 3.1, a gradient echo is created from an initial RF excitation pulse; however, an additional gradient is used to encode data in a direction orthogonal to the readout axis. In this case, gradients of different amplitudes are used over a series of acquisitions to define spatial position along this phase encoding axis. The resolution (matrix dimension) along this axis (below) is typically proportional to the number of steps used in this encoding process.

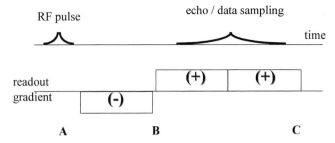

Figure 3.3. Schematic representation of the process for reading out gradient echo information. The initial RF excitation pulse tips the magnetization vector into the transverse plane (position A). At this point, all spins are in-phase and coherent. By applying the negative readout gradient, spins dephase and the overall transverse signal is temporarily lost (location at position B). Phase coherence can be recalled with the application of a positive readout gradient (first plus sign), leading to a gradient recalled echo. The amplitude of this echo is always less than the initial signal because local dephasing effects (i.e., magnetic field inhomogeneity or T2* effects) cannot be compensated with a simple gradient reversal. Further application of the readout gradient (the second plus sign) causes further dephasing and signal loss (final position C). Because the readout gradient is on during the data sampling, we are able to determine spatial positions based on the returning frequency. Because moving spins are not at the same location for the gradient application at A, B, and C, their ability to rephase (refocus) is impaired. The result may be that moving blood may rephase at different times (and blur) or fail to rephase (and show a loss of signal, or flow void). By keeping the duration of A, B, and C as short as possible, this effect is minimized.

than TE times. The readout gradient FE time tends to be the most critical in MRA because it is on for the largest portion of the sequence.

A number of factors are under the influence of TE; both T2 and T2* decay, magnetic field susceptibility, and the phase relation between fat and water vectors (see Fig. 3.3). FE time will largely determine the phase characteristics of moving spins. For example, it may be beneficial merely to add time between the excitation RF pulse and the beginning of the first readout gradient event to have fat and water vectors opposed. That is, the FE time would be the same, but merely shifted later in time. This may often be the case when sequences are modified from a high-field MR scanner (fat/water are opposed at 6.6 msec for 1.5 Tesla) to a lower magnetic field (at 1.0 Tesla, where fat/water are opposed at 9.9 msec).

The phase of a group of stationary spins is the sum of the base magnetic field plus the contribution of the gradient field times the duration and the gyromagnetic ratio,

$$\Phi_{stationary} = \gamma^* [B_0 + xG_x] * t$$

where, Φ is the phase from stationary tissues, γ the gyromagnetic ratio, Bo is the base magnetic field (including local inhomogeneities), x is position along gradient

G_x, and t is the duration of gradient on-time. In gradient echo imaging, the phase dispersal from the dephasing gradient lobe is balanced by the net phase from the rephasing lobe, resulting in a net zero phase for stationary protons.

For moving spins, this phase calculation is complicated by the fact that position x is changing with time. The phase of a constant velocity spin group is a function of the velocity of movement along the gradient and the duration of the gradient event squared,

$$\Phi_{velocity} = \Phi_{stationary} + \gamma/2 * [VG_x] * t^2$$

From this, we see the accumulated phase (Φ) depends on the square of the gradient on-time duration (t^2) more than its amplitude (G_x). Unless corrected or minimized, this additional phase accumulation can introduce dephasing within the voxel. Intravoxel dephasing results in a self-cancellation within and loss of signal for the voxel. This is observed clinically when a focal stenosis produces a downstream poststenotic lesion, or "jet," that is far larger than the lesion itself. Phase accumulations may not self-cancel and result in a nonzero phase vector that, when added to the phase, shift from the 2-D and 3-D encoding process to produce a series of vascular "ghosts."

The phase is further modified for nonconstant velocities or accelerating spins. Another term is introduced that is the product of acceleration, the gradient amplitude, and the third power of the duration of the gradient event. Accelerating spins may also produce additional signal losses and/or introduce artifact if not corrected, and may be seen clinically as pulsatility ghosts. Given the strong phase dependence on the duration of gradient events, shorter FE (and TE) times with their reduced dephasing are generally preferred (21,22).

An additional gradient lobe may be introduced to reduce the dephasing effects of constant velocity flow. By using three gradient events, the sequence can minimize dephasing by nulling both the first moment (velocity) as well as the zeroth (stationary). This strategy is referred to as *gradient moment refocusing* (GMR) (or GMN, gradient moment nulling) and is widely used for both MR angiographic and imaging studies. Additional gradient lobes may be introduced to compensate for higher orders of motion (acceleration and jerk) (23–25), but have been impractical given their longer TEs (26,27). The advent of faster rise times and higher amplitude gradient instrumentation will permit higher-order motion correction with minimal time penalties.

The physical parameters of the MR scanners present limits on sequence options. Gradients may turn on and off only so quickly and may have only limited peak performance. Using modified acquisition and reconstruction methods to minimize these limits, reduced TEs may be possible (28). One often-used method merely shifts the echo center earlier toward the RF pulse (29). Reducing the dephasing lobe duration shifts the echo closer to the RF pulse and produces both a shorter TE and FE in a gradient echo sequence. For complex Fourier reconstructions this introduces a first-order phase roll across the image, but is not apparent with typical magnitude image reconstruction. If the sampling asymmetry is too extensive (i.e., the ratio of the time before the peak to that after is less than 1:3) and not corrected, the abrupt truncation of one echo side may introduce a "ringing" artifact in the frequency encoding direction. This artifact may be reduced significantly if, prior to the standard reconstruction, a windowing, or cosine filter function is applied to more gently roll-off the abbreviated side of the echo (30). On the other hand a Half-Fourier (conjugate synthesis) reconstruction strategy may be used where the "missing" portion of the echo signal is calculated. With Half-Fourier reconstruction, blurring effects can be minimized at regions where high and low intensities have a sharply defined border. This more complicated reconstruction can be costly and has the potential for introducing additional motion artifact (31,32). Another potential solution for shorter TEs is using non-GMR sequences (i.e., sequences with only a dephasing and rephasing lobe). In one study, Schmallbrook compared short TE without GMR (3.1 msec) and with GMR (4.5 msec) in visualizing focal stenoses. The shorter echo time was effective in reducing susceptibility effects and some dephasing, but suffered in comparison to the flow compensated later echo for reducing dephasing (33).

Improved gradient performance, discussed later, offers the potential for even shorter TEs with gradient refocusing and clinically appropriate spatial resolution.

Cardiac MRI

As discussed briefly earlier, the MR image is a composite of hundreds of samples. Although each of the samples are taken in only a few milliseconds, the resulting image typically requires hundreds of seconds to acquire. Should the anatomy move during this acquisition, the MR images will contain artifacts that will distort or obscure features. In MRI, the phase of the returning proton signal is subtly varied along one or two dimensions so that the data set may be transformed into a complete model of the organ. When physiologic motion changes the position and dimensions of the organs during the acquisition, the returning phase no longer represents the intended MR-encoded signal of spatial position. Modulation of this encoding process by cardiac motion, flow, respiratory excursions, and involuntary motion all produce the familiar ghosting or smearing of the image.

One simple way to overcome periodic motion, such as the contracting heart, is to synchronize the acquisition of data with a consistent point in the cardiac cycle. By sampling at the same point in the cyclic motion, tissues return to the same location and artifact is greatly reduced. As long as motion is cyclic and regular, and the anatomy returns to a consistent location, the method works well, albeit inefficiently. On the other hand, another strategy is to continue to acquire data when the anatomy is largely in a nonmoving state. Scanning techniques that require long acquisition windows (>100 msec) often image during diastole to minimize motion artifact. Another example of this is respiratory gating, where data is acquired only during the quiescent period of breathing and the remaining portion of the respiratory cycle is ignored.

Coronary MRI

Imaging of the coronary arteries has long been a goal and a technical challenge in MRI. The goal has been to provide a clinical service that could reliably visualize the proximal coronary branches in a noninvasive manner. The obstacles to successful coronary images seem technically daunting in comparison to MRI of other areas of the body. The vessels themselves are small in caliber, they are subject to high flow rates and pulsatility, are prone to focal constriction, contain variations in surface roughness along their length, travel along many tortuous, nonplanar pathways, and are both upon and within a beating surface. In addition, the patient contributes additional complications. The heart rate may vary during the acquisition, EKG signals or beats may be missed, the diaphragm moves with each respiratory excursion (34), the patients may have limited ability to cooperate for the MR exam, and a strong lipid or fat signal may dominate the imaging field.

Because of these technical and physiologic problems, the field of coronary MRI has developed somewhat more slowly than other areas of the body. From the earliest clinical reports, researchers have observed that coronary arteries were visible on routine images as incidental findings. Almost from the beginning of clinical MR usage, reports noted anecdotally that spin-echo images of the aortic base depicted the proximal tree as structures with signal loss corresponding to flow. Although encouraging, these findings were not consistent enough to provide visualization of the vessels reliably. Thus, coronary MRI remained a research interest with limited clinical usefulness for some time.

One could characterize the evolution of coronary MRI as progressing through three phases or generations. First, there were a series of modifications to the basic 2-D imaging sequences to substantially reduce imaging times. By completing the MR image within one breath-hold, the problem of respiratory motion is greatly reduced and consistent results, so critical for clinical studies, are possible (35). Second, there were a generation of techniques that were longer (minutes to tens of minutes), but offered volumetric acquisitions and a means to eliminate respiratory motion via mathematical correction models that include a separate data sampling of body position (navigator). This second generation offered improved resolution and coverage as well as a technique that may not require as much operator–patient interaction. The third is a generation that makes use of higher-performance MR systems (notably the gradients) to produce volumetric acquisitions in very fast imaging times (seconds). This latest generation is still evolving, but it holds the promise of improving resolution, coverage, and consistency.

In the development of new techniques, the set of requirements is wide and almost contradictory. Any useful method must be robust to provide reliable and clinically useful data on even the sickest of patients. At a minimum, the method must cover at least the proximal coronary branches and potentially image all major vessels. The method must be very easy to use, not requiring a dedicated expert radiologist or cardiologist on-hand, but should allow further benefit if one is available. The method should ideally be simple with a vessel contrast pattern that is understandable and with minimal artifact. The resulting data from the acquisition should allow further refinement and postprocessing to extract additional information. Where possible the method should also provide information that is both comple-

mentary to existing methods, yet compatible with those methods so that results can be compared.

It is in this environment and against a backdrop of general MRI improvements that progress in coronary MRA has been made.

First Generation: 2-D Breathhold Acquisition Schemes

In 1991 Atkinson and Edelman reported a fast imaging method that allowed multiphase cardiac imaging to be performed in one breathhold (36). This modification eliminated the problem of respiratory motion by reducing the imaging time 7- to 15-fold and producing a complete multiphase series of cardiac motion. Their technique employed a different strategy for encoding the spatial information for MR. Prior to that, each phase-encoding line was acquired with one R-wave (see Figs. 3.4 and 3.5). Thus, a 128 × 256 matrix that required 128-

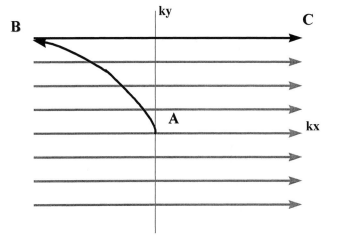

Figure 3.5. *K*-space representation for a simple phase encoding process. The phase-encoding gradient passes through a number of steps with each TR, or re-excitation of the spins. In doing so, these steps help to define the *k*-space data used to encode spatial positions along both readout and phase-encoding axes. Like Figure 3.4 (left), the initial RF excitation pulse produces coherent spins (position A). In this case, however, the transition from point A to B moves along both read and phase axes as both are applied simultaneously. There, as the readout gradient is reversed, the *k*-space trajectory moves from the left to the right (from B to C). After the TR interval, the next RF pulse again returns to point A. The phase-encoding gradient strength is then reduced slightly and the next lower line is gathered. This process is repeated over and over until an adequate amount of *k*-space has been covered and an image may be created by performing a 2-D Fourier transform of the data. In general, the central portions of *k*-space (near A) define the large features, or the low spatial frequencies, within the image. The outer portions define the details or high spatial frequencies. In the standard implementation, each line of *k*-space represents one R-R interval (e.g., a 128-line image requires 128 heartbeats or about 2 minutes). For cineangiographic cardiac imaging, each phase or time-point after the R-wave would have its own data set.

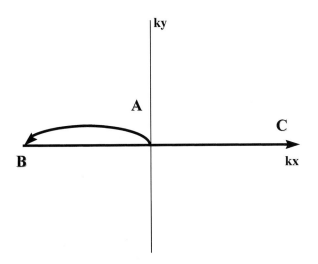

Figure 3.4. *K*-space representation of the gradient recalled echo process. The initial RF pulse leaves the spins with a coherent resonance. This is point A, at the origin of *kx* (readout axis) and *ky* (phase-encoding axis). The application of the negative readout gradient pulse causes dephasing along that axis and moves our position in *k*-space to the left to position B. This dephasing process is reversed with the application of the first positive gradient interval and the *k*-space position is returned to point A. The second plus readout gradient interval subsequently moves the position further to the right to position C, indicative of further dephasing along the readout direction. Note that because no additional gradients were applied orthogonal to the readout, there was no movement along the *ky* direction.

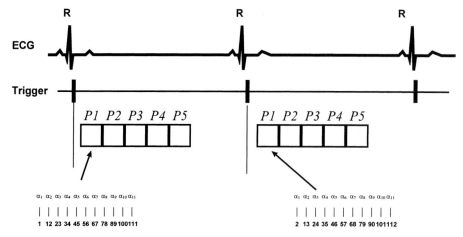

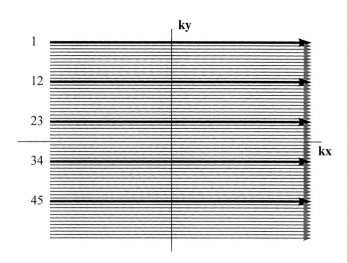

Figure 3.6. Data acquisition process for segmented *k*-space multiphase imaging (11 lines/R-wave). With each R-wave, data is encoded via a series of rapid gradient recalled echos (GRE). Rather than merely encode one line per R–R interval, segmented *k*-space encodes multiple lines (in this case 11 lines). The result is a much more rapid acquisition process (e.g., instead of requiring 110 heartbeats to record a 110 × 256 matrix, segmented *k*-space can do this in 10 heartbeats). Segmented *k*-space rests on the assumption that the data acquisition window (the time necessary to encode 11 lines) is rapid enough that cardiac motion is not significant. In fact, multiple cardiac phases may be encoded with this strategy. Five phases (P1–P5) are acquired, each with its own *k*-space map. Because heart rates vary from one individual to another and the need for systolic detail may change, most MR systems offer a range of segments and data acquisition windows. Thus, for faster heart rates, shorter acquisition times are needed requiring fewer lines per segment. Slower heart rates allow more time per data acquisition window, which allow for more encodings. This enables either a shorter overall scan time (fewer heartbeats are needed to acquire the same spatial resolution) or increased spatial resolution for the same number of R–R intervals.

phase encode steps, would last 128 beats or, typically, about 2 minutes. They modified the method by acquiring multiple phase-encodings with each R-wave, substantially reducing the scan time (Figs. 3.6 and 3.7). This method of breaking up the acquisition or segmenting *k*-space used an interleaved approach wherein subsequent R–R lines filled in spaces between previous segments. By interleaving the acquisitions, small signal variations due to slight R–R changes, body position, or flow signal were minimized.

Edelman and others further modified the method by increasing the number of phase encodings per R-wave, adding flow compensation and fat suppression to opti-

mize the process for single slice, single phase coronary imaging (37) (see Figs. 3.8 and 3.9). These changes and a modified scanning protocol dramatically improved the visualization of the coronaries. By emphasizing the peak flow during the relatively quiet diastolic portion of the cardiac cycle, suppressing the myocardial and pericardial fat signal, and by improving the spatial resolution, this method represented a significant improvement over the initial multiphase technique. This technique also offered the first realistic opportunity for routine clinical coronary MRI. With good technical features, such as very short scan times, strong flow signal, and the wide commercial acceptance by manufacturers,

Figure 3.7. *K*-space representation of the imaging process. In the example, 11 *k*-space lines were acquired per R–R interval. Data from the segmented acquisition process can fill *k*-space either sequentially (i.e., from the top down in order) or interleaved. The interleaving process is preferred as it produces fewer artifacts, and improved image quality. Over the course of the data acquisition, subtle changes occur. These may be due to heart rate changes, T1 relaxation effects, inflow, or some cardiac motion. By interleaving, the data is spread out so that data from early in the acquisition process is placed high above in *k*-space and the later data below. The result is not sharp transitions. By filling in *k*-space sequentially (e.g., fill in lines 1–11, then 12–22, etc.), there are abrupt changes from adjacent segments (e.g., lines 11 and 12 would be acquired at different times within their data acquisition windows) and ghosting.

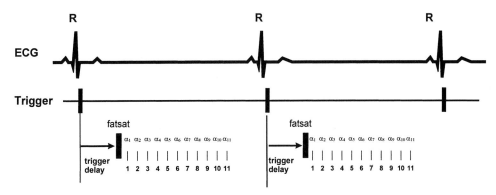

Figure 3.8. Data acquisition process for conventional segmented *k*-space MRA (11 lines/segment). This process is different from the preceding multiphase example in that all of the acquired data is used to create one data set. By focusing on acquiring that data over the relatively quiescent diastole and increasing the number of phase encodes per R-wave, this method could be optimized for 2-D breathhold coronary imaging. For coronary imaging, the delay would be set to begin acquisition after systole (> 300 msec), at which time the fat suppression pulse would be applied (MT as well if desired). Multiple phase-encoding lines would subsequently be acquired with a simple, flow-compensated gradient echo sequence. With this strategy, a 220 × 256 matrix could be acquired in 20 heartbeats.

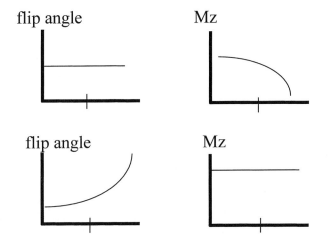

Figure 3.9. Principle of incremented flip angle imaging. In this schematic, the flip angle for each phase-encoding line remains the same (upper left) for each phase-encoding line (horizontal axes). The result (upper right) is that the longitudinal magnetization remaining (Mz) diminishes with each pulse, as the short TR and high flip angle do not allow adequate time for full T1 recovery before the next pulse is applied. Left uncorrected, this diminished signal later in the acquisition process reduces the available signal and will produce a loss of spatial resolution and/or artifact. One solution would be to reduce these flip angles further to minimize the Mz differences; however, the result would be diminished overall signal and poorer image quality. An alternate solution is to vary the flip angle during the acquisition. The lower left graph shows the process where the excitation angle starts low and increases with each phase encoding. The last flip angle optimally would be 90 degrees because it would tip all remaining magnetization into the transverse plane to be encoded. With this scheme (lower right), the magnetization remains more constant and at a higher level than the constant flip angle process. *Note:* This process does not work with multiphase imaging (e.g., in Fig. 3.6) where subsequent phases begin immediately thereafter.

this early technique was been optimized and widely disseminated.

Second Generation: 3-D Volumetric Acquisitions

Although fast, widely available, and able to represent flowing blood, the 2-D breathhold method was not without limitations. One significant problem was that the tortuous vessels tended to leave the imaging plane, requiring a cooperative patient and multiple parallel scans to cover the artery fully with some confidence. Multiple scans were not sufficient to image vessels when subsequent breathholds did not exactly duplicate (<1–5 mm) the diaphragmatic position and alignment of segments was not possible (38). Furthermore, not all patients tolerated the 10–25-second breathholding period well. In fact, more often the scan quality was reduced in those patients least able to perform the test but most likely to benefit from it. Venous and arterial structures were hard to differentiate because veins lie in close proximity to the arteries and have overlapping tortuous pathways. Because the method relies on inflow regardless of direction, the method did not reliably separate the two.

For these reasons and others, volumetric or 3-D acquisitions were offered as an alternative means to image the coronaries. Volumetric imaging is performed in much the same manner as the 2-D methods except that the slice (or slab) is much thicker and it is divided into multiple thin, contiguous partitions (images) via a second phase-encoding process. Modern MR systems perform 3-D imaging routinely for brain, knee, or angiographic studies elsewhere in the body. These 3-D protocols have the advantage over 2-D imaging that the slices are contiguous and that, for the same length of scan time, offer improved S/N. What complicates the application of 3-D imaging for the coronaries is that encoding of the third dimension requires additional time. For each partition created an additional phase-encoding pass is needed (e.g., a four partition 3-D scan takes four times longer than the equivalent single slice 2-D approach, and a 32 partition scan takes 32 times longer). This quickly takes 3-D imaging out of the realm of simple breath-holding and into a regime where scan times can be several minutes and respiratory blur a problem (39).

One proposed method for overcoming respiratory motion problems with long acquisition times has been to provide feedback to the patient to coach him/her to perform the proper breathing maneuvers. The intent would be that in a well-motivated and responsive patient, the diaphragm (and heart) could reliably be returned to the same location, allowing additional data without misregistration. With consistent positioning of the heart, scan times could be quite long and would allow for improved spatial resolution (40). This method is in effect a multiple breathhold examination that attempts to improve on nonfeedback inconsistencies. One implementation of the method acquired data over eight R–R intervals (plus two initial beats to re-establish T1 recovery patterns) per breathhold. This protocol used 16 lines per segment, which allowed a 32-partition × 128 × 256 matrix to be acquired over a 32-breathhold scan time (about 10 minutes). With proper feedback, diastolic heart position was within 2 mm. One major drawback with the method is the degree of cooperation required from the patient. In cooperative volunteers with good breathholding ability, the method can demonstrate significant image quality improvement with good visualization of the proximal and distal vessel branches. The more typical cardiac diseased patient, however, is less cooperative and less able to hold his/her breath, leading to reduced image quality and vessel depiction.

An alternative to overcoming this motion problem is to use the MRI process itself to help limit the effects of respiratory motion. This concept uses a secondary data acquisition to identify the position of diaphragm from which that information is used later to correct for the position of the heart (see Figs. 3.10 and 3.11). Because this process uses a second acquisition (echo) to reposition the data, it is often referred to as a navigator echo technique (41). As was briefly illustrated in Figures 3.1 and 3.2, the MRI process makes use of the Fourier transform to extract spatial information from temporal data acquisitions. Routine imaging employs a readout gradient to define a frequency range corresponding to the spatial FOV. As data is acquired during this readout period, local spatial information (i.e., frequency information) is retrieved after the Fourier transform of the time-domain samples. This process occurs thousands of times

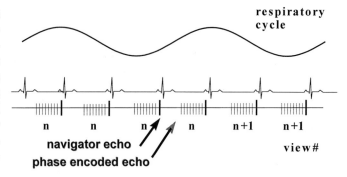

Figure 3.10. Overview of navigator imaging. Similar to the examples shown earlier, this figure demonstrates segmented *k*-space data acquisition with each R-wave. With each segment, one additional sample (echo) is taken to identify the position of the diaphragm. Based on this position taken from the navigator echo, the reconstruction can determine whether the sample is correct as is, out of range and unusable, or within a range that can be corrected. This assumption works well when the respiratory cycle is long relative to the cardiac cycle and the diaphragmatic position is considered stable throughout the segment.

during a normal MRI scan. Should something move between adjacent samples, or phase-encoding lines, the mismatch results in a discontinuous sampling of the body. After the image transform, this produces ghosts in the direction of encoding. We have all seen these in

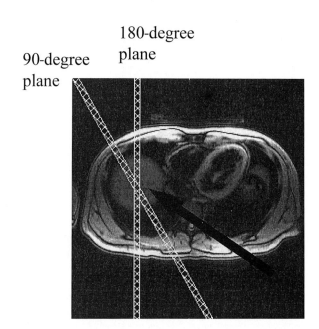

Figure 3.11. Positioning of the navigator echo location. One means to identify a column of tissue uniquely in the body is to use a simple spin echo experiment. Spin echos are produced when a plane of excited protons (from the 90-degree pulse) intersect with a refocusing plane (from the 180-degree pulse). The result is a small sliver of tissue that has high-density liver tissue on one end and low-density, low-signal lung parenchyma on the other (large arrow).

body imaging where subcutaneous fat appears repetitively across the image, ghosting in and out of the body. If the motion can be identified reliably, it can be fixed and image quality improved.

MR data acquired during the readout period is sampled for both amplitude and phase. These samples allow the system both to calculate the frequency shift (spatial position) as well as the contribution from the phase-encoding process. The Fourier transformed image that is usually produced represents merely the magnitude of the signal, not the phase. In the context of MRI, the Fourier transform has a theorem that a spatial displacement represents the linear shift of phase, and vice versa. This Fourier shift theorem states that the spatial representation of an object can be moved by linearly shifting the phase of the sampled time-domain data (42). Ehman and Felmlee have used this concept to correct for abdominal and shoulder imaging (43). For cardiac

imaging, this opens up the possibility that large data sets, collected over long periods of time could be corrected back to a position where the respiratory motion is eliminated if only the degree of displacement were known (Figs. 3.11 and 3.12). This has lead to a variety of novel methods to sample the heart's position, both directly and indirectly, to assess the degree of motion (44,45). Of course, one could use the navigator merely to assess the position of the diaphragm and determine if the data is within an acceptable range. This go–no go collection of data improves the overall image quality, but it may be very inefficient when patients move during the scan, have abrupt breathing patterns, or inconsistent breathing motion.

Over the years, multiple groups including Stanford, Mayo Clinic (44), Mallinckrodt Institute of Radiology (46), the National Heart, Lung and Blood Institute (47), and the Beth Israel/Deaconess Medical Center (48), have all reported progress with these areas. The Emory group and others have reported success with using the same navigator concept to 2-D TOF imaging to allow additional scan time and improved image quality when compared with simple breathholds (49).

Third Generation: Fast Breathheld Volumetric Acquisitions

The concept of sampling data and "navigating" it back to its proper position is a sound one (50). Breathhold time constraints are removed, higher resolution matrixes are possible, and the additional time necessary to sample the diaphragm is minimal. The 3-D volume can be reformatted to follow tortuous coronary vessels without requiring further data acquisition. Given these advantages, it would appear that navigator methods would be the method of choice for all coronary imaging.

These second-generation navigator-based methods are not without limitations. For each direction of motion, a navigator sample needs to be taken. For simple diaphragmatic respiratory travel, one navigator can correct a major source of artifact by translating the raw data back to its assumed position; however, the diaphragm (and heart) move in a complicated 3-D realm and simple 1-D corrections cannot adequately compensate for all motions. There can be a wide variation in the nature of breathing patterns from individual to individual, or even within one individual as he/she sleeps or becomes anxious or restless. Additional navigators are possible along multiple directions to correct for these motions, but they come at the cost of more time spent detecting the heart position and less imaging the coronary arteries. In addition the optimal position of the navigators is as close as possible to the heart (if not in the heart itself), further complicating set up and possibly

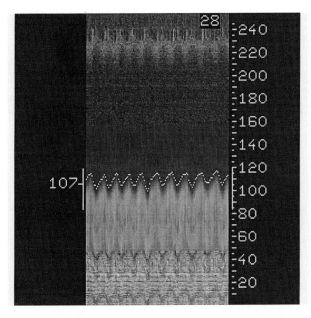

Figure 3.12. Graph of superior-inferior motion of the diaphragm over time. The horizontal scan represents time (total left-to-right coverage is about 30 seconds) and the vertical axis represents spatial information. This graph is the result of using the 90–180-echo configuration over the diaphragm. The low-density lung is represented by low signal above the number 107, and the liver signal is below. Over the 30 seconds, there are about 10 respiratory cycles. This information is important to the other imaging parameters that ensure each part of the respiratory motion is adequately covered. In this case, a semi-automated algorithm has determined that the best estimate for the lung–liver edge is about the number 107 (a column number out of 256 columns). It has then set its local threshold for acceptance about this figure, indicating what would have been acceptable on this initial, scout run. A subsequent graph can be produced after the acquisition to aid in understanding the process and to help should the images not appear correctly.

saturating blood signal. Navigators do well to correct for translation motion. The twisting, rotational motion of the myocardium during contraction and relaxation are much more difficult to correct and may be beyond the potential of navigators. Finally, navigator technology entails an additional level of operator training, further limiting the pool of potential uses and opening up possibilities of errors (e.g., navigating on pulmonary artery signal, not diaphragm motion or missing a window of acceptable motion).

To overcome these problems, newer techniques are incorporating the advantages of both breathhold acquisitions and 3-D volumetric scanning. As seen with the first-generation methods, breathholding can substantially improve image quality and lead to a more robust study. Volumetric acquisitions address the limit of vessel continuity and can improve vessel detail. These two methods combined present a next generation of coronary techniques.

In the first-generation techniques, simple single slice 2-D acquisitions were doable with common, state-of-the-art circa 1988 technology. The simple gradient echo acquisitions rarely required gradients in excess of 10 mT/m and seem to benefit little from further technical improvements over the last few years (51). Navigator techniques did not initially require expanded gradient power. The strategy in both cases was to use the relatively quiescent 300–600 msec of diastole to image as much of k-space (i.e., complete the acquisition) as possible. (Imaging during systole was an option (52), but it was typically avoided because motion from residual myocardial and chamber signal could often obscure the vessels.) Later, evolutionary progress in gradient performance allowed the navigator methods to go much faster and/or image with much higher resolution; however, the ability of the navigator process itself to correct motion has set an upper limit on overall image quality, robustness, and clinical acceptance.

In 1995, Wielopolski and Bomert introduced a technique that combined the benefits of the 3-D volumetric method with a fast, breathheld acquisition (53,54). Their advance rested on the inclusion of a new imaging method, echo-planar imaging (EPI). EPI was first reported more than 20 years ago during MRI's infancy (55), and had been used for limited coronary imaging in two dimensions (56). EPI differs from the simple gradient echo described earlier in one critical facet. For conventional gradient echo imaging, each echo requires one RF pulse; in EPI, this is not true. The distinction is an important one. The inclusion of an RF pulse adds a considerable amount of "overhead" to the data acquisition process (e.g., 30–60% of the time between samples may be due to this).

How, then, does one begin to make an image from just one RF excitation? For the first echo (or first line of k-space), the imaging process is identical (57). The RF pulse tips magnetization into the transverse plane, where the phase-encoding gradient distorts phase in one direction and the combination of a negative–positive pulse pair produces an echo. This is so far identical to conventional imaging; however, if the readout gradient again reverses polarity, another echo will be produced, close in amplitude to the first. If a small amount of phase encoding can be applied between the first and second echos, this second echo can then fill up another line of k-space. If the readout can be reversed quickly, dozens of echos (i.e., data samples) can be acquired before T2* signal loss eliminates the residual signal. Encoding of the third dimension along the slice selection is similar to that within the plane with a slight change in encoding gradient strength from one acquisition to the next. This process can be broken into subparts or segments so that some of the acquisition may be done during subsequent R–R intervals. Although the principle of imaging via multiple echos is simple, numerous technical issues need to be addressed to make EPI successful. The result has been a long latency between Mansfield's first work and the clinical acceptance of the method within the later part of this decade.

In general, EPI performance depends upon the MR system gradient's performance—faster, stronger gradients make better images (see Table 3.1). One key development of engineering over the years has been the expanded performance of the MR gradient system, both in terms of peak amplitude and rise time. Current clinical MR scanners, compared with earlier systems, have gradient systems that can produce amplitudes two to three times larger, with rise times three to five times faster and much more overall stability and reliability. Echo planar imaging has expanded the role of MR applications in the body and is offered on every commercial high-field MR scanner today. Full implementation of these rapid 3-D imaging methods is still some time away because further technical refinements are needed for commercial implementation.

The Future of Coronary MR

Detailed elsewhere in this book by other authors is their view of the progress in coronary MR. As briefly described, these first-, second-, and third-generation techniques define a baseline standard against which further progress will be judged. Numerous groups across the commercial and academic spectra are working on improvements to our techniques and knowledge base. It's an open question how these improvements will be integrated and improved. At this time there are a number of exciting possibilities for coronary MR in the immediate future.

Table 3.1. Comparison of gradient progress for commercially available whole body imagers.

	Circa 1990	Circa 1995	Current	Dedicated
Peak amplitude	10 mT/m	25 mT/m	20 mT/m	~40 mT/m
Rise time	1000 μsec	600 μsec	400 μsec	~150 μsec
Slew rate (mT/m/ms)	10	40	50	220
Linearity	5%	8%	5%	+/−15%
Field-of-view	50 cm	50 cm	50 cm	40 cm
Duty cycle	100%	100%	100%	100%
Inner diameter	60 cm	60 cm	60 cm	60 cm

Early MR devices used relatively slow gradients with limited amplitude. As the number of available techniques increased and cardiac imaging became a priority, gradient performance increased considerably (whereas MR system costs remained about the same). Future devices in test, such as a dedicated cardiac scanner, will have improved performance. This may come at the cost of slightly worse linearity and reduced imaging FOV. Note that the requirement for high duty cycle is still a relevant concern as the fast imaging methods use considerably more of the overall imaging time. The requirement for a large, 60-cm patient bore is also a concern because patient comfort and access are important issues for cardiac studies.

Spiral Scanning

Current fast scanning methods fill k-space in a manner described in the preceding figures, sweeping across k-space line-by-line. This method works well with most studies where structures are unmoving. For highly mobile areas of the body (e.g., the coronaries), alternate means of covering k-space may be preferable. One strategy is to cover k-space by starting at the center point and spiraling out with an Archemedian trajectory (58). By starting at the center of k-space and moving out spirally, flow misregistration can be reduced and the vessel lumen better identified. For some types of gradients, the requirement of an oscillation with ever-increasing amplitude is possible and may be preferable. Spiral imaging is amenable to both 2-D and 3-D methods, as well as single-shot or segmented (multishot) acquisitions. Off-resonance effects (fat–water or field inhomogeneities) cause a characteristic blurring or ghosting in traditional cartesian k-space coverage. In spiral, this pattern is different because the blurring effect is radial and may be outside the workable FOV. Work to date from Stanford and other groups has shown great promise for the technique (59).

Improved Signal-to-Noise

In general, MR techniques eventually become limited by the available S/N as imaging times grow shorter and voxel dimensions shrink. For example, current users report a voxel size of less than 5 mm^3 (60), increasing their diagnostic confidence in small proximal lesions and stenoses in more distal sections. To compensate for reduced S/N, current users employ multichannel array coils tailored to scan only selected parts of the body. The multiple channels can be combined to give an improvement of up to 40% in the available S/N without requiring additional scanning time. On the other hand, one could use multiple coils to substantially reduce the imaging time without significant S/N penalty. In one implementation of this multisurface coil image process (SMASH) (61), researchers at the Beth Israel/Deaconess Medical Center used individual coils to encode along the main axis of the magnet. For small, dedicated areas of the body (e.g., the coronary arteries) multiple coils across the chest can have similar S/N. If these coils are sampled separately, it is possible to use their data to synthesize the phase-encoding process along the main axis without taking time to apply additional gradient pulses. Their results have sped the image acquisition process four- to eightfold, with no reduction in image quality, while using conventional MR equipment.

Higher Gradient Performance

Although echo-planar imaging produces images more quickly than conventional spin echo or gradient echo methods, it is also more prone to artifacts from flow (62), overall motion, T2* blurring, fat–water misregistration, and inhomogeneity within the magnetic field. To overcome these problems, researchers have been investigating the use of third-generation acquisitions, but with conventional gradient echo sequences. By providing an RF pulse with every echo and using a very short TE (1 msec, or less), the problems of T2* blurring, flow artifact, fat–water misregistration, and inhomogeneity are reduced or eliminated. If the scan protocols are short enough, however, the entire volume may be accomplished in one breathhold.

The problem with these fast turboFLASH acquisitions is that typical ToF contrast no longer exists during these short data acquisition periods. Fast flow blood normally causes a continual replacement of saturated spins and a sharp vessel–lumen contrast is possible. With RF pulses applied every 3–4 msec, there is little time for T1 signal recovery, and the blood signal is quickly reduced to background. To overcome this, researchers have begun to use the MR contrast agent gadolinium to enhance the blood signal. The result is a fast acquisition, good spatial and temporal resolution, and minimal artifact that may represent a major step forward in clinical protocol design (63–67). Further improvements may come from the use of macromolecular, intravascular agents that preferentially enhance only the vessels and not background myocardium. In one report, Li reported signal enhancement of 96 to 276% over pre-contrast signal (68).

Although these methods seem to offer an exciting clinically useful protocol, further evolutionary trends point to even more improved gradient performance over the next few years. Faster gradients (shorter rise times) will minimize the wasted time switching from one gradient application to the next. Higher amplitudes will offer reduced FOV and/or higher spatial matrixes.

Real-Time Imaging

Finally, gradient performance and overall system performance improvements may alter the way we perform MR studies. By using fast gradients, high-speed computers, and rapid data links, it is now possible to scan tissues quickly and immediately view the results. Both Siemens and General Electric have begun to implement these fluorolike imaging techniques commercially on their scanners (69,70). The fast, real-time nature of these devices may revive first-generation methods because their performance is more like an ultrasound device, giving interactive feedback to the operator *during* the scan [One report from Holland et al. demonstrated over a series of volunteers and patients that our notion of a breathhold may be wrong. Using 1-D positional projection measurements, they calculated that the average total diaphragm displacement during a 20-second breathhold at end-inspiration was 11 mm, and even at end-expiration it was 3 mm (71)]. With constant feedback from a real-time scanner and a more interactive operator and patient, imaging of the coronary arteries becomes more feasible.

In the end, perhaps, a combination of all of these techniques will be necessary to promote a widespread use of coronary MRA (72).

References

1. Anderson CM, Edelman RR, Turski PA. Clinical magnetic resonance angiography. New York: Raven Press, 1993.
2. Keller PJ, Hunter WW, Schmalbrock P. Multislice fat-water imaging with chemical shift selective presaturation. Radiology 1987;164:539–41.
3. Haase A, Frahm J, Hanicke W, Matthaei D. 1H NMR chemical shift selective (CHESS) imaging. Phys Med Biol 1985; 30:341–44.
4. Wolff SD, Balaban RS. Magnetization transfer contrast (MTC) and tissue water proton relaxation in vivo. Magn Reson Med 1989;10:135–44.
5. Wolf SD, Eng J, Balaban RS. Magnetization transfer contrast: method for improving contrast in gradient recalled echo images. Radiology 1991;179:133–37.
6. Hu BS, Conolly SM, Wright GA, Nishimura DG, Macovski A. Pulsed saturation transfer contrast. Magn Reson Med 1992;26:241.
7. Atkinson DJ, Brant-Zawadzki M, Gillan G, et al. Improved MR angiography: magnetization transfer suppression with variable flip angle excitation and increased resolution. Radiology 1994;190:890–94.
8. Pachot-Clouard M, Darrasse L. Optimization of T2 selective binomial pulses for magnetization transfer. Magn Reson Med 1995;34:462–65.
9. Edelman RR, Ahn SS, Chien D, et al. Improved time-of-flight angiography of the brain with magnetization transfer contrast. Radiology 1992;184:395.
10. McGowan JC, Schnall MD, Leigh JS. Magnetization transfer imaging with pulsed off-resonance saturation: variation in contrast with saturation duty cycle. J Magn Reson Imag 1994;4:79–83.
11. Pike GB, Hu BS, Glover GH, Enzmann DR. Magnetization transfer time-of-flight magnetic resonance angiography. Magn Reson Med 1992;25:372.
12. Kojima F, Miyazaki M, Makita J, et al. A slice selective off-resonance sinc pulse (SORS) for saturation transfer contrast in 3D TOF MR angiography. Proceedings of the Society of Magnetic Resonance in Medicine. San Francisco. 1993, p. 567.
13. Nishimura DG, Macovski A, Pauly JM. Considerations of magnetic resonance angiography by selective inversion recovery. Magn Reson Med 1988;7:472–84.
14. Wang JS, Hu BS, Macovski A, Nishimura DG. Coronary angiography using fast selective inversion recovery. Magn Reson Med 1991;18:417–23.
15. Edelman RR, Chien D, Atkinson DJ, Sandstrom J. Fast time-of-flight MR angiography with improved background suppression. Radiology 1991;179:867–70.
16. Li D, Haacke EM, Mugler JP, Berr S, Brookeman JR, Hutton MC. Three-dimensional time-of-flight MR angiography using selective inversion recovery RAGE with fat saturation and ECG-triggering: application to renal arteries. Magn Reson Med 1994;31:414–22.
17. Richardson DB, Bampton AEH, Riederer SJ, MacFall JR. Magnetization-prepared NR angiography with fat suppression and venous saturation. J Magn Reson Imag 1992; 2:653–64.
18. Edelman RR, Siewert B, Adamis M, Gaa J, Laub G, Wiepolski P. Signal targeting with alternating radiofrequency (STAR). Magn Reson Med 1994;31:233–38.
19. McConnell MV, Goldfarb JW, Manning WJ, Edelman RR. High-resolution black-blood coronary MR imaging using navigator gating. Processing of ISMRM 1997 Conference.
20. Arai AE, Bove KE. Coronary angiography with double IR FSE. ISMRM 1998, p. 848.
21. Wielopolski P, Zisk J, Patel M, Edelman RR. Evaluation of ultra-short echo time MR angiography with a whole body echo-planar imager. Proceedings of the Society of Magnetic Resonance in Medicine. San Francisco. 1993, p. 384.

22. Sebok NR, Sebok DA, Wilkerson D, Mezrich RS, Zatina M. In-vitro assessment of the behavior of magnetic resonance angiography in the presence of constrictions. Invest Radiol 1993;28:604–10.

23. Pattany PM, Chiu LC, Lipcamon JD, et al. Motion artifact suppression (MAST) for magnetic resonance imaging. JCAT 1987;11:369–77.

24. Xiang QS, Nalcioglu O. A formalism for generating multiparametric encoding gradients in NMR tomography. IEE Trans Med Imag 1987;MI-6:14–20.

25. Durek JL, Simonetti OP, Hurst GC. Modified gradients for motion suppression: variable echo time and variable bandwidth. Magn Reson Imag 1990;8:141–51.

26. Ruggeri PM, Laub GA, Masaryk TJ, Modic MT. Intracranial circulation: pulse sequence considerations in three dimensional (volume) MR angiography. Radiology 1989;171:785–91.

27. Urchuk SN and Plewes DB. Mechanisms of flow-induced signal loss in MR angiography. J Magn Reson Imag 1992;2:453–62.

28. Lian Zhi-Pei, Boada FE, Constable RT, Haacke EM, Lauterbur PC, Smith MR. Constrained reconstruction methods in MR imaging. Rev Magn Reson Med 1992;4:67–185.

29. Nishimura DG, Macovski A, Jackson JL, Hu RS, Stevick CA, Axel L. Magnetic resonance angiography by selective inversion recovery using a compact gradient echo sequence. Magn Reson Med 1988;8:96–103.

30. Mugler JP, Brookeman JR. Evaluation of a simple method for reconstructing asymetrically sampled echo data. J Magn Reson Imag 1991;1:487–91.

31. Margozian P and Lenz G. Reconstruction of gradient echo MR measurements with very short TE by half Fourier methods. Proceedings of the Society of Magnetic Resonance in Medicine. 1987; p. 446.

32. MacFall JR, Pelc NJ, Vavrek RM. Correction of spatially dependent phase shifts for partial Fourier imaging. Magn Reson Imag 1988;6:143–55.

33. Schmallbrook P, Yuan C, Chakeres DW, Kohli J, Pelc NC. Volume MR angiography: methods to achieve very short echo times. Radiology 1990;175:861–65.

34. Wang Y, Riederer SJ, Ehman RL. Respiratory motion of the heart: kinematics and the implications for the spiral resolution of coronary imaging. Magn Reson Med 1995:34;713–19.

35. Hofman MB, vanRossum AC, Sprenger M, Westerhof N. Assessment of flow in the right coronary artery by MR phase contrast velocity measurement: effects of cardiac and respiratory motion. Magn Reson Med 1996;35:521–31.

36. Atkinson DJ, Edelman RR. Cineangiography of the heart in a single breath-hold with a segmented TurboFLASH sequence. Radiology 1991;178:359–62.

37. Edelman RR, Manning W, Burstein D, Paulin S. Coronary arteries: breath-hold MR angiography. Radiology 1991;181:641–43.

38. Liu YL, Riederer SJ, Rossman PJ, Grimm RC, Debbins JP, Ehman JP. A monitoring, feedback, and triggering system for reproducible breath-hold MR imaging. Magn Reson Med 1993;30:507–11.

39. Wang Y, Grist T, Korosec RF, et al. Respiratory blur in 3D coronary imaging. Magn Reson Med 1995;33:541–48.

40. Wang Y, Grimm RC, Rossman PJ, et al. 3D Coronary MR angiography in multiple breath-holds using a respiratory feedback monitor. Magn Reson Med 1995;34:11–16.

41. Ehman RL, Felmlee JP. Adaptive technique for high-definition MR imaging of moving structures. Radiology 1989;173:255–63.

42. Wang Y, Grimm RC, Felmlee JP, Riederer SJ, Ehman RL. Algorithims for extracting motion information from navigator echos. Magn Reson Med 1996;36:117–23.

43. McGee KP, Grimm RC, Felmlee JP. The shoulder: adaptive motion correction of MR images. Radiology 1997;205:541–45.

44. Wang Y, Riederer SJ, Ehman RL. Respiratory motion of the heart: kinematics and the implications for the spatial resolution in coronary imaging. Magn Reson Med 1995;33:713–19.

45. Li D, Kaushikkar S, Haacke EM, et al. Coronary arteries: 3D MR imaging with retrospective gating. Radiology 1996;201:857–63.

46. Li D, Kaushikar S, Haacke EM, et al. Coronary arteries: three dimensional MR imaging with retrospective gating. Radiology 1996;201(3):857–63.

47. Foo TK, Hot VB, King KF. Three-dimensional double-oblique coronary artery MR imaging using real-time respiratory navigator and linear phase shift processing. ISMRM 1998, p. 323.

48. Chuang ML, Chen MH, Kasgiwala VC, McConnell, Edelman RR, Manning W. Adaptive correction of imaging plane position in segmented k-space cine cardiac MRI. J Magn Reson Imag 1997;7:811–14.

49. Oshinski JN, Hofland L, Mukundan S, Dixon WT, Parks WT, Pettigrew RI. 2D coronary MR angiography without breath-holding. Radiology 1996;20:737–43.

50. Wang Y, Rossman PJ, Grimm RC, Riederer SJ, Ehman RL. Navigator-echo-based real-time respiratory gating and triggering for reduction of respiration effects in three-dimensional coronary MR angiography. Radiology 1996;198:55–60.

51. Bradley WG, Atkinson DJ, Chen DY. Using High Performance Gradients. *In*: Bradley WG, Bydder GM, eds. Advanced MR imaging techniques, 1st ed. London: Martin Dunitz, 1997.

52. Duerinckx A, Atkinson DJ. Coronary MR angiography during peak-systole: works in progress. J Magn Reson Imag 1997;7:979–86.

53. Bomert P, Jensen D. Coronary artery imaging at 0.5 T using segmented 3D echo planar imaging. Magn Reson Med 1995;34:779–85.

54. Wielopolski PA, Manning WJ, Edelman RR. Single breath-hold volumetric imaging of the heart using magnetization prepared 3-dimensional echo planar imaging. J Magn Reson Imag 1995;4:403–9.

55. Mansfield P. Multiplanar image formation using NMR spin echos. J Phys C 1977;10:L55.

56. Poncelet BP, Weiskoff RM, Wedeen VJ, Brady TJ, Kantor H. Time of flight quantification of coronary flow with echo-planar MRI. Magn Reson Med 1993;30:447–57.

57. Atkinson DJ, Edelman RR, Bradley WGB. Echo planar imaging. *In*: Bradley WG, Stark DD, eds. Magnetic resonance imaging, *3rd ed.* St. Louis: Mosby, 1999.

58. Meyer CH, Hu BS, Nishimura DG, Macovski A. Fast spiral coronary artery imaging. Magn Reson Med 1992;28:202–13.

59. Pat GT, Meyer CH, Nishimura D. Effects of vessel motion in coronary MRA. ISMRM (abstracts) 1997:837.

60. Woodard PK, Li D, Haacke EM, et al. Detection of coronary stenoses on source and projection images using 3D MR angiography with retrospective gating: preliminary experience. Am J Roentgenol 1998;170:883–88.

61. Sodickson DK, Manning WJ. Simultaneous acquisition of spatial harmonics (SMASH): fast imaging with radiofrequency coil arrays. Magn Reson Imag 1997;38:591–603.

62. Butts K and Riederer SJ. Analysis of flow effects in echo planar imaging. J Magn Reson Imag 1992;2:285–93.

63. Goldfarb JW, Edelman RR. Coronary arteries: breath-hold, gadolinium enhanced, 3D MR angiography. Radiology 1998;206:830–34.

64. Zheng J, Li D, Bae KT, Haacke EM, Woodard PK. 3D gadolinium enhanced coronary MRA: initial experience. Proc Soc Magn Res Med 1998.

65. Gotoh M, Sakuma H, Kawada N, et al. 3D coronary MRA: effect of gadodiamide administration. Proc Soc Magn Res Med 1998.

66. Kessler W, Achenbach S, Moshage W, Ropers D, Laub G. Coronary arteries: 3D breath-hold MRA using a gadolinium enhanced ultrafast gradient echo technique. Proc Soc Magn Reson Med 1998.

67. Piotr A, Wielopolski RJM, van Geuns PJ, de Feyter MO. Breathhold coronary MR angiography with volume targeted imaging. Radiology 1998;209:209–29.

68. Li D, Dolan RP, Walovitch RC, Lauffer RB. Three dimensional MRI of coronary arteries using an intravascular contrast agent. Magn Reson Med 1998;39:1014–18.

69. Riederer SJ, Tasciyan T, Farzaneh F, Lee JN, Wright RC, Herfkens RJ. MR fluoroscopy: technical feasibility. Magn Reson Med 1988;8:1–15.

70. Hardy CJ, Darrow RD, Pauly JM, et al. Interactive coronary MR. Magn Reson Med 1998;40:105–10.

71. Holland A, Goldfarb JW, Barentsz JO, Edelman RR. Diaphragm motion during suspended breathing: implications for MR imaging of the heart. Proc ISMRM, 1998.

72. Meyer CH, Hu BS, Kerr AB, et al. High-resolution multislice spiral coronary angiography with real-time interactive localization. Proc ISMRM, 1997.

4
History of Coronary MRA

André J. Duerinckx

Early Attempts

When reviewing the history of coronary magnetic resonance angiography (MRA), there is an extensive prehistory. It was noted early on that almost any cardiac-gated magnetic resonance imaging (MRI) pulse sequence applied to thoracic imaging was occasionally able to show small segments of native coronary vessels and bypass grafts (1–4), similar to what happens with computed tomography (CT) scanning of the chest. Using conventional ECG-gated spin-echo techniques Lieberman et al. (1) reported in 1984 that they were able to visualize portions of the native coronary arteries in 7 of 23 patients. In 1987 Paulin et al. (3) reported that they were able to identify prospectively the presence and origin of the left main coronary artery in six subjects and the right coronary artery ostium in four of six subjects. It was obvious to everybody, however, that this was not a reliable technique to visualize native coronary arteries. In the early 1990–1991 period several coronary MRA techniques that were not too reliable or reproducible were experimented with and then abandoned. These techniques took advantage of averaging over multiple respiratory cycles during a very long acquisition or pseudorespiratory gating (5,6). A very interesting early approach described in 1991 by Wang et al. (7) used fast selective inversion recovery and projection imaging with some success. In retrospect this is very similar to the projectional techniques and 3-D rendering used with the latest third-generation coronary MRA techniques (see Chap. 20).

Although not very successful for imaging of native coronary artery imaging, the early cardiac-gated spin-echo and gradient-recalled-echo imaging techniques were much more successful in the evaluation of coronary bypass graft patency (see also historical overviews in Chaps. 10 and 11). These early successes in evaluating bypass graft patency have been reviewed extensively in several review articles and book chapters (8–10). Most of this early work was limited by the fact that bypass graft patency was only evaluated in a single point, thus making it impossible to comment on lesions elsewhere or lesion severity. More recently developed techniques using 3-D contrast-enhanced MRA have significantly improved the value of MRI for coronary bypass evaluation.

First-Generation Coronary MRA

The history of coronary MRA really started, at least in the published literature, in February 1991 with the first article where Atkinson and Edelman (11) described a new EKG-triggered k-space segmented pulse sequence for cardiac imaging. This was followed in December 1991 by a second article by Edelman et al. (12) that described its application to coronary artery MRI. EKG-triggered k-space segmented techniques allow a significant reduction of the total acquisition time for 2-D imaging such that images can be acquired within a single breathhold. These techniques will be referred to as the "first-generation coronary MRA techniques." They are now available on most commercial MRI scanners. The concept of k-space segmentation is widely used in many MRI applications (13), including the newer cardiac MRI techniques (14,15). This same technique has since been shown also to work with nonrectangular k-space sampling schemes (e.g., spiral scanning) (16). Spiral coronary MRA has some advantages over the traditional approach, but is not yet routinely available on most commercial MRI scanners. Typical examples of coronary MRA obtained with this technique are shown in Figures 1.1 and 1.2. There are, however, several problems with these first-generation techniques. First, although it is adequate for 2-D coronary MRA, breathholding cannot easily be extended to 3-D acquisitions (17,18). Second, the duration of the total examination can be long because of the need to acquire many sequential 2-D images, each requiring one breathhold. Thus, inconsistent breathholding and image misregistration problems can happen (19). Third, the technique requires a significant amount of user experience, skill, and familiarity with the cardiac and coronary anatomy to produce good results. With some training and practice, most technologists, radiologists, and/or cardiologists can learn how to perform these studies (see Chap. 5).

It has also been demonstrated that the first-generation techniques can provide relatively good image quality for cardiac imaging and some coronary imaging by relying on signal averaging when patients cannot cooperate with breathholding commands (20). Hands-on cardiac MRI courses have been organized to teach these coronary MRA techniques. One such 2-day cardiac MRI seminar was offered in Leuven, Belgium, October 3–4, 1997. Several of the images that will be shown in Chapter 5 were acquired during this course, using participants of the course as volunteers. We hope that this book will help to popularize these techniques. Initial clinical results with first-generation techniques have been very promising with the sensitivity for significant coronary lesion detection ranging from 56% to 100% (10,21–23) (see Chap. 12). Initial clinical results have also been very successful in imaging bypass grafts, coronary stents (24,25), and coronary artery variants, such as anomalous origin or proximal course of the coronary vessels (26–29) or aneurysms as in Kawasaki disease (30,31).

With the development of these 2-D single breathhold techniques there was also an interest in extending this to 3-D imaging. Three-dimensional imaging offers the advantage of higher signal-to-noise ratio, shorter echo times, more isotropic pixel resolution, and the ability to examine the data set with a multiplanar reformatting technique. The initial attempts at using signal averaging (without breathholding) for 3-D coronary imaging did not produce very good results (17,18,32,33). Another 3-D coronary MRA technique, developed by Scheidegger et al., used a brief coached breathholding strategy that only required a 1-second breathhold in every 4 seconds (with the respiratory cycle typically lasting four heartbeats) (34–38). The results were very good and have inspired others to continue in this direction. Scheidegger et al. were the first to use sophisticated 3-D imaging display technology for coronary MRA (see Chap. 23). This and other pioneering work on 3-D coronary MRI formed the basis for the development of the second-generation techniques and has been reviewed in detail elsewhere (39).

Second-Generation Coronary MRA

The second-generation techniques for coronary MRA require much less training to perform, can provide higher-spatial resolution, are more patient-friendly, as they require no breathholding ("free breathing"), and appear very promising. These techniques are referred to as the "navigator" techniques. They allow higher-resolution 2-D and low or high-resolution 3-D data acquisitions. These techniques were first described in 1993–1994 (40–42), but they are still undergoing constant improvements because the initial proposed implementations had severe shortcomings (43,44). The initial implementations of these second-generation techniques, which are now available on some commercial MR scanners, use visual feedback or real-time or retrospective respiratory gating to compensate for respiratory motion. They rely upon a navigator pulse to determine motion of the diaphragm (breathing motion). By either providing feedback to the patient (as to when to hold his/her breath) for repeated breathholds, or by feeding information back to the MRI computer, respiratory motion and/or inconsistency in repeated breathholding are eliminated. This allows more time to acquire image data (as one is not limited to a single breathhold), and thus allows for acquisition of 3-D data sets or higher-resolution 2-D data sets. The technique can also be used with a spiral data acquisition scheme (45). An example of this technique is illustrated in Figure 1.3. The navigator pulse most often determines the motion of the diaphragm, but in some implementations it directly monitors the motion of portions of the left ventricular wall. For the repeated breathholding versions, inconsistent breathholding is no longer a problem because the patient receives feedback as to when to stop breathing. For the nonbreathhold (or "free breathing") versions, the regularity of the breathing pattern during the long-scan acquisition (sometimes up to 15 minutes) is important.

Several recommendations have been made to improve these techniques: The navigator echo (NE) window should be placed around end-expiratory position; subjects should not sleep; scan efficiency should be monitored and, if needed, the NE window needs to be repositioned throughout the scan duration (46). Because of these and similar recommendations many adaptations and improvements to this navigator scheme have been made to improve its efficacy, including adaptive windowing (to correct for upward creep of the diaphragm in the supine position after 15–20 minutes) and the use of three orthogonal navigator echoes (to minimize motion in all three directions). Once implemented, this technique requires less expertise and training because a 3-D transaxial slab covering the top of the heart and aortic root can be acquired and images can be analyzed later. In this sense it is very similar to electron-beam computed tomography (EB-CT) acquisitions for coronary calcium determination.

There are potential problems with this second-generation coronary MRA technique because it is now implemented on some of the commercial MRI scanners. First, each acquisition takes much longer than with first-generation techniques (up to 12 to 15 minutes in some cases vs. a single 10 to 15-second breathhold) before the first images are generated. Second, it has been recognized that the initial implementation of the navigator techniques sometimes did not work in up to 50% of normal volunteers (for a variety of unknown reasons) (47), can be very noisy, and are very much a function of the regularity and the type of breathing pattern. Navigator pulse-correction techniques have also been used with the first-generation coronary MRA techniques to avoid slice misregistration when consecutive 2-D images are acquired during consecutive breathholds (44,48,49). The navigator techniques have also been used to acquire small volume scan acquisitions (thin 3-D slabs) oriented along the right coronary artery (RCA) (50). The initial clinical results with a 3-D navigator technique have shown sensitivities for coronary artery lesion detection from 65% to 87% (see Chap. 12).

Third-Generation Coronary MRA and Other Technique Improvements

Third-generation coronary MRA techniques have been developed that combine the user-friendliness of the second-generation techniques with the speed, reliability, and flexibility of the first-generation techniques. They could be labeled the "one-breathhold multiple slice" acquisitions. Many approaches to attain this goal have been experimented with over the years, and Chapter 20 will cover this ever-expanding field of investigation. We will briefly summarize the more important techniques that can be classified as "third generation."

One ideally wants to acquire the entire cardiac anatomy in a single breathhold with isotropic spatial resolution. A precursor of this concept was first described in 1995 by Wielopolski, who used segmented echoplanar imaging (EPI) (22,51). Wielopolski et al. have since proposed small-volume scan acquisitions (thin 3-D slabs) oriented along the coronaries, which is a technique referred to as the volume coronary arteriography using targeted scans (VCATS) technique (52–54). Other groups have developed similar pulse sequences (55,56). An example of a 3-D data set obtained with this technique is shown in Figure 1.4. The small volume acquisitions use fat-suppressed 3-D segmented TurboFLASH with EKG-gating and fast acquisitions times to allow breathholding. These are EKG-triggered fast implementations of the by-now established dynamic contrast-enhanced MRA techniques (see description in next paragraph). These new pulse sequences are now being implemented by some vendors for use on the next generation software release for commercial MR scanners.

Real-time cardiac imaging has recently become possible (57–64). This may have a dramatic effect on how we will perform coronary MRA in the future and on which techniques will prevail. Having real-time interactive imaging as an integral component allows quick location of oblique coronary scan planes prior to high-resolution coronary MRA. This offers another very powerful approach to overcoming problems inherent with first-generation techniques.

Other techniques, like SMASH (62, 65–71) and sensitivity encoding (SENSE) (72), have also been introduced to speed up acquisitions. Sensitivity encoding (SENSE) is based on the fact that receiver sensitivity generally has an encoding effect complementary to Fourier preparation by linear field gradients. Thus, by using multiple receiver coils in parallel, scan time in Fourier imaging can be considerably reduced.

Black-Blood and Bright-Blood Imaging

Spin-echo (SE) based techniques are considered "black-blood" techniques and are ideal to observe the vessel lumen. On the contrary, gradient-recalled echo (GRE) based techniques provide, in general, the opposite contrast by making use of the signal enhancement possible from inflow of non-saturated blood to the region of interest to produce "bright-blood" images. Half-Fourier acquired single-shot turbo spin echo (HASTE), a single shot modification of fast-SE, is extensively used for abdominal imaging (73) but can also be EKG-gated to provide black-blood imaging. With cardiac-gated HASTE cardiac anatomy and bypass graft patency have been studied (74,75). However, most coronary MRA sequences utilize a bright-blood approach. It is yet unclear how this choice will affect imaging of the coronary vessel wall and plaque.

Hybrid Techniques

Hybrid approaches using navigator echoes can be incorporated in first (2-D) and third (3-D) generation techniques to make it possible to collect data over multiple breathholds and to improve inter-slice (2-D) or inter-slab (3-D) correlation (43,44).

MR Contrast Agents

The use of MR contrast agents will have a dramatic effect on coronary MRA techniques, just as dynamic contrast-enhanced MRA has totally changed the way thoracic and body MRA are performed today. Dynamic contrast-enhanced MRA was first described by Prince in 1993 and can now be performed during short breathhold periods of 7–23 seconds for carotid MRA and pulmonary MR. Acquisition times for 3-D MRA have become so short that breathholding may no longer be needed for some applications. The same non–EKG-triggered techniques have been used to image native coronary arteries (76) and coronary artery bypass grafts (CABG) (74,75,77–79). By adding cardiac gating and reducing the amount of data acquired these 3-D breathhold EKG-triggered MRA techniques become what is described in this book as "third-generation coronary

MRA techniques" (55) (see earlier). More information will be provided in Chaps. 15, 16, and 20.

Other Ways to View the History of Coronary MRA Development

There are other ways to categorize the existing coronary MRA techniques. For example, based solely on the complexity of patient set-up procedures, the techniques can be subdivided into three groups: 2-D approaches using a single breathhold or multiple breathholds; 3-D approaches that use averaging over multiple breathholds or imaging within a breathhold; and projectional approaches using tagging and subtraction within a breathhold. Direct respiratory feedback or navigator pulses with real-time or retrospective feedback allow for performing 2-D and 3-D coronary MRA without breath-holding, thus also providing the potential for higher spatial resolution and improved patient comfort.

In this book we have opted for a classification based on a combination of complexity of the study, patient comfort, and how much information is acquired within one data acquisition (80).

References

1. Lieberman LM, Botti RE, Nelson AD. Magnetic Resonance of the heart. Radiol Clin North Am 1984;22:847–58.
2. Kessler W, Laub G, Achenbach S, Ropers D, Moshage W, Daniel WG. Coronary arteries: MR angiography with fast contrast-enhanced three-dimensional breath-hold imaging—initial experience. Radiology 1999;210(2):566–72.
3. Paulin S, vonSchulthess GK, Fossel E, Krayenbuehl HP. MR imaging of the aortic root and proximal coronary arteries. Am J Roentgenol 1987;148:665–70.
4. Gomes A, Lois J, Drinkwater D, Corday S. Coronary artery bypass grafts: visualization with MR imaging. Radiology 1987;162:175–79.
5. Dumoulin C, Souza S, Darrow R, Adams W. A method of coronary MR angiography (technical note). J Comput Assist Tomogr 1991;15(4):705–10.
6. Cho Z, Mun C, Friedenberg R. NMR angiography of coronary vessels with 2-D planar image scanning. Magn Reson Med 1991;20:134–43.
7. Wang S, Hu B, Macovski A, Nishimura D. Coronary angiography using fast selective inversion recovery. Magn Reson Med 1991;18:417–23.
8. Stanford W, Galvin JR, Skorton DJ, Marcus ML. The evaluation of coronary bypass graft patency: direct and indirect techniques other than coronary arteriography (review article). Am J Roentgenol 1991;156:15–22.
9. Buser PT, Higgins CB. Coronary artery graft disease: diagnosis of graft failure by magnetic resonance imaging. In: Lüscher TF, Turina M, Braunwald E, eds. Coronary artery graft disease: mechanisms and prevention. Berlin: Springer-Verlag, 1994:99–112.
10. Danias PG, Edelman RR, Manning WJ. Coronary MR angiography. Cardiol Clin 1998;16(2):207–25.
11. Atkinson D, Edelman R. Cineangiography of the heart in a single breathhold with a segmented TurboFLASH sequence. Radiology 1991;178:359–62.
12. Edelman R, Manning W, Burstein D, Paulin S. Coronary arteries: breath-hold MR angiography. Radiology 1991; 181(3):641–43.
13. Mezrich R. A perspective on k-space. Radiology 1995; 195:297–315.
14. Bluemke DA, Boxerman JL, Mosher T, Lima JA. Segmented k-space cine breath-hold cardiovascular MR imaging: part 2. Evaluation of aortic vasculopathy. Am J Roentgenol 1997;169(2):401–7.
15. Bluemke DA, Boxerman JL, Atalar E, McVeigh ER. Segmented k-space cine breath-hold cardiovascular MR imaging: part 1. Principles and technique. Am J Roentgenol 1997;169(2):395–400.
16. Meyer CH, Hu BS, Nishimura DG, Macovski A. Fast spiral coronary artery imaging. Magn Reson Med 1992;28(2): 401–6.
17. Paschal C, Haacke E, Adler L, Finelli DA. Magnetic resonance coronary artery imaging. Cardiovasc Intervent Radiol 1992;15:23–31.
18. Paschal CB, Haacke EM, Adler LP. Three-dimensional MR imaging of the coronary arteries: preliminary clinical experience. J Magn Reson Imag 1993;3(3):491–501.
19. Duerinckx AJ, Atkinson DP, Mintorovitch J, et al. Two-dimensional coronary MR angiography: limitations and artifacts. Eur Radiol 1996;6(3):312–25.
20. Duerinckx AJ, Lewis BS, Louie HW, Urman MK. MRI of pseudoaneurysm of a brachial venous coronary bypass graft. Catheter Cardiovasc Diag 1996;37:281–86.
21. Duerinckx AJ. MRI of coronary arteries. Int J Card Imag 1997;13(3):191–97.
22. Wielopolski PA, van Geuns RJ, de Feyter PJ, Oudkerk M. Coronary arteries. Eur Radiol 1998;8(6):873–85.
23. Duerinckx AJ. Coronary MR angiography (invited article). In: Cardiac Radiology, Boxt LM, ed. The radiological clinics of North America. Philadelphia: W.B. Saunders, 1999;37(2):273–318.
24. Duerinckx AJ, Atkinson D, Hurwitz R, Mintorovitch J, Whitney W. Coronary MR angiography after coronary stent placement (case report). Am J Roentgenol 1995; 165(3):662–64.
25. Duerinckx AJ, Atkinson D, Hurwitz R. Assessment of coronary artery patency after stent placement using magnetic resonance angiography. J Magn Reson Imag 1998;8: 896–902.
26. Post JC, vanRossum AC, Bronzwaer JGF, et al. Magnetic resonance angiography of anomalous coronary arteries: a new gold standard for delineating the proximal course? Circulation 1995;92:3163–71.
27. McConnell MV, Ganz P, Selwyn AP, Li W, Edelman RR, Manning WJ. Identification of anomalous coronary arteries and their anatomic course by magnetic resonance coronary angiography. Circulation 1995;92:3158–62.
28. Manning WJ, Li W, Cohen SI, Johnson RG, Edelman RR. Improved definition of anomalous left coronary artery by magnetic resonance coronary angiography. Am Heart J 1995;130(3 pt 1):615–17.
29. Duerinckx AJ, Bogaert J, Jiang H, Lewis BS. Anomalous origin of the left coronary artery: diagnosis by coronary

MR angiography (case report). Am J Roentgenol 1995; 164:1095–97.

30. Duerinckx AJ, Takahashi M. Coronary MR angiography in Kawasaki disease (abstr.). Radiology 1996;201(P):274.

31. Duerinckx AJ, Troutman B, Allada V, Kim D. Coronary MR angiography in Kawasaki disease: a case report. Am J Roentgenol 1997;168:114–16.

32. Hofman MBM, Paschal CB, Li D, Haacke M, vanRossum AC, Sprenger M. MRI of coronary arteries: 2D breath-hold vs 3D respiratory-gated acquisition. J Comput Assist Tomogr 1995;19(1):56–62.

33. Li D, Kaushikkar S, Haacke EM, et al. Coronary arteries: three-dimensional MR imaging with retrospective respiratory gating (technical development and instrumentation). Radiology 1996;201:857–63.

34. Scheidegger M, deGraaf R, Doyle M, Vermeulen J, vanDijk P, Pohost G. Coronary artery MR imaging during multiple brief (1 sec) expiratory breathholds (abstr.). In: Proceedings of the Eleventh Annual Scientific Meeting of the Society of Magnetic Resonance Imaging (SMRM). Berlin, Germany, August 8–14;1992, p. 602.

35. Doyle M, Scheidegger MB, DeGraaf RG, Vermeulen J, Pohost GM. Coronary artery imaging in multiple 1-sec breath holds. Magn Reson Imag 1993;11:3–6.

36. Scheidegger MB, Müller R, Boesiger P. Magnetic resonance angiography: methods and its applications to the coronary arteries. Tech Health Care 1994;2:255–65.

37. Scheidegger MB, Boesiger P. Coronary MR imaging. In: Lanzer P, Rösch J, eds. Vascular diagnosis. Berlin: Springer-Verlag, 1994:415–20.

38. Scheidegger MB, Stuber M, Boesiger P, Hess OM. Coronary artery imaging by magnetic resonance. Herz 1996; 21(2):90–96.

39. Duerinckx AJ. Coronary MR angiography. In: Cardiac MR imaging. Boxt LM, guest ed. MRI clinics of North America. Philadelphia: W.B. Saunders, 1996;4(2):361–418.

40. Liu YL, Riederer SJ, Rossman PJ, Grimm RG, Debbins JF, Ehman RL. A monitoring, feedback, and triggering system for reproducible breath-hold MR imaging. Magn Reson Med 1993;30:507–11.

41. Liu YL, Rossman PJ, Grimm RC, Debbins JP, Ehman RL, Riederer SJ. Comparison of two breath-hold feedback techniques for reproducible breath holds in MRI (abstr.). In: Printed program of the First Meeting of the Society of Magnetic Resonance (SMR). Dallas, March 5–9, 1994; J Magn Reson Imag 1994;4 (P):61.

42. Wang Y, Rossman PJ, Grimm RC, Riederer SJ, Ehman RL. Navigator-echo-based real-time respiratory gating and triggering for reduction of respiration effects in three-dimensional coronary MR angiography. Radiology 1996; 198:55–60.

43. Danias PG, McConnell MV, Khasgiwala VC, Chuang ML, Edelman RR, Manning WJ. Prospective navigator correction of image position for coronary. Radiology 1997; 203(3):733–36.

44. McConnell MV, Khasgiwala VC, Savord BJ, et al. Prospective adaptive navigator correction for breath-hold MR coronary angiography. Magn Reson Med 1997;37(1):148–52.

45. Sachs TS, Meyer CH, Irazzabal P, Hu BS, Nishimura DG, Macovski A. The diminishing variance algorithm for real-time reduction of motion artifacts in MRI. Magn Reson Med 1995;34:412–22.

46. Taylor AM, Jhooti P, Wiesmann F, Keegan J, Firmin DN, Pennell DJ. MR navigator-echo monitoring of temporal changes in diaphragm position: implications for MR coronary angiography. J Magn Reson Imag 1997;7(4):629–36.

47. Stehling M. Coronary arteries: experience with navigator echoes (abstr.). In: VIII International Workshop on Magnetic Resonance Angiography. Rome, Italy; Oct. 16–19, 1996.

48. McConnell MV, Khasgiwala VC, Savord BJ, et al. Comparison of respiratory suppression methods and navigator locations for MR coronary angiography. Am J Roentgenol 1997;168(5):1369–75.

49. Oshinski JN, Hofland L, Mukundan S, Dixon WT, James WJ, Pettigrew RI. Two-dimensional MR coronary angiography without breath holding. Radiology 1996;201: 737–43.

50. Oshinski JN, Hofland L, Dixon WT, Pettigrew RI. Magnetic resonance coronary angiography using navigator echo gated real-time slice following. Int J Card Imag 1998;14(3):191–99.

51. Wielopolski PA, Manning WJ, Edelman RE. Single breath-hold volumetric imaging of the heart using magnetization-prepared 3-dimensional segmented echo-planar imaging. J Magn Reson Imag 1995;5(4):403–9.

52. Wielopolski PA, VanGeuns RJ, DeFeijter PJ, DeBruin HG, Bongaerts AH, Oudkerk M. Comparison of breath-hold 3D and retrospectively respiratory gated 3D MR coronary angiography with conventional coronary angiography (abstr). In: 1997 Scientific Program of the 83rd Scientific Assembly and Annual Meeting of the Radiological Society of North America (RSNA). Nov 30–Dec 5, 1997; Chicago, 1997; Radiology; 205(P):154.

53. Wielopolski PA, vanGeuns RJM, deFeyter PJ, Oudkerk M. VCATS (volume coronary arteriography using targeted scans), MR coronary angiography using breath-hold volume targeted acquisitions (abstr). In: Proceedings of the Sixth Scientific Meeting of the International Society for Magnetic Resonance in Medicine (ISMRM). April 18–24, 1998 (paper #14). Sydney, Australia, 1998.

54. Wielopolski P, vanGeuns RJ, deFeyter PJ, Oudkerk M. Breath-hold coronary MR angiography with volume targeted imaging. Radiology 1998;209:209–20.

55. Kessler W, Laub G, Achenbach S, Ropers D, Moshage W, Daniel WG. Coronary arteries: MR angiography with fast contrast-enhanced three-dimensional breath-hold imaging—initial experience. Radiology 1999;210(2):566–72.

56. Goldfarb JW, Edelman RR. Coronary arteries: breath-hold, gadolinium-enhanced, three-dimensional MR angiography. Radiology 1998;206(3):830–34.

57. Stehling M, Howseman A, Chapman B, et al. Real-time NMR imaging of coronary vessels (letter). Lancet 1987; 2(8566):964–65.

58. Hardy CJ, Curwen RW, Darrow RD. Robust coronary MRI by spiral fluoroscopy with adaptive averaging (abstr.). In: Proceedings of the Sixth Scientific Meeting of the International Society for Magnetic Resonance in Medicine (ISMRM), April 18–24, 1998 (paper #22). Sydney, Australia, 1998 (in press).

59. Hardy CJ. Real-time cardiovascular MR imaging. In:

Reiber JHC, vanderWall EE, eds. What's new in cardio-vascular imaging? Dordrecht: Kluwer Academic Publishers, 1998: 207–19.

60. Hardy CJ, Darrow RD, Pauly JM, et al. Interactive coronary MRI. Magn Reson Med 1998;40(1):105–11.

61. Chien D, Heid O, Simonetti O, Laub G. New developments in ultrafast and interactive cardiac MR by Siemens Medical Systems (abstr). *In*: Twenty-sixth Annual Meeting of the North American Society for Cardiac Imaging. Dallas, 1998.

62. Sodickson DK, Stuber M, Botnar RM, Kissinger KV, Manning WJ. SMASH real-time cardiac imaging at echocardiographic frame rates (abstr.). *In*: Book of abstracts and proceedings of the Seventh Meeting of the International Society of Magnetic Resonance in Medicine (ISMRM). Philadelphia, May 22–28, 1999.

63. Bundy JM, Laub G, Kim R, Finn JP, Simonetti OP. Real-time data acquisition for LV function (abstr.). *In*: Book of abstracts and proceedings of the Seventh Meeting of the International Society of Magnetic Resonance in Medicine (ISMRM). Philadelphia, May 22–23, 1999.

64. Weiger M, Pruessmann KP, Boesiger P. High performance cardiac real-time imaging using SENSE (abstr.). *In*: Book of abstracts and proceedings of the Seventh Meeting of the International Society of Magnetic Resonance in Medicine (ISMRM). Philadelphia, May 22–23, 1999.

65. Jakob PM, Griswold MA, Edelman RR, Manning WJ, Sodickson DK. Cardiac imaging with SMASH (abstr.). *In*: Proceedings of the Sixth Scientific Meeting of the International Society for Magnetic Resonance in Medicine (ISMRM), April 18–24, 1998 (paper #16). Sydney, Australia, 1998.

66. Jakob PM, Griswold MA, Edelman RR, Sodickson DK. AUTO-SMASH: a self-calibrating technique for SMASH imaging. SiMultaneous Acquisition of Spatial Harmonics [in process citation]. Magma 1998;7(1):42–54.

67. Sodickson DK, Manning WJ. Simultaneous acquisition of spatial harmonics (SMASH): fast imaging with radiofrequency coil arrays. Magn Reson Med 1997;38(4):591–603.

68. Sodickson DK, Stuber M, Botnar RM, Kissinger KV, Manning WJ. Accelerated coronary MR angiography in volunteers and patients using double-oblique 3D acquisitions combined with SMASH (abstr.). *In*: Society for Cardiovascular Magnetic Resonance, Second Meeting, January 22–24, 1999. Atlanta, Georgia. 1999:81.

69. Sodickson DK, Griswold MA, Jakob PM. SMASH imaging. Magn Reson Imag Clin N Am 1999;7(2):237–54, vii–viii.

70. Griswold MA, Jakob PM, Chen Q, et al. Resolution enhancement in single-shot imaging using simultaneous acquisition of spatial harmonics (SMASH). Magn Reson Med 1999;41(6):1236–45.

71. Sodickson DK, Griswold MA, Jakob PM, Edelman RR, Manning WJ. Signal-to-noise ratio and signal-to-noise efficiency in SMASH imaging. Magn Reson Med 1999; 41(5):1009–22.

72. Pruessmann KP, Weiger M, Scheidegger MB, Boesiger P. SENSE: sensitivity encoding for fast MRI [in process citation]. Magn Reson Med 1999;42(5):952–62.

73. Regan F. Clinical applications of half-Fourier (HASTE) MR sequences in abdominal imaging. Magn Reson Imag Clin North Am 1999;7(2):275–88.

74. Kalden P, Kreitner KF, Wittlinger T, et al. [The assessment of the patency of coronary bypass vessels with a 2D T2-weighted turbo-spin-echo sequence (HASTE) in the breath-hold technique]. *Rofo Fortschr Geb Rontgenstr Neuen Bildgeb Verfahr* 1999;170(5):442–48.

75. Wittlinger T, Voigtlander T, Grauvogel K, et al. [Noninvasive evaluation of coronary bypass grafts by magnetic resonance imaging. Comparison of the Haste and Fisp-3-D sequences with the conventional coronary angiography]. Z Kardiol 2000;89(1):7–14.

76. Ho VB, Foo TKF, Arai AE, Wolff SD. Gadolinium-enhanced two-dimensional coronary MR angiography using an automated contrast bolus detection algorithm (MR smartprep) (abstr.). *In*: Proceedings of the Sixth Scientific Meeting of the International Society for Magnetic Resonance in Medicine (ISMRM), April 18–24, 1998 (paper #19). Sydney, Australia, 1998.

77. van Rossum AC, Galjee MA, Post JC, Visser CA. A practical approach to MRI of coronary artery bypass graft patency and flow. Int J Card Imag 1997;13(3):199–204.

78. Vrachliotis TG, Bis KG, Aliabadi D, Shetty AN, Safian R, Simonetti O. Contrast-enhanced breath-hold MR angiography for evaluating patency of coronary artery bypass grafts. Am J Roentgenol 1997;168(4):1073–80.

79. Wintersperger BJ, Engelmann MG, von Smekal A, et al. Patency of coronary bypass grafts: assessment with breath-hold contrast-enhanced MR angiography—value of a non-electrocardiographically triggered technique. Radiology 1998;208(2):345–51.

80. Wielopolski PA, van Geuns RJ, de Feyter PJ, Oudkerk M. Coronary arteries. Eur Radiol 2000;10(1):12–35.

5

2-D and 3-D Breathhold Coronary MRA: How Do I Do It?

André J. Duerinckx

Introduction

Coronary magnetic resonance angiography (MRA) can routinely visualize the proximal and middle portion of most coronary arteries and some coronary artery branches. Coronary MRA can and should be used for noninvasive imaging in a variety of clinical situations (e.g., in the evaluation of congenital coronary artery anomalies, in the follow up of proximal coronary lesions after angioplasty, and in the noninvasive determination of the patency of bypass grafts and coronary stents). The use of coronary MRA for blind prospective detection of coronary lesions is now being evaluated, and coronary MRA techniques may become an integral part of the clinical evaluation and screening of patients with ischemic heart disease.

With the development of a new group of ultrafast imaging sequences reliable and reproducible MRA of the coronary arteries has become possible. A first generation of coronary MRA techniques was first described in 1991 and is now commercially available on most clinical magnetic resonance imaging scanners. These techniques rely upon a combination of segmental acquisition in *k*-space of the data to minimize cardiac motion and the use of a single breathhold to minimize respiratory motion artifacts (see also Chaps. 3 and 15). Second- and third-generation techniques have since been developed; however, because only the first-generation coronary MRA techniques are now universally available on most commercial MR imagers, we will devote this chapter on clinical practice and applications to these techniques. However, because both first (2-D) and third (3-D) generation techniques acquire image data during sequential breathholds, the practical aspects of image plane selection, instructions to the patients, and coverage of the coronary artery territory are very similar.

Thus, the guidelines given in this chapter for first-generation techniques (sequential 2-D images) also apply, with minor modifications, to the third-generation breathhold techniques (sequential thin slabs of 3-D image data). More detailed description of the third-generation technique can be found in Chapter 20.

This chapter will provide an understanding of these techniques, and discuss their use for MRI of normal coronary anatomy. We refer the reader to future chapters for discussions of more specialized applications (Chaps. 7–12) or more detailed reviews of techniques (Chaps. 3, 15, and 20).

Principles Underlying Breathhold Coronary MRA Pulse Sequence Design

A detailed review of this topic has been provided elsewhere by Duerinckx (1,2) and others (3,4). We will only very briefly review how the anatomy and physiology of coronary arteries is dealt with when designing coronary MRA pulse sequences.

Temporal Resolution

Image sharpness of coronary MRA is greatly influenced by cardiac motion and temporal resolution. Coronary MRA requires the avoidance of motion (cardiac and respiratory motion) and compensation for pulsatile blood flow, all of which degrade the image quality by causing ghosting and image blurring.

Cardiac Motion
EKG triggering synchronizes data acquisition to the cardiac cycle and allows a better depiction of the heart and surrounding structures. The heart shows a highly variable motion pattern, which is most pronounced during systole and early diastole, but nearly absent during mid- and late diastole. Because coronary flow decreases from early to late diastole, mid- to late diastole appears optimally suited for coronary MRA.

Partially adapted from a chapter published in Magnetic resonance of the heart and great vessels: clinical applications. *In*: Medical Radiology—Diagnostic Imaging and Radiation Oncology. Bogaert J, Duerinckx AJ, Rademakers FE, eds. Berlin: Springer-Verlag, 1999.

Respiratory Motion

Breathholding and/or respiratory compensation/feedback schemes are used to eliminate this type of motion.

Spatial Resolution

Temporal resolution is a key factor that indirectly determines the size of the acquisition matrix. For a given field-of-view (FOV), this then determines the spatial resolution. The spatial resolution and signal-to-noise in coronary MRA can be further improved by either switching to nonbreathhold techniques (thus eliminating some of the time constraints needed for breathhold techniques) or by using better coil designs and faster gradients.

Flow-to-Background Noise Contrast Ratio

Coronary arteries are usually embedded in fat, which has high signal intensity on T1 weighted images. Suppression of the high signal from fat offers improved coronary vessel detection with MRA. This technique is called *fat-saturation* and is essential in coronary MRA to suppress the signal from the peri- and epicardial fat.

Timing of Data Acquisition Within Each Heart Cycle

Because of the complex pattern of cardiac motion and the biphasic flow patterns in the coronary vessels, it would appear that mid- to late diastole offers the best compromise when imaging coronary vessels (5,6).

Practical Aspects of Breathhold Coronary MRA

Patient set up, instruction, and image plane selection are quite different for single breathholding, repeated breathhold (with feedback), and nonbreathholding sequences. The nonbreathhold sequences are much simpler because they require virtually no patient instructions beside a recommendation to breathe regularly and to keep still during the scan. Most of what follows specifically applies to single breathhold techniques.

Breathhold Instructions for Sequential Repeated Breathholding

Patient set up and scanning protocols for 2-D breathhold sequences have been discussed at length in a previous publication (1) and will only be summarized here. For the breathhold techniques the patient should be instructed on how to hold his/her breath during a nonforced, normal end-expiration for the duration of each scan. These maneuvers should be practiced for several minutes prior to the start of the scan. It is important to work on this with the patient prior to starting the MR scan to obtain breathholding that is as consistent as possible. Because patient cooperation is so essential it is virtually impossible to apply these techniques to children under 14 years old because even though healthy young children can easily hold their breaths for 14 seconds they often fail to do it in a consistent way.

The question often arises as to whether or not it is best to acquire image data during end-expiration or end-inspiration. In the cardiac imaging community many (if not most) people traditionally use end-expiration based on personal evidence that the quality of the breathholds was better than it was during end-inspiration. Others, mostly in the abdominal imaging community, where breathhold MRI has also become important, argue that it may be easier and more comfortable for sick patients to hold their breath at end-inspiration. With the development of the second generation coronary MRA techniques, and the need for adaptive repositioning of the navigator echo window, several investigators have started to quantitate diaphragm motion during normal breathing in a supine position, during sleep periods, and even during breathholding. Holland et al. (7) reported that breathholding does not eliminate motion of the diaphragm. Based on a study of 10 healthy normal volunteers (five men, five women; mean age: 31.9 years) they calculated that the average total diaphragm displacement during a 20-second breathhold at end-inspiration was 11 mm. At end-expiration the average total diaphragm displacement was only 3 mm, with an average diaphragm velocity of 0.15 mm/second (range: 0.01 to 0.3 mm/second). During both end-inspiration and end-expiration there was a gradual upward creep of the diaphragm during the short 20-second period of breathholding. It was a linear and gradual motion at end-expiration for all volunteers. At end-inspiration, however, it was more irregular, with time varying velocities in some of the volunteers.

The implications for coronary artery imaging are very important. Even though these findings need to be validated in patients, they confirm what most cardiac imagers already knew from comparing end-expiration and end-inspiration. End-expiratory breathholding is definitively better, and most patients, even very ill ones, can tolerate it just as well as end-inspiratory breathholding.

Dealing with Breathhold Difficulties

The quality of breathholding may be confirmed by the use of posteriorly placed EKG leads (when patients are in prone position) with loss of respiratory variation in the EKG baseline. If the patient occasionally cannot hold his/her breath, one just repeats the image acquisitions as needed.

However, if this problem persists, one has to be prepared to adapt the breathhold coronary MRA exam to each individual patient and his/her ability to cooperate. If the patient has trouble holding his/her breath for the required duration (12–16 seconds), one can lower the matrix size (e.g., to 126 × 254) or increase the number of views per *k*-space segment (e.g., increase from 9 to 11 views or phase step acquisitions per heartbeat).

For sedated patients with regular breathing patterns, one can average several data sets obtained with the 2-D techniques without breathholding and sometimes still obtain diagnostic-quality images (e.g., for aneurysm or pseudoaneurysm imaging) (8). Even in pediatric patients where compliance with breathholding is not the best, these techniques appear to produce acceptable images of larger vessels, such as the aorta (9).

Dealing with Poor Cardiac Triggering

The set up for cardiac triggering was reviewed by Box in a comprehensive review article (10). We refer to this very good article, and will only discuss a few extra points.

In very heavy patients and patients with severe arrhythmias, it may be difficult to obtain adequate data acquisition because of the following reasons. In very heavy patients whose body almost totally fills the internal diameter of the magnet, it is often difficult to obtain a relatively noise-free EKG trigger signal. In patients with arrhythmia, it is difficult to get 16 consecutive heartbeats without intervening arrhythmia. Because of these reasons it is sometimes impossible to obtain good cardiac triggering with these patients.

There are fortunately sometimes solutions for these difficult cases. The MRI system can pseudotrigger and provide adequate image quality, although this only rarely happens. For large-size patients with very noisy cardiac triggering when in a prone position (i.e., lying on a surface coil), reverting to a supine position and using the body coil will reduce the noise of the cardiac trigger signal enough to make scanning possible. This will reduce the spatial resolution, but the significantly improved image quality compensates for this decreased spatial resolution.

One also has to adjust the time delay (TD) depending upon the patient's heart rate. For example, if the R–R interval is 1000 msec (a slow heart rate) a TD ≈ 600 to 700 msec would be optimal. If the heart rate is much faster, the time delay should be lowered appropriately (e.g., to TD ≈ 350 msec or less). For the single breathhold coronary MRA performed at our institution the temporal resolution of 117 msec can become inadequate for patients with fast heart rates and R–R intervals of less than 500 msec. For most patients, unfortunately, reducing the seg-

mental acquisitions to six or eight views (or phase encodings) per *k*-space segment would increase the duration of the image acquisition too much. Even though patients may initially be able to tolerate this for a few breathholds they will soon tire, and not enough time will be available to complete a high-quality coronary MRA study. This compromise between somewhat suboptimal time resolution and realistic breathholding durations needs to be made for each individual patient by the radiologist performing the procedure.

Typical Image Acquisition Sequences

The image acquisition sequence for 2-D techniques is typically as follows. Beginning at the level of the aortic sinus transaxial images are obtained along the aortic root over a vertical distance from 2 to 3 cm with an overlap of 2–3 mm. Single- and double-oblique images are subsequently obtained in planes positioned in the right atrioventricular and interventricular grooves to visualize the right coronary artery (RCA) and the left anterior descending (LAD) coronary artery. No systematic attempt is made to visualize the circumflex coronary artery because it is located too posteriorly in the chest wall to be well visualized with a surface coil. Total imaging time ranges from 45 minutes to 1 hour 30 minutes per patient.

For the 3-D techniques the approach is different because a 3-D slab covering the proximal portions of the coronary arteries is acquired in one sitting. Subsequent data processing (e.g., multiplanar reconstruction, segmentation, etc.) can then be used to visualize the vessels. Total imaging times range from one breathhold for 3-D segmented echo planar imaging (EPI) or turboFLASH to 12–15 minutes for 3-D techniques with retrospective respiratory gating.

Another excellent discussion of this topic is provided by Wielopolski et al. from (11).

Surface Coils

There still is no final word on which surface coils are best to use. The circular polarized body array coils, which are available on most MRI scanners, allow more homogeneous coverage of the heart and coronary vessels. They also increase patient comfort, as the patient can be in a supine position. The early work on coronary MRA using the first-generation techniques was almost all performed with the patient in a supine position on a spine surface coil, with the heart positioned close to the coil (3,5,6,12–15). It is important to realize that this may still occasionally be the best approach because the fat-suppression algorithms do not always provide homogeneous fat-suppression with the body array coils. Fat suppression is essential for good coronary artery contrast. Whenever inhomogeneous fat-suppression becomes a problem it is often more efficient to reposition the patients in a prone position and proceed the study with a different surface coil (e.g., a spine phased-array coil).

Optimal Selection of Imaging Planes

For 3-D transaxial plane acquisitions with navigator echo techniques this is not an issue, and one should follow the same guidelines as given for coronary calcium screening protocols using EB-CT. For 2-D breathhold acquisitions (first-generation technique), however, or for the newer targeted thin-slab 3-D breathhold techniques (third-generation technique) this is an important issue. One has to find the main axis of the heart. This is well known to cardiologists and people performing echocardiography. It does not always seem so easy to radiologists starting out in this field.

For 2-D breathhold coronary MRA, several approaches have been described to select the best imaging planes to visualize the coronary arteries (16–19). There are basically two approaches: the iterative approach and the direct anatomical approach. We will briefly describe both.

The iterative approach works as follows. One can first localize the aortic root and then acquire sequential transaxial images throughout the lowest portion of the aortic root. This usually allows visualization of the left main coronary artery, the proximal LAD and circumflex coronary arteries, and—on the lowest cuts—the origin of the RCA. Using this approach, one can then interactively try to find the right atrioventricular groove and continue imaging the RCA. A similar approach with multiangle double-obliqued imaging planes can be used to image the more distal LAD (20).

Duerinckx et al. (21) have suggested an anatomical approach. Their approach is based on the a priori knowl-

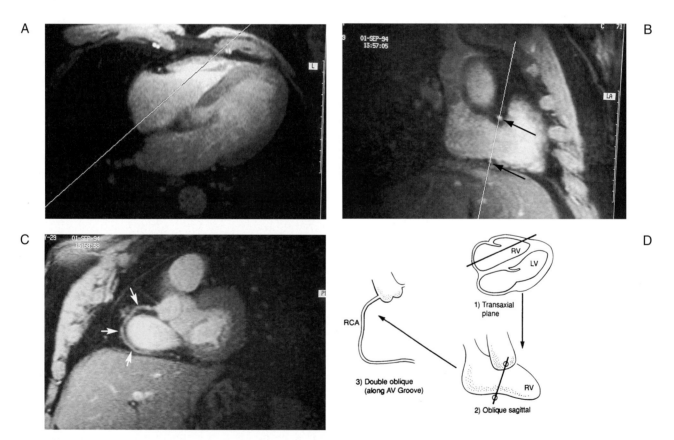

Figure 5.1. Optimal image plane selection sequence to image the RCA. (A) Transaxial view through the left ventricle. This image is used to determine the orientation of the long-axis of the heart projected onto a transaxial plane. It is then used to select the orientation of the next imaging plane (as indicated by line). (B) Oblique coronal plane through the right ventricle, which transects the right coronary artery in two points (arrows). This image is used to select a plane located in the anterior atrio-ventricular groove, which contains the RCA (indicated by line). It also gives an idea as to the orientation of the cardiac long-axis in an obliqued coronal plane. (C) Plane located in the anterior atrioventricular groove shows a large segment of the RCA (arrows). This plane corresponds to a conventional angiogram, left anterior oblique view with caudal angulation. (D) Schematic drawing of the method used for optimal selection of imaging planes for coronary MR angiography depiction of RCA. Also shown are: RV = Right ventricle; and LV = Left ventricle. (B,C from Duerinckx AJ. MRA of the coronary arteries. Top MRI, 1995;7(4): 267–85.) (Reprinted with permission from Duerinckx (2)).

edge of the cardiac anatomy and course of the coronary vessels. Imaging planes are selected comparable to those obtained with conventional X-ray coronary angiography and echocardiography. Imaging plane selection for cardiac MRI can be relatively easy and fast for some of the coronary vessels, and has been previously described (22,23). A quick start for RCA imaging is to use a transverse image at the level of the left ventricle (short-axis view) to prescribe a sagittal oblique slice through the middle of the left ventricle (long-axis view). From this, one can then easily acquire images along the atrioventricular groove. Using this anatomical approach, imaging of the RCA can easily and reliably be performed (see Fig. 5.1). Sakuma et al. reported a similar anatomical approach to LAD imaging where they used multiangle epicardial tangential views for better visualization of the distal LAD (20). Furthermore, the use of cine display can improve recognition of the continuity of the coronary artery tree (17).

New interactive MRI plane selection techniques are being developed to facilitate the selection of optimal section orientations (24). When they become commercially available they may have a dramatic effect on the total duration of coronary MRA and cardiac MR examinations.

Typical Coronary MRA

Typical 2-D coronary MRAs are shown in Figures 5.2, 5.3, and 5.4. In most volunteers and a significant number of patients who can cooperate with breathholding commands, large portions of the proximal coronary arterial tree can be imaged.

Coronary MRA studies done mostly in normal volunteers (13,15,20,25–27) and several studies done in patients only (14,28) have measured the length of the coronary arteries typically visualized with the coronary MRA technique. These findings are summarized in Table 5.1.

We have included data from a transesophageal study (TEE) of proximal coronary artery lesions for comparison (30). The difference in measured lengths between the different studies may be explained by a different approach to the selection of imaging planes.

Flow in the diagonal branches of the LAD was visible in 80% of the subjects in a study by Manning et al. (13). In a study of 15 patients by Duerinckx et al., however, the branch vessels were seldom visualized, except for the acute marginal and diagonal branches. Moreover, the proximal circumflex artery was poorly visualized due to the use of a surface coil and prone positioning (25).

The frequency of significant lesions in the LCx is relatively low. Because of this 2-D coronary MRA, even with its limitation of poor visualization of the LCx, may

still be a valuable noninvasive screening tool for coronary artery disease.

Artifacts and Limitations of First-Generation Techniques

The most important limitation of today's coronary MRA is the great variation in the appearance of significant (>50%) coronary lesions and the large number of image artifacts that can be misinterpreted as representing lesions. It can be very tempting to interpret an artifactual change in the signal intensity of flow in a vessel as representing a lesion, especially if the artifact just happens to be located in the vicinity of the real lesion. Such erroneous overinterpretation of artifacts as lesions will increase the sensitivity for lesion detection, as will be explained and illustrated in the next section. If done consistently, it would unfortunately also significantly reduce the specificity of the technique, thus ultimately reducing its clinical impact. Issues relating to "lesion" appearance on MR will be discussed in the next section. The discussion here will be limited to general artifacts and limitations as seen in healthy normal volunteers without coronary lesions.

The Anatomical Approach to Imaging of the RCA with a 2-D or 3-D Breathhold Technique

As most clinical users only have access to the first-generation coronary MRA techniques we will discuss practical aspects of the use of these breathhold techniques, specifically as they relate to image plane selection for RCA imaging. Third-generation (3-D) techniques, with their ability to acquire thin 3-D data stacks to cover a tortuous RCA, will make the selection of the imaging planes somewhat less critical (11). The need to acquire multiple 2-D images to cover tortuous vessels usually disappears with the 3-D techniques. The risk of misinterpreting an out-of-plane vessel segment as a lesion also decreases with the 3-D technique. Nevertheless, if one becomes very good at selecting imaging planes for the 2-D breathhold technique, one will have few problems with the less critical image plane (or 3-D image slab) selections for 3-D breathhold techniques. Therefore we will provide multiple examples of image plane selection for the 2-D breathhold techniques.

The anatomical approach to imaging of the right coronary artery was already shown in Figure 5.1 and can be very easily applied. The learning curve for this technique is relatively reasonable. The key requirements to performing this type of study are the ability

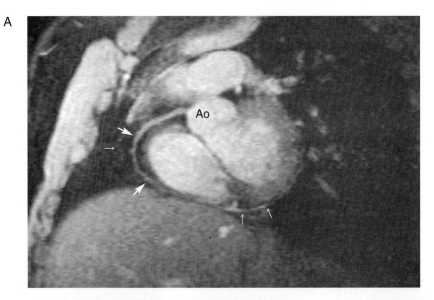

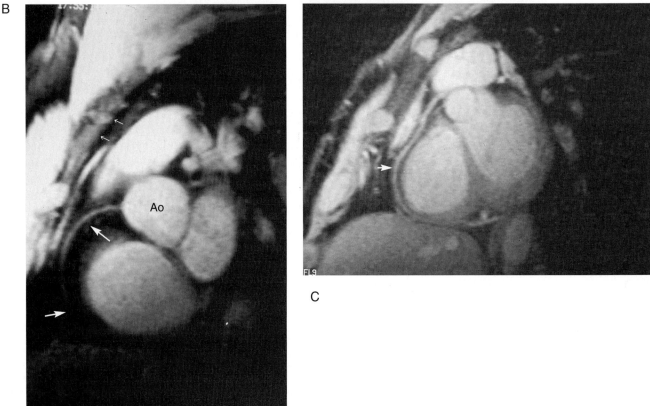

Figure 5.2. The right coronary artery. The RCA lies in the anterior atrioventricular groove. Large portions of the RCA can usually be visualized with a single imaging plane through the anterior atrioventricular groove, as demonstrated in three different volunteers (A–C). (A) The origin, proximal, and mid-RCA are all shown. (B) The proximal and middle RCA are shown; the distal RCA was seen in adjacent parallel plane. (C) The origin, proximal, and mid-RCA are shown. Also shown are: the pericardial sac (thin arrows); Ao = ascending aorta. The figures shown here illustrate how subtle changes in orientation can allow the visualization of both the proximal and ostial portion of RCA in some patients. This is not always the case, however, as illustrated in Figure 1.1, where a slightly different orientation of the imaging plane in the atrioventricular groove allows the visualization of the mid- and distal RCA, but then requires a separate oblique transaxial plane to see the origin of the RCA. (Reprinted with permission from Duerinckx (2).)

A

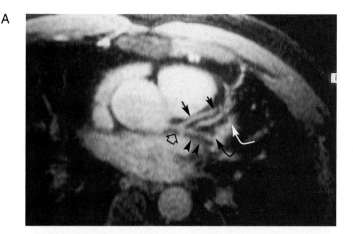

B

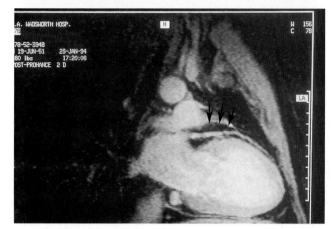

Figure 5.3. Left coronary artery system is relatively complex and requires multiple imaging planes to visualize. (A) Oblique transaxial plane shows the left main (open arrow) LAD (arrows) and several diagonal branches (arrowheads) and the great cardiac vein (curved arrow). (B) Two-chamber view demonstrates a large portion of the LAD (arrows).

to be able to determine the direction of the long axis of the right ventricle and/or left ventricle quickly. One starts off with the transaxial image for the left ventricle followed by an oblique sagittal image to get the second component of the axis of the heart. Using that information a short-axis view can be obtained that shows its position of the level of the anterior atrioventricular groove, and, therefore, visualizes the RCA. This is the equivalent of a caudal left anterior oblique (LAO) view in conventional X-ray coronary angiography.

Because of the necessity to recognize the cardiac axis and be able to determine the orientation of the heart, this requires either specialized training of and/or practice by the MR technologist or the presence of a physician familiar with cardiac anatomy. This is unlike the 3-D coronary MRA techniques using navigator pulses where minimal training is required.

We will now detail variations encountered when

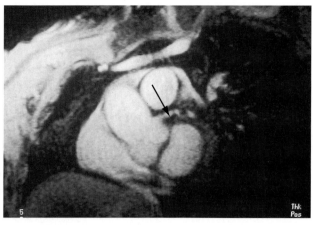

Figure 5.4. Left main coronary artery (arrow). The optimal plane for imaging of the left main coronary artery is often an oblique coronal plane, as shown here. This corresponds to a left anterior oblique orientation in conventional coronary angiography. Also shown are: Ao = ascending Aorta; PA = pulmonary artery; RA = right atrium. (Reprinted with permission from Duerinckx (2).)

imaging the proximal and middle RCA with a single breathhold 2S technique. The images shown are from real volunteers scanned during the 2-day cardiac MRI seminar held in Leuven, Belgium, October 3–4, 1997. MRI studies were performed on volunteers within a small class group of 5–10 radiologists. Each one of these acquisitions was performed in 4–7 minutes time.

Figure 5.5 shows a straightforward case where the RCA is relatively straight in its middle course (Case #1). Figure 5.6 illustrates what happens when there is mild out-of-plane tortuosity of the RCA (Case #2). During mid- and late diastole, due to dilatation of the heart, the RCA is stretched out and almost completely lies within a single plane (i.e., the anterior or right A-V groove), as illustrated in Figures 5.1 and 5.5. Figure 5.7 illustrated a moderate amount of image degradation due to very slight motion artifacts. Even when there is perfect breathholding, there could be up to 3 mm of upward creep of the diaphragm during a 20-second breathhold (see earlier discussion) Figure 5.8 illustrates what happens when there is severe out-of-plane tortuosity of the RCA (Case #4). This case clearly illustrates how for a very tortuous RCA additional image acquisitions need to be obtained in order to follow that vessel with the 2-D coronary MRA techniques. If not done correctly, one could easily misinterpret these gaps and areas of low signal as representing coronary lesions. Figure 5.9 illustrates what happens when there is mild in-plane tortuosity of the RCA (Case #5). Figure 5.10 illustrates what happens when there is a combination of mild in-plane and mild out-of-plane tortuosity of the RCA (Case #6).

Table 5.1. Comparison of the length of coronary arteries visualized by coronary MRA.

	n	RCA	LM	LAD	LCX
2-D: Manning et al., 1993 (Ref. 13)	25	58 (24–122)	10 (8–14)	44 (28–93)	25 (9–42)
2-D: Pennell et al., 1993 (Ref. 15)	26	53.7 ± 27.9	10.4 ± 5.2	46.7 ± 22.8	26.3 ± 17.5
2-D: Duerinckx et al., 1994 (Ref. 14)	21	65 ± 23	12 ± 3	53 ± 19	19 ± 12
2-D: Sakuma et al., 1994 (Ref. 20)	18	65 ± 23	n/a	62 ± 10	23 ± 11
2-D: Duerinckx et al., 1994 (Ref. 25)	15	78.4	13.9	54.9	14.7
2-D: Hofman et al., 1995* (Ref. 27)	10	55 ± 11	8 ± 2	42 ± 14	16 ± 12
3-D: Li et al.** (Ref. 29)	?	3 to 7**	n/a	5 to 50 **	5 to 50**
3-D: Paschal et al.* (Ref. 26)	7	34 (12–50)	5 (4–14)	24 (5–47)	24 (8–64)
3-D: Hofman et al., 1995* (Ref. 27)	10	37 ± 14	7 ± 3	37 ± 9	11 ± 12
3-D gated: Hofman et al., 1995* (Ref. 27)	10	46 ± 10	8 ± 4	37 ± 11	17 ± 14
2-D: Post et al. (Ref. 28)	35	89 ± 32	9 ± 4	62 ± 16	21 ± 9
TEE: Samdarshi et al., 1992 (Ref. 30)	111	7 ± 2	9.3 ± 1	8.2 ± 8	6.7 ± 9

Data are from 1992–1995.
From: Duerinckx AJ, Coronary MR angiography, MRI Clin North Am 1996;4:361–418, with permission.
Results are expressed in millimeters, and depending on the study as: mean ± standard deviation or mean (range: min–max). n = number of subjects; RCA = right coronary artery; LM = left main stem artery; LAD = left anterior descending artery and LCx = left circumflex artery.
*Not all vessels could be visualized in each subject;
**range reflects the most frequently measured lengths, not the full range.

These techniques can also be used to image the left coronary artery system. Imaging of the left coronary artery system, however, requires a much more sophisticated level of interactivity. Many different schemes have been developed. The idea is basically to start with a semitransaxial plane through the aortic root to localize the left main coronary artery and then follow the LAD. Different approaches to this can be used. One consists of tracking down the LAD along the interventricular groove and obtaining planes transaxial to the cardiac surface that contains both the LAD and the great cardiac vein.

The Need for Postprocessing

Representation of 3-D vascular structures is a complex task that often requires significant postprocessing that is not routinely available at clinical sites. The best-known techniques are maximum-intensity projection (MIP) as used with traditional MRA acquisitions, surface rendering after segmentation (which has become very popular with helical CT angiography), and multiplanar reconstruction from 3-D data sets. We will not discuss these options in detail given their limited availability at the present time.

Figure 5.5. Most typical case where the RCA is relatively straight in its middle course. (A) The initial transaxial image visualizes a cross-section of the RCA. (B) Oblique coronal plane through the right ventricle intersects the RCA in two points. The cross-section of the proximal right coronary artery in this particular case has the shape of a comma. This comma shape most likely presents a cross-section of the RCA and either partial voluming of the more distal portion of the RCA and/or the beginning of a side-branch. (C) Plane located in the anterior atrioventricular groove. The origin of the RCA and proximal RCA are clearly shown. (D) One additional imaging plane was obtained perpendicular to the atrioventricular groove plane. The mid-RCA is also shown, providing an orthogonal view of the vessel (when compared with image C). (E,F) Schematic drawing of the RCA superimposed on a schematic representation of the cardiac chambers (as in Fig. 2.1B) where the circle represents the atrioventricular grooves and the loop represents the interventricular grooves). (A–D) (Reprinted with permission from Duerinckx (39).)

A

B

C

D

E

F

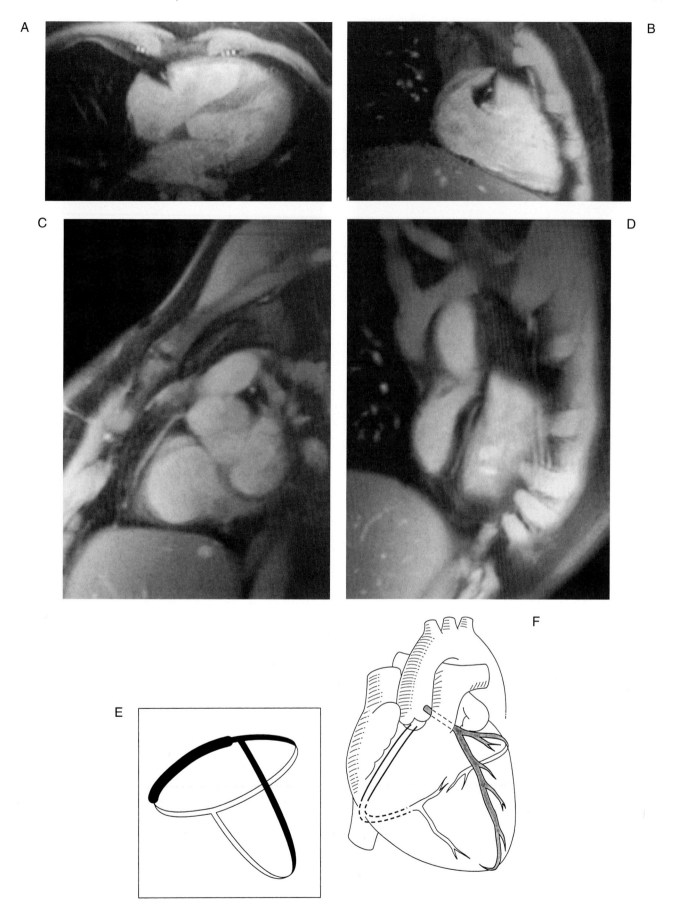

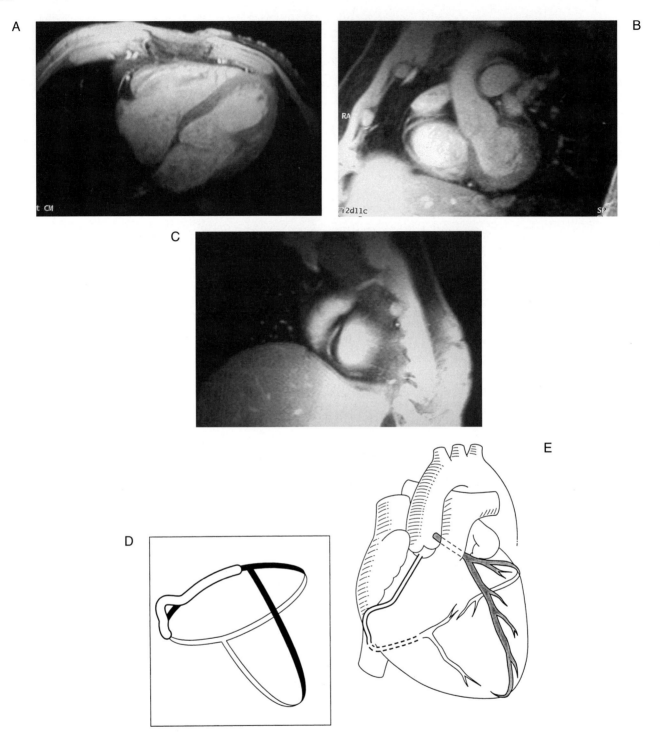

Figure 5.6. Mild out-of-plane tortuosity of the RCA. (A) Transaxial image shows dotlike cross-section of the RCA. (B) Plane located in the right atrioventricular (V) groove only shows portions of the RCA. A small fragment of the mid-RCA is not seen. (C) Plane providing 90-degree view (perpendicular to image plane shown in C). The mid-RCA courses posteriorly over a short segment. This explains the interrupted appearance of the RCA as seen on the AV groove plane; it was due to mild tortuosity of the RCA. (D,E) Schematic drawing of the RCA superimposed on a schematic representation of the cardiac chambers (as in Fig. 2.1B), where the circle represents the atrioventricular grooves and the loop represents the interventricular grooves). (A–C) (Reprinted with permission from Duerinckx (39).)

A
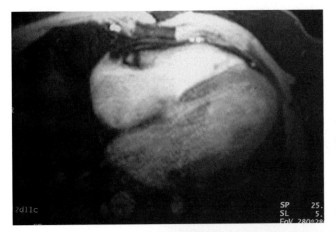

B
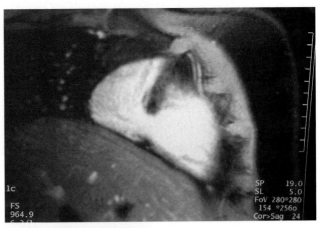

C
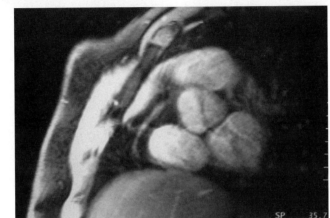

Figure 5.7. Image degradation due to suboptimal breathholding. (A) Transaxial image shows dotlike cross-section of the RCA. (B) Oblique coronal plane through the right ventricle should normally intersect the right coronary artery in two dotlike points; this is not the case here. In this particular case the atrioventricular groove is clearly seen as an area of low signal intensity. The coronary MRA sequences rely on fat suppression. The low-signal area seen is the pericardial fat and subpericardial fat surrounding the right coronary artery. The cross-sections of the RCA on this oblique coronal image, however, are not clearly seen, but the orientation of the AV groove can easily be determined. By selecting the imaging plane through this right atrioventricular groove (as done in Figs. 5.1, 5.5, and 5.6) one still obtains the usual image of the right coronary artery. (C) Plane located in the right atrioventricular (V) groove shows RCA. The RCA image is somewhat blurred again due to lack of total complete breathholding or other slight motion artifact. (Reprinted with permission from Duerinckx (39).)

Three-dimensional rendering of coronary arteries is one type of postprocessing that requires segmentation of the data (31,32). To execute this 3-D rendering routine, "seeds" are placed in both the left- and right-coronary vessels, and thresholds are set to discriminate individual coronary vessels from adjacent structures (31). Segmentation of the left-coronary system with its many branches is much more involved than the RCA segmentation.

Edelman et al. (33) have also described a technique to render projection MRAs that depict a substantial length of human coronary arteries from sequential 2-D breathhold images. They applied the technique to 5 normal volunteers and 10 patients.

Other aspects of postprocessing were discussed in the April 1998 issue of the *Journal of Roentgenology* (34–38) (see further discussion on this topic in Chap. 22).

The Future of Breathhold Coronary MRA

Breathhold techniques hold great potential because they provide either 2-D or 3-D image data at a rapid pace, with almost instantaneous feedback (unlike the free-breathing navigator-based techniques; see Chap. 6). The first-generation 2-D techniques have now reached a level of stability and commercial implementation such that most MR users can and should use them. The new targeted breathhold thin-slab 3-D techniques developed

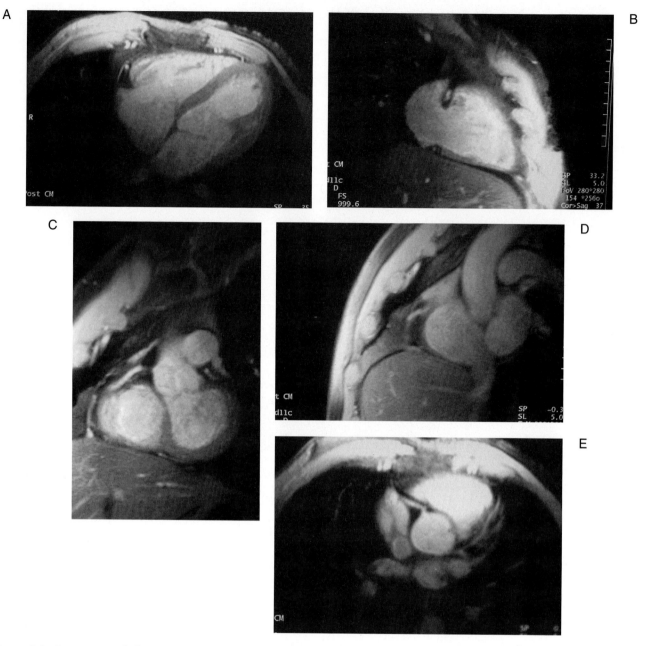

Figure 5.8. Severe out-of-plane tortuosity of the RCA. (A) Transaxial image shows dotlike cross-section of the RCA. Portions of the mitral valve are shown. (B) Oblique coronal plane through the right ventricle intersects the right coronary artery in two dotlike points. (C) Plane located in the right atrioventricular (V) groove only shows portions of the RCA. A small fragment of the mid-RCA is not seen. Only a small portion of the proximal RCA is shown. (D) Plane parallel to the right atrioventricular (V) groove plane in (C), but displaced posteriorly. The missing portion of the RCA is now shown. (E) Transaxial image through the aortic root. (F,G) Schematic drawing of the RCA superimposed on a schematic representation of the cardiac chambers (as in Fig. 2.1B) where the circle represents the atrioventricular grooves and the loop represents the interventricular grooves). (A–E) (Reprinted with permission from Duerinckx (39).)

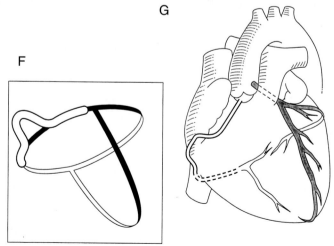

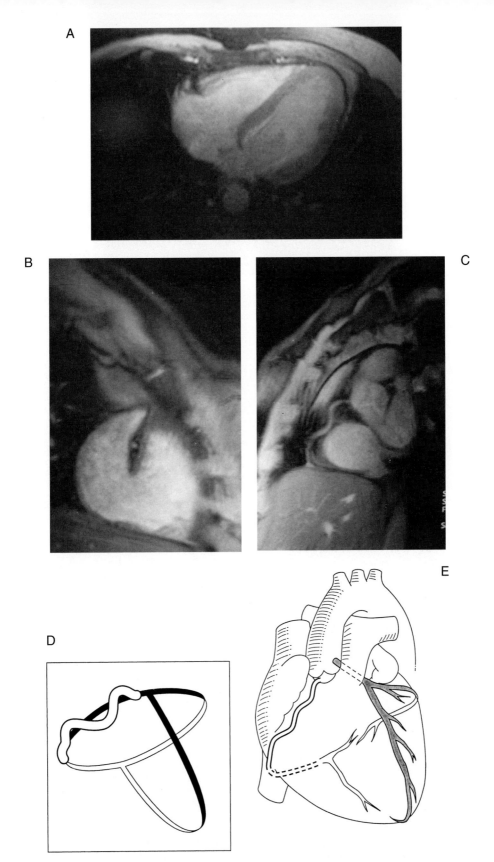

Figure 5.9. Mild in-plane tortuosity of the RCA. (A) Transaxial image shows dotlike cross-section of the RCA. (B) Oblique coronal plane through the right ventricle intersects the right coronary artery in two points. The proximal cross-section of the RCA is clearly shown, but the distal one is only faintly seen. The right AV groove, however, is clearly visible and allows selection of the plane through the right atrioventricular groove. (C) Plane located in the right atrioventricular (V) groove shows a tortuous RCA. A long portion of the RCA is clearly seen; it is very tor-tuous, but it almost totally lies within a single plane with no anterior or posterior displacement. In this particular description, anterior and posterior refer to two displacements toward the base or apex of the heart. (D,E) Schematic drawing of the RCA superimposed on a schematic representation of the cardiac chambers (as in Fig. 2.1B) where the circle represents the atrioventricular grooves and the loop represents the interventricular grooves. (A–C) (Reprinted with permission from Duerinckx (39).)

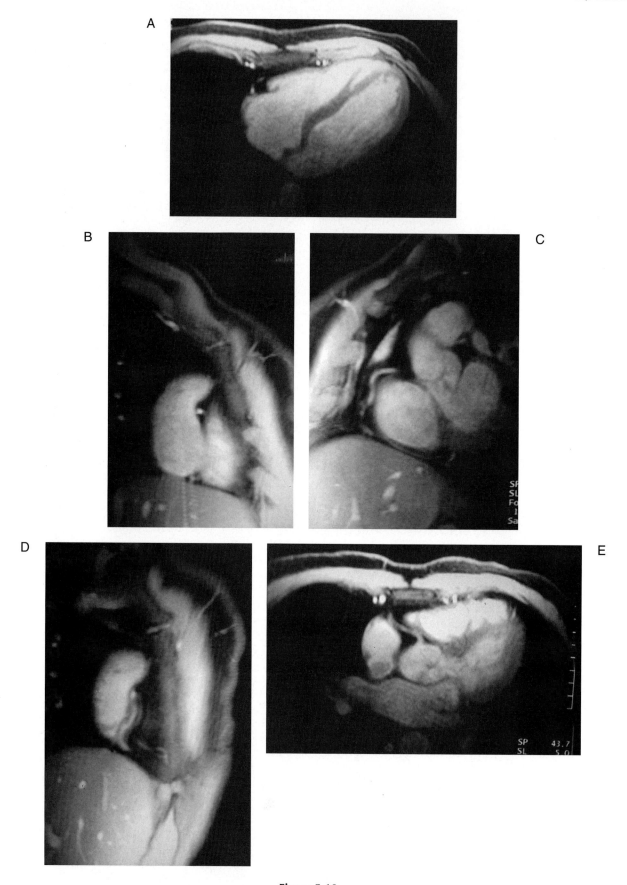

Figure 5.10.

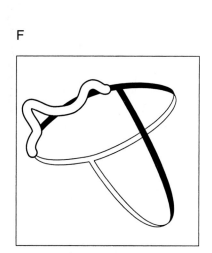

F

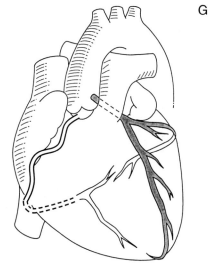

G

Figure 5.10. Mild in-plane and out-of-plane tortuosity of the RCA. (A) Transaxial image shows dotlike cross-section of the RCA. (B) Oblique coronal plane through the right ventricle intersects the RCA in two points. (C) Plane located in the right atrioventricular groove shows a tortuousity (in-plane) with missing segments more distally (due to out-of-plane tortuosity). There is also no signal seen in the proximal RCA ostium. (D) An image plane perpendicular to (c). The mid- to distal RCA is clearly seen, as is a right ventricular branch. (E) An obliqued transaxial plane clearly shows the ostium (see also Fig. 5.1). (F,G) Schematic drawing of the RCA superimposed on a schematic representation of the cardiac chambers (as in Fig. 2.1B) where the circle represents the atrioventricular grooves and the loop represents the interventricular grooves. (A–E) (Reprinted with permission from Duerinckx (39).)

show great promise and require similar skills to select the imaging planes or slabs (11). Changes in technique development have been and continue to be so fast that there has been no time or interest for in-depth large-scale clinical testing of any of the coronary MRA techniques, except for the first-generation coronary MRA techniques.

Coronary flow reserve assessment by MRI, which will be discussed later in Chapters 13 and 14, can be added to the evaluation of coronary anatomy. Such combined noninvasive MR study of anatomy and flow may become the ultimate cost-effective coronary screening tool. Despite their current limitations (discussed in more detail in Chap. 15) first-generation MRA techniques can help in many clinical applications (e.g., in the identification of congenital coronary anatomy variants), and in the noninvasive follow up of patients who have undergone coronary angioplasty, coronary stent placement, or bypass grafting.

References

1. Duerinckx AJ. Review: MR angiography of the coronary arteries. Top Magn Reson Imag 1995;7(4):267–85.
2. Duerinckx AJ. Coronary MR angiography. *In*: Cardiac MR imaging, Boxt LM, guest ed. MRI Clin North Am 1996; 4(2):361–418.
3. Manning W, Edelman R. Magnetic resonance coronary angiography. Magn Reson Q 1993;9(3):131–151.
4. Pearlman JD, Edelman RE. Ultrafast magnetic resonance imaging: segmented TurboFLASH, echo-planar, and real-time nuclear magnetic resonance. Radiol Clin North Am 1994;32(3):593–612.
5. Duerinckx AJ. Coronary MR angiography (letter) (response-to-letter-to-the-editor). Radiology 1995;195(3):876.
6. Manning WJ, Edelman RR. Coronary MR angiography (letter-to-the-editor). Radiology 1995;195(3):875.
7. Holland AE, Goldfarb JW, Edelman RR. Diaphragmatic and cardiac motion during suspended breathing: preliminary experience and implications for breath-hold MR imaging. Radiology 1998;209(2):483–89.
8. Duerinckx AJ, Lewis BS, Louie HW, Urman MK. MRI of pseudoaneurysm of a brachial venous coronary bypass graft. Catheter Cardiovasc Diag 1996;37:281–86.
9. Hernandez RJ, Aisen AM, Foo TKF, Beekman RH. Thoracic cardiovascular anomalies in children: evaluation with a fast gradient-recalled-echo sequence with cardiac-triggered segmented acquisition. Radiology 1993;188: 775–80.
10. Boxt LM. How to perform cardiac MR imaging. *In*: Cardiac MR imaging, Boxt LM, guest ed. MRI Clin North Am 1996;4(2):191–216.
11. Wielopolski P, vanGeuns RJ, deFeyter PJ, Oudkerk M. Breath-hold coronary MR angiography with volume targeted imaging. Radiology 1998;209:209–20.
12. Manning WJ, Li W, Edelman RR. A preliminary report comparing magnetic resonance coronary angiography with conventional angiography. N Engl J Med 1993;328: 828–32.

13. Manning WJ, Li W, Boyle NG, Edelman RE. Fat-suppressed breath-hold magnetic resonance coronary angiography. Circulation 1993;87:94–104.
14. Duerinckx AJ, Urman M. Two-dimensional coronary MR angiography: analysis of initial clinical results. Radiology 1994;193:731–38.
15. Pennell DJ, Keegan J, Firmin DN, Gatehouse PD, Underwood SR, Longmore DB. Magnetic resonance imaging of coronary arteries: technique and preliminary results. Br Heart J 1993;70(4):315–26.
16. Duerinckx AJ, Urman M. Optimal imaging planes for MR coronary angiography (abstr.). *In*: Book of abstracts of the Eleventh Annual Scientific Meeting of the European Society for Magnetic Resonance in Medicine and Biology. Vienna, Austria, April 20–24, 1994:83.
17. Sakuma H, Caputo GR, Steffens J, Shimakawa A. Breath-hold MR angiography of coronary arteries with optimal double-oblique imaging planes and cine display (abstr.). *In*: Seventy-ninth Scientific Assembly and Annual Meeting of the Radiological Society of North America (RSNA). Chicago, November 28–December 3, 1993. Radiology 1993; 189(P):278.
18. Post JC, vanRossum AC, Hofman MB, Valk J, Visser CA. A protocol for two-dimensional magnetic resonance coronary angiography, studied in three-dimensional magnetic resonance data sets. Am Heart J 1995;130(1):167–73.
19. Gates ARC, Huang CL-H, Crowley JJ, et al. Magnetic resonance imaging planes for the 3-dimensional characterization of human coronary arteries. J Anat 1994;185:335–46.
20. Sakuma H, Caputo GR, Steffens JC, et al. Breath-hold MR cine angiography of coronary arteries in healthy volunteers: value of multiangle oblique imaging planes. Am J Roentgenol 1994;163(3):533–37.
21. Duerinckx AJ, Urman MK, Atkinson DJ, Simonetti OP, Sinha U. Optimal imaging planes for coronary MR angiography (abstr.). *In*: Printed program of the First Meeting of the Society of Magnetic Resonance (SMR). Dallas, 1994. J Magr Reson Imag;P(4):123.
22. Axel L. Efficient methods for selecting cardiac magnetic resonance image locations. Invest Radiol 1992;27:91–93.
23. Burbank F, Parish D, Wexler L. Echocardiographic-like angled views of the heart by MR imaging. J Comput Assist Tomogr 1988;12:181–95.
24. Hangiandreou NJ, Debbins JP, Rossman PJ, Riederer SJ. Interactive selection of optimal section orientations using real-time MRI. J Magn Reson Imag 1995;34:114–19.
25. Duerinckx AJ, Urman MK, Atkinson DJ, Simonetti OP, Sinha U, Lewis B. Limitations of MR coronary angiography (abstr.). *In*: Printed Program of the First Meeting of the Society of Magnetic Resonance (SMR). Dallas, March 5–9, 1994; J Magn Reson Imag 1994;4:81.
26. Paschal CB, Haacke EM, Adler LP. Three-dimensional MR imaging of the coronary arteries: preliminary clinical experience. J Magn Reson Imag 1993;3(3):491–501.
27. Hofman MBM, Paschal CB, Li D, Haacke M, vanRossum AC, Sprenger M. MRI of coronary arteries: 2D breath-hold vs 3D respiratory-gated acquisition. J Comput Assist Tomogr 1995;19(1):56–62.
28. Post JC, vanRossum AC, Hofman MBM, Valk J, Visser CA. Clinical utility of two dimensional breathhold MR angiography in coronary artery disease (abstr.). *In*: Book of Abstracts of the Third Meeting of the Society of Magnetic Resonance (SMR) and the Twelfth Annual Scientific Meeting of the European Society for Magnetic Resonance in Medicine and Biology (ESMRMB). Nice, France, August 20–25, 1995.
29. Li D, Paschal CB, Haacke EM, Adler LP. Coronary arteries: three-dimensional MR imaging with fat saturation and magnetization transfer contrast. Radiology 1993;187:401–6.
30. Samdarshi T, Nanda N, Gatewood R, et al. Usefulness and limitations of transesophageal echocardiography in the assessment of proximal coronary artery stenosis. J Am Coll Cardiol 1992;19:572–80.
31. Doyle M, Scheidegger MB, DeGraaf RG, Vermeulen J, Pohost GM. Coronary artery imaging in multiple 1-sec breath holds. Magn Reson Imag 1993;11:3–6.
32. Börnert P, Jensen D. Coronary artery imaging at 0.5 T using segmented 3D echo planar imaging. Magn Reson Med 1995;34:779–85.
33. Edelman RR, Manning WJ, Pearlman J, Wei L. Human coronary arteries: projection angiograms reconstructed from breath-hold two-dimensional MR images. Radiology 1993;187(3):719–22.
34. Rogers LF. The heart of the matter: noninvasive coronary artery imaging (editorial). Am J Roentgenol 1998;170:841.
35. Duerinckx AJ, Lipton MJ. Noninvasive coronary artery imaging using CT and MR imaging [comment]. Am J Roentgenol 1998;170(4):900–2.
36. Achenbach S, Moshage W, Ropers D, Bachmann K. Curved multiplanar reconstructions for the evaluation of contrast-enhanced electron beam CT of the coronary arteries. Am J Roentgenol 1998;170:895–99.
37. Woodard PK, Li D, Haacke EM, et al. Detection of coronary stenosis on source and projection images using three-dimensional MR angiography with retrospective respiratory gating: preliminary experience. Am J Roentgenol 1998;170:883–88.
38. Shimamota R, Suzuki J-i, Nishikawa J-i, et al. Measuring the diameter of coronary arteries on MR angiograms using spatial profile curves. Am J Roentgenol 1998;170:889–93.
39 Duerinckx AJ. Coronary MR angiography. Radiol Clin North Am 1999;37(2):273–318.

6

3-D Free-Breathing (Navigator) Coronary MRA: How Do I Do It?

Pamela K. Woodard and Debiao Li

Even though contrast-enhanced cardiac-gated three-dimensional (3-D) techniques can now be performed in a single breathhold (1), 3-D navigator respiratory-gated methods offer an alternative to patients unable to hold their breath. Moreover, whereas cardiac-gated 3D breathhold sequences for coronary magnetic resonance angiography (MRA) are not yet available on most magnetic resonance imaging (MRI) systems, several of the major MR system manufacturers offer navigator respiratory-gated as part of their commercially available cardiac MR software.

Along with eliminating breathhold requirements, advantages to respiratory-gated 3-D coronary MRA include better signal than short breathhold sequences, which allow the study to be performed without the administration of contrast material. In addition, because a relatively large volume may be covered, navigator techniques often require less precise set up than many breathhold methods and a detailed knowledge of coronary artery anatomy is less necessary, allowing a competent technologist to perform the examination.

Three-dimensional navigator methods, however, also have some shortcomings. As the patient breathes throughout the examination, respiratory gating techniques may not entirely eliminate artifacts caused by respiratory motion. This is especially true for patients with erratic breathing patterns. Because 3-D data acquisition requires 4–15 minutes of imaging time, it is more difficult for patients to keep a consistently regular breathing pattern throughout the entire examination.

Respiratory Gating Techniques

Because of the incompatibility of MR software between manufacturers, and because most MR research laboratories are limited to the MR system of one supplier, a number of different respiratory gating techniques have been developed for coronary artery imaging. These techniques include retrospective respiratory gating, prospec-

tive respiratory gating, respiratory feedback, and the diminishing variance algorithms.

Retrospective Respiratory Gating

With retrospective respiratory gating, two excitation bands are placed at either the right or left hemidiaphragm. One band is excited by a 90-degree flip angle radiofrequency (rf) pulse; the second has a 180-degree flip angle rf pulse (2,3). Together these rf pulses create a vertical navigator spin echo beam that measures diaphragmatic motion in the superior–inferior direction corresponding to each in-plane phase-encoding line for each heartbeat (Fig. 6.1). A fixed number of repeated measurements are acquired for each phase-encoding line. A histogram is created after data acquisition. This measures phase-encoding lines as a function of diaphragmatic position. The most common position of the diaphragm is determined (i.e., usually end-expiration) and chosen as the gating center. For a given line in k-space, only data acquired when the position of the diaphragm falls within a range (usually $+/- 1$ mm) from the gating center are used for image reconstruction. With this 3-D technique (2–5) a 3.2–4.0-cm slab, composed of 16–20 partitions of 2 mm each, is acquired in each scan with the center of the slab set by the operator. In the most recent version of the software, partitions are automatically interpolated to 1 mm in the z-axis. In-plane resolution is on the order of 1×1 mm^2. When contrast agents are used, in-plane resolution can be improved by turning off the posterior channels of the phased array coil and decreasing the field-of-view. Depending on the heart rate of the patient, each sequence takes 4–8 minutes to acquire. This is the technique currently marketed by Siemens Medical Systems (Erlangen, Germany).

Real-Time Respiratory Gating and Feedback

Investigators using real-time respiratory gating employ a two-dimensional (2-D) selective pulse to excite a lon-

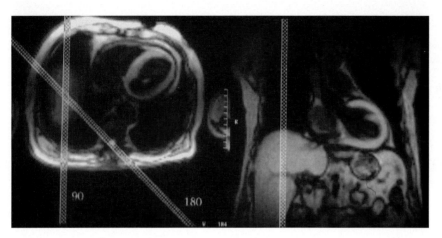

Figure 6.1. (A) Transaxial scout image at the position of the diaphragm demonstrates crossed position of the excitation bands at the right hemidiaphragm. One of these excitation bands has a flip angle of 90 degrees and the second has a flip angle of 180 degrees. (B) Together these two bands create a vertical navigator SE which measures diaphragmatic motion.

gitudinal cylindrical beam that is positioned through the diaphragm to monitor its motion (Fig. 6.2) (6). As image data is collected, navigator echoes are acquired immediately before and after the image data readout train in every cardiac cycle. This technique differs from retrospective respiratory gating in that the decision to reject or accept each segment of data is made prospectively or in "real-time." When the position of the diaphragm sampled by these navigator echoes falls within a specified range, image data are accepted and image collection moves on to the next line of data. If, however, the diaphragm is not in the gate window, the same segment of data is reacquired during the next heartbeat (6). This method has been employed by both users of the General Electric (Milwaukee, Wisconsin) and Philips MR systems (Best, Netherlands). Another sequence available on the Philips system uses a cylindrical excitation pulse that is placed directly through the

heart (7,8). A component of adaptive motion correction is coupled with this type of navigator echo acquisition. This feature automatically factors in a superior–inferior displacement correction for the portion of the heart being imaged.

Respiratory triggering or feedback is a method of optimizing the real-time respiratory-gating process, shortening the data acquisition process by obtaining a navigator profile and then visually prompting the patient to hold his or her breath in a consistent location based on the navigator information (9,10). Coaching the patient in this fashion, fewer lines of data need to be reacquired. Although this technique is helpful in shortening the overall scan time, use of this technique requires an alert and cooperative patient.

Diminishing Variance Algorithm

The diminishing variance algorithm combines the advantages of both prospective and retrospective gating methods (11). With retrospective gating, the acceptance window is flexible and the number of acquisitions is fixed. With prospective gating the acceptance window is fixed and the number of acquisitions is flexible. With the diminishing variance algorithm, however, both the acceptance window and number of acquisitions are flexible. This allows for the most efficient collection of data within the gate window. Nevertheless, to perform the diminishing variance algorithm adequately a fast computer is required to update the histogram of diaphragmatic displacements in real-time, after each data acquisition.

Practical Considerations

Patient Positioning and Cardiac Triggering

For most coronary MRI, the patient is positioned supine with EKG leads placed either on the anterior or posterior chest wall. To reduce cardiac motion, EKG triggering is required and data are collected during diastole.

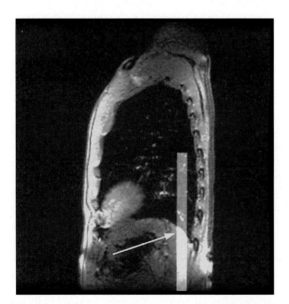

Figure 6.2. Cylindrical beam using a 2-D excitation pulse. The navigator beam is positioned through the posterior left diaphragm. (Reproduced with permission from Wang et al. (8).)

Posterior lead placement has been suggested by some researchers as being preferable because posterior placement limits EKG signal noise secondary to lead motion caused by respiration.

At our institution, we usually place the leads anteriorly, in a square, on the lower left chest wall over the heart. This can be done with either individual leads or with a commercially available "quatrode"-type set up. Leads with graphite tips are often useful to avoid susceptibility artifact. More recently, optical EKG leads have been developed to reduce gradient-induced gating interference.

Although not routinely used, peripheral pulse gating may occasionally offer some advantages if one expects changes in the R–R interval throughout the examination. This is because of the differences in the ordering of trigger delay (TD) and data acquisition. The TD comes first with EKG triggering before data acquisition; however, the TD comes second with peripheral gating, after the data acquisition. If the R–R interval becomes longer for any reason, with EKG gating, the next cardiac cycle is skipped. With peripheral gating, however, the extra time required for the new extended R–R interval merely cuts into the TD and the next cardiac cycle can immediately trigger the next data acquisition. This would hypothetically permit more efficient data acquisition.

In order to increase signal-to-noise, patients are positioned with their thorax between the anterior and posterior plates of a four-channel phased-array coil (Fig. 6.3). Two of these channels are located in the anterior plate, and the second two are located in the posterior plate. A phased-array body surface coil is currently available from most MR manufacturers. When a phased-array body surface coil is unavailable, some researchers have used the spine coil placed at the anterior chest wall (12). The lack of a posterior coil, however, limits the signal reception of the posterior heart. If contrast agents are not used, this lack of posterior signal can make the circumflex artery, which is already difficult to assess, even less visible. In addition, with the spine coil, patients must be placed in the prone position, which may be uncomfortable for some patients.

Image Plane Placement

Although scanning the coronary arteries can be performed in any plane in which the right or left coronary artery systems run, a transaxial plane for left coronary arteries and the oblique sagittal plane for the right coronary artery are the most useful. With 3-D imaging, because the regions acquired with one scan are relatively thick, the transaxial plane is the most expedient for coronary artery imaging, allowing for rapid coverage of the entire heart. Three, and occasionally four, slabs are usually necessary for complete coverage. Each scan is set up to overlap with adjacent slabs by about 30% in order to avoid an artifactual low signal band between the two slabs. This artifact will be discussed in more detail later in the chapter, but it is caused by a decrease in signal at the boundary of each slab of data acquired (Fig. 6.4). In addition, the transaxial plane is the easiest to set up, requiring the least user expertise. Because the first scan is acquired at the aortic root, precise knowledge of coronary artery anatomy is not necessary. Multiple overlapping scans can then be "queued-up" with relative ease by the MR technologist without physician intervention.

Nevertheless, whereas the transaxial scan images the left coronary artery system in plane, the transaxial scan images much of the right coronary artery (RCA) in cross-section. An oblique sagittal scan orientation is useful if one wishes to acquire an image of most of the RCA in a single scan with the least artifact. With this orientation, if set up properly, the RCA can be seen from the ostium to quite nearly its entrance to the posterior descending

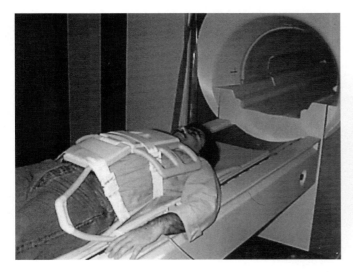

Figure 6.3. Volunteer lying supine between the anterior and posterior plates of a phased-array body surface coil.

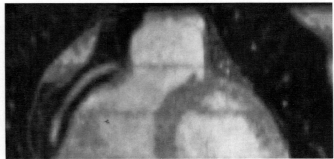

Figure 6.4. Multiplanar reconstruction (MPR) image of a normal RCA. Three slabs (representing three consecutive acquisitions) are stacked together. Despite approximately 30% overlap, a low signal band can be seen between each region.

A
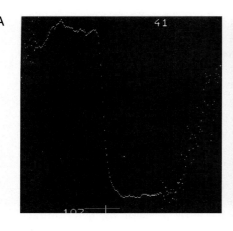
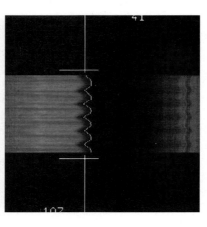
B

Figure 6.5. (A) A 1-D reconstruction from a set of navigator scout data demonstrates the amplitude of the navigator image (represented by the dotted line) as a function of the cranial–caudal position. The steep slope indicates a sharp liver/lung interface. (B) The bright signal is indicative of liver and the dark region indicative of lung. The undulating white line between the two is the diaphragmatic interface. Because of the patient's even and regular respiration, this would be the ideal patient to scan with the retrospective respiratory gating technique.

artery (PDA). If desired, an oblique sagittal orientation can also be used to look at the left main and proximal portions of the left anterior descending (LAD).

The Ideal Patient

The breathing pattern of patients plays an important role in determining the image quality and time efficiency of studies acquired with respiratory gating methods. Here we focus on our experience with retrospective respiratory gated imaging. With this technique, prior to data acquisition, a scout echo image is obtained to examine the navigator echo position, respiratory pattern, and to assess the range in which the lung–liver boundary is located. A navigator echo image will be displayed at the console. This can be quite useful in determining whether respiratory gating or a breathhold technique will be the most expedient for imaging that particular patient. A suitable patient to scan with a respiratory gating technique should demonstrate even, regular diaphragmatic excursion without dramatic superior–inferior diaphragmatic movement. The graph of the one-dimensional (1-D) reconstruction from the set of navigator echoes demonstrates the signal amplitude of the navigator echo line as a function of the cranial–caudal position. A steep slope indicates a sharp liver–lung interface necessary for appropriate motion detection (Fig. 6.5).

Although it is not impossible to scan patients with erratic breathing patterns, one must remember that the longer the breathing cycle, the more likely it is that certain phase-encoding lines will not be acquired within the gate window. This results from the fact that only five repeated measurements are acquired consecutively for each phase-encoding line. If the breathing cycle is longer than the five cardiac cycles, the five acquisitions of the same phase-encoding lines will only cover a portion of the breathing cycle. This increases the likelihood that these phase-encoding lines may provide no data acquired within the desired gate window. A simple solution to this problem might be to either increase the number of acquisitions or to change the order of data collection so that k-space is covered entirely before the next repetition. With retrospective respiratory gating, if enough lines of data in the gating window are not available, lines of data outside of that range will also be used for image reconstruction. This residual motion will then create image artifacts.

Obstacles to Effective Scanning and Methods of Overcoming Them

There are a few obstacles that occasionally occur and which could prevent the acquisition of a diagnostic examination. Patients with sleep apnea, erratic breathing, or very deep diaphragmatic excursion (Fig. 6.6) are par-

A
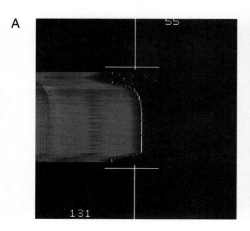
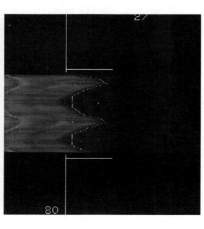
B

Figure 6.6. (A) Navigator scout demonstration of the diaphragmatic position (white line) in a patient with sleep apnea. Note that respiration is suspended for a period of time only to fluctuate dramatically as the patient awakens. (B) Demonstration of deep diaphragmatic excursion. Both of these breathing patterns increase the difficulty of obtaining a good-quality examination.

Figure 6.7. (A) Breathing patterns in the same patient pre- and posttraining. (B) Note, also, the improvement of image quality in the prone position.

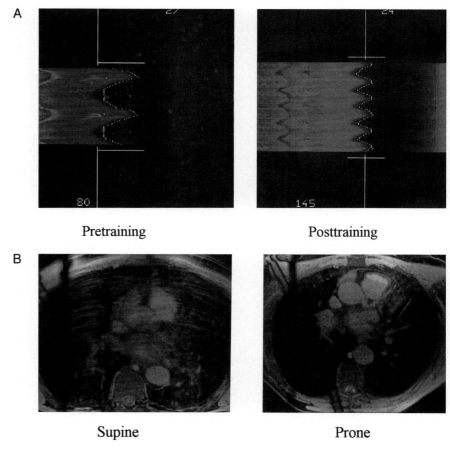

Pretraining   Posttraining

Supine   Prone

ticularly difficult to scan with effective gating. In patients with sleep apnea, we have found it helpful to attempt to keep the patient awake throughout the 4–8 minutes of scan time. We do this by announcing to the patient, at minute intervals, the time left until the end of the scan. A number of techniques have been helpful in patients with erratic breathing patterns. If the patient is alert and oriented, we have found it possible to train a patient to breathe in a regular fashion by mentally counting to himself. In patients with deep diaphragmatic excursion, scanning the patient prone occasionally has proved useful (Fig. 6.7).

Another problem can be uneven saturation of epicardial fat. This is especially a problem if the fat immediately adjacent to a coronary artery is unevenly saturated. Because both the vessel and the unsaturated fat are bright, the vessel is obscured. Depending upon the severity of the problem and the manufacturer of the MR system, one can employ a number of simple corrective procedures. Certain systems allow manual shimming of the magnetic field. Another, more-serious problem is that if the subject contains a significant amount of fat tissue in the sensitive region of the coil, fat frequency may be selected in frequency adjustment. In this case water and soft tissue, instead of fat, are saturated by the frequency selective rf pulse.

Different methods of overcoming this problem can be used depending upon the vendor of the imaging system. On the Siemens systems at our institution, we change the imaging frequency by steps of 20 Hz, by either adding or subtracting, until satisfactory fat saturation is obtained.

Finally, myocardium can obscure adjacent coronary arteries. Researchers have attempted various methods of suppressing myocardial signal, including inversion recovery, magnetization transfer (13), and T2 preparation prepulse methods (8).

Processing and Image Display

Questions have arisen as to the best method of image display. Should individual partitions of 3-D data sets be read alone, or should some effort be made to present the data as projection images? Methods of possible image display include individual partitions (Fig. 6.8), multiplanar reconstruction (MPR), maximum intensity projection images (MIPs), or volume-rendered images (Fig. 6.9). Individual partitions can be filmed, assessed on a workstation, or presented in cine format. For assessment of projection images, removal of myocardium certainly enhances the visibility of the more distal vessels in 3-D projections, but when performed manually is relatively

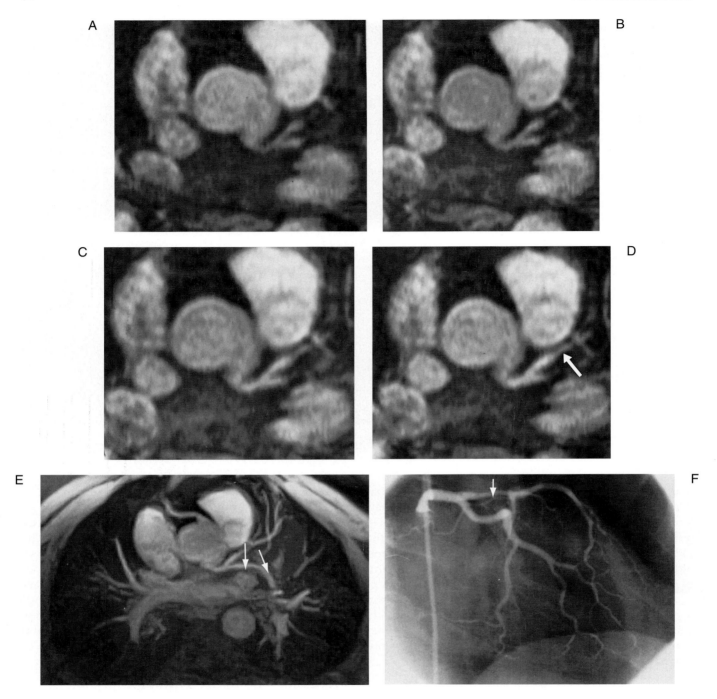

Figure 6.8. (A–D) Four individual partitions (interpolated to 0.5-mm intervals) in a patient with an LAD stenosis (arrow). (E) Filtered maximium intensity projection image on the same patient. Manual removal of the left ventricular myocardium was performed to permit visibility of the LAD more distally. Again, the LAD stenosis can be seen (arrow). On the conventional angiogram (F), this lesion (arrow) was clinically read as a 50–70% stenosis. (Reprinted with permission from Li et al. (2,22).)

time consuming. Although no truly efficient postprocessing system for the creation of projection images is currently available, development of more automatic postprocessing software is under way and will be necessary if projection images are to be used routinely. Volume-rendered images are not commonly used, but they could be performed on a computer workstation using commercially available software. Volume-rendered images have an advantage of being easily created, without removal of myocardium. A disadvantage to volume-rendered images is that the adjacent cardiac blood pool is of the same signal as the coronary arteries, will be

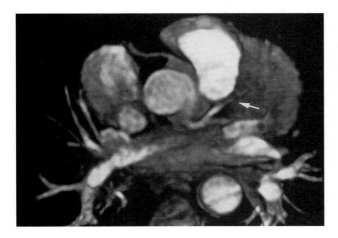

Figure 6.9. Volume-rendered image created from data on patient in Figure 6.8. An arrow points to the site of stenosis. Volume-rendered images do not require manual removal of the left ventricular myocardium and are, thus, easier to create. (Courtesy of Robert P. Dolan, Ph.D., EPIX, Inc., Cambridge, MA.)

seen in the final image, and has the potential to obscure the coronary arteries.

Assessment of each data set at the console by the clinician interpreting the data quite likely will permit the most accurate interpretations. With this method, MPRs can be performed through areas of questionable stenosis. In the future, quick methods of creating suitable projection or volume-rendered images would ideally also be readily available at the system console.

Interpretive Pitfalls—Our Own Experience

We and others have identified a number of interpretive pitfalls in 3D coronary artery MR. Some of these are as follows (5).

First, consider banding between stacked slabs. This banding occurs in the creation of 3-D projection images between stacked slabs. This signal decrease is caused by signal inhomogeneity in image acquisitions most peripheral from the center of the slab and can be decreased by overlap of slabs. We usually overlap adjacent slabs by 30%; however, decreased signal may still occur and the reader should be aware of the phenomenon in order to avoid mistaking the decrease in signal for stenoses. On the other hand, banding between stacked slabs can occur because of slab misregistration. An additional method of overcoming this problem is to obtain images of all vessels in plane.

Second, signal distal to a complete occlusion caused by retrograde flow secondary to collateral artery formation. We studied two patients with a 100% stenosis in the proximal right coronary artery, where this problem occurred. On cardiac catheterization, both of these patients demonstrated no contrast distal to the stenoses initially, but contrast could be identified later in the run in the distal vessel as it became partially reconstituted secondary to collateral vessels. On MR, however, whereas the stenosis could be seen, signal persisted distal to the stenosis likely caused by the retrograde flow. This phenomenon has been observed with both 2-D and 3-D methods. If retrograde flow is suspected, the direction of flow in the vessel can be determined by phase contrast images obtained above and below the stenosis, or possibly by the placement of flow saturation bands.

Third, tortuous vessels, entering in and out of plane on individual 3-D partitions can simulate stenoses. This can be ameliorated by thorough assessment of prior and subsequent images obtained in the same data set, or it may be rectified by the assessment of projection images or MPR images.

Fourth, volume averaging with surrounding structures such as adjacent pericardium can mask stenoses. We have observed this phenomenon on oblique sagittal 3-D projection images of the RCA (Fig. 6.10), which likely occurs secondary to cardiac motion. This can sometimes be compensated for by obtaining additional images in an alternate orientation.

Fifth, on projection images, adjacent structures can obscure stenoses. Again, in our experience pericardium has been a culprit. To rectify this, individual images can be viewed. MPR images may also be useful.

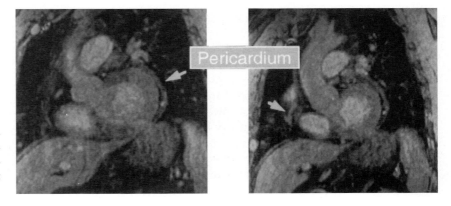

Figure 6.10. Example of a patient with pericardial thickening. Because of volume averaging with the adjacent vessel, this pericardial thickening obscures a 70% eccentric mid-RCA stenosis.

Intravascular Contrast Agents

Intravascular contrast agents are currently being explored as a means of increasing signal-to-noise ratio (SNR) (14–16). If successful, they will likely be of more benefit to 3-D imaging in comparison to 2-D methods. This is because, as mentioned earlier, 2-D images already demonstrate better contrast-to-noise (CNR) in comparison to 3-D images, secondary to high blood inflow signal. The additional SNR provided by the intravascular contrast agent will permit increased resolution and, hypothetically, permit increased visibility of stenoses.

Clinical Trials

Navigator echo gating has been applied in several small clinical trials for the assessment of proximal coronary artery stenoses. To date, most clinical trials have employed the retrospective respiratory gating technique. These trials (with patient numbers ranging from 10 to 36) using 3-D methods described sensitivities of 38–83% with relatively high specificities (greater than 90%) (3–5). It is of note that at least one large multicenter trial using the Boston Cookbook protocol for 3-D free-breathing methods on Philips MR Scanners is in progress (22).

Summary

It must be remembered that 3-D MRA techniques for the assessment of coronary arteries are still evolving and much can be done in the way of improving them. To obtain adequate sensitivity for detection of coronary artery stenoses, in-plane resolution will need to be increased, and the window of acquisition could be decreased to avoid image blur. As described earlier, improved spatial resolution could be facilitated by intravascular contrast agents that would increase SNR.

Methods of increasing efficiency might include a software package that could allow for faster and more automated processing of projection images, or workstations that could provide applications of volume rendering. Permitting radiologists actively to assess the data sets with MPR at the system console is another factor that may decrease the number of false positives and may possibly increase sensitivity.

Whereas screening for coronary artery stenoses is the ultimate goal, 3-D techniques are already suitable for use in the assessment of anomalous coronaries and are especially suited to young children (17,18). Other clinical uses for coronary artery MRA that have been explored and are currently under investigation include assessment of stenoses postangioplasty and assessment of coronary graft patency after bypass (19,20). Several additional technical and clinical advances using 3-D navigator techniques and autocorrelation techniques have been described (21–26).

References

1. Wielopolski PA, van Geuns RJ, de Feyter PJ, Oudkerk M. Breath-hold coronary MR angiography with volume-targeted imaging. Radiology 1998;209:209–19.
2. Li D, Kaushikkar S, Haacke EM, Woodard PK, Dhawale P, Kroeker RM, et al. Three-dimensional magnetic resonance imaging of coronary arteries with retrospective respiratory gating. Radiology 1996;201:857–63.
3. Post JC, van Rossum AC, Hofman MBM, Valk J, Visser CA. Three-dimensional respiratory-gated MR angiography of coronary arteries: comparison with conventional coronary angiography. Am J Roentgenol 1996;166:1399–404.
4. Müller MF, Fleish M, Kroeker R, Chatterjee T, Meier B, Vock P. Proximal coronary artery stenosis: three-dimensional MRI with fat saturation and navigator echo. J Magn Reson Imag 1997;7:644–51.
5. Woodard PK, Li D, Haacke EM, Dhawale PJ, Kaushikkar S, Barzilai B, et al. Detection of coronary stenoses on source and projection images using 3D MR angiography with retrospective respiratory gating: preliminary experience. Am J Roentgenol 1998;170:883–88.
6. Wang Y, Rossman PJ, Grimm RC, Riederer SJ, Ehman RL. Navigator-echo-based real-time respiratory gating and triggering for reduction of respiration effects in three-dimensional coronary MR angiography. Radiology 1996; 198:55–60.
7. McConnell MV, Khasgiwala VC, Savord BJ, Chen MH, Chaung ML, Edelman RR, et al. Comparison of real-time navigator gating to other respiratory motion suppression techniques for magnetic resonance coronary artery angiography (abstr.). Proc ISMRM, Fourth Scientific Meeting, New York, 1996:450.
8. Botnar RM, Stuber M, Danias PG, Kissinger KV, Manning WJ. Improved coronary artery definition with T2-weighted, free-breathing, three-dimensional coronary MRA. Circulation 1999;99:3139–48.
9. Wang Y, Grimm RC, Rossman PJ, Debbins JP, Riederer SJ, Ehman RL. 3D coronary MR angiography in multiple breath-holds using a respiratory feedback monitor. Magn Reson Med 1995;34:11–16.
10. Wang Y, Christy PS, Korosec FR, Alley MT, Grist TM, Polzin JA, et al. Coronary MRI with a respiratory feedback monitor: the 2D imaging case. Magn Reson Med 1995;33:116–21.
11. Sachs TS, Meyer CH, Irarrazabal P, Hu BS, Nishimura DG, Macovski A. Diminishing variance algorithm for real-time reduction of motion artifacts in MRI. Magn Reson Med 1995;34:412–22.
12. Pennell DJ, Keegan J, Firmin DN, Gatehouse PD, Underwood SR, Longmore DB. Magnetic resonance imaging of coronary arteries: technique and preliminary results. Br Heart J 1993;70:315–26.
13. Li D, Paschal CB, Haacke EM, Adler LP. Coronary arteries: three-dimensional MR imaging with fat saturation and magnetization transfer contrast. Radiology 1993;187:401–6.

14. Dolan RP, Prasad PV, Wielopolski PA, Li W, Walovitch RC, Edelman RR, et al. First pass myocardial imaging with MS-325, a new intravascular magnetic resonance contrast agent (abstr. P3). *In*: Abstracts for the Scientific Conference on Current and Future Application of Magnetic Resonance in Cardiovascular Disease, AHA Symposium, San Francisco, January 14–16, 1996.

15. Walovitch RC, Parmelee DJ, Dolan HS, Oullet HS, Lauffer RB. MR angiography and pharmacokinetics of MS-325 (abstr). Proc ISMRM, Fourth Scientific Meeting, New York, 1996:77.

16. Peters DC, Frayne R, Kosorsec FR, Polzin JA, Grist TA, Wedding KL, et al. Simulation of contrast enhanced single breathhold multiphase 3D coronary artery imaging (abstr.). Proc ISMRM, Fourth Scientific Meeting, New York, 1996:670.

17. McConnell MV, Ganz P, Selwyn AP, Li W, Edelman RR, Manning WJ. Identification of anomalous coronary arteries and their anatomic course by magnetic resonance coronary angiography. Circulation 1995;92:3158–62.

18. Post JC, van Rossum AC, Bronzwaer JGF, de Cock CC, Hofman MBM, Valk J, et al. Magnetic resonance angiography of anomalous coronary arteries: a new gold standard for delineating the proximal course? Circulation 1995;92:3163–71.

19. Debatin JF, Strong JA, Sostman HD, Negro-Vilar R, Paine SS, Douglas JM, et al. MR characterization of blood flow in native and grafted internal mammary arteries. J Magn Reson Imag 1993;3:443–50.

20. White RD, Caputo GR, Mark AS, Modin GW, Higgins CB. Coronary artery bypass graft patency: noninvasive evaluation with MR imaging. Radiology 1987;164:681–86.

21. Manning W, Danias P, Kissinger K, Stuber M, Botnar R, et al. MR coronary artery multi-center study with the Boston Cookbook protocol (abstr.). *In*: Book of Abstracts of the First International Workshop on Coronary MR & CT Angiography. Organized and Published by the North American Society for Cardiac Imaging. Lyon, France, Oct 1–3, 2000:1.

22. Haacke EM, Li D, Kaushikkar S. Cardiac MRI: concepts and techniques. Top Magn Reson Imag 1995;7:200–17.

23. Ikonen AE, Manninen HI, Vainio P, et al. Repeated 3D coronary MR angiography with navigator echo gating: technical quality and consistency of image interpretation. J Comput Assist Tomogr 2000;24(3):375–81.

24. Manduca A, McGee KP, Welch EB, Felmlee JP, Grimm RC, Ehman RL. Autocorrection in MR imaging: adaptive motion correction without navigator echoes. Radiology 2000;215(3):904–9.

25. Sardanelli F, Molinari G, Zandrino F, Balbi M. Three-dimensional, navigator-echo MR coronary angiography in detecting stenoses of the major epicardial vessels, with conventional coronary angiography as the standard of reference. Radiology 2000;214(3):808–14.

26. Wang Y, Ehman RL. Retrospective adaptive motion correction for navigator-gated 3D coronary MR angiography. J Magn Reson Imag 2000;11(2):208–14.

7
Clinical Applications Today

André J. Duerinckx

Most of the clinical applications of coronary magnetic resonance angiography (MRA) have been validated using first-generation techniques with breathholding. For a clinician thinking about ordering a coronary MRA it is important to know when such a study can add value to the work up of a patient, and what the confidence level is for obtaining a definitive clinical diagnosis, and answer. It is equally important to know when coronary MRA is the only modality that can provide the answer, as it is in certain cases of congenital coronary anatomy. This chapter provides a brief review of the existing literature of proven clinical applications of coronary MRA. We will point out along the way which applications are easy to perform, which are more difficult, and which are still somewhat experimental. More detailed discussions on specific applications will be provided in Chapters 8–12.

Clinical applications of 2-D coronary MRA include coronary lesion detection (1–6), the delineation of congenital coronary artery anomalies (7–13), the characterization of previously known coronary lesions (5,14), coronary bypass graft patency (15–20) and complications of coronary bypass surgery (21), vessel patency and evaluation after coronary stent placement (22–24), coronary anatomy after heart transplantation (25,26), and coronary flow reserve quantification (27–30).

Imaging Coronary Artery Lesions

The detection of coronary artery lesions by MR is probably the most talked about application of coronary MRA. It is interesting that it is the least mature and most experimental application. We will discuss it in great detail later in the book (Chap. 12); however, because of its universal appeal, as it represents the "holy grail" of cardiac magnetic resonance imaging (MRI) (31–35), we will briefly mention it here. It was originally hoped that coronary MRA could become a noninvasive screening tool for the detection of coronary artery lesions. This is still a dream today. After 6 years of preclinical trials of coronary MRA, no technique has yet emerged that can provide a sensitivity and specificity for coronary lesion detection that compares with traditional contrast coronary angiography. It may be that herein lies the real problem with some of the research: We should not expect from a noninvasive imaging technique (i.e., coronary MRA) to perform as well as a very invasive alternative (i.e., contrast X-ray coronary angiography). Nobody expects this from nuclear cardiology or exercise stress-testing. It is hoped that by reassessing the unrealistic expectations we originally had for the role of coronary MRA in the work up of patients with ischemic heart disease we will soon find a worthwhile place for this technology. More discussions on this topic follow in Chapter 12.

Imaging Congenital Anomalies of the Coronary Arteries

Until a few years ago there were only isolated reports on the use of MRI to determine the origin or proximal course of an anomalous coronary artery (see introduction to Chap. 8). For example, Doory et al. reported on five patients with anomalous coronary artery (36). In all 5 patients, magnetic resonance imaging provided definitive confirmation of the courses of the anomalous left and right coronary arteries. This study was performed using T1 weighted spin-echo sequences in multiple planes on the 1.5 Tesla GE Signal Scanner. No coronary MRA technique was used. More recently several new case reports appeared that described the use of coronary MRA to evaluate such anomalous vessels (7–9). Then, in the December 1, 1995, issue of *Circulation*, two major articles were published that established coronary MRA as the technique of choice for the delineation of the origin and proximal course of anomalous coronary arteries (10,11). Each one of these publications will be discussed in more detail later. Since then the use of MRI and/or coronary MRA for the detection of coronary artery aneurysms or AV-fistulae has also been well documented (12,13,37–39) (see also Chap. 9). All of these studies are easy-to-perform applications. Most radiologists should be able to reproduce the results shown in the literature with the existing first-generation coronary MRA techniques.

In a first 1995 article in *Circulation* by McConnell et al. (10) from the Cardiovascular Divisions, Beth Israel Hospital and Brigham and Women's Hospital, a total of 16 patients (nine men, seven women; age 44–81 years) with anomalous aortic origins of the coronary arteries by conventional X-ray angiography were studied with coronary MRA. Multiple images of the major epicardial coronary arteries were obtained by use of a first-generation breathhold technique (a fat suppressed, segmented *k*-space gradient-echo pulse sequence) in a blinded fashion by the investigators who were blinded to previous X-ray angiography data. The anomalous coronary pathology as determined by the X-ray coronary angiography included right-sided left main coronary artery ($n = 3$), right-sided left circumflex artery ($n = 6$), separate left-sided left anterior descending and left circumflex arteries ($n = 2$), left-sided right coronary artery ($n = 4$), and an anteriorly displaced right coronary artery ($n = 1$). Coronary MRA correctly identified the anomalous coronary vessels in 14 or 15 patients. The anomalous vessel was incorrectly identified in only one patient, and the course of the anomalous vessel was not clearly seen in two patients; one of these was a nondominant anomalous right coronary artery. We concluded that coronary MRA is a useful technique for the noninvasive identification of anomalous coronary arteries and their anatomic course.

In a second article Post et al. (11), from the Free University Hospital and the Institute for Cardiovascular Research of the Free University, Amsterdam/InterUniversity Cardiology Institute of the Netherlands, Utrecht, reported on a study of 38 patients of which 19 had an anomalously originating coronary artery. The specifically asked question was: Is coronary MRA of the anomalous coronary arteries the new gold standard for delineating the proximal course of these vessels? Both the origin and the proximal course of the coronary arteries were defined. After separate analysis of the MRI and conventional X-ray angiography studies, a final consensus result was defined for each patient. Successful MR coronary angiography was performed in 37 of 38 patients. An X-ray coronary angiogram was available in 36 of the 38 patients. Sensitivity and specificity for detecting anomalous coronary arteries and delineating the proximal course in this second study were 100%. The data in this study suggests that coronary MRA is highly accurate in determining the origin and in delineating the proximal course of anomalous coronary arteries, even in those cases in which X-ray coronary angiographic diagnosis was difficult or even erroneous. Differences of opinion existed in three patients about the proximal course (but not the origin) of the anomalous artery. After a joint review of three cases, however, it was unanimously decided that MRA unambiguously delineated the proximal course of these anomalous arteries, whereas conventional X-ray angiography interpretation of this course had been erroneous or at least difficult.

Imaging of Coronary Artery Bypass Grafts

Patients having one or more coronary artery bypass graft (CABG) operations constitute an important part of the practice of cardiac radiology. Because CABG is performed in a very large number of Americans annually, and follow-up studies have shown a rather significant number of postoperative occlusions, there is a great interest in providing imaging techniques for CABG occlusion. It has been shown that 10–30% of grafts are occluded one to 2 years and 45–55% are occluded 10–12 years after grafting. There are major differences in occlusion rates between the saphenous vein and internal mammary artery graft, with occlusion rates in the first postoperative year of 20% and 5%. To date, the gold standard for evaluating graft patency in CABG patients is still coronary angiography, which is an invasive and costly procedure that is not risk free. There are other direct methods such as ultrasound, computed tomography (CT), electron-beam computed tomography (EB-CT), MR imaging, and Doppler sonography. Indirect imaging methods include radionuclide ventriculopathy, Thallium-201 scintigraphy, and position imaging tomography.

In addition to the gold standard of X-ray–based coronary angiography, the other direct imaging modalities (e.g., transthoracic echocardiography, Doppler sonography, and CT) have some limitations. The great disadvantage of transthoracic echocardiography is that it requires considerable expertise and it is difficult to differentiate the graft flow signal from that generated by the aorta and pulmonary arteries. The technique is also less applicable for circumflex grafts that are located more posteriorly. Published sensitivities and specificities for the technique run from 83 to 92% and from 56 to 100%, respectively (40). Conventional and ultrafast CT offer another alternative. Ultrafast CT has shown considerable promise in imaging bypass graft. A multicenter study by Stanford et al. (41) has shown a sensitivity of 93% for detecting angiographically patent grafts and a specificity of 89% for determining angiographic closed grafts. The overall accuracy was 92%. The number of technically adequate studies was more than 94%. Many other published studies have reported results from the use of ultrafast CT for coronary bypass graft patency determination (40). An example of CABG imaged with ultrafast CT is shown in Figure 7.1.

Magnetic resonance imaging (MRI) offers an important alternative approach to imaging of coronary artery bypass grafting. Bypass grafts are relatively stationary when compared to native coronary arteries. This explains why cardiac-gated spin-echo (dark blood) and

A

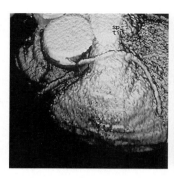 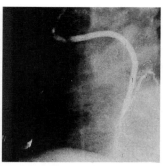

B **Figure 7.1.** Coronary artery bypass graft is imaged with electron-beam CT (EB-CT). (A) Volume rendered EB-CT angio-gram of a bypass graft to the left anterior descending (LAD). (B) Corresponding selective coronary X-ray angiogram. (Reprinted with permission from Achenbach et al., Non-invasive coronary angiography by contrast-enhanced electron-beam computer tomography. Clin Cardiol 1998;21: 323–330.)

gradient-recalled-echo (bright blood) MRI techniques to evaluate graft patency have had relatively good success rates. It also explains the relative success of the other noninvasive imaging techniques. Figure 7.2 shows the typical locations of saphenous vein bypass grafts. The more proximal portions of the grafts are subjected to less cardiac motion than the distal anastomosis to the native vessels. In the early days the MRI technique focused on determining graft patency by imaging a small portion of the bypass graft. In fact, a single cross-section of the graft in one or two transaxial planes is all that was usually imaged. These techniques used traditional EKG-gated MR pulse sequences: cardiac-gated spin-echo T1-weighted imaging where patent grafts appeared as flow void (dark blood) , and cine MR where a patent graft shows up as a high signal area (bright

blood). We refer the reader to several excellent reviews of the literature on this early use of MRI for graft patency (15,40,42). Table 7.1 summarizes these early results, which at this point in time are more of historical than practical clinical value (see also Chap. 4). Although one might have hoped that coronary MRA would be very helpful for this application, this has not been the case. The first-generation coronary MRA techniques require pretest knowledge of the position of the blood vessels. The location of native coronary vessels with respect to the heart is relatively well known, thus allowing easy selection of appropriate imaging planes (as discussed in Chap. 5); however, following the course of bypass grafts, without clear landmarks inside the chest cavity, can be more difficult. This explains why no extensive studies using a first-generation coronary MRA technique to image large sections of bypass grafts have been performed. Studies to image internal mammary artery grafts have been performed (43) because the course of these vessels is more predictable, as shown in Figure 7.3. The distal graft anastomosis is also somewhat easier to image with coronary MRA because it is located close to an easy to visualize cardiac surface (see later discussions).

Given the great challenges of interactively tracking the course of a bypass graft through the chest cavity with no clear landmarks, the advent of new contrast-enhanced 3-D MRA techniques with short acquisition times (within a single breathhold, thus eliminating breathing motion) has made a dramatic change in our ability to image these vessels. These new noncardiac-gated 3-D MRA techniques are adequate to image the proximal and middle portion of grafts, but not the distal anastomosis where cardiac motion is still a problem. Since their first description in 1993 by Prince et al. (50), enormous progress has been made with these 3-D dynamic Gadolinium enhanced MRA techniques (51–53). The duration of 3-D slab acquisitions has decreased from several minutes in 1993 to time periods under 8 seconds for carotid MRA in 1998. These contrast-enhanced 3-D noncardiac-gated MRA approaches are now being routinely used to image the thoracic aorta, renal arteries, and the abdominal aorta, and they are starting to be used for imaging of the carotid arteries (54,55) and the pulmonary arteries (56,57). Its use most recently has been used for CABG imaging (18–20). These techniques nicely comple-

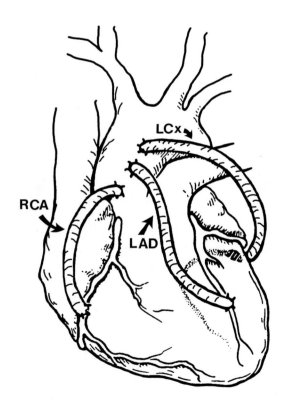

Figure 7.2. Typical location of saphenous vein bypass grafts coming off the proximal ascending aorta and anastomosing the native coronary arteries.

Table 7.1. Summary of 1987–1996 MRI studies evaluating traditional cardiac-gated MRI techniques (spin-echo and gradient echo) for the assessment of graft patency after aortocoronary bypass grafting.

	Number of patients	Number of grafts	Patent (%)	Sensitivity (%)	Specificity (%)
Spin-echo					
White et al., 1987, Ref. 44	25	72	69	86	72
Rubinstein et al., 1987, Ref. 45	20	47	62	90	72
Jenkins et al., 1988, Ref. 46	16	41	63	89	73
Galjee et al., 1996, Ref. 16	47	84	74	98	85
Gradient echo					
White et al., 1988, Ref. 47	28	28	52	93	86
Aurigemma et al., 1989, Ref. 48	45	45	73	88	100
Galjee et al., 1996, Ref. 16	47	84	74	98	88
Flow mapping					
Hoogendoorn et al., 1995, Ref. 49	17	22	77	100	88

The newer noncardiac-gated contrast-enhanced 3-D MRA and half-Fourier acquired single-shot turbo spin-echo (HASTE) techniques are discussed in the text.
Modified from Danias et al., Ref. 42.

ment the cardiac-gated coronary MRA techniques that offer direct visualization of native coronary arteries, small segments and the distal anastomosis of a CABG, and internal mammary arteries and veins (16,43), as illustrated in Figure 7.3. Moreover, the capability for 3-D visualization and 3-D reconstruction from MRA data has tremendously improved the visualization of much longer portions of coronary bypass grafts. It should be noted that metal artifact due to sternal sutures, surgical clips, or stents do not usually interfere with visualization of a graft. They only obscure the graft in very small focal ar-

eas and still allow clear visualization of the majority of the largest portion of the graft. We will now review the more promising recently published approaches to CABG imaging (see also Chaps. 10 and 11). Most of these should be easily reproducible on any clinical MRI scanner.

In a first study, published in the April 1997 issue of the *American Journal of Roentgenology* by Vrachliotis et al. (18), a total of 45 grafts (29 saphenous vein bypass grafts; 12 left internal mammary artery grafts; 4 right internal mammary artery grafts) were evaluated in 15 patients. These 15 patients underwent 3-D breathhold

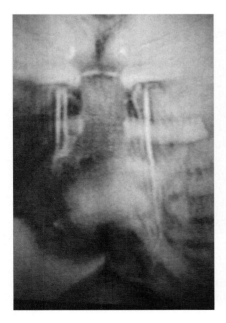
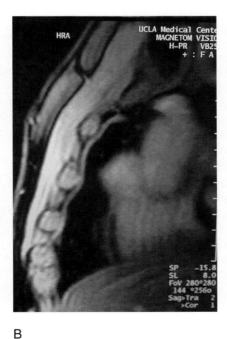
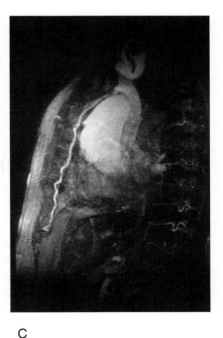

A   B   C

Figure 7.3. Typical appearance of the internal mammary vessels (arteries and veins) as seen on first-generation coronary MRA. (A) Coronal image obtained along the anterior chest wall, with the patient prone on a standard spine coil. (B) Sagittal image of the right/left mammary vessels. Unlike saphenous vein grafts these vessels are easy to track and follow (see text). (C) Sagittal image of the mammary vessel during a dynamic contrast-enhanced MRA.

EKG-triggered contrast enhanced MRA on a 1.5 Tesla commercial scanner (Magnetom Vision Scanner, Siemens Medical Systems, Iselin, NJ) with 25 mT/m gradients and 600-μsec rise time. These MRA studies were performed within 24 hours of the conventional coronary angiography studies. MRA was in agreement with the coronary angiography in 42 of the 44 grafts, after exclusion of one saphenous vein graft that was revealed as occluded by X-ray coronary angiography but was patent by MRA. Additional information on this work is provided in Chap. 10.

In a second study by Wintersperger et al. (19,20) breathhold contrast-enhanced MRA was also evaluated as a tool to assess coronary bypass graft patency. Examples of CABG imaged by this group are shown in Chapter 11. These authors set out to demonstrate the feasibility and reliability of the contrast-enhanced MRA technique in the assessment of venous and internal mammary artery graft patency after CABG surgery, using X-ray coronary angiography as a reference standard. The study included 27 patients with a total of 76 (48 venous/28 internl mammary artery (IMA) coronary bypass grafts. These patients were examined 26.5 ± 5.8 months after surgery with both MRA and X-ray angiogram within 12.6 ± 10.5 hours. MRA was performed on a 1.5 Tesla whole-body scanner (Magnetom Vision Scanner, Siemens Medical Systems, Germany) using the same contrast-enhanced 3-D gradient echo sequence; that is, a 3-D FLASH sequence without EKG triggering with the following parameters: TR = 4.4 ms, TE = 1.8 ms, and 40-degree flip angle; matrix size of 512 with field-of-view (FOV) of 500 mm. The rectangular FOV was used as needed. The 3-D volume slab had a thickness of 96 mm subdivided into the 26–40 partitions with an acquisition time of about 30 seconds. The typical slice thickness was 3 mm. A single bolus of 20 cc gadopentetate dimeglumine (Magnevist, Schering AG, Germany) followed by a saline flush was used. Arrival time of the bolus was also calculated using a test bolus. We found that coronary MRA and traditional X-ray coronary angiography were in agreement in 70 of 76 grafts. Sensitivity was 95% for venous grafts, 96% for IMA grafts, and 95% overall. Specificity was 85% for venous graft and 67% for IMA grafts. These authors concluded that with contrast-enhaced MRA, which is a reliable assessment of CABG patency, is possible.

In the preceding studies, the following definitions of sensitivity, specificity, and predicted values were used. An occluded (by coronary angiography) graft was defined as true positive (occluded, diseased). On the other hand, a patent (by coronary angiography) graft was defined as true negative. In these studies, no specific attempt is made at determining focal lesions, focal stenosis, or anastomotic problems. Although these newer studies visualize larger portions of the graft, they still only look at patency; therefore, no attempt is ever made

to evaluate underlying stenosis or partial thrombus. As the high sensitivity in most of the studies illustrates, MRI is a relatively good tool at detecting a totally occluded graft; however, the relatively lower specificity also means that a significant proportion of patent grafts (by X-ray coronary angiography) are erroneously labeled as being occluded by MRI. This is because MRI failed to visualize the graft or failed to visualize flow in the patent portion of the graft. Calcifications, metal clips, thickened pericardium, and small pericardial collections of fluid can mimic the signal void of flowing blood on spin-echo images. Flowing blood on gradient echo images is depicted as a bright signal. Because of this it has been suggested that the specificity of MRI for graft patency will be improved with gradient-recalled echo (GRE) techniques.

As mentioned before these noncardiac-gated 3-D contrast-enhanced MRA techniques cannot visualize the distal CABG anastomosis. For visualization of distal anastomosis, EKG-triggered techniques are needed. Preliminary success with an EKG-triggered approach has been described by Vrachliotis et al. (18) as well as in two case reports (21,58). An example of the use of a first-generation coronary MRA technique to visualize a bypass graft is shown in Figure 7.4. (see also Chap. 8). Warner et al. (58) describes how magnetic resonance coronary artery imaging was useful when planning a redo of a coronary bypass graft operation. This specifically was the case of a 57-year-old man who had undergone triple vessel coronary artery vessel bypass grafting. Because the previous saphenous vein graft to the left anterior descending coronary artery (LAD) was

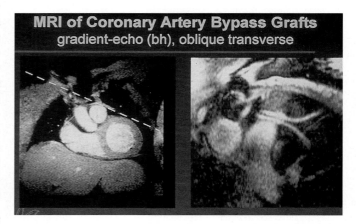

Figure 7.4. Imaging of coronary artery bypass graft using single breathhold segmented *k*-space gradient-echo technique. (A) Coronal scout view used for selection of the oblique transaxial plane. (B) Oblique transaxial image with partial in-plane view of two bypass grafts overriding the pulmonary artery. The most anterior graft deflects toward the LAD, whereas the most posterior graft is directed toward the circumflex perfusion area. (Reprinted with permission from van Rossum et al., A practical approach to MRI of coronary artery bypass graft patency and flow. Int J Card Imag 1997;13:199–204.)

aneurysmal, there was very poor opacification of the distal LAD during a repeat X-ray coronary angiogram. In this particular case, the coronary MRA technique clearly showed the distal LAD to be a sufficient quality to be able to redo the bypass surgery. In another case report by Duerinckx et al. (21) a 74-year-old man with a saphenous vein graft to the LAD also had an area of aneurysmal dilatation in the graft. Although the major problems after CABG surgery are graft stenosis, pseudoaneurysms do occur and MRI offers a good modality to visualize these grafts, as shown in Figure 7.5. This case report is another example where MRI can significantly help with the cardiologist when the amount of contrast available via conventional contrast-enhanced coronary X-ray angiography is insufficient and needs further clarification. It also illustrates how these coronary MRA sequences can occasionally be used without breathholding and still produce relatively good results.

Another, very different approach to bypass graft evaluation is the combination of traditional imaging of patency of the graft with flow profile analysis. Several papers have addressed this. Galjee et al. looked at 47 patients with previous history of coronary artery bypass grafting who underwent angiography and both spin-echo and cine phase velocity imaging (16). Twenty-three grafts were patent; twenty-five were occluded. The typical flow pattern was a balance biphasic for a floor pattern. The ultimate role of adding flow measurement is unknown but appears very promising (59–63).

MRA and flow quantification of the internal mammary artery graft after minimally invasive direct coronary artery bypass have also been successfully performed (64). Six patients who had undergone minimally invasive direct coronary artery bypass surgery were examined to evaluate an MRI protocol that provided information about cardiac function, bypass graft patency, and flow characteristics with a single examination. Preliminary results by Miller et al. suggest that the imaging protocol allows accurate followup of patients after minimally invasive direct coronary artery bypass surgery (64). Bypass graft patency was correctly determined in all patients. In four patients, anastomoses were visualized by MRA, and flow measurements revealed a volume range of 28–84 ml/min (native and grafted internal mammary arteries) and a trend for the flow values of bypass grafts to be lower than those of native vessels. Interobserver reproducibility was good ($r = .99$; slope, .98).

Cardiac-gated coronary MRA for imaging of bypass grafts has also been described. As stated earlier, first-generation techniques require time-consuming interactive search patterns, with one 2-D image per breathhold, to locate the grafts, and can thus be time consuming (65). The third-generation techniques, with thin slabs 3-D breathhold scans, are easier to use for this purpose because the 3-D slabs cover larger volumes. The second-generation navigator-based techniques offer an even easier approach as they cover larger 3-D slabs (66–68). Using a retrospective navigator-based second-generation coronary MRA technique, Kessler et al. reported the results on 7 patients with CABGs within a large study on coronary artery stenosis detection, correctly classifying 4 occluded and 13 of 15 patent grafts (67).

Another approach for CABG imaging uses cardiac-gated breathhold black-blood fast spin-echo HASTE (69–71). Kalden et al. evaluated the patency of coronary artery bypass grafts with a 2-D T2-weighted breathhold turbo spin-echo sequence HASTE. The HASTE technique has been well described elsewhere (72–75). Kalden et al. studied 38 patients with 97 grafts (19 internal mammary artery and 78 saphenous vein grafts) and a total of 120 distal anastomoses at 1.5 Tesla in supine position using a phased array body coil (69). An ECG-gated 2-D T2-weighted breathhold turbo-spin-echo sequence HASTE was performed. Reference method was selective coronary angiography. The image material was evaluated independently by two radiologists (observer one, a radiological fellow, and the second a staff radiologist). Observer one reached a sensitivity of 96% (72/75) and a specificity of 91% (20/22), positive predictive value was 97%, negative predictive value 87%. Seventy-nine of the 97 (81%) patent distal anastomoses were correctly identified. Observer two achieved a sensitivity of 92% (69/75) and a specificity of 82% (18/22), positive and negative predictive values were 95% and 75% respectively. From 97 patent distal anastomoses 59 (61%) were recognized. The interobserver agreement was good (Cohen's kappa = 68%, p-value [McNemar] = 58%). Alden et al. concluded that the HASTE sequence makes a reliable assessment of graft patency possible and that this sequence is a helpful tool for planning flow measurements and 3-D MRA (69). In addition, HASTE can be a great compliment to noncardiac-gated 3-D MRA (described earlier) because its shorter acquisition times allows better imaging of the distal graft anastomosis.

Imaging of Coronary Artery Stents

Another potentially important application of coronary MRA is determining the patency of coronary vessels after stent placement. Because stents are metallic objects and cause a major image artifact on the MRI, they are very easy to localize. Coronary MRA can then be used to determine flow in the vessels proximal and distal to the stent and thus determine vessel patency. Lesion severity or partial thrombosis cannot be assessed presently. Only total occlusion versus (total or partial) patency can be assessed (22–24,76). The clinical implications of this are that conventional X-ray angiography techniques are still better than MRI, depending on what the clinical question is. When clinical suspicion is low,

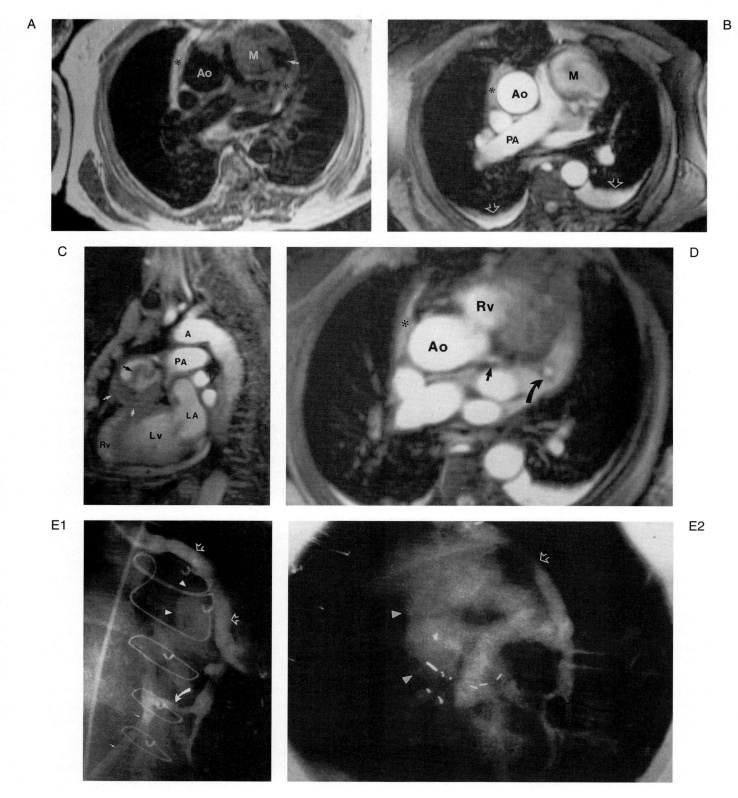

however, and the clinician prefers an initial noninvasive imaging study, coronary MRA could provide a very good initial imaging step.

Newer stents made of nickel-titanium, tantalum, and other new materials in which the metal stent artifact may no longer be a problem have already been tested in humans (77,78). These newer stents may offer great potential for the imaging of partial thrombosis stenosis within this stent, as suggested by preliminary reports.

Patients are routinely given anticoagulants for 30 days after stent deployment. During this 30-day window, cardiologists are reluctant to perform angiography because anticoagulation must first be reversed. Thus, when patients present acutely after stent placement with signs and/or symptoms suggestive of stent thrombosis but a clinical picture that is not clear, they would benefit from a noninvasive imaging technique to evaluate stent patency. A self-imposed 8-week waiting period for MRI after stent placement has been suggested by the stent manufacturers (79). Until MRI can be recommended for imaging during the immediate poststent placement period, the only alternative will remain a repeat coronary angiogram. These conventional contrast coronary angiograms can definitively establish patency of the stent, but they are invasive and somewhat contraindicated in the acute stage. In addition, the location of the stents cannot always easily be established by angiography, as stainless steel stents are radiolucent, and one widely used version of stent (the Palmaz-Schatz™

stent) is barely visible by fluoroscopy (80). There is a great interest, therefore, in newer noninvasive imaging methods, such as CT and MRI, which could be used to offer additional insight in those circumstances.

Coronary MRA of stents is a safe and noninvasive imaging procedure. Coronary artery stents are not significantly influenced by the magnetic fields that are used for imaging in clinical MRI systems at 1.5 T (81); thus, routine MRI of patients with coronary or saphenous vein graft stents should not cause significant motion of the prosthesis (22,79,82). A possible explanation is the relatively low ferromagnetic nature of the metals used for the manufacture of coronary stents. Shellock et al. evaluated safety during MRI (i.e., magnetic field interactions, heating, and artifacts) for metallic stents (83). Different types of metallic stents were tested for magnetic field interactions, heating, and artifacts using a 1.5-T MR system. Magnetic field-related translational attraction and torque were assessed using previously described techniques. Heating was evaluated using an infrared thermometer to record temperatures immediately before and after performing MRI using a whole-body-averaged specific absorption rate of 1.3 W/kg. Artifacts were assessed by placing the stents inside a fluid-filled phantom and performing MRI using fast spoiled gradient-echo and T1-weighted spin-echo pulse sequences. For the 10 different stents evaluated, Shellock et al. found no magnetic field interactions (83), and the artifacts involved signal voids that would not

---

Figure 7.5. A 74-year-old white male with a history of coronary artery disease presented with hypertension, severe chest pain possibly consistent with angina pectoris, and back pain. Fifteen years prior to this admission, the patient had undergone coronary artery bypass grafting, at which time a vein graft taken from his arm was used as a Y graft, with one limb going to the left anterior descending (LAD) artery and the second to the first obtuse marginal branch (OM1) of the circumflex. MRI study with multiple images at the level of the pseudoaneurysm (A–D). Because of the patient's inability to hold his breath while sedated, the usual coronary MRA protocol was performed without breath-holding. Thus, the coronary MRA portion of the study was suboptimal when compared with a "cooperative nonsedated" patient who can hold his/her breath. (A) Spin-echo MRI in the transaxial plane. A large vascular mass (M) is noted, which compresses the lower portion of the RVOT. Due to relatively slow flow the signal density in most of the mass is of medium intensity. There is an area of dark signal (short white arrow) corresponding to a region of increased flow velocity, possibly indicating the site of connection with the pericardial space. Respiratory motion artifacts obscure the bilateral pleural effusions. A pericardial effusion is present (*, asterisk). (B) Transaxial GRE image shows the bilateral pleural effusion as areas with high signal (open arrows). (C) Oblique sagittal GRE image. The vascular mass has a complex substructure that is now clearly demonstrated. A serpentine low signal line (short black arrow) runs throughout the middle portion of the mass, indicating either a complex flow pattern or a thin membrane. There is significant thrombus (white arrows) formation along the anterior and inferior portion of the mass. In this imaging plane the left ventricle is superimposed upon portions of the right ventricle, creating the impression of an enlarged LV. The inferior extent of the pericardial effusion is clearly demonstrated (*, asterisk). (D) GRE image in oblique transaxial plane showing the origin of the native left coronary artery system (short black arrow) that continues in a large circumflex coronary artery (not shown). Also noted is a high signal intensity focus corresponding to a cross-section of the bypass graft leading to the OM1 branch (curved black arrow). Also shown in this scan are: ascending aorta (Ao); left ventricle (Lv); left atrium (LA); right ventricle (Rv); pulmonary artery (PA); pericardial effusion (*, asterisk). (E) Conventional coronary angiography views after selective injection of bypass graft showing the area of leakage into the pseudoaneurysm. (E1) RAO view of the selective injection of the brachial venous graft (open arrows). There is leakage shown into the cavity (arrowheads). The contrast then continues into the second portion of the graft with retrograde flow into the proximal OM1 (curved arrow) and circumflex coronary artery (thin arrows). (E2) Left anterior oblique (LAO) view of the same selective injection of the graft (open arrow) showing the extent and complex anatomy of the cavity in more detail (arrowheads). This corresponds to what was demonstrated on the MRI scan (Fig. 7.2C), where a membranelike structure in the middle of the cavity suggested a complex internal structure. (Reprinted with permission from Duerinckx et al. (46).)

A
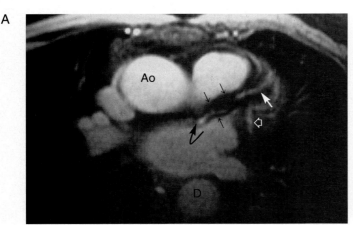
B
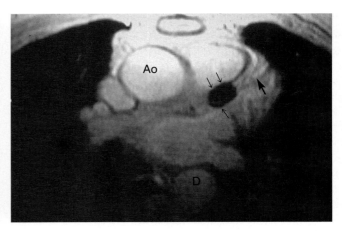

Figure 7.6. A 55-year-old man with a single stent in the proximal left anterior descending artery (LAD). The proximal LAD is shown in two perpendicular planes. (A) Oblique transaxial images with fat-suppression. The proximal LAD (curved black arrow), mid-LAD (white arrow), and great cardiac vein (open arrow) are shown. An area of signal void due to the susceptibility artifact of the stent is visualized (thin arrows). Also shown are: Ao = Ascending aorta; D = Descending aorta. (B) Oblique transaxial images without fat suppression. The area of signal void due to the susceptibility artifact of the stent is better visualized (thin arrows). The mid-LAD is only faintly seen (arrow). Also shown are: Ao = Ascending aorta; D = Descending aorta. (C) 4-chamber view with fat-suppression. The proximal and mid-LAD are shown (arrows). In this fat-suppressed image, the stent appears as an area of flow interruption (thin arrows) with flow signal seen in the vessel proximal and distal to the stent. LV = Left ventricle; RV = right ventricle. (D) Four-chamber view without fat-suppression. The area of signal void due to the susceptibility artifact clearly localizes the stent (thin arrows), and corresponds to the area of signal void seen in (C). The proximal and mid-LAD are only faintly seen. (Reprinted with permission from Duerinckx et al. (76).)

create diagnostic problems as long as the area of interest was not positioned exactly where a particular stent was located. Strohm et al. examined 14 different coronary stents from seven manufacturers in 1.0 Tesla and 1.T Tesla systems (84). They demonstrated no evidence of stent motion or measurable change in temperature in explanted pig hearts. Kramer et al. have also assessed safety of stents during MRI early after stent placement for acute myocardial infarction (85,86). They reported no significant safety problems. Schroeder et al. also confirmed that MRI seems safe in patients with intracoronary stents (87).

A recent case report described how ultrafast CT enabled the clear detection of a Palmaz-Schatz™ stent with-

A
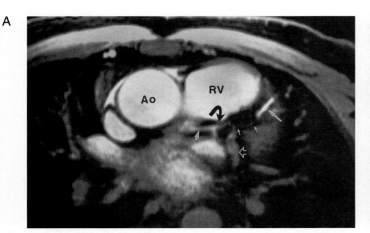
B
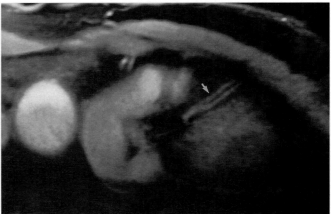

Figure 7.7. A 52-year-old man with a single stent in the proximal LAD. This case illustrates how slight changes in imaging plane orientation can significantly improve visualization of the coronary vessel distal to the stent and, thereby, confirm patency of the vessel after stent placement. (A) Image in an oblique transaxial plane with fat suppression. Shown are the left main coronary artery (short arrow), the LAD proximal to the stent (curved arrow) and distal to the stent (arrow), and a portion of the great cardiac vein (open arrow). Also shown is a portion of the circumflex coronary artery. (B) In a slightly more oblique transaxial plane, a much larger portion of the distal LAD is seen (arrow), as is the adjacent great cardiac vein.

out artifacts and was valuable in confirming its location (80). Another report discussed the use of ultrafast CT to evaluate a stent after a patient developed chest pain following bypass grafting, and later implementation of a Gianturco-Roubin stent (88). Schmermund et al. describe the use of electron-beam computed tomography (EB-CT) to assess coronary vessel patency after stent imaging in 22 patients (89,90). Quantitative analysis of densitometric curves in a region of interest distal to the stented vessel segment was performed to establish patency or occlusion. Another case report described how MRI localized a Palmaz-Schatz stent in the right coronary artery (RCA) and showed vessel patency distal to the stent (22).

The first study on the assessment of coronary artery patency following stent placement using coronary MRA was published by Duerinckx et al. (76). In this study, the authors studied 16 patients with 26 stents. The study

was performed on a 1.5 Tesla Siemens Scanner. The distribution of stent locations was: 10 in the RCA, 10 in the LAD, 2 in the circumflex coronary artery (Circ), and 4 in the saphenous vein graft (SVG) to RCA. One patient had two RCA and two LAD stents, one had three RCA and one LAD stent, and one had three SVG stents and two had double RCA stents. The authors concluded that coronary MRA is safe for noninvasive imaging of coronary artery stents, and that in the proper clinical setting it can be used to help suggest patency; however, it cannot exclude partial occlusion of partial thrombosis. Representative examples of such coronary stent images are shown in Figures 7.6, 7.7, and 7.8.

A follow up report by De Cobelli et al. confirmed similar findings about stent patency assessment by MRI in 13 stented coronary vessels with 18 stents 1 day to 8 months after stent placement (23,24,91). Different types

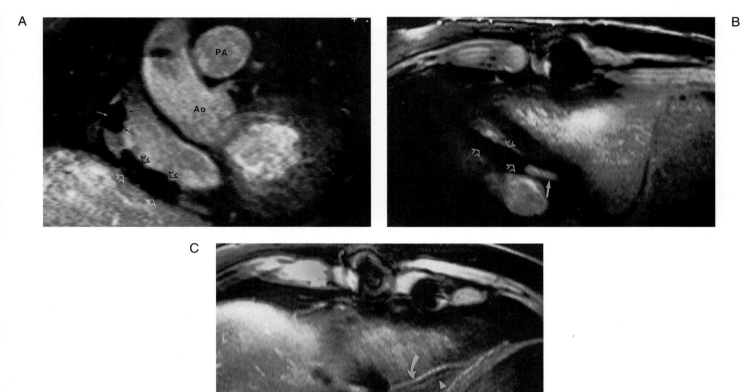

Figure 7.8. A 54-year-old man with three stents in an SVG to the posterior descending artery (PDA). (A) In an imaging plane oriented along the proximal course of the SVG two areas of apparent flow interruption are noted. The first one (closed arrows) corresponds to the first stent and is 15 mm long. The second one (open arrows) is twice as long and corresponds to two adjacent stents placed during a very complicated interventional procedure. Also shown are: Ao = Ascending aorta; PA = pulmonary artery. (B) Imaging plane along the distal course of the bypass graft and parallel to the basal inferior wall of the heart. The area of interrupted flow due to the double stent is again noted (open arrows) with a bright flow signal in the distal SVG (arrow) continuing past the distal portion of the stent. (C) Image plane parallel to the inferior wall of the right ventricle. The continuation of the distal bypass graft into the PDA (curved arrow) is shown. An oval-shaped flow void artifact is seen at the location of a surgical clip at the anastomosis of the distal SVG and the PDA. Also shown is the middle cardiac vein running parallel to the PDA (arrowheads).

of stents were evaluated: Palmatz-Schatz ($n = 6$), Multilink ($n = 6$), Crossflex ($n = 5$) and Wiktor ($n = 1$). The study was performed on a 1.5 Tesla GE scanner. Both studies (24,61) confirmed the safety of the MRI studies.

Amano et al. have described artifacts of coronary stents (92). MR flow measurements after stent placement are possible (93) as are other applications (94–96).

Imaging in Postsurgical Patients

The use of coronary MRA in postsurgical patients or after interventional procedures is increasing. Rapid heart rates, sternal wires, and altered cardiac orientation do not prevent coronary MRA in heart transplant recipients (26,97). Artifacts from bypass graft markers or clips can interfere with complete visualization of a graft, and could simulate stenosis in a graft. Sternal wires do not interfere with imaging of the majority of native coronary arteries and bypass grafts.

Post- and Preangioplasty Follow Up

Although existing coronary MRA pulse sequences may not be adequate to replace conventional coronary angiography for screening and detecting of coronary arterial lesions, they can play a significant role in the evaluation and follow up of known proximal coronary artery lesions. If and when a proximal coronary arterial lesion can be detected with coronary angiography, it is relatively easy and totally noninvasive to study the anatomy of this lesion periodically with MRI as needed (e.g., after interventional procedures such as angioplasty (98).

Duerinckx et al. have described the usefulness of coronary MRA prior to angioplasty (98). The range of indications for percutaneous transluminal coronary angioplasty (PTCA) has increased greatly since the procedure was initially introduced. The success rate depends on the anatomy and length of the occlusion and on the state of the distal vessel. Duerinckx et al. presented a case where the use of magnetic resonance angiography (MRA) allowed to evaluate the length of a subtotal occlusion prior to PTCA, and thus could have had an impact on therapeutic decisions (99). This capability may further expand the clinical use of MR technology in the practice of cardiology.

Coronary Blood Flow and Flow Reserve

The ability to also measure blood flow is a major advantage of coronary MRA over coronary X-ray angiography. This will be discussed in more detail in Chapters 13 and 14. The clinical significance of determining coronary flow reserve and changes in velocity and flow in coronary vessels cannot be understated. Early work (i.e., before the advent of breathhold velocity-encoded cine MRI) has concentrated on flow measurements in mammary arteries, as they are subjected to much less respiratory motion than the native vessels (100–102). More recent work using the breathhold velocity-encoded cine MRI has shown promising initial results in native vessels (27–30), bypass grafts, and mammary arteries (60). The results obtained so far have unfortunately been limited to small portions of proximal coronary artery territory. The reproducibility in other laboratories has not yet been established (103). The preliminary results are nevertheless extremely encouraging and point us into the right direction. More basic and applied clinical work will be needed to validate these techniques. One can think of many theoretical reasons why none of the MRI-based techniques used to quantitate coronary flow could possibly work (104). Nevertheless most experimental data seem to suggest otherwise. Our MRI techniques may not yet be good enough to measure the actual coronary flow, but at least some of us can already measure coronary flow reserve.

References

1. Manning WJ, Li W, Edelman RR. A preliminary report comparing magnetic resonance coronary angiography with conventional angiography. N Engl J Med 1993;328: 828–32.
2. Duerinckx AJ, Urman M. Two-dimensional coronary MR angiography: analysis of initial clinical results. Radiology 1994;193:731–38.
3. Post JC, vanRossum AC, Hofman MB, Valk J, Visser CA. Three-dimensional respiratory-gated MR angiography of coronary arteries: comparison with conventional coronary angiography. Am J Roentgenol 1996;166(6):1399–404.
4. Hundley WG, Clarke GD, Landau C, et al. Noninvasive determination of infarct artery patency by cine magnetic resonance angiography. Circulation 1995;91:1347–353.
5. Pennell DJ, Bogren HG, Keegan J, Firmin DN, Underwood SR. Assessment of coronary artery stenosis by magnetic resonance imaging. Heart 1996;75:127–33.
6. Post JC, van Rossum AC, Hofman MB, de Cock CC, Valk J, Visser CA. Clinical utility of two-dimensional magnetic resonance angiography in detecting coronary artery disease. Eur Heart J 1997;18(3):426–33.
7. vanCampen LC, deCock C, Bronzwaer JG, vanRossum AC. Single coronary artery: morphological and functional evaluation by MRI (letter). Eur Heart J 1995;16(12): 2003–4.
8. Duerinckx AJ, Bogaert J, Jiang H, Lewis BS. Anomalous origin of the left coronary artery: diagnosis by coronary MR angiography (case report). Am J Roentgenol 1995; 164:1095–97.
9. Manning WJ, Li W, Cohen SI, Johnson RG, Edelman RR. Improved definition of anomalous left coronary artery by magnetic resonance coronary angiography. Am Heart J 1995;130(3, pt. 1):615–17.

10. McConnell MV, Ganz P, Selwyn AP, Li W, Edelman RR, Manning WJ. Identification of anomalous coronary arteries and their anatomic course by magnetic resonance coronary angiography. Circulation 1995;92:3158–62.

11. Post JC, vanRossum AC, Bronzwaer JGF, et al. Magnetic resonance angiography of anomalous coronary arteries: a new gold standard for delineating the proximal course? Circulation 1995;92:3163–71.

12. Duerinckx AJ, Troutman B, Allada V, Kim D. Coronary MR angiography in Kawasaki Disease: a case report. Am J Roentgenol 1997;168:114–16.

13. Duerinckx AJ, Perloff JK, Currier JW. Arteriovenous fistulae of the circumflex and right coronary arteries with drainage into an aneurysmal coronary sinus. Circulation 1999;99:2827–28.

14. Briffa NP, Clarke S, Kugan G, Coulden R, Wallwork J, Nashef SA. Surgical angioplasty of the left main coronary artery: follow-up with magnetic resonance imaging. Ann Thor Surg 1996;62(2):550–52.

15. Buser PT, Higgins CB. Coronary artery graft disease: diagnosis of graft failure by magnetic resonance imaging. In: Lüscher TF, Turina M, Braunwald E, eds. Coronary artery graft disease: mechanisms and prevention. Berlin: Springer-Verlag, 1994: 99–112.

16. Galjee MA, vanRossum AC, Doesburg T, vanEenige MJ, Visser CA. Value of magnetic resonance imaging in assessing patency and function of coronary artery bypass grafts. An angiographically controlled study. Circulation 1996;93(4):660–66.

17. Schmidt HC, Voigtlaender T, Kreitner KF, Wittlinger T, Meyer J, Thelen M. Assessment of patency of bypass grafts to the left anterior descending coronary artery: correlation of MR imaging with coronary angiography (abstr.). Radiology 1996;201(P):273.

18. Vrachliotis TG, Bis KG, Aliabadi D, Shetty AN, Safian R, Simonetti O. Contrast-enhanced breath-hold MR angiography for evaluating patency of coronary artery bypass grafts. Am J Roentgenol 1997;168(4):1073–80.

19. Wintersperger BJ, von Smekal A, Engelmann MG, et al. [Contrast media enhanced magnetic resonance angiography for determining patency of a coronary bypass. A comparison with coronary angiography]. Rofo. Fortschritte auf dem Gebiete der Rontgenstrahlen und der Neuen Bildgebenden Verfahren 1997;167(6):572–78.

20. Wintersperger BJ, Engelmann MG, von Smekal A, et al. Patency of coronary bypass grafts: assessment with breath-hold contrast-enhanced MR angiography—value of a non-electrocardiographically triggered technique. Radiology 1998;208(2):345–51.

21. Duerinckx AJ, Lewis BS, Louie HW, Urman MK. MRI of pseudoaneurysm of a brachial venous coronary bypass graft. Cath Cardiovasc Diagn 1996;37:281–86.

22. Duerinckx AJ, Atkinson D, Hurwitz R, Mintorovitch J, Whitney W. Coronary MR angiography after coronary stent placement (case report). Am J Roentgenol 1995; 165(3):662–64.

23. DeCobelli F, Rosanio S, Vanzulli A, Mellone R, Chierchia S, DelMaschio A. Breathhold cine coronary MR angiography: patency assessment after stent placement (abstr.). In: 1997 Scientific Program of the Eighty-third Scientific Assembly and Annual Meeting of the Radiological Society of North America (RSNA). Nov 30–Dec 5, 1997, Chicago. Radiology 1997;205(P):154.

24. DeCobelli F, Guidetti D, Vanzulli A, Mellone R, Chierchia S, Del Maschio A. [Magnetic resonance angiography of coronary arteries: assessment in patients with coronary stenosis and control after stent positioning]. Radiologia Medica 1998;95(1–2):54–61.

25. Mohiaddin RH, Bogren HG, Lazim F, et al. Magnetic resonance coronary angiography in heart transplant recipients (abstr.). In: Book of Abstracts of the Fourth Meeting of the International Society of Magnetic Resonance in Medicine (ISMRM). New York, April 27–May 3, 1996; Vol. 2: 671.

26. Davis SF, Kannam JP, Wielopolski P, Edelman RR, et al. Magnetic resonance coronary angiography in heart transplant recipients. J Heart Lung Transplant 1996;15(6):580–86.

27. Clarke GD, Eckels R, Chaney C, et al. Measurement of absolute epicardial coronary artery flow and flow reserve with breathhold cine phase-contrast magnetic resonance imaging. Circulation 1995;91(10):2627–34.

28. Sakuma H, Blake LM, Amidon TM, et al. Coronary flow reserve: noninvasive measurement in humans with breath-hold velocity-encoded cine MR imaging. Radiology 1996;198:745–50.

29. Hofman MBM, vanRossum AC, Sprenger M, Westerhof N. Assessment of flow in the right human coronary artery by magnetic resonance phase contrast velocity measurements: effects of cardiac and repiratory motion. Magn Reson Med 1996;35:521–31.

30. Hundley WG, Lange RA, Clarke GD, et al. Assessment of coronary arterial flow and flow reserve in humans with magnetic resonance imaging. Circulation 1996; 93(8):1502–8.

31. Caputo GC. Coronary arteries: potential for MR imaging (editorial). Radiology 1991;181(3):629–30.

32. Caputo RC. Coronary MR angiography: a clinical perspective (editorial). Radiology 1994;193(3):596–98.

33. Rogers LF. The heart of the matter: noninvasive coronary artery imaging (editorial). Am J Roentgenol 1998;170: 841.

34. Dinsmore RE. Noninvasive coronary arteriography— here at last ? [comment]. Circulation 1995;91(5):1607–8.

35. Goldsmith MF. Realizing potential of MR coronary angiography may ease patients' test load and diagnosis costs (editorial). JAMA 1994;271(4):256.

36. Doorey AJ, Wills JS, Blasetto J, Goldenberg EM. Usefulness of magnetic resonance imaging for diagnosing an anomalous coronary artery coursing between aorta and pulmonary trunk. Am J Cardiol 1994;74:198–99.

37. Bisset GS, Strife JL, McCloskey J. MR imaging of coronary artery aneurysms in a child with Kawasaki disease. Am J Roentgenol 1989;152:805–7.

38. Duerinckx AJ, Takahashi M. Coronary MR angiography in Kawasaki disease (abstr.). Radiology 1996;201(P):274.

39. Hwang SW, Yucel EK, Bernard S. Aortic root abscess with fistula formation. Chest 1997;111(5):1436–38.

40. Stanford W, Galvin JR, Skorton DJ, Marcus ML. The evaluation of coronary bypass graft patency: direct and indirect techniques other than coronary arteriography (review article). Am J Roentgenol 1991;156:15–22.

41. Stanford W, Brundage B, MacMillan R, et al. Sensitivity and specificity of assessing coronary bypass graft patency with ultrafast computed tomography: results of a multicenter study. J Am Coll Cardiol 1988;12(1):1–7.

42. Danias PG, Edelman RR, Manning WJ. Coronary MR angiography. Cardiol Clin 1998;16(2):207–25.

43. Duerinckx AJ, Grieten M, Atkinson D, Altamirano J. Breathhold MR angiography of the internal mammary arteries (abstr). In: Book of abstracts and Proceedings of the Fifth Meeting of the International Society of Magnetic Resonance in Medicine (ISMRM). Vancouver, B.C., Canada, April 12–18, 1997; Vol 2: 840.

44. White R, Caputo G, Mark A, Modin G, Higgins C. Coronary artery bypass graft patency: noninvasive evaluation with MR imaging. Radiology 1987;164(3):681–86.

45. Rubinstein R, Askenase A, Thickman D, Feldman M, Agarwal J, Helfant R. Magnetic resonance imaging to evaluate patency of aortocoronary bypass grafts. Circulation 1987;76(4):786–91.

46. Jenkins J, Love H, Foster C, Isherwood I, Rowlands D. Detection of coronary artery bypass graft patency as assessed by magnetic resonance imaging. Br J Radiol 1988; 61:2–4.

47. White R, Pflugfelder P, Lipton M, Higgins C. Coronary artery bypass grafts: evaluation of patency with cine MR imaging. Am J Roentgenol 1988;150:1271–74.

48. Aurigemma G, Reichek N, Axel L, Schiebler M, Harris C, Kressel H. Noninvasive determination of coronary artery bypass graft patency by cine magnetic resonance imaging. Circulation 1989;80:1595–602.

49. Hoogendoorn LI, Pattynama PM, Buis B, van der Geest RJ, van der Wall EE, de Roos A. Noninvasive evaluation of aortocoronary bypass grafts with magnetic resonance flow mapping. Am J Cardiol 1995;75(12):845–48.

50. Prince MR, Yucel EK, Kaufman JA, Harrison DC, Geller SC. Dynamic Gadolinium-enhanced three-dimensional abdominal MR Arteriography. J Magn Reson Imag 1993; 3:877–81.

51. Prince MR, Narisimham DL, Stanley JC, et al. Breath-hold Gadolinium-enhanced MR angiography of the abdominal aorta and its major branches. Radiology 1995;197:785–92.

52. Prince MR, Narasimham DL, Stanley JC, et al. Gadolinium-enhanced magnetic resonance angiography of abdominal aortic aneurysms. J Vasc Surg 1995;21:656–69.

53. Prince MR, Narasimham DL, Jacoby WT, et al. Three-dimensional Gadolinium-enhanced MR angiography of the thoracic aorta. Am J Roentgenol 1996;166:1387–97.

54. Cloft HJ, Murphy KJ, Prince MR, Brunberg JA. 3D gadolinium-enhanced MR angiography of the carotid arteries. Magn Reson Imag 1996;14(6):593–600.

55. Kim JK, Farb RI, Wright GA. Test bolus examination in the carotid artery at dynamic gadolinium-enhanced MR angiography. Radiology 1998;206(1):283–89.

56. Meaney JF, Prince MR, Nostrant TT, Stanley JC. Gadolinium-enhanced MR angiography of visceral arteries in patients with suspected chronic mesenteric ischemia. J Magn Reson Imag 1997;7(1):171–76.

57. Duerinckx AJ, Grant EG, Bakhda RK, To SY, Peters G, Shaaban A. A Phase II study of the use of a new blood pool agent (NC100150) for pulmonary angiography (abstr). Radiology 1998;209(P):494.

58. Warner OJ, Ohri SK, Pennell DJ, Smith PLC. Magnetic resonance coronary artery imaging for redo coronary operations (a case report). Ann Thorac Surg 1996;62:1513–16.

59. Schreiber WG, Voigtländer T, Kreitner K-F, et al. Measurement of flow reserve in coronary bypass grafts (abstr.). In: Book of abstracts and Proceedings of the Seventh Meeting of the International Society of Magnetic Resonance in Medicine (ISMRM). Philadelphia, May 22–23, 1999.

60. Sakuma H, Globits S, O'Sullivan M, et al. Breath-hold MR measurements of blood flow velocity in internal mammary arteries and coronary artery bypass grafts. J Magn Reson Imag 1996;6(1):219–22.

61. van Rossum AC, Bedaux WL, Hofman MB. Morphologic and functional evaluation of coronary artery bypass conduits. J Magn Reson Imag 1999;10(5):734–40.

62. Voigtlander T. Coronary artery and bypass flow measurement—Basic methodology and current status. Magma 1998;6(2–3):96–7.

63. Walpoth BH, Muller MF, Genyk I, et al. Evaluation of coronary bypass flow with color-Doppler and magnetic resonance imaging techniques: comparison with intraoperative flow measurements. Eur J Cardiothorac Surg 1999;15(6):795–802.

64. Miller S, Scheule AM, Hahn U, et al. MR angiography and flow quantification of the internal mammary artery graft after minimally invasive direct coronary artery bypass. Am J Roentgenol 1999;172(5):1365–69.

65. van Rossum AC, Galjee MA, Post JC, Visser CA. A practical approach to MRI of coronary artery bypass graft patency and flow. Int J Card Imag 1997;13(3):199–204.

66. Wielopolski PA, van Geuns RJ, de Feyter PJ, Oudkerk M. Coronary arteries. Eur Radiol 2000;10(1):12–35.

67. Kessler W, Achenbach S, Moshage W, et al. Usefulness of respiratory gated magnetic resonance coronary angiography in assessing narrowings > or = 50% in diameter in native coronary arteries and in aortocoronary bypass conduits. Am J Cardiol 1997;80(8):989–93.

68. Molinari G, Sardanelli F, Zandrino F, Balzan C, Masperone MA. Magnetic resonance assessment of coronary artery bypass grafts. Rays 1999;24(1):131–39.

69. Kalden P, Kreitner KF, Wittlinger T, et al. [The assessment of the patency of coronary bypass vessels with a 2D T2-weighted turbo-spin-echo sequence (HASTE) in the breath-hold technique]. Rofo Fortschr Geb Rontgenstr Neuen Bildgeb Verfahr 1999;170(5):442–48.

70. Kalden P, Kreitner KF, Wittlinger T, et al. Assessment of coronary artery bypass grafts: value of different breathhold MR imaging techniques. Am J Roentgenol 1999; 172(5):1359–64.

71. Wittlinger T, Voigtlander T, Grauvogel K, et al. [Noninvasive evaluation of coronary bypass grafts by magnetic resonance imaging. Comparison of the Haste and Fisp-3-D sequences with the conventional coronary angiography]. Z Kardiol 2000;89(1):7–14.

72. Regan F. Clinical applications of half-Fourier (HASTE) MR sequences in abdominal imaging. Magn Reson Imag Clin North Am 1999;7(2):275–88.

73. Laub G, Simonetti O, Nitz W. Single-shot imaging of the heart with HASTE (abstr.). In: Book of Abstracts of the 3rd Meeting of the Society of Magnetic Resonance (SMR)

and the Twelfth Annual Scientific Meeting of the European Society for Magnetic Resonance in Medicine and Biology (ESMRMB). Nice, France, August 20–25, 1995;Vol 1:246.

74. Duerinckx AJ, Yu WD, El-Saden S, Kim D, Wang JC, Sandhu HS. MR imaging of cervical spine motion with HASTE. Magn Reson Imag 1999;17(3):371–81.

75. Aerts P, VanHoe L, Bosmans H, Oyen R, Marchal G, Baert AL. Breath-hold MR urography using the HASTE technique. Am J Roentgenol 1996;(166):543–45.

76. Duerinckx AJ, Atkinson D, Hurwitz R. Assessment of coronary artery patency after stent placement using magnetic resonance angiography. J Magn Reson Med 1998;8: 896–902.

77. Teitelbaum GP, Raney M, Carvlin MJ, Matsumoto AH, Barth KH. Evaluation of ferromagnetism and magnetic resonance imaging artifacts of the tantalum vascular stent. Cardiovasc Intervent Radiol 1989;12:125–27.

78. Laissy JP, Grand C, Mator C, Struyven J, Berger JF, Schounan-Claeys E. Magnetic resonance angiography of intravascular endoprosthesis: investigation of three devices. Cardiovasc Intervent Radiol 1995;18:360–66.

79. Kotsakis A, Tan KH, Jackson G. Is MRI a safe procedure in patients with coronary stents in situ? (editorial). Int J Clin Prac 1997;51(6):349.

80. Yamaoka O, Ikeno K, Fujioka H, et al. Detection of Palmaz-Schatz stent by ultrafast CT. J Comput Assist Tomogr 1995;19(1):128–30.

81. Scott NA, Pettigrew RI. Absence of movement of coronary stents after placement in a magnetic resonance imaging field. Am J Cardiol 1994;73:900–1.

82. Friedrich MG, Kivelitz D, Strohm O, et al. Intracoronary stents are safe during MR imaging of the heart (abstr.). In: Society for Cardiovascular Magnetic Resonance, Second Meeting, January 22–24, 1999. Atlanta, 1999:36.

83. Shellock FG, Shellock VJ. Metallic stents: evaluation of MR imaging safety. Am J Roentgenol 1999;173(3):543–47.

84. Strohm O, Kivelitz D, Gross W, et al. Safety of implantable coronary stents during 1H-magnetic resonance imaging at 1.0 and 1.5 T. J Cardiovasc Magn Reson 1999; 1(3):239–45.

85. Kramer CM, Rogers WJ, Mankad SV, Pakstis DL, Vido D, Reichek N. Short and long-term safety of magnetic resonance imaging soon after stenting for acute myocardial infarction (abstr.). In: Society for Cardiovascular Magnetic Resonance, Second Meeting, January 22–24, 1999. Atlanta, GA:1999;99.

86. Kramer CM, Rogers WJ, Pakstis DI. Absence of adverse outcomes after magnetic resonance imaging early after stent placement for acute myocardial infarction: a preliminary study. J Cardiovasc Magn Reson 2000;2(4):257–62.

87. Schroeder AP, Houlind K, Pederson EM, Thuesen L, Nielsen TT, Egleblad H. Magnetic resonance imaging seems safe in patients with intracoronary stents. J Cardiovasc Magn Reson 2000;2(1):43–9.

88. Nyman MA, Schwartz RS, Breen JF, Garratt KN, Holmes DR. Ultrafast computed tomographic scanning to assess patency of coronary artery stents in bypass grafts. Mayo Clinic Proc 1993;68:1021–23.

89. Schmermund A, Haude M, Sehnert C, et al. [Noninvasive evaluation of the patency of coronary vessel stents using electron beam tomography segment images with administration of contrast media]. Zeitschrift für Kardiologie 1995;84(11):892–97.

90. Schmermund A, Haude M, Baumgart D, et al. Noninvasive assessment of coronary Palmaz-Schatz stents by contrast enhanced electron beam computed tomography. Eur Heart J 1996;17(10):1546–53.

91. De Cobelli F, Cappio S, Vanzulli A, Del Maschio A. MRI assessment of coronary stents. Rays 1999;24(1):140–48.

92. Amano Y, Ishihara M, Hayashi H, et al. Metallic artifacts of coronary and iliac arteries stents in MR angiography and contrast-enhanced CT. Clin Imag 1999;23(2):85–9.

93. Nagel E, Hug J, Bunger S, et al. Coronary flow measurements for evaluation of patients after stent implantation. Magma 1998;6(2–3):184–85.

94. Baum F, Vosshenrich R, Fischer U, Castillo E, Grabbe E. Stent artifacts in 3D MR angiography: experimental studies. Rofo Fortschr Geb Rontgenstr Neuen Bildgeb Verfahr 2000;172(3):278–81.

95. Lenhart M, Volk M, Manke C, et al. Stent appearance at contrast-enhanced MR angiography: in vitro examination with 14 stents. Radiology 2000;217(1):173–78.

96. Manke C, Nitz WR, Lenhart M, et al. Magnetic resonance monitoring of stent deployment: in vitro evaluation of different stent designs and stent delivery systems. Invest Radiol 2000;35(6):343–51.

97. Mohiaddin RH, Bogren HG, Lazim F, et al. Magnetic resonance coronary angiography in heart transplant recipients. Cor Art Dis 1996;7(8):591–97.

98. Pennell DJ, Bogren HG, Keegan J, Firmin DN, Underwood SR. Detection, localization and assessment of coronary artery stenosis by magnetic resonance imaging (abstr.). In: Book of Abstracts and Proceedings of the Second Meeting of the the Society of Magnetic Resonance (SMR). San Francisco, August 6–12, 1994;Vol. 1: 369.

99. Duerinckx AJ, Laughrun D, Lewis BS. Usefulness of coronary MR angiography prior to angioplasty. Int J Card Imag 1999;15(6):533–40.

100. Debatin J, Strong J, Negro-Vilar R, Sostman H, Pelc N, Herfkens R. MR characterization of blood flow in native and grafted internal mammary arteries (abstr.). In: Proceedings of the RSNA Seventy-eighth Scientific Assembly and Annual Meeting. Chicago, 1992;185(P):102.

101. Debatin JF, Strong JA, Sostman HD, et al. MR Characterization of Blood Flow in Native and Grafted Internal Mammary Arteries. J Magn Reson Imag 1993;3(3):443–51.

102. Duerinckx AJ. Coronary hemodynamics in patients with artery bypass grafts using phase contrast MRI (abstr.). In: Sixteenth Annual Meeting of Society for Cardiac Angiography and Interventions. San Antonio, May 18–22, 1993.

103. Nitz WR, Kessler W, Stingl D, Moshage W, Laub G. Can we trust breath-hold MR velocity measurements of coronary blood flow? (abstr.) Radiology 1996;201(P):166.

104. Frayne R, Polzin JA, Mazaheri Y, Grist TM, Mistretta CA. Effect of and correction for in-plane myocardial motion on estimates of coronary-volume flow rates. J Magn Reson Imag 1997;7(5):815–28.

8
MRA of Anomalous Coronary Arteries

Johannes C. Post and Albert C. van Rossum

Clinical Significance of Anomalous Coronary Arteries

Major coronary artery anomalies are found in 0.3–0.8% of the population (1–4). Although the majority of these anomalies will not have serious sequelae, some types of anomalous origin and proximal course of the coronary arteries are associated with myocardial infarction and sudden death. In particular, the pattern with proximal coronary artery segments crossing between the aorta and the pulmonary trunk has been reported to be potentially lethal (5–11). In contrast to the increased risk associated with this interarterial course, serious sequelae occur only rarely with other courses. These low-risk courses include aberrant arteries that have their origin in the contralateral aortic sinus and subsequently run a septal (through the floor of the right ventricular infundibulum), a posterior (behind the aorta), or an anterior free wall course (over the free anterior wall of the right ventricular infundibulum) to cross over to their perfusion area. Because the proximal course of an aberrant coronary artery is of major importance in defining the associated risk on myocardial infarction or sudden cardiac death, unambiguous visualization of this course is important.

Rationale for MRA

With the current standard technique for the assessment of coronary artery anatomy (i.e., conventional X-ray coronary angiography) the exact proximal course of anomalous coronary arteries may sometimes be difficult to determine (7,8,12–15). Differentiation between an increased-risk interarterial and a low-risk septal course of an anomalous artery has particularly been reported to be often incorrect (13,14). Misdiagnosis has been reported to occur in up to 50% of cases (13). Even experienced angiographers may have difficulty in delineating the proximal course of anomalous coronary arteries on a con-

ventional X-ray coronary angiogram. Conventional angiography provides a two-dimensional (2-D) projection view of a complex three-dimensional (3-D) structure. In addition, with selective visualization of the coronary arteries, relating these arteries to their surroundings (e.g., pulmonary trunk, myocardial septum) is difficult. Furthermore, the limited possibilities of angulation inherent to the technique preclude obtaining views perpendicular to the aortic root, which would be very useful to visualize the relationship of an anomalous coronary artery to the great arteries. The placement of right-sided catheters (7,8), simultaneous right ventriculography during coronary injection (12), the recognition of specific patterns or hall-marks (13,14), or angulated views (3) have all been suggested as an aid to differentiate between the various proximal courses, but even then correct delineation of the proximal course may be difficult.

Magnetic resonance (MR) coronary angiography has proven to be accurate in the imaging of proximal coronary anatomy in patients (16–19). It is a tomographic technique that is potentially better in elucidating 3-D anatomy than is a projection technique. It provides anatomic information of surrounding structures, concomitantly with the coronary anatomy. The free choice of the imaging plane is an advantage over the limited possibilities of angulation in conventional coronary angiography. These features are of particular value in the imaging of anomalous coronary anatomy.

In initial reports of the capability of magnetic resonance imaging (MRI) techniques to demonstrate anomalously originating coronary arteries conventional "black blood" spin-echo techniques were used to document incidental cases (20–22). Other authors have reported the imaging of coronary artery aneurysms (23,24) and fistulas (24–26) with MR techniques. After the introduction of gradient-echo techniques for coronary artery imaging in 1991 (27–31), a rapid further development of these "bright blood" MR coronary angiographic techniques has occurred. In two studies the successful diagnostic application of a fast segmented gradient echo technique to a series of patients with coronary anomalies was reported (32,33). An excellent sensitivity and specificity in detecting aberrant coronary arteries and localizing their origins was found. The technique appeared to be superior to conventional X-ray angiography in delineating their proximal course.

Imaging Protocol

Successful visualization of the proximal coronary anatomy, including the localization of anomalous origins and the delineation of aberrant proximal courses, can be obtained following a relatively simple imaging protocol.

1. Acquire a coronal localizer image of the heart.
2. Plan a series of transverse images around the aortic root. Care should be taken to include the complete anomalous proximal coronary anatomy. The most cranial slice should be above the level of the proximal anterior interventricular groove, and imaging should proceed caudad until the transition of the left ventricle into the aortic root has been completely imaged. In most cases a diagnosis can be made solely from this set of transverse images.
3. An alternative or additional approach is to obtain a similar set of images with an orientation parallel to the aortic valve plane.
4. Perpendicular to the previous sets of images, oblique images can be obtained along the main axis of the visualized anomalous vessel. Although in our experience these orientations are not essential to make the diagnosis, they do provide illustrative images.

Annotated examples are shown in Figure 8.1 to Figure 8.6.

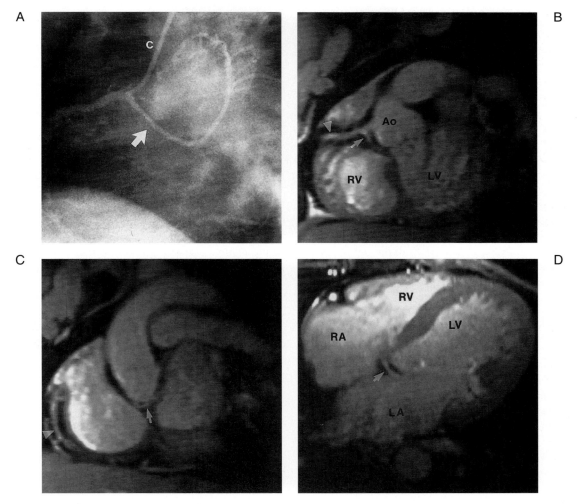

Figure 8.1. (A) shows a conventional X-ray coronary angiography showing a left main coronary artery (LMCA; arrow) anomalously originating from the right aortic sinus. (B) and (C) are from an oblique series of MR angiographic images. (B) shows the origin of the anomalous LMCA (arrow) from the proximal right coronary artery (RCA) (arrowhead). In (C), which is posterior to (B), the LMCA (arrow) is seen to pass caudally and posteriorly from the aortic root to the left. A middle segment of the RCA (arrowhead) is also seen in this section. Transverse image (D) is pathognomonic for all left coronary arteries originating from the right aortic sinus and taking a retroaortic course to the left. A coronary segment is seen to cross over just caudal and posterior to the origin of the aorta from the left ventricle.

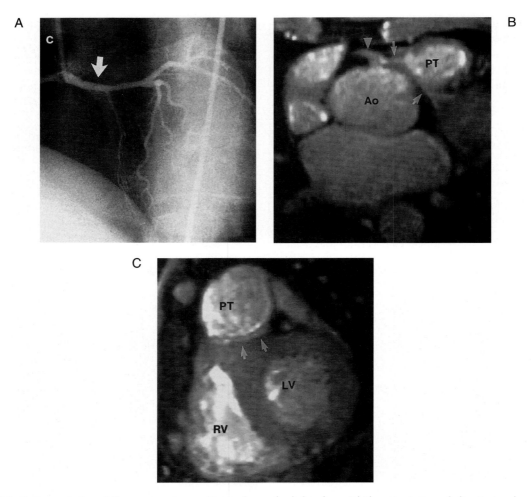

Figure 8.2. (A) is the conventional X-ray coronary angiography showing an anomalous LMCA originating from the right aortic sinus. (B) is a transverse MRI depicting the LMCA (arrows) arising together with the RCA (arrowhead) from the right aortic sinus. The LMCA runs between the aorta and pulmonary trunk to the left, where it bifurcates into an left anterior descending (LAD) and left circumflex (LXc). (C) is perpendicular to (B), along the main axis of the interarterial segment, and depicts this interarterial segment (arrows) in an oblique orientation.

The Clinical Value of MRA

Indications for magnetic resonance angiography (MRA) of anomalous coronary anatomy may include: (1) patients that have undergone conventional X-ray contrast coronary angiography and in which uncertainty exists concerning the precise delineation of the course of an aberrant coronary artery; (2) investigation of patients in which total proximal occlusion or congenital absence of a major epicardial coronary artery is suspected, but where an anomalous origin of the artery cannot be excluded; (3) a primary investigation in adolescent and young patients who present with angina, arrhythmias, or syncope on severe exercise; (4) work up before cardiac surgery of patients with an uncertain course of an anomalous coronary artery to avoid the risk of trauma to the aberrant artery (34,35); (5) the screening of certain subgroups of individuals that in case of the presence of an interarterially coursing aberrant coronary artery would run an especially increased mortality risk (e.g., highly competitive athletes) (36).

Conclusions

Although conventional X-ray angiography is still the standard technique for imaging coronary arteries and quantifying stenoses, delineating the proximal course of anomalous coronary arteries in relation to the great arteries can be difficult or even erroneous. MRA is capable of unambiguously defining this proximal course. The technique is a very useful adjunct to conventional coronary angiography and might even be considered a new clinical standard for delineating the prognostically important proximal course of anomalous coronary arteries.

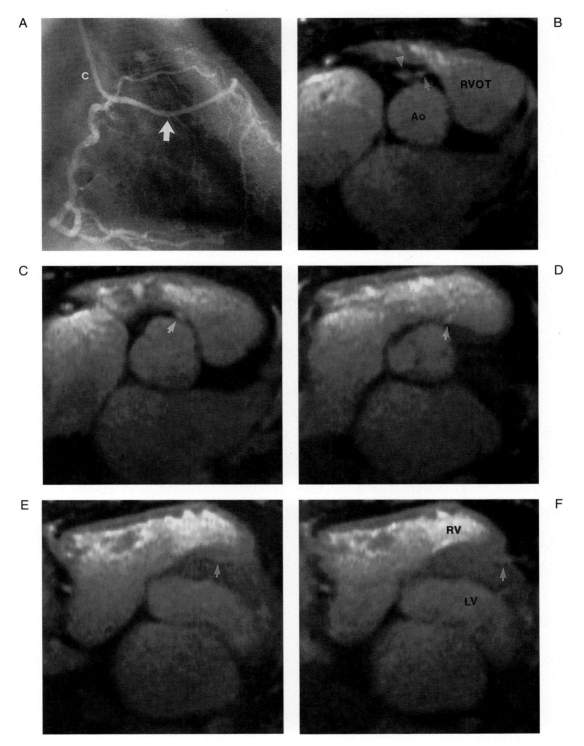

Figure 8.3. (A) from the conventional X-ray coronary angiography, shows an anomalous LAD, originating from the right aortic sinus. (B) through (F) are from a series of contiguous MR sections visualizing the anomalous LAD (arrow) arising with the RCA (arrowhead) from the right aortic sinus (B) and subsequently descending and entering the interventricular myocardial septum (D), where it runs through the septum (E) to reappear in the interventricular groove (F). Apprehension of the contiguity can be optimized by mounting the images in a cine loop.

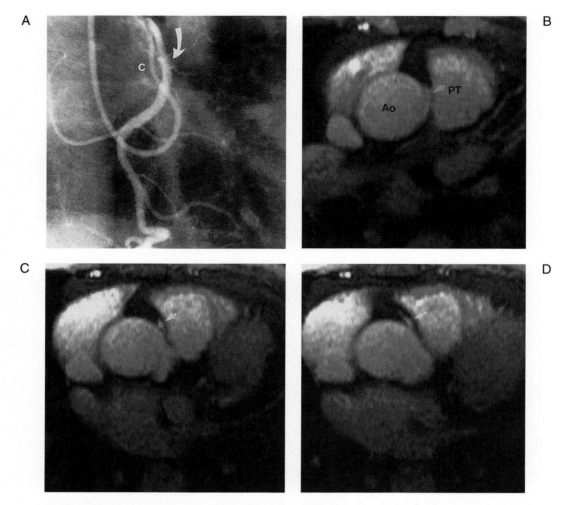

Figure 8.4. (A) from the conventional X-ray coronary angiography, shows an RCA (arrow) anomalously originating from (above) the left aortic sinus. (B) through (D) illustrate the proximal RCA (arrow) originating from above the left aortic sinus adjacent to the commissure and running between the aorta and pulmonary trunk to the right atrioventricular groove.

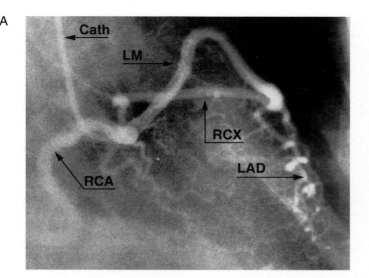

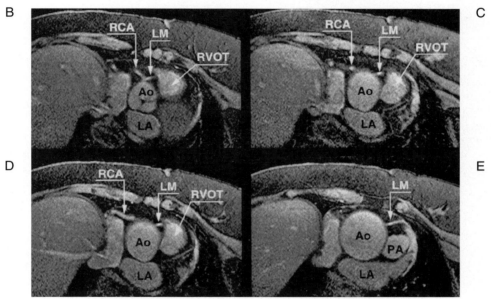

Figure 8.5. (A) shows the conventional angiogram. (B) through (E) are images from an oblique transverse series and illustrate the anomalous origin of an LMCA from the right aortic sinus and its subsequent anterior course over the wall of the right ventricular outflow tract. (Ao indicates aorta; c, catheter; LA, left atrium; LV, left ventricle; PT, pulmonary trunk; RA, right atrium; RV, right ventricle; and RVOT, right ventricular outflow tract. Figs. 8.1–8.4 with permission from Reference 32; Fig. 8.5 is courtesy of HW Vliegen, the Netherlands).

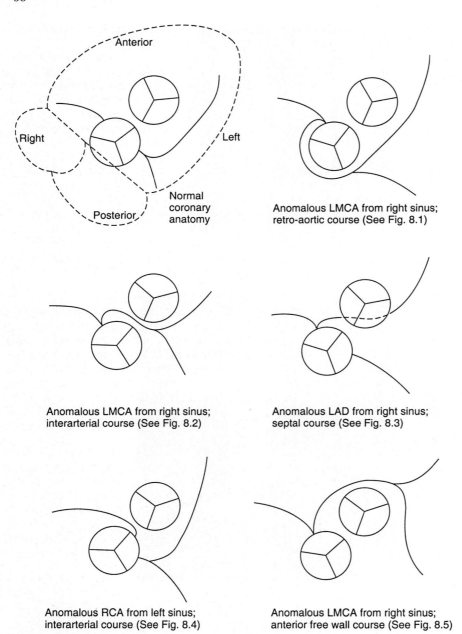

Figure 8.6. The coronary anomalies from the previous examples are summarized in a diagram. The different courses that an anomalously originating artery can take are illustrated here.

Normal coronary anatomy

Anomalous LMCA from right sinus; retro-aortic course (See Fig. 8.1)

Anomalous LMCA from right sinus; interarterial course (See Fig. 8.2)

Anomalous LAD from right sinus; septal course (See Fig. 8.3)

Anomalous RCA from left sinus; interarterial course (See Fig. 8.4)

Anomalous LMCA from right sinus; anterior free wall course (See Fig. 8.5)

References

1. Chaitman BR, Lespérance J, Saltiel J, Bourassa MG. Clinical, angiographic, and hemodynamic findings in patients with anomalous origin of the coronary arteries. Circulation 1976;53:122–31.
2. Kimbiris D, Iskandrian AS, Segal BL, Bemis CE. Anomalous aortic origin of coronary arteries. Circulation 1978; 58:606–15.
3. Click RL, Holmes DR, Vlietstra RE, Kosinski AS, Kronmal RA, CASS participants. Anomalous coronary arteries: location, degree of atherosclerosis and effect on survival— a report from the Coronary Artery Surgery Study. J Am Coll Cardiol 1989;13:531–37.
4. Yamanaka O, Hobbs RE. Coronary artery anomalies in 126,595 patients undergoing coronary arteriography. Cathet Cardiovasc Diag 1990;21:28–40.
5. Jokl E, McClellan JT, Ross GD. Congenital anomaly of left coronary artery in young athlete. JAMA 1962;182:572–73.
6. Cheitlin MD, De Castro CM, McAllister HA. Sudden death as a complication of anomalous left coronary origin from the anterior sinus of Valsalva: a not-so-minor congenital anomaly. Circulation 1974;50:780–87.
7. Liberthson RR, Dinsmore RE, Fallon JT. Aberrant coronary artery origin from the aorta: report of 18 patients, review of literature and delineation of natural history and management. Circulation 1979;59:748–54.
8. Moodie DS, Gill C, Loop FD, Sheldon WC. Anomalous left main coronary artery originating from the right sinus of Valsalva: pathophysiology, angiographic definition, and

surgical approaches. J Thorac Cardiovasc Surg 1980;80: 198–205.

9. Roberts WC, Siegel RJ, Zipes DP. Origin of the right coronary artery from the left sinus of Valsalva and its functional consequences: analysis of 10 necropsy patients. Am J Cardiol 1982;49:863–68.

10. Isner JM, Shen EM, Martin ET, Fortin RV. Sudden unexpected death as a result of anomalous origin of the right coronary artery from the left sinus of Valsalva. Am J Med 1984;76:155–58.

11. Kragel AH, Roberts WC. Anomalous origin of either the right or left main coronary artery from the aorta with subsequent coursing between aorta and pulmonary trunk: analysis of 32 necropsy cases. Am J Cardiol 1988;62: 771–77.

12. Hobbs RE, Millit HD, Raghavan PV, Moodie DS, Sheldon WC. Congenital coronary artery anomalies: clinical and therapeutic implications. *In*: Vidt D, ed. Cardiovascular therapy. Philadelphia: FA Davis; 1982:43–58.

13. Ishikawa T, Brandt PWT. Anomalous origin of the left main coronary artery from the right anterior aortic sinus: angiographic definition of anomalous course. Am J Cardiol 1985;55:770–76.

14. Serota H, Barth CW III, Seuc CA, Vandormael M, Aguirre F, Kern MJ. Rapid identification of the course of anomalous coronary arteries in adults: the "dot and eye" method. Am J Cardiol 1990;65:891–98.

15. Giannoccaro PJ, Sochowski RA, Morton BC, Chan KL. Complementary role of transoesophageal echocardiography to coronary angiography in the assessment of coronary artery anomalies. Br Heart J 1993;70:70–74.

16. Manning WJ, Li W, Edelman RR. A preliminary report comparing magnetic resonance coronary angiography with conventional angiography. N Engl J Med 1993;328: 828–32.

17. Pennell DJ, Keegan J, Firmin DN, Gatehouse PD, Underwood SR, Longmore DB. Magnetic resonance imaging of coronary arteries: technique and preliminary results. Br Heart J 1993;70:315–26.

18. Duerinckx AJ, Urman MK. Two-dimensional coronary MR angiography: analysis of initial clinical results. Radiology 1994;193:731–38.

19. Post JC, van Rossum AC, Hofman MBM, Valk J, Visser CA. Respiratory-gated three-dimensional MR angiography of coronary arteries and comparison with x-ray contrast angiography. Am J Roentgenol 1996;166:1399–404.

20. Douard H, Barat JL, Mora B, Baudet E, Broustet JP. Magnetic resonance imaging of an anomalous origin of the left coronary artery from the pulmonary artery. Eur Heart J 1988;9:1356–60.

21. Machado C, Bhasin S, Soulen RL. Confirmation of anomalous origin of the right coronary artery from the left si-

nus of valsalva with magnetic resonance imaging. Chest 1993;104:1284–86.

22. Doorey AJ, Wills JS, Blasetto J, Goldenberg EM. Usefulness of magnetic resonance imaging for diagnosing an anomalous coronary artery coursing between aorta and pulmonary trunk. Am J Cardiol 1994;74:198–99.

23. Bisset GS III, Strife JL, McCloskey J. MR imaging of coronary artery aneurysms in a child with Kawasaki disease. Am J Roentgenol 1989;152:805–7.

24. Pucillo AL, Schechter AG, Moggio RA, Kay RH, Baum SJ, Herman MV. MR imaging in the definition of coronary artery anomalies. J Comput Assist Tomogr 1990;14:171–74.

25. Boxer RA, LaCorte MA, Singh S, Ishmael R, Cooper R, Stein H. Noninvasive diagnosis of congenital left coronary artery to right ventricle fistula by nuclear magnetic resonance imaging. Pediatr Cardiol 1989;10:45–47.

26. Kubota S, Suzuki T, Murata K. Cine magnetic resonance imaging for diagnosis of right coronary arterial-ventricular fistula. Chest 1991;100:735–37.

27. Edelman RR, Manning WJ, Burstein D, Paulin S. Coronary arteries: breath-hold MR angiography. Radiology 1991; 181:641–43.

28. Burstein D. MR imaging of coronary artery flow in isolated and in vivo hearts. J Magn Reson Imag 1991;1:337–46.

29. Cho ZH, Mun CW, Friedenberg RM. NMR angiography of coronary vessels with 2-D planar image scanning. Magn Reson Med 1991;20:134–43.

20. Dumoulin CL, Souza SP, Darrow RD, Adams WJ. A method of coronary MR angiography. J Comput Assist Tomogr 1991;15:705–10.

31. Wang SJ, Hu BS, Macovski A, Nishimura DG. Coronary angiography using fast selective inversion recovery. Magn Reson Med 1991;18:417–23.

32. Post JC, van Rossum AC, Bronzwaer JGF, de Cock CC, Hofman MBM, Valk J, et al. Magnetic resonance angiography of anomalous coronary arteries: a new gold standard for delineating the proximal course? Circulation 1995;92:3163–71.

33. McConnell MV, Ganz P, Selwyn AP, Li W, Edelman RR, Manning WJ. Identification of anomalous coronary arteries and their anatomic course by magnetic resonance coronary angiography. Circulation 1995;92:3158–62.

34. Hallman GL, Cooley DA, Singer DB. Congenital anomalies of the coronary arteries: anatomy, pathology, and surgical treatment. Surgery 1966;59:133–44.

35. Roberts WC, Morrow AG. Compression of anomalous left circumflex coronary arteries by prosthetic valve fixation rings. J Thorac Cardiovasc Surg 1969;57:834–38.

36. Pelliccia A, Spataro A, Maron BJ. Prospective echocardiographic screening for coronary artery anomalies in 1,360 elite competitive athletes. Am J Cardiol 1993;72:978–79.

9
Coronary Artery Variants and Adult Congenital Heart Disease

André J. Duerinckx, Akram Shaaban, Anthony Lewis, Joseph Perloff, and Hillel Laks

Introduction

There are both congenital and acquired anomalies of the coronary arteries. The most common congenital anomaly involves an abnormal origin and/or abnormal course of the proximal portion of the coronary arteries. Other anomalies include aneurysms of the coronary arteries and arteriovenous fistulae. This chapter presents a few case reports of such anomalies as well as a selected review of recent literature.

As discussed in Chapter 7, until a few years ago there were only isolated reports on the use of magnetic resonance imaging (MRI) to determine the origin or proximal course of an anomalous coronary artery (see introduction to Chap. 8). For example, Doory et al. reported on five patients with anomalous coronary artery (1). In all five patients, magnetic resonance imaging provided definitive confirmation of the courses of the anomalous left and right coronary arteries. This study was performed using T1-weighted spin-echo sequences in multiple planes on the 1.5 Tesla GE Signal Scanner. No coronary magnetic resonance angiography (MRA) technique was used. Several new case reports appeared more recently that describe the use of coronary MRA to evaluate such anomalous vessels (2–4). In the December 1, 1995, issue of *Circulation*, two major articles were published that established coronary MRA as the technique of choice for the delineation of the origin and proximal course of anomalous coronary arteries (5,6). Each one of these publications is discussed in more detail in Chapters 7 and 8.

The use of MRI and/or coronary MRA for the detection of coronary artery aneurysms or AV-fistulae since then has also been well documented (7–11). Kawasaki disease, a generalized vasculitis of unknown etiology, is a leading cause of acquired heart disease in children in the United States and has widespread cardiovascular involvement, including coronary arterial aneurysms (12). Coronary arteriovenous fistulae are

malformations of the coronary circulation. Prior to surgical or interventional therapy the anatomy of these complex vascular structure needs to be imaged. Coronary MRA offers a noninvasive imaging approach to these coronary anomalies. Sequential transaxial two-dimensional (2-D) breathhold coronary MR angiograms can be obtained. Three-dimensional (3-D) volume renderings can then be obtained from these 2-D transaxial images. The 3-D reconstructions visualize all abnormally enlarged coronary arteries and the proximal portions of the normal coronary artery anatomy in most cases. All of these studies are easy to perform applications of coronary MRA. Most radiologists should be able to reproduce the results with existing first-generation coronary MRA techniques.

The remainder of this chapter will present a detailed review of two case reports that illustrate how easy it is to apply these new MRI techniques with commercial MR scanners and first-generation coronary MRA pulse sequences.

Case Report 9.1: Coronary MRA in Kawasaki Disease*

Introduction

Kawasaki disease, a generalized vasculitis of unknown etiology, is a leading cause of acquired heart disease in children in the United States. This acute and severe febrile illness, principally of young children, has widespread cardiovascular involvement, including coronary arterial aneurysms, myocardial infarction, myocarditis, pericarditis, and valvulitis (13). Coronary arterial

---

*Modified, with permission, from Duerinckx et al. (9).

aneurysms may precipitate thrombosis or evolve into segmental stenosis that may cause myocardial ischemia. Rupture of aneurysms and inflammation of the conduction system may also cause death. Echocardiography is the primary noninvasive imaging tool for evaluation and follow up of coronary arterial abnormalities in these patients (14). We report on the use of an alternative noninvasive imaging technique, coronary MRA, to reveal and localize areas of aneurysmal dilatation in a patient diagnosed with Kawasaki disease.

Case Report

In December 1994 a 9-year-old Asian-American boy presented with fever and symptoms that fit Kawasaki disease. An echocardiogram revealed both right and left coronary arterial dilatation, with the right coronary artery (RCA) measuring approximately 7 mm, and the left anterior descending (LAD) coronary artery approximately 8 mm. The distal extent of the areas of dilatation could not be established. The patient was treated medically and his systemic symptoms improved. Follow-up echocardiograms done 2 months later and in August 1995 revealed no significant changes from prior echocardiograms, except for a gradual increase in the diameter of the dilated RCA from 7 to 9 mm. An exercise stress test showed normal exercise tolerance and no electrocardiographic (EKG) changes or left ventricular wall abnormalities. In January 1996 the patient underwent a noninvasive coronary MRA to better reveal the extent of the coronary arterial dilatation.

Coronary MRA was done using a 2-D breathhold MR technique that requires breathholding (up to 14 seconds at a time) and cardiac gating. MRI was done with a conventional 1.5 Tesla Vision whole-body imager with 25 mT/m gradients (Siemens Medical Systems, Inc., Iselin, NJ). This first-generation coronary MRA technique is further described in Chapters 3, 5, and 21.

Image planes were selected according to a standard coronary MRA protocol developed to minimize the time required for selection of echocardiographic anatomical planes (15). Images were obtained in planes located in the right atrioventricular groove (Fig. 9.1A) as well as in or tangential to the interventricular groove (Figs. 9.1B–D). Coronary MRAs of the RCA showed a fusiform and segmented aneurysm of the proximal and middle RCA (Fig. 9.1A) that was 40 mm long and 11 mm at its largest diameter. The extent of this RCA aneurysm was not revealed on echocardiography. Coronary MRAs of the left main coronary artery and proximal LAD appeared to show vessels of normal caliber, except for two small focal saccular aneurysms in the proximal and mid-LAD (Figs. 9.1C and D) that were not revealed on earlier echocardiograms. The first LAD aneurysm was 14-mm long and 7 mm at its largest diameter; the second aneurysm was 10-mm long and 4 mm in diameter. Due to the tortuosity of the proximal and middle LAD, the areas of saccular aneurysmal dilatation are only partially revealed in each 2-D imaging plane, with partial volume effects caused by in- and out-of-plane vessel motion.

Discussion

The noninvasive evaluation of aneurysmal dilatation of the coronary arteries in patients with Kawasaki disease is very important, both at the time of initial clinical evaluation and during long-term follow up. Based on the latest "guidelines for long-term management of patients with Kawasaki disease," approved by the Scientific Advisory Committee of the American Heart Association in 1993, long-term management of these patients should be based on risk stratification (16). This risk stratification is based on the relative risk of myocardial ischemia and allows for patient management to be individualized, including the indications for invasive coronary angiography. Stratification in risk levels (levels 1 to 5) is based on the presence or absence of coronary artery changes. Another study on coronary arterial aneurysms in patients with Kawasaki disease grouped 210 patients based on maximum diameter of the largest aneurysm and the total length of aneurysms (17). All aneurysms with a diameter greater than 9 mm became stenotic during a multiyear follow up (average follow up, 7.8 years). Aneurysms of 5–9 mm in diameter, with a length greater than 15 mm for the LAD or greater than 30 mm for the RCA, also became progressively stenotic.

Based on this risk stratification for long-term follow up, our patient with Kawasaki disease was categorized as risk level 4. The recommended regimen included long-term antiplatelet aspirin therapy, a pediatric cardiology reevaluation with echocardiogram, and perhaps an electrocardiogram and chest radiograph at 1-year intervals (16). Stress testing to evaluate myocardial function was also performed because the patient is more than 10 years of age. Because the noninvasive studies did not suggest myocardial dysfunction, cardiac catheterization with selective coronary angiography was not performed. Based on the study by Suzuki et al. (17) our patient, who has an RCA aneurysm with a diameter greater than 9 mm and longer than 30 mm, is at very high risk for progressive stenosis of the RCA.

Although echocardiography is the primary tool for the evaluation and follow up of such coronary arterial abnormalities, revealing the coronary arteries becomes progressively more difficult as young patients grow. Echocardiography also has serious limitations for revealing stenosis and thrombosis. In addition, because such aneurysms heal by two different pathological processes (marked intimal proliferation and massive

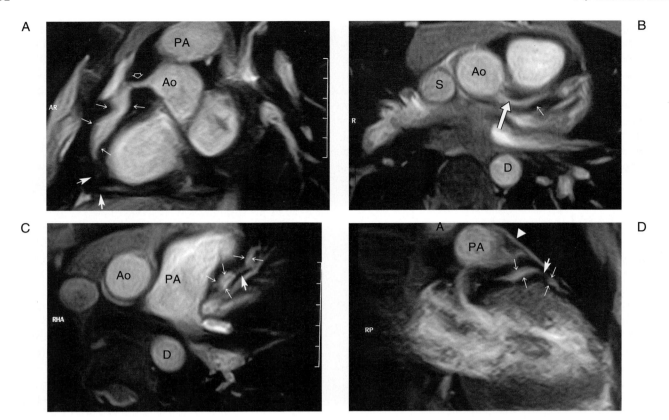

Figure 9.1. An 11-year-old boy with 3-year history of clinically stable Kawasaki disease. (A) Coronary MRA of RCA with the imaging plane in right atrioventricular groove reveals ostium and proximal RCA within normal limits (open arrow). Note that proximal RCA then widens into fusiform and segmented aneurysm (short arrows). The more distal RCA, which is partially revealed (curved arrows), appears of normal caliber. Ao = ascending aorta; PA = pulmonary artery. (B,C) Coronary MRAs in two oblique transaxial planes with slightly different angula-

tion show normal left main coronary artery (open arrow) and proximal left anterior descending artery (arrow) that has two smaller aneurysms (thin arrows). Ao = ascending aorta; PA = pulmonary artery; D = descending aorta; S = superior vena cava. (D) Coronary MRA in plane equivalent to vertical two-chamber view reveals a 90-degree view of mid-LAD (arrow) with two areas of aneurysmal dilatation (thin arrows). Also shown is portion of the pericardium (arrowhead). A = Aortic arch; PA = pulmonary artery.

thrombosis), the use of conventional contrast-based coronary angiography has limitations because the technique may not specifically show intramural changes in the coronary artery (13). Thus, an alternative noninvasive study, such as MRI, which can detect flow, thrombus, and fibrous tissue at any age of a patient, may be needed, especially when planning aggressive antithrombolytic therapy (18). MRI can both visualize the patent coronary lumen and visualize areas of intimal proliferation and/or thrombus formation.

Early cardiac-gated MR studies have occasionally been able to reveal coronary artery vessels (19), including dilated or aneurysmal coronary vessels such as seen in patients with Kawasaki disease (7). More reliable coronary MRA techniques, however, have been developed and evaluated in adult populations with ischemic heart disease (15,20,21). The greatest clinical success so far has been achieved with the breathhold 2-D technique used on our patient. During a typical 1-hour coronary MRA study, large portions of the coronary arterial tree

can be revealed, including much more distal coronary territory than is possible with echocardiography. In adults, coronary MRA can typically reveal the first 5–11 cm of the RCA, the full left main artery, the first 4–8 cm of the LAD (15), and the very proximal portion of the left circumflex artery. Due to the requirement of repeated, consistent breathhold periods, its applicability in the pediatric population has been limited. With older children, however, such as our patient, breathhold practice before the MR study made the task much easier.

Conclusions

Coronary MRA offers great promise as an alternative noninvasive imaging technique for revealing coronary artery anomalies in patients with Kawasaki disease. MRI offers an ideal complement to echocardiography, and may provide additional clinical information that may affect risk stratification for long-term management of these patients. As described in this case, MRI offers improved visualization of more distal coronary aneurysms and allows better measurement of the total length of long aneurysms, which also improves the accuracy of risk stratification. The combination of coronary MRA with other cardiac-triggered MR techniques may also permit revealing thrombus, thus accomplishing a completely noninvasive evaluation (7,18). Further work is needed, however, to establish the role of MRI versus echocardiography and angiography in the evaluation of these patients, both during initial presentation and long-term follow up.

Case Report 9.2: 3-D MRI of Coronary Arteriovenous Fistula

Coronary arteriovenous fistulae are uncommon, but they represent the most prevalent of the hemodynamically significant congenital malformations of the coronary circulation that permit adult survival (22). When the coronary arteries arise normally from the aorta, but then communicate directly with a cardiac chamber, coronary sinus, or other vascular structure, this represents a fistula and a left-to-right cardiac shunt. Patient survival into adulthood depends on the amount of blood flowing through the communication, and the myocardial ischemia that may result from the fistulous bypass (coronary steal). It is a relatively uncommon malformation of the heart, but it allows adult survival, although the life span is not normal. These coronary arteriovenous fistulae are sometimes initially detected by echocardiography during a work up for unrelated problems or after detection of a cardiac murmur. Due to incremental use of intravascular procedures, such as percutaneous transluminal coronary angioplasty (PTCA), endomyocardial biopsy, and permanent transvenous pacing, more acquired fistulae are now being reported (23).

We will report on the use of an alternate noninvasive imaging technique, coronary MRA, to reveal and localize the areas of coronary artery dilatation and occasional coronary artery aneurysm formation in two patients with coronary arteriovenous fistulas.

Materials and Methods

Study Patients

Two adult patients with known coronary arteriovenous fistulae were referred to our medical center for evaluation and surgical treatment. Determination of the complex 3-D anatomy of these coronary arteriovenous fistulae from the selective coronary and X-ray coronary angiograms was difficult because of the multiple overlapping structures and very dilated vessels and coronary sinus. An MRI study was performed in each case to better delineate this complex anatomy.

Case 1

JC, a 44-year-old asymptomatic male, presented with a history of nonsustained atrial fibrillation for the past 8 years. At age 37, a transthoracic echocardiogram disclosed an enlarged left ventricle (diastolic dimension 7.4 cm, ejection fraction 56%) and a very large coronary sinus with Doppler color flow evidence of diastolic and systolic turbulence, consistent with entry of a coronary arteriovenous fistula. A selective coronary angiogram visualized a dilated circumflex and right coronary arteries, both of which entered aneurysmal coronary sinus.

Case 2

MP, a 65-year-old woman, presented with a murmur first detected at age 21 that had been followed by her family physician and several cardiologists. At age 40, while in treatment by her gynecologist, she was sent for an echocardiogram that suggested mitral valve prolapse. A repeat echocardiogram performed 4 years later confirmed the same findings. Approximately 4 months prior to her visit to our hospital a repeated Doppler echocardiogram suggested a ruptured sinus of valsalva aneurysm. A follow-up transesophageal echocardiogram suggested the presence of an aortic sinus aneurysm. An X-ray coronary angiogram was then performed that revealed an RCA fistula draining into the coronary sinus, and aneurysmal dilatation of the proximal portion of the RCA.

MRI

Coronary MRA was done using a 2-D breath-hold MR technique that requires breath-holding (up to 14 seconds at a time) and cardiac gating. MRI was done with a conventional 1.5 Tesla Vision whole-body imager with 25 mT/m gradients (Siemens Medical Systems, Inc., Iselin, NJ). This first-generation coronary MRA technique is further described in Chapters 3, 5, and 21.

Image planes were selected according to a standard coronary MRA protocol developed to minimize the time required for selection of echocardiographic anatomical planes (24). Images were obtained in planes located in the right atrioventricular groove as well as in or tangential to the interventricular groove. In addition, consecutive transaxial slices with 5-mm slice interspace were acquired throughout the heart. A 3-D volume reconstruction was performed on a stand-alone 3-D workstation (ISG, Allegro, Mountain View, CA).

Results

Coronary MRAs were successfully performed in both patients and confirmed the findings from previous echocardiograms and X-ray coronary angiograms. In Case 9.1, selective coronary angiography visualized dilated circumflex and right coronary arteries, both of

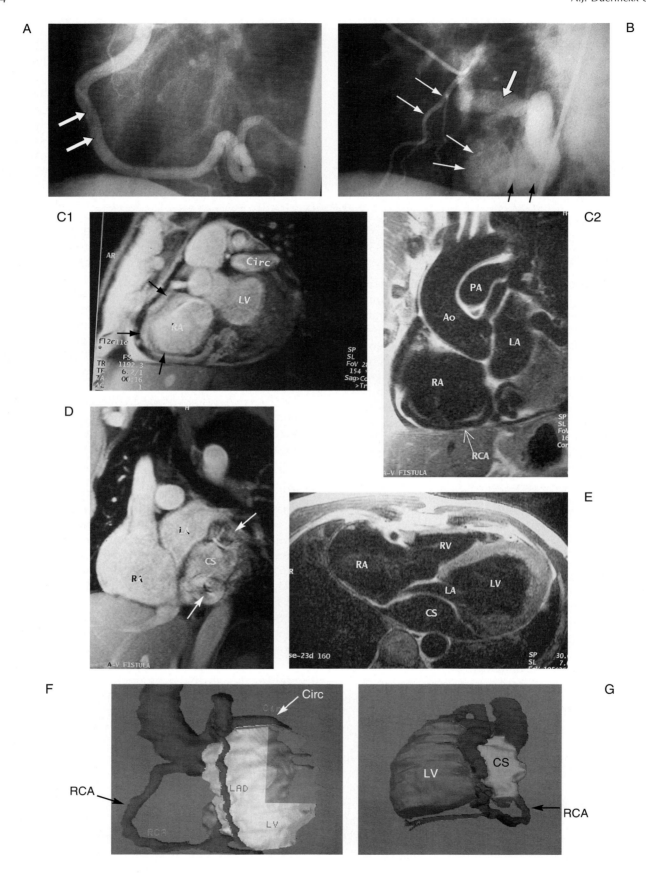

which entered an aneurysmal coronary sinus (Fig. 9.2A,B). The coronary MRAs confirmed ectasia of several coronary vessels. The diameter of the proximal right coronary artery was 10 mm (Fig. 9.2C), and the diameter of the left main coronary artery was 11 mm. The circumflex artery was 11 mm in its proximal diameter, then abruptly widened to 18–20 mm and became very tortuous. The LAD artery, by contrast, was 5–6 mm in diameter. The enlarged coronary sinus measured 8.5 × 4.5 × 3.5 cm (Fig. 9.2C,D) and compressed the inferior portion of the left atrium. The 3-D volume renderings provide an overview of this complex anatomy (Figs. 9.2F,G). These images assisted in planning surgical closure of the coronary arteriovenous fistulae, at which time the right atrial appendage and a portion of the enlarged right atrium were excised, and a Maze procedure was performed. Two months after the operation, the left ventricular diastolic dimension was 6.1 cm (vs. 7.4-cm preop), and the ejection fraction was 45% (vs. 56% preop). Six months after the operation, the left ventricular diastolic dimension was 5.4 cm, and the ejection fraction was 63%. An exercise radionuclide myocardial perfusion scan was normal.

In Case 9.2, selective coronary angiography visualized a dilated RCA with a proximal aneurysm that entered an aneurysmal coronary sinus (Fig. 9.3A). The left coronary artery system was normal. Coronary MRAs were obtained before and after surgical repair. The preoperative coronary MRA delineated: the proximal RCA aneurysm which measured 4 × 4 × 3 cm (Fig. 9.3B); the tortuous course of the proximal RCA entering and exiting the aneurysm; the dilated RCA measuring 12 mm; and the enlarged coronary sinus that measured 4 × 3 × 7 cm (Figs. 9.3C,D). The patient underwent a partial resection of the area of aneurysmal RCA dilatation and distal closure of the fistula. The procedure was well tolerated. The coronary MRA after surgical repair shows the postsurgical appearance of the dilated RCA (Figs. 9.3E,F).

Discussion

Three-dimensional visualization of complex anatomical structures can assist in better understanding complex relationships and can help plan for interventions. We will illustrate the use of 3-D volume rendering based on transaxial breathhold coronary MRAs in two patients with coronary arteriovenous fistulae.

A review of the world literature on coronary arteriovenous fistulae reported on a total of 76 subjects with 96 congenital and acquired coronary arteriovenous fistulae during the 1985 to 1995 period, plus six new patients with eight fistulae (23). In this group the number of acquired, as opposed to congenital, coronary arteriovenous fistulae reported had increased from a previously reported frequency of 0% [in a 1975 review (25)] to 36%. The majority (78%) of all patients were treated medically. Surgical techniques consisting of ligation of the fistula were used in 10% of the reviewed subjects, whereas percutaneous transcatheter embolization (PTE) was performed in 12%.

Under age 20, the congenital coronary arteriovenous fistulae are generally asymptomatic, but symptoms and complications increase appreciably with age. The complications include congestive heart failure, myocardial ischemia, infarction, sudden death, and infective endocarditis. The management of asymptomatic patients with coronary arteriovenous fistulae remains controversial. Several management options are now available. Said et al. recommend that small asymptomatic fistulae be managed conservatively because they may close spontaneously (23), and 78% of the cases in their review were managed medically. They recommend that surgery or PTE should be reserved for larger (left-to-right shunt ≥ 1.5) fistulae. They recommend PTE as the future treatment of choice provided that the lesion has an amenable anatomy (26). Since 1983 the surgical motility was already relatively low at 1–2%; thus, even asymptomatic patients could undergo surgical repair (27). The preintervention assessment requires selective

---

Figure 9.2. Coronary arteriovenous fistula in a 44-year-old man obtained just prior to surgical correction. (A) LAO view of the RCA. Contrast enters from the dilated RCA (large arrows) into the coronary sinus. (B) Craniocaudal LAO view of the left coronary system. The LAD (medium-sized arrows) is of normal caliber. The circumflex coronary artery (large arrows) is very tortuous and dilated. Contrast in the enlarged coronary sinus is superimposed on the distal circumflex structure (small arrows). (C) Coronary MRA of the RCA in an LAO equivalent view. Large portions of the right coronary artery are clearly seen (arrows) (LV = left ventricle, Circ = circumflex coronary artery). (D) Transaxial MRI cross-section of the heart showing the four cardiac chambers and the enlarged coronary sinus, which indents the left atrium (RA = right atrium; LA = left atrium; RV = right ventricle; LV = left ventricle; CS = coronary sinus). (E) Coronal MRI through the posterior portion of the heart during breathhold acquisition using a standard 2-D cardiac-triggered magnetic resonance angiographic technique. The coronary sinus (CS) is strikingly enlarged, and indents the left atrium. Entry points of the dilated circumflex and right coronary arteries are shown as "fish-mouths" (arrows). The circumflex coronary artery enters the upper portion of the dilated coronary sinus (upper arrow), and the RCA enters the lower portion (lower arrow) (LA = left atrium; RA = right atrium). (F,G) A 3-D volume rendering with an anterior (E) and posterior (F) view shown. A dilated, tortuous circumflex (CIRC) and the dilated RCA arterio-venous fistulae enter an aneurysmal coronary sinus (CS) (LAD = left anterior descending artery; Ao = ascending aorta; LV = left ventricle). (Reprinted with permission from Duerinckx et al. (11).)

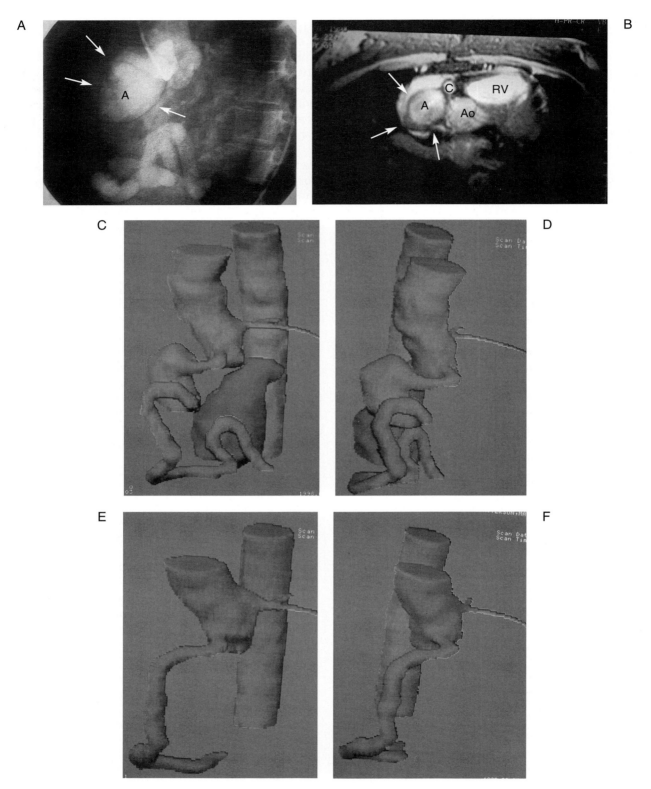

coronary arteriography to determine the extent of myocardium served by the feeder vessel of the fistula. The potential to jeopardize the myocardium by occluding the distal runoff (either by proximal fistula ligation or subsequent thrombosis) must be considered.

Imaging techniques used for noninvasive diagnosis of coronary arteriovenous fistulae include Doppler color flow mapping (28), Doppler echocardiography (29), computed tomography (29), and MRI (30–32). Compared with echocardiography, both CT and MRI provide a more global overview of dilated coronary structures and coronary aneurysms. CT imaging, however, requires iodinated contrast materials and X-ray radiation. MRI offers a noninvasive technique without X-ray radiation or the need for iodinated contrast material injections.

Coronary MRA has been shown to be a value in imaging of coronary artery variants (2,5,6,33), after coronary artery bypass grafting (34,35), after coronary stent placement (36), and even for the detection of coronary lesions (37). Three-dimensional acquisitions of coronary MRAs using navigator pulse-echo techniques are possible, but they require longer acquisition times and are sometimes unreliable. The sequential acquisition of breathhold 2-D coronary MRA images followed by a 3-D volume rendering is an alternative way of obtaining 3-D information. The breathhold 2-D coronary MRA pulse sequences are now available on almost all new commercial MRI scanners and can easily be applied. The use of 3-D workstations is also becoming more widespread, and the combination of the two can help almost any imager to transform 2-D data into valuable 3-D volume renderings for use during clinical evaluations of this group of patients. More studies are needed before we will know if the systematic use of these techniques on larger groups of patients with complex coronary malformations will have an impact on the treatments offered to these patients.

Other Published Case Reports of Congenital and Acquired Anomalies of the Coronary Arteries

Several other important case reports have recently been published. Flacke et al. also described coronary aneurysms in Kawasaki disease detected by Coronary MRA (38).

Kobayashi et al. described a giant coronary aneurysm of Kawasaki disease developing during postacute phase (39). Velasco et al. described multiple coronary aneurysms in a young man (40). Voigtlander et al. described ectasia and aneurysm of the right coronary artery resulting from a shunt to the coronary sinus (32). Le Breton et al. described aneurysms and pseudo-aneurysms of saphenous vein coronary artery bypass grafts (41).

Duerinckx et al. described MRI of pseudoaneurysm of a brachial venous coronary bypass graft (42). Gilkeson et al. described a pseudoaneurysm of aortic cannulation site after coronary artery bypass grafting and its evaluation with gadolinium-enhanced MR angiography (43). Holland et al. described the preoperative MRA assessment of the coronary arteries in an ascending aortic aneurysm (44).

Coronary MRA in Patients with Adult Congenital Heart Disease (Grown-up Congenital Heart Disease)

Taylor et al. described coronary artery imaging in grown-up congenital heart disease and the complementary role of magnetic resonance and X-ray coronary angiography (45). There is a high incidence of anomalous coronary arteries in subjects with congenital heart disease. These abnormalities can be responsible for myocardial ischemia and sudden death or be damaged during surgical intervention. It can be difficult to define the proximal course of anomalous coronary arteries with the use of conventional X-ray coronary angiography. Magnetic resonance coronary angiography (MRCA) has been shown to be useful in the assessment of the 3-dimensional relationship between the coronary arteries and the great vessels in subjects with normal cardiac morphology but has not been used in patients with congenital heart disease. Taylor et al. studied 25 adults with various congenital heart abnormalities (45). X-ray coronary angiography and respiratory-gated MRCA were performed in all subjects. Coronary artery origin and proximal course were assessed for each imaging modality by separate, blinded investigators. Images were then compared and a consensus diagnosis was reached. With the consensus readings for both magnetic resonance and X-ray coronary angiography, it was possible to identify the origin

---

Figure 9.3. Coronary arteriovenous fistula in a 65-year-old woman obtained prior to and after surgical correction. (A) Craniocaudal left anterior oblique (LAO) view of the right coronary system. The proximal RCA enters a large aneurysm, and then continues its more distal turtuous course. Due to the overlap of the very tortuous structures, interpretation is difficult. (B) Coronal MRI that demonstrates the RCA aneurysm (arrows). (C,D) A 3-D volume rendering of the preoperative appearance of the RCA. The LAO (C) and lateral (D) views are shown. The coro- nary MRA was obtained during mid- to late diastole, during which the RCA of the cardiac chambers are most dilated, thereby stretching out some of the tortuous RCA. The enlarged coronary sinus is shown in green. (E,F) A 3-D volume rendering of the postoperative appearance of the RCA. The LAO (E) and lateral (F) views are shown. The postoperative course shows good repair with no to minimal kinking of the proximal RCA. (Reprinted with permission from Duerinckx et al. (46).)

and course of the proximal coronary arteries in all 25 subjects: 16 with coronary anomalies and 9 with normal coronary arteries. Respiratory-gated MRCA had an accuracy of 92%, a sensitivity of 88%, and a specificity of 100% for the detection of abnormal coronary arteries. The MRCA results were more likely to agree with the consensus for definition of the proximal course of the coronary arteries (p < 0.02). Taylor et al. concluded that for the assessment of anomalous coronary artery anatomy in patients with congenital heart disease, the use of the combination of MRCA with X-ray coronary angiography improves the definition of the proximal coronary artery course. MRCA provides correct spatial relationships, whereas X-ray angiography provides a view of the entire coronary length and its peripheral run-off. Furthermore, respiratory-gated MRCA can be performed with breathholding and with only limited subject cooperation.

References

1. Doorey AJ, Wills JS, Blasetto J, Goldenberg EM. Usefulness of magnetic resonance imaging for diagnosing an anomalous coronary artery coursing between aorta and pulmonary trunk. Am J Cardiol 1994;74:198–99.

2. Duerinckx AJ, Bogaert J, Jiang H, Lewis BS. Anomalous origin of the left coronary artery: diagnosis by coronary MR angiography (case report). Am J Roentgenol 1995;164:1095–97.

3. vanCampen LC, deCock C, Bronzwaer JG, vanRossum AC. Single coronary artery: morphological and functional evaluation by MRI (letter). Eur Heart J 1995;16(12):2003–4.

4. Manning WJ, Li W, Cohen SI, Johnson RG, Edelman RR. Improved definition of anomalous left coronary artery by magnetic resonance coronary angiography. Am Heart J 1995;130(3 Pt 1):615–17.

5. McConnell MV, Ganz P, Selwyn AP, Li W, Edelman RR, Manning WJ. Identification of anomalous coronary arteries and their anatomic course by magnetic resonance coronary angiography. Circulation 1995;92:3158–62.

6. Post JC, vanRossum AC, Bronzwaer JGF, et al. Magnetic resonance angiography of anomalous coronary arteries: a new gold standard for delineating the proximal course? Circulation 1995;92:3163–71.

7. Bisset GS, Strife JL, McCloskey J. MR imaging of coronary artery aneurysms in a child with Kawasaki disease. Am J Roentgenol 1989;152:805–7.

8. Duerinckx AJ, Takahashi M. Coronary MR angiography in Kawasaki Disease (abstr.). Radiology 1996;201(P):274.

9. Duerinckx AJ, Troutman B, Allada V, Kim D. Coronary MR angiography in Kawasaki disease: a case report. Am J Roentgenol 1997;168:114–16.

10. Hwang SW, Yucel EK, Bernard S. Aortic root abscess with fistula formation. Chest 1997;111(5):1436–38.

11. Duerinckx AJ, Perloff JK, Currier JW. Arteriovenous fistulae of the circumflex and right coronary arteries with drainage into an aneurysmal coronary sinus. Circulation 1999;97:2827–28.

12. Chung CJ, Stein L. Kawasaki disease: a review. Radiology 1998;208(1):25–33.

13. Amplatz K, Moller JH. Kawasaki disease. In: Amplatz K, Moller JH, eds. Radiology of congenital heart disease. St. Louis: Mosby, 1993:1093–98.

14. Capannari TE, Daniels SR, Meyer RA, Schwartz DC, Kaplan S. Sensitivity, specificity and predictive value of two-dimensional echocardiography in detecting coronary artery aneurysms in patients with Kawasaki disease. J Am Coll Cardiol 1986;7:355–60.

15. Duerinckx AJ. Coronary MR angiography. In: Cardiac MR imaging, Boxt LM, guest ed. MRI Clin North Am 1996;4(2):361–418.

16. Dajani AS, Taubert KA, Takahashi M, et al. Guidelines for long-term management of patients with Kawasaki disease. Report from the Committee on Rheumatic Fever, Endocarditis, and Kawasaki Disease, Council on Cardiovascular Disease in the Young, American Heart Association. Circulation 1994;89(2):916–22.

17. Suzuki A, Kamiya T, Arakaki Y, Kinoshita Y, Kimura K. Fate of coronary arterial aneurysms in Kawasaki disease. Am J Cardiol 1994;74:822–24.

18. Tsubata S, Ichida F, Hamamichi Y, Miyazaki A, Hashimoto I, Okada T. Successful thrombolytic therapy using tissue-type plasminogen activator in Kawasaki disease. Pediatr Cardiol 1995;16:186–89.

19. Paulin S, vonSchulthess GK, Fossel E, Krayenbuehl HP. MR imaging of the aortic root and proximal coronary arteries. Am J Roentgenol 1987;148:665–70.

20. Manning WJ, Li W, Edelman RR. A preliminary report comparing magnetic resonance coronary angiography with conventional angiography. N Engl J Med 1993;328:828–32.

21. Duerinckx AJ, Urman M. Two-dimensional coronary MR angiography: analysis of initial clinical results. Radiology 1994;193:731–38.

22. Perloff JK. Congenital anomalies of the coronary circulation. In: Perloff JK, ed. The clinical recognition of coronary heart disease. Fourth ed. Philadelphia: W.B. Saunders Company, 1994:738.

23. Said SAD, ElGamal MIH, vanderWerf T. Coronary arteriovenous fistulas: collective review and management of six cases—changing etiology, presentation and treatment strategy. Clin Cardiol 1997;20:748–52.

24. Duerinckx AJ. Coronary arteries: how do I image them? In: Bogaert J, Duerinckx AJ, Rademakers F, eds. Magnetic resonance of the heart and great vessels: clinical applications. Berlin: Springer-Verlag, 1999: 223–43.

25. Rittenhouse EA, Doty DB, Ehrenhaft JL. Congenital coronary artery-cardiac chamber fistula. Review of operative management. Ann Thorac Surg 1975;20:468–85.

26. Reidy JF, Anjos RT, Qureshi SA, Baker EJ, Tynan MJ. Transcatheter embolization in the treatment of coronary artery fistulas. J Am Coll Cardiol 1991;18:187–92.

27. Urrutia SCO, Falaschi G, Ott DA, Cooley DA. Surgical management of 56 patients with congenital coronary artery fistulas. Ann Thorac Surg 1983;35:300–7.

28. Shakudo M, Yoshikawa J, Yoshida K, Yamamura Y. Non-invasive diagnosis of coronary artery fistula by Doppler color flow mapping. J Am Coll Cardiol 1989;13:1572–77.

29. Slater J, Lighty GW, Winer HE, Kahn ML, Kronzon I, Isom W. Doppler echocardiography and computed tomography in diagnosis of left coronary arteriovenous fistula. J Am Coll Cardiol 1984;4:1290–93.

30. Aydogan U, Onursal E, Cantez T, Barlas C, Tanman B, Gürgan L. Giant congenital coronary artery fistula to left superior vena cava and right atrium with compression of left pulmonary vein simulating cor triatriatum—diagnostic value of magnetic resonance imaging. Eur J Cardiothorac Surg 1994;8:97–99.
31. Sato Y, Ishikawa K, Sakurai I, et al. Magnetic resonance imaging in diagnosis of right coronary arteriovenous fistula—a case report. Jap Circ 1997;61:1043–46.
32. Voigtländer T, Roberts HC, Otto M, et al. Images in cardiovascular medicine. Ectasia and aneurysm of the right coronary artery resulting from a shunt to the coronary sinus. Circulation 1998;97(22):2276–77.
33. Vliegen HW, Doornbos J, de Roos A, Jukema JW, Bekedam MA, van der Wall EE. Value of fast gradient echo magnetic resonance angiography as an adjunct to coronary arteriography in detecting and confirming the course of clinically significant coronary artery anomalies. Am J Cardiol 1997;79(6):773–76.
34. van Rossum AC, Galjee MA, Post JC, Visser CA. A practical approach to MRI of coronary artery bypass graft patency and flow. International J Card Imag 1997;13(3):199–204.
35. Vrachliotis TG, Bis KG, Aliabadi D, Shetty AN, Safian R, Simonetti O. Contrast-enhanced breath-hold MR angiography for evaluating patency of coronary artery bypass grafts. Am J Roentgenol 1997;168(4):1073–80.
36. Duerinckx AJ, Atkinson D, Hurwitz R. Assessment of coronary artery patency after stent placement using magnetic resonance angiography. J Magn Reson Med 1998;8:896–902.
37. Duerinckx AJ. MRI of coronary arteries. Int J Card Imag 1997;13(3):191–97.
38. Flacke S, Setser RM, Barger P, Wickline SA, Lorenz CH. Coronary aneurysms in Kawasaki's disease detected by magnetic resonance coronary angiography. Circulation 2000;101(14):E156–57.
39. Kobayashi T, Sone K, Shinohara M, Kosuda T. Images in cardiovascular medicine. Giant coronary aneurysm of Kawasaki disease developing during postacute phase. Circulation 1998;98(1):92–3.
40. Velasco M, Zamorano JL, Almeria C, Ferreiros J, Alfonso F, Sanchez-Harguindey L. [Multiple coronary aneurysms in a young man. A diagnostic approach via different technics]. Rev Esp Cardiol 1999;52(1):55–8.
41. Le Breton H, Pavin D, Langanay T, et al. Aneurysms and pseudoaneurysms of saphenous vein coronary artery bypass grafts. Heart 1998;79(5):505–8.
42. Duerinckx AJ, Lewis BS, Louie HW, Urman MK. MRI of pseudoaneurysm of a brachial venous coronary bypass graft. Cathet Cardiovasc Diagn 1996;37:281–86.
43. Gilkeson RC, Clampitt MS, Stewart RM, Laden NS. Pseudoaneurysm of aortic cannulation site after coronary artery bypass grafting: evaluation with gadolinium-enhanced MR angiography. Am J Roentgenol 1999;172(3):843–44.
44. Holland AE, Barentsz JO, Skotnicki S, Ruijs SH, Goldfarb JW. Preoperative MRA assessment of the coronary arteries in an ascending aortic aneurysm. J Magn Reson Imag 2000;11(3):324–26.
45. Taylor AM, Thorne SA, Rubens MB, et al. Coronary artery imaging in grown up congenital heart disease: complementary role of magnetic resonance and x-ray coronary angiography. Circulation 2000;101(14):1670–78.
46. Duerinckx AJ, Shaaban A, Lewis A, Perloff J, Laks H. 3-D MR imaging of coronary arteriovenous fistulas. Eur Radiol 2000;10(9):1459–63.

10
MR Assessment of Coronary Artery Bypass Graft Patency

Thomas G. Vrachliotis and Kostaki G. Bis

Introduction

The development of a noninvasive imaging method for the evaluation of patency of coronary artery bypass grafts (CABG) is of major clinical importance because increasing numbers of patients have undergone coronary artery bypass surgery. The gold standard examination in the evaluation of these patients is presently coronary angiography, which is an invasive and expensive procedure that carries the inherent risks of any angiographic procedure. Because patients that have undergone CABG surgery will need follow-up studies to assess the anatomic integrity of their grafts, the importance of developing a noninvasive method for their evaluation is apparent.

Anatomy and Course of Coronary Artery Bypass Grafts

The vessels used to bypass narrowed segments of native coronary arteries are either saphenous veins, internal mammary arteries, or both. Saphenous vein bypass grafts (SVBG) are anastomozed to the anterior aspect of the ascending aorta several centimeters cephalad to the coronary sinuses (1,2). Vein grafts to the right coronary artery (RCA) are anastomozed along the right or along the lateral surface of the ascending aorta. They subsequently course caudally in a vertical fashion parallel to the atrioventricular groove to reach the site of anastomosis on the RCA (1,3,4). Saphenous vein grafts to the left coronary circulation are anastomozed to the ascending aorta cephalad to the ones that supply the RCA. Grafts that supply the left circumflex coronary artery (LCx) territory are the most cephalad ones, whereas the grafts that supply the left anterior descending coronary artery (LAD) are found caudal to the ones anastomozed

to the LCx territory. The sequence, therefore, of proximal anastomozes on the ascending aorta in a patient with three saphenous vein grafts to the corresponding three coronary artery territories is to the LCx, to the LAD, and to the RCA when viewed from superior to inferior, respectively (Fig. 10.1). Saphenous vein grafts to the left coronary artery (LAD and LCx) subsequently course over the main pulmonary artery toward the left side of the cardiac surface.

When internal mammary arteries are used to bypass the native coronaries, they are dissected away from the posterior surface of the upper seven ribs and separated from their terminal branches (5,6). The right internal mammary artery (RIMA) is used to bypass the right coronary artery or the left anterior descending artery. The left internal mammary artery (LIMA) is used to bypass the left anterior descending or the left circumflex artery (7).

Noninvasive Evaluation of Coronary Artery Bypass Graft Parency

Postoperative angina may occur because of progression of disease in the native coronaries or graft occlusion. The frequency of postoperative angina has been estimated to be 30% in the first year after CABG surgery (8). Graft occlusion occurs in 10–30% of grafts in the first 1–2 years after surgery, and 45–55% of the grafts are occluded by 10–12 years after surgery (9–11). In a patient with postoperative angina, determination of graft patency does not exclude the presence of stenosis nor does it obviate the need for coronary angiography. In the symptomatic patient during the early postoperative period, however, it is important to establish graft patency because occlusion is likely due to acute thrombosis rather than to chronic atherosclerotic disease.

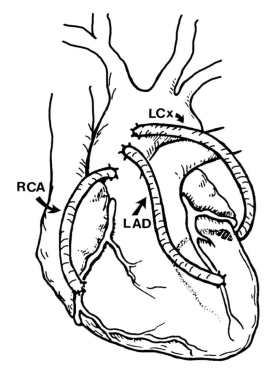

Figure 10.1. Graphic representation of three saphenous vein bypass grafts. The LCx graft is seen most cephalad followed by the LAD and RCA (most inferior) grafts.

Graft patency can be assessed by indirect or direct methods. The gold standard against which other methods are judged is coronary angiography. Indirect methods assume patency or occlusion by changes in regional myocardial perfusion or by myocardial wall contraction patterns. These indirect methods include rest and exercise radionuclide ventriculography, echocardiography, thallium-201 and Tc99m-sestamibi scintigraphy, and positron emission tomography. Direct methods include conventional computed tomography (CT), ultrafast CT, digital subtraction angiography, Doppler sonography, and magnetic resonance imaging (MRI) (12).

MRI

In 1983 Herfkens et al. (13) first reported imaging a coronary artery bypass graft on an axial MRI of the chest. The use of magnetic resonance as a noninvasive imaging method for evaluating patency of coronary artery bypass grafts was subsequently explored by several investigators (14–23) using various MR techniques.

Overview of MR Techniques

Spin Echo Techniques

Flowing blood on spin-echo images is seen as a signal void area because the excited protons move out of the imaging plane. Early investigators (14–16) used this MR principle to study patients with bypass grafts. Their results showed high sensitivity and moderate specificity in detecting graft patency. With the spin-echo techniques, however, flow void can be mimicked by the presence of calcifications, metal artifacts, thickened pericardium, and small pericardial fluid collections. Furthermore, slow flow within patent grafts will present with higher signal intensity, mimicking thrombus, thereby decreasing the methods' specificity. In addition to these considerations, issues such as lengthy presence of the patient within the bore of the magnet were also addressed.

Gradient-Echo Techniques

Flowing blood on gradient-recalled echo techniques (GRE) appears bright because of the flow related enhancement phenomenon. The use of GRE techniques was implemented by various investigators (16,20–22). The reported sensitivity and specificity rates were very high (20). Long scanning times, imaging at multiple levels, and in-plane saturation effects, however, may compromise the practical application of the technique. In addition, due to prolonged echo times of > 6 msec, there are pronounced magnetic susceptibility artifacts from metallic clips.

The implementation of velocity-encoded cine MRI or dynamic phase contrast techniques (21,24–26) to quantitate flow velocities and volumes in bypass grafts have been described for measuring CABG function. This technique should supplement the anatomic imaging of CABG evaluation and provide baseline flow information following surgery. The reassessment of CABG flow with anatomic (magnetic resonance angiography, MRA) imaging when a patient is symptomatic should enhance the sensitivity and specificity for CABG disease. The current limitations of phase contrast techniques when imaging CABGs are limited spatial resolution and respiratory motion artifacts. In addition, temporal resolution is suboptimal with breathhold sequences employing segmented gradient-echo technology. The implementation of higher matrixes, more acquisitions, and navigator echo respiratory compensation techniques should improve the nonbreathhold phase contrast sequences. Furthermore, improved gradient performance and echo-sharing techniques should also improve the temporal resolution of breathhold acquisitions. The implementation of respiratory three-dimensional (3-D) navigator echo-based MRA (27), a time of flight technique, has been applied to study CABG patency. This technique eliminates the misregistration of two-dimensional (2-D) techniques; however, because of the saturation effects on the blood pool, consistent high vascular-to-background signal is not achieved. This technique, however, may be more robust with the implementation of blood pool contrast agents.

MR Angiography

EKG-Triggered 3-D Contrast Enhanced MRA

The most recently reported (23) MRA method employs a breathheld 3-D contrast-enhanced technique that is performed in a single breathhold. Sensitivity and specificity for the detection of graft patency are 93% and 97%, respectively. With further improvements in the technique, it is expected that the usefulness of this method will be significantly increased. As this is the most recent MR technique as well as the one that is readily available in the evaluation of patency of coronary artery bypass grafts, a brief description of the technique will be presented. MR imaging is performed at 1.5 Tesla. Patients are imaged in the supine position with a body phased-array coil centered at the midsternal level. ECG triggering is used through an external monitor. Four leads are attached to the patients' anterior chest wall and six turbo-fast-low-angle shot (turbo-FLASH) localizing images are obtained in the three orthogonal planes during a breathhold in deep inspiration. From the coronal localizers, five transverse turbo-FLASH localizing images are obtained to encompass an area from the mid-aortic arch to the level of the cardiac apex. The axial image at the level of the greatest transverse diameter of the heart is used to optimally position the 3-D MRA slab in the sagittal plane. The sequence used is a 3-D fast-imaging in-steady-state-precession (3-D-FISP), EKG-triggered, contrast-enhanced, gradient-recalled echo sequence (28). Artifacts related to breathing are eliminated with breathholding, and sensitivity to cardiac motion and vascular pulsation is minimized with EKG-triggering. The parameters are TR/TE, 5/2 msec; flip angle, 14 degrees; matrix, 96×256 to 124×256; slab thickness, 100–110 mm; 30–34 partitions; and partition thickness, 2.94–3.67 mm. In-plane resolution ranges from 2.02×1.56 mm to 2.82×1.56 mm with a rectangular field of view ranging from 350 to 450 mm.

The sequence is triggered to every R wave, and all lines of any given partition are filled in one R–R interval. The number of partitions, therefore, dictates the number of heartbeats required to complete the acquisition. The duration of the breathhold period after hyperventilation varies from 21 to 30 seconds. A trigger time delay of 50–250 msec is used to drive the acquisition toward diastole. The sum of time delay and the number of lines multiplied by TR should always be kept slightly less than one R–R interval to avoid missing a heartbeat. The 3-D slab is placed in the sagittal plane and the right cardiac border is always included in the slab because a graft to the right coronary artery territory is expected to traverse this area. The apical area may not be included in its entirety as the distal 1.5–2 cm of the cardiac apex is not an area where grafts are en-

countered. Noncontrast imaging always precedes the contrast-enhanced sequence to ascertain parameter optimization and patient compliance. Contrast material is loaded into the IV line prior to injection. After the patient hyperventilates by breathing in and out five times, 0.1–0.2 mmol/kg of gadopentetate dimeglumine (Magnevist; Berlex Laboratories, Wayne, NJ) is hand-injected at a rate of 2–3 ml/sec, and scanning commences 10 seconds after the start of the injection through an antecubital vein. Higher graft contrast-to-noise is achieved by doubling the dose of contrast using this sequence and by increasing the rate of injection (currently 3 cc/sec). Two back-to-back measurements are performed with an interscan delay of 8 seconds, during which the patient exhales and then inhales and holds his/her breath.

The second sequence measurement is used in the event of a slow circulation time and lack of graft enhancement on the first measurement. Axial multiplanar reconstruction (MRP) images are generated from the sagittal 3-D data of the immediate acquisitions, and image evaluation is performed on the scanner's console. The normal anatomy of saphenous vein grafts (Figs. 10.2, 10.3, and 10.4) and internal mammary artery grafts (Fig. 10.5) are demonstrated.

Criteria for patency include the following: a saphenous vein graft is considered patent if its course can be followed on the individual partitions and MPR images as an enhancing small round or linear structure from the aortotomy site to the heart. Likewise, an internal mammary artery graft is considered patent if it can be seen and followed as an enhancing area coursing toward the cardiac epicardial surface. In cases in which artifacts from surgical clips may obscure the enhancing graft (Figs. 10.2 and 10.3), its reappearance at a subsequent partition or MPR image is evidence of patency. A graft is considered occluded if no enhancement is seen along the expected course of the graft to the cardiac epicardial surface (Fig. 10.6). Care should be taken on the postcontrast images when there is the appearance of an enhancing graft; a thrombosed graft may be of high signal intensity in the precontrast partitions. It may also appear with high signal intensity following contrast administration (Fig. 10.7). Therefore, studying the precontrast partitions will prevent a false-negative result. Finally, vein graft stenosis can also be demonstrated with this technique (Fig. 10.8).

Current 3-D Contrast-Enhanced MRA Techniques

The EKG-triggered FLASH sequence described earlier is certainly a robust technique for imaging bypass grafts without or with very few pulsation artifacts. With improved gradient performance, however, where gradient rise times of 300 μsec can be achieved, the repetition

Figure 10.2. Normal anatomy of three coronary artery saphenous vein grafts. Sagittal EKG-triggered contrast-enhanced MRA partitions are demonstrated in a patient with three saphenous vein coronary artery bypass grafts from their aortotomy sites to their respective target sites. Several contiguous 3.7-mm partitions are demonstrated. (A) Two contiguous partitions near the aortic aortotomy site demonstrate the left circumflex (LCx), left anterior descending (LAD), and right coronary artery (RCA) vein grafts (AAo: ascending aorta; Ra: right atrium; La: left atrium; r: right pulmonary artery). (B) Two additional more lateral 3-D partitions reveal the LCx graft (arrow) and RCA graft (arrowheads); however, the LAD graft is not identified (open arrow) due to the superimposed magnetic susceptibility artifact from an adjacent surgical clip (AAo: ascending aorta; Ra: right atrium; La: left atrium; r: right pulmonary artery). (C) On the subsequent more lateral 3-D partitions, just lateral to the RCA saphenous vein graft, the LCx (arrows) is identified and the LAD (curved arrows) graft reappears, free from metallic artifact obscuration (Ra: right atrium; La: left atrium; r: right pulmonary artery).

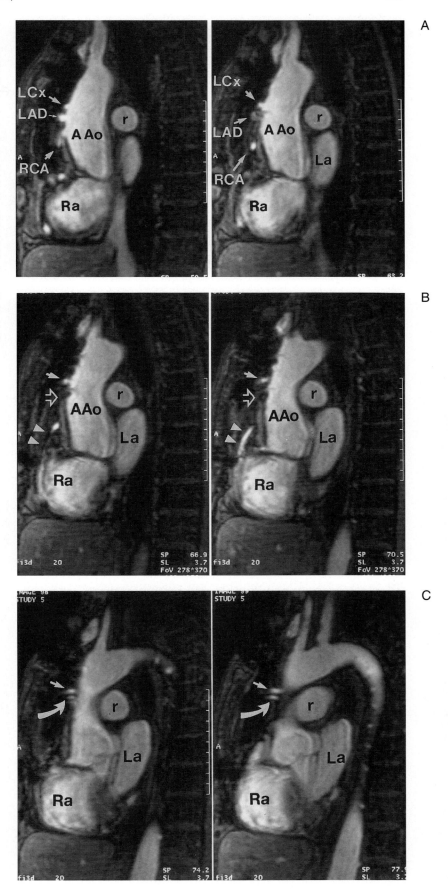

D

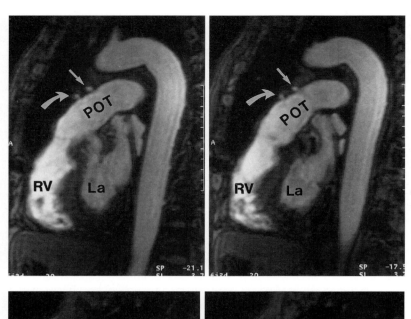

E

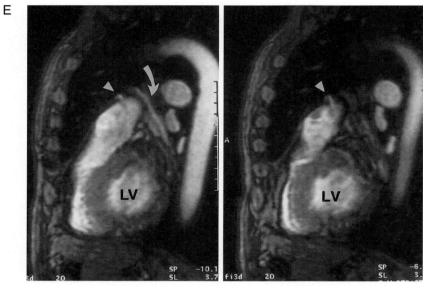

F

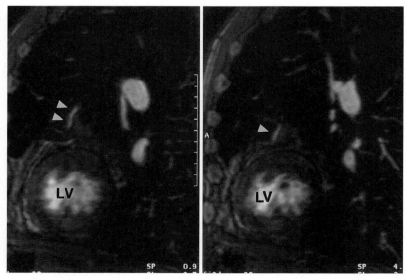

Figure 10.2. *Continued.* (D) Two additional 3-D partitions at the level of the pulmonary outflow tract (POT) demonstrate the ventral relationship of the LCx (arrows) and LAD (curved arrows) grafts (La: left atrium; RV: right ventricle). (E) Lateral to the pulmonary outflow tract, the LCx (curved arrow) graft is identified coursing to its target site. Immediately ventral to it, the LAD graft (arrowheads) is seen in cross-section (LV: left ventricle). (F) Finally, the most lateral 3-D partitions reveal the LAD graft (arrows) as it courses towards its target site into the native LAD coronary distribution (LV: left ventricle).

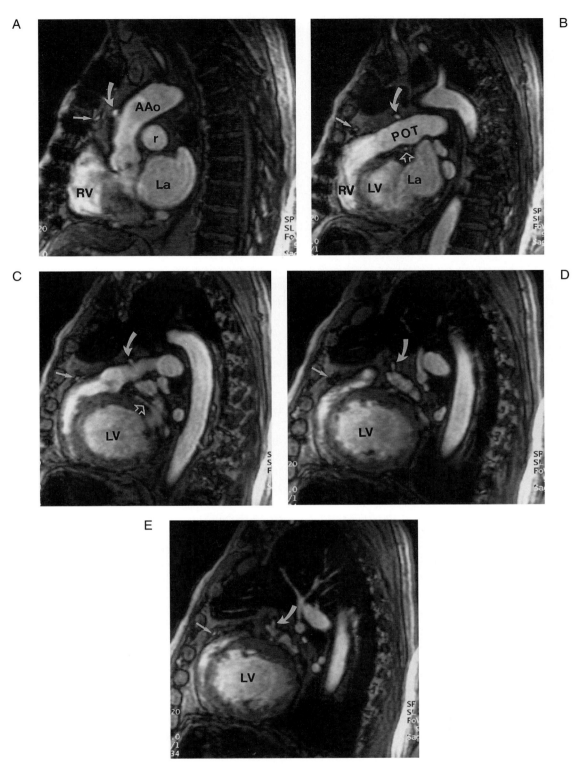

Figure 10.3. Normal anatomy of a saphenous and an internal mammary artery graft. Sagittal EKG-triggered contrast-enhanced 3-D partitions in a patient with a saphenous vein graft to the LCx artery and a left internal mammary (LIMA) artery graft to the LAD. (A) A 3-D sagittal partition through the ascending aorta reveals the more anterior LIMA graft (arrow) and the LCx vein graft (curved arrow) at its aortotomy site (AAo: ascending aorta; RV: right ventricle; La: left atrium; r: right pulmonary artery). (B) On a more lateral sagittal 3-D partition at the level of the pulmonary outflow tract (POT), the LCx coronary artery graft (curved arrow) is seen over the pulmonary outflow tract posteriorly and the LIMA graft (arrow) is seen more anteriorly. It is of note that the native LAD (open arrow) is seen in cross-section (RV: right ventricle; LV: left ventricle; La: left atrium). (C) On a more lateral 3-D partition, the LCx (curved arrow) and LIMA (arrow) grafts are identified, as is the native LCx coronary artery (open arrow) (LV: left ventricle). (D,E) Two more lateral 3-D partitions show obscuration of the LIMA graft (arrow) due to superimposed metallic artifact from an adjacent clip and the more posterior LCx tract (curved arrow). The LIMA graft (arrow) appears on a more lateral section (E) indicating its patency just prior to its entry into the LAD target site. The LCx vein graft (curved arrow) is again noted posteriorly as it courses toward its target site (LV: left ventricle).

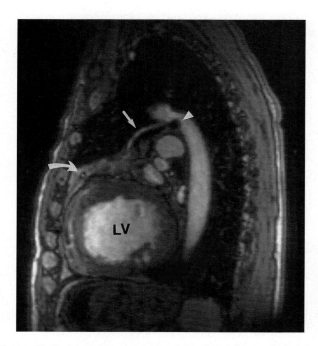

Figure 10.4. Atypical vein graft arising from the interior aortic arch. A sagittal EKG-triggered contrast-enhanced 3-D partition in a patient with a LIMA graft (curved arrow) and a vein graft arising from an atypical location (arrow). The vein graft is arising from the inferior aspect of the distal aortic arch and subsequently, was grafted into the LCx coronary artery. Focal metallic clip artifact (arrowhead) (LV: left ventricle).

time (TR) and echo-time (TE) can be decreased to 3.2 and 1.2 msec, respectively. Furthermore, when the data in the Fourier domain is sync interpolated, the number of partitions is doubled, whereby individual 3-D partitions are reconstructed with a 50% overlap. This slice interpolation process significantly improves the maximum intensity projection (MIP) resolution in all projections. Furthermore, the reduction of TR allows for a reduction in the imaging time for one 3-D acquisition. This is important in reducing the amount of contrast while preserving high vascular-to-background contrast. With the EKG-triggered 3-D-FLASH sequence described earlier, although 0.1 mmol/kg of contrast can be employed, higher vascular-to-background contrast was achieved with a double dose injection (0.2 mmol/kg). The time for acquiring 30–40 2–3 mm 3-D partitions interpolated to 60–80 partitions is approximately 8–10 seconds when using a matrix of 256 × 100 to 256 × 150. With this rapid acquisition, multiple 3-D-data sets can be obtained over time using a 0-second intermeasurement delay. The typical protocol with this slice interpolation and short TR and TE technique involves the injection of a single (0.1 mmol/kg) dose of contrast (3 cc/second injection rate) at the time patients are instructed to hold their breath.

Simultaneous with the contrast injection (via a power injector) and breathhold command, the sequence is started to acquire three 3-D data sets over time. Each 3-D data set is between 8 and 10 seconds in length, resulting in a breathhold time of 24–30 seconds. Images are calculated after acquiring all 3-D data sets. The first 3-D data set serves as a mask. The second and third 3-D data sets demonstrate contrast enhancement of the aorta. The mask, which contains the pulmonary arterial and right ventricular phase, is then subtracted from the subsequent data sets. Subtractions are subsequently subjected to maximum intensity projection and targeted maximum intensity projection processing, as well as to axial multiplanar reformation. The subtraction process eliminates the background fat and muscle signal, as well as pulmonary arteries (Fig. 10.9). Enhanced vascular-to-background contrast of CABGs (Fig. 10.10) is achieved with this new method. It should be noted that the vascular-to-background contrast is also significantly enhanced by acquiring a single 3-D data set during the bolus phase of contrast injection. The bolus phase of a rapid (3 cc/second) injection of 0.1 mmol/kg of contrast typically lasts approximately 10–15 seconds. The imaging time of 8–10 seconds for one 3-D data set, therefore, is centered over this bolus phase. Finally, the short TE of 1.2 msec results in a moderate reduction of pulsation artifacts. As such, the acquisition is not EKG-triggered allowing for a simple and more rapid protocol for CABG imaging compared with EKG-triggered acquisitions. For optimal contrast-to-noise, the flip angle at a TR of 3.2 msec was optimized with the Bloch equation at 25 to 30 degrees.

Figures 10.9 and 10.10 demonstrate the normal internal mammary arteries with this short TR/TE, slice interpolation, subtraction, contrast enhanced 3-D MRA technique. The small internal mammary artery grafts are demonstrated with very high conspicuity. This is certainly an advantage over the EKG-triggered study, where imaging of the internal mammary artery grafts was somewhat more difficult compared with saphenous vein bypass grafts. Furthermore, the multiplanar reformation capabilities (Fig. 10.11) for displaying CABGs using this 3-D sequence is more robust given the initial sync interpolation of the data.

Figure 10.12 demonstrates yet another 3-D contrast-enhanced technique, whereby a 512 × 200 matrix MRA study is obtained in a 24-second breathhold period. The higher matrix is certainly advantageous for imaging small CABGs.

Conclusion

Noninvasive CABG imaging with MRI and MRA techniques are certainly robust and can significantly guide the clinical management of patients with CABG surgery

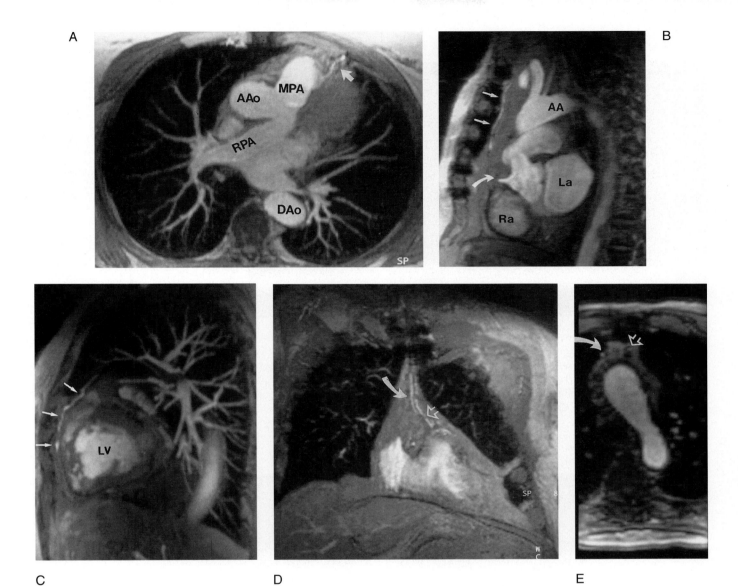

Figure 10.5. Normal internal mammary artery grafts with EKG-triggered contrast-enhanced 3-D MRA. (A) An axial targeted maximum intensity projection of a LIMA graft (arrow) is well-delineated as it courses to the LAD distribution (MPA: main pulmonary artery; RPA: right pulmonary artery; AAo: ascending aorta; DAo: descending aorta). (B) A sagittal targeted maximum intensity projection of a LIMA graft (arrows) in another patient demonstrates its course ventral to the mediastinal fat (Ra: right atrium; La: left atrium; AA: aortic arch; curved arrow: ostium of RCA). (C) A sagittal targeted maximum intensity projection of a LIMA graft (arrows) distally at its target site (LV: left ventricle). (D) A coronal targeted MIP image in a patient with a LIMA (open arrow) and a RIMA (curved arrow) demonstrate the near parallel and close relationship of the two mammary grafts. (E) An axial multiplanar reformation of the data from the patient displayed in Fig. 10.5D reveals the enhancing RIMA (curved arrow) and LIMA (arrow) in the anterior mediastinum ventral to the aortic arch.

A
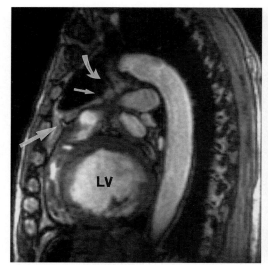
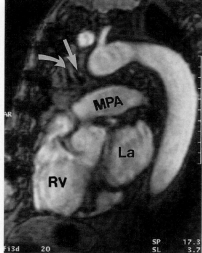
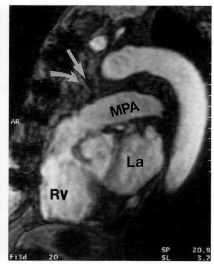
B

Figure 10.6. Saphenous vein bypass graft occlusions. (A) A sagittal EKG-triggered contrast-enhanced 3-D partition in a patient with occlusion of the LCx and LAD saphenous vein grafts is noted. The nonenhancing LCx graft is seen posteriorly (curved arrow), and the more anterior LAD vein graft (small arrow) appears as an unenhancing dark round structure. Of incidental note, the patent LIMA graft is seen over the right ventricular outflow tract anteriorly (large arrow) (LV: left ventricle). (B) Two contiguous EKG-triggered contrast-enhanced 3-D partitions reveal, in a different patient, nonenhancing LCx (arrows) and LAD (curved arrows) grafts (MPA: main pulmonary artery; RV: right ventricle; La: left atrium).

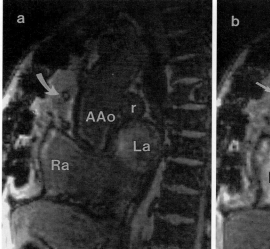
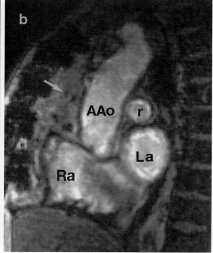

Figure 10.7. False-positive diagnosis of CABG patency. Pre- (A) and post- (B) contrast-enhanced 3-D sagittal partitions demonstrate apparent enhancement of a vein graft (arrow) on the postcontrast study. The vein graft, however, is of high signal on the precontrast study (curved arrow) and did not show an increase of signal-to-noise postcontrast, which indicates the presence of thrombosis. (AAo: ascending aorta; La: left atrium; Ra: right atrium; r: right pulmonary artery.)

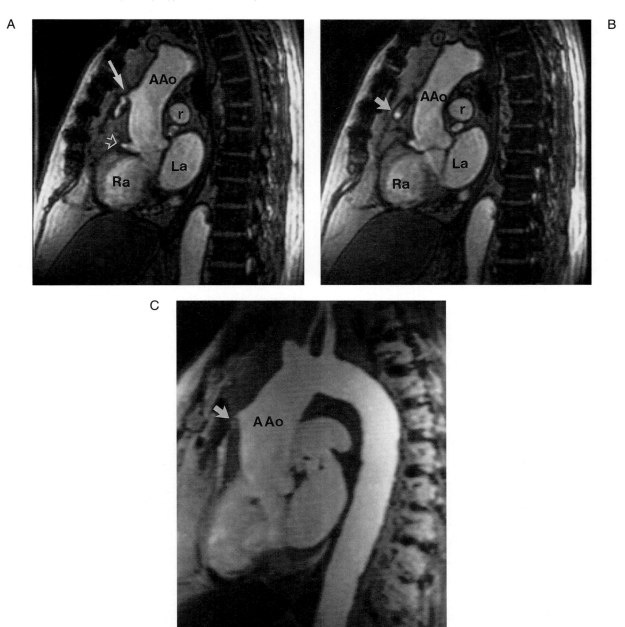

Figure 10.8. Saphenous vein stenosis. Two contiguous EKG-triggered 3-D contrast-enhanced partitions in a patient with a single saphenous vein graft reveals proximal stenosis (arrow) immediately beyond the aortotomy site in (A). Immediately laterally, the vein graft is seen as a punctate area (arrow) of enhancement (B). A maximum intensity projection (C) demonstrates the saphenous vein graft to the right coronary artery. The proximal stenosis (arrow) is well depicted. It should be noted that this vein graft could not be opacified at cardiac catheterization despite several attempts to engage the vein graft orifice. Its patency, however, was proven at surgery (Open arrow: ostium of RCA; AAo: ascending aorta; Ra: right atrium; La: left atrium; r: right pulmonary artery).

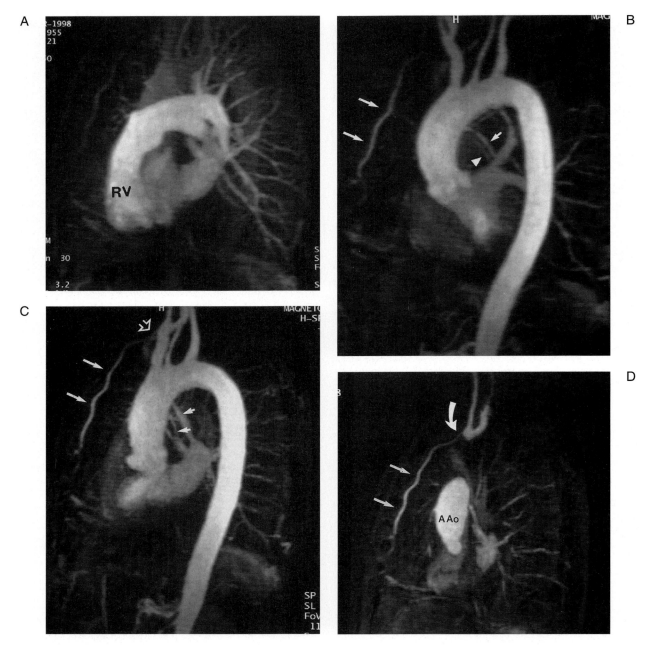

Figure 10.9. Breathhold contrast-enhanced 3-D MRA with slice interpolation (TR/TE 3.2/1.2 msec). (A) The sagittal MIP image during the first 3-D acquisition obtained over 10 seconds immediately after onset of injection of 0.1 mmol/kg of contrast at a rate of 3 cc/second reveals the right ventricular and pulmonary arterial phase with some enhancement of the left atrium and pulmonary veins (RV: right ventricle). (B) A sagittal MIP image is demonstrated during the second 10 seconds of data acquisition. The partitions obtained during this second 3-D measurement were subjected to a subtraction process by subtracting the initial pulmonary arterial phase demonstrated earlier from this phase. It should be noted that the pulmonary arterial phase is not identified on this and on the subsequent (C) MIP image. The patient's native right internal mammary artery (arrows) is identified. The known LIMA graft is not identified due to occlusion. The patient's LCx (small arrows) and LAD (arrowhead) vein grafts are faintly visualized (curved arrows). (C) Different MIP images nicely portrays the origin (open arrow) and course of the right internal mammary artery (arrows) with lack of visualization of the LIMA graft. The patient's LCx and LAD saphenous vein grafts are also seen (small arrows). (D) A single 3-D partition after the subtraction process best delineates the native right internal mammary artery (arrows) and its origin (curved arrow) (AAo: ascending aorta).

A   B

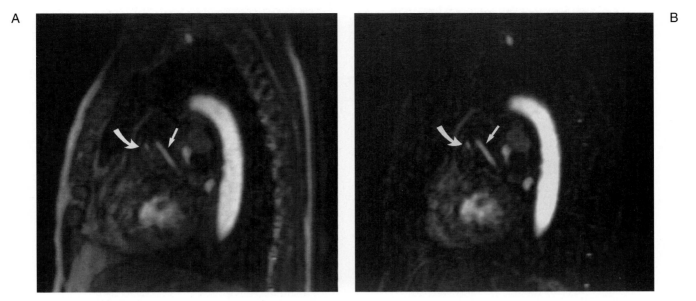

Figure 10.10. Subtraction process in 3-D contrast-enhanced MRA. (A) A single 3-D contrast-enhanced partition before subtraction process reveals the LCx graft (curved arrow) and LAD (arrow) graft. The subcutaneous fat and musculature is noted. (B) A 3-D partition showing improved vascular-to-background contrast following subtraction of the initial "mask."

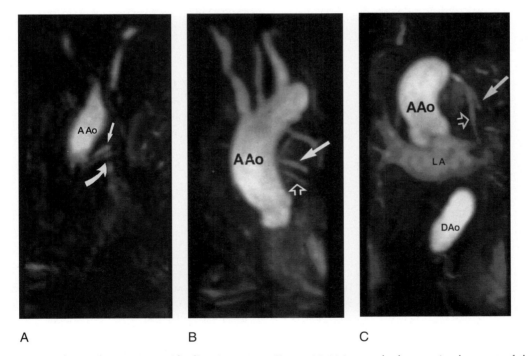

A   B   C

Figure 10.11. Contrast-enhanced 3-D MRA with slice interpolation techniques allow for exquisite multiplanar reformations (MPR) in any orientation with subsequent maximal intensity projection. (A) A single coronal 3-D MPR from a sagittally acquired study shows two small vein grafts (LCx: arrow; LAD: curved arrow) (AAo: ascending aorta). (B) A targeted coronal MIP image from coronal 3-D multiplanar reformations demonstrated in

Figure 10.11A reveals the proximal aspect of the LCx (arrow) and LAD (open arrow) saphenous vein grafts (AAo: ascending aorta). (C) A targeted maximum intensity projection of the coronal multiplanar reformations just posterior to that shown in Figure 10.11B reveals the continuation of the two vein grafts. LCx (arrow) and LAD (open arrow) saphenous vein grafts (AAo: ascending aorta; DAo: descending aorta; LA: left atrium).

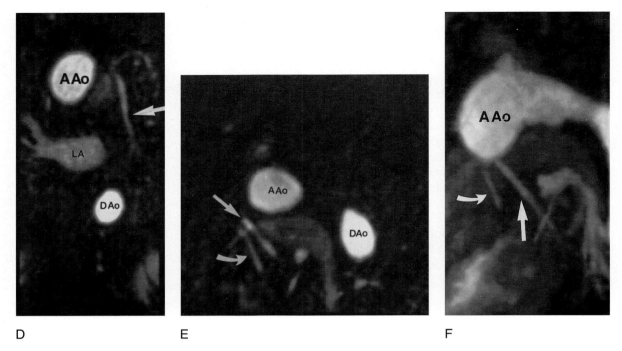

D   E   F

Figure 10.11. *Continued.* (D) Immediately posteriorly, the LCx coronary artery graft (arrow) is seen on a single 3-D partition (AAo: ascending aorta, DAo: descending aorta, LA: left atrium). (E) Oblique sagittal multiplanar reformation reveals the LCx (ar- row) and LAD (curved arrow) vein grafts and on (F), a maxi- mum intensity projection of these two grafts is noted (AAo: as- cending aorta; DAo: descending aorta; LA: left atrium).

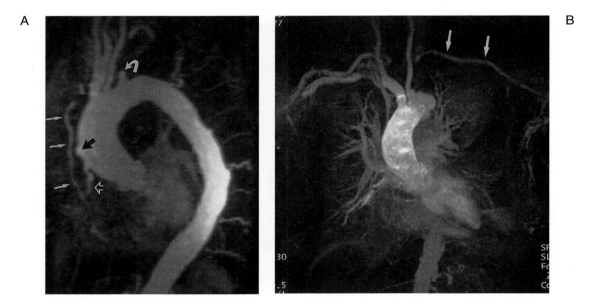

Figure 10.12. Breathhold high-resolution 3-D contrast- enhanced MRA of CABG artery disease. Employing a breath- hold 3-D contrast-enhanced MRA acquisition utilizing a 512 × 200 matrix and a double dose (0.2 mmol/kg) contrast bolus, the sagittal maximum intensity projection (A) reveals the patient's right internal mammary artery anteriorly (arrow), an occluded saphenous vein graft at its aortotomy site (open arrow), and an additional occluded saphenous vein graft (curved arrow) a few centimeters beyond its origin. It should be noted that there is a long segment occlusion of the left proximal subclavian artery (curved arrow). This involves the take-off of the patient's known LIMA graft used for LAD grafting. A coronal MIP image (B) re- veals reconstitution of the subclavian artery (arrows) via thyro- cervical trunk branches.

that present with chest pain. The rapid noninvasive procedure can provide an anatomical map to reduce catheterization times and iodinated contrast loads to patients. In addition, a negative or normal study may significantly reduce the need for invasive and costly work ups with cardiac catheterization. Rapid 3-D MRA with contrast enhancement using a variety of techniques can display, in a noninvasive manner, the anatomy of bypass grafts. Although metallic artifacts from surgical clips have been minimized with the reduction of TEs, metallic clip artifact can and frequently results in focal signal loss of patent grafts. As such, anatomical imaging should be supplemented with flow quantification for physiologic and functional information of the graft status. Current techniques are robust; however, in the future flow quantification techniques should significantly improve whereby spatial and temporal resolution are enhanced, especially with breathhold acquisitions. In addition, promising results with blood pool agents should allow for more time to image the vein and mammary grafts, and this should allow one to further improve the spatial resolution of coronary artery bypass graft imaging with MRA.

References

1. Favaloro RG. Saphenous vein graft in the surgical treatment of coronary artery disease. J Thorac Cardiovasc Surg 1969;58:178–85.
2. Spencer FC. Surgical management of coronary artery disease. *In*: Sabiston DC, Spencer FC, eds. Gibbon's surgery of the chest, fourth ed. Philadelphia: Saunders 1983; 1424–51.
3. Baltaxe HA, Carlson RG, Lillehei CW. Roentgenographic appearance of aorto-coronary artery bypass using a reversed saphenous vein. Am J Roentgenol 1970;110:734–38.
4. Guthaner DF, Wexler L. The radiologic evaluation of patients with coronary bypass. Curr Prob Diag Radiol 1976; 6:3–32.
5. Green GE, Simon HS, Gordon RB, Tice DA. Anastomosis of the internal mammary artery to the distal left anterior descending coronary artery. Circulation 1970(Suppl. 2): 79–85.
6. Kittredge RD, Kemp HG, Jr. Left internal mammary artery-coronary artery bypass anatomy. Am J Roentgenol 1977;128:395–401.
7. Jahnke EJ, Love JW. Bypass of the right and circumflex coronary arteries with the internal mammary artery. J Thorac Cardiovasc Surg 1976;71:58–63.
8. CASS principal investigators and their associates. Coronary artery surgery study (CASS): a randomized trial of coronary artery bypass surgery—quality of life in patients randomly assigned to treatment groups. Circulation 1983;68:951–60.
9. Campeau L, Enjalbert M, Lesperance J, Viaslic C, Grodin CM, Bourassa MG. Atherosclerosis and late closure of aortocoronary saphenous vein grafts: sequential angiographic studies at two weeks, one year, five to seven years,

and ten to twelve years after surgery. Circulation 1993 (Suppl. II):II-1–11-7.
10. Loop FD. Progress in surgical treatment of coronary atherosclerosis (part I). Chest 1983;84:611–622.
11. Laurie GM, Morris GE, Jr, Chapman DW, et al. Patterns of patency of 596 grafts up to seven years after aortocoronary bypass. J Thorac Cardiovasc Surg 1977; 73:443–48.
12. Stanford W, Galvin JR, Skorton DJ, Marcus ML. The evaluation of coronary bypass graft patency: direct and indirect techniques other than coronary arteriography. Am J Roentgenol 1991;156:15–22.
13. Herfkens RJ, Higgins CB, Hricak H, et al. Nuclear magnetic resonance imaging of the cardiovascular system: normal and pathologic findings. Radiology 1983;147(3): 749–59.
14. Gomes AS, Lois JF, Drinkwater DC, Corday SR. Coronary artery bypass visualization with MR imaging. Radiology 1987;162:175–79.
15. Rubinstein RI, Askenase AD, Thickman D, Feldman MS, Agrarwal JB, Helfant RAH. Magnetic resonance imaging to evaluate patency of aortocoronary bypass grafts. Circulation 1987;76:786–91.
16. White RD, Caputo GR, Mark AS, Modin GW, Higgins CB. Coronary artery bypass graft patency: noninvasive evaluation with MR imaging. Radiology 1987;164:681–86.
17. Jenkins JPR, Love HG, Foster CJ, Isherwood I, Rowlands DJ. Detection of coronary artery bypass graft patency is assessed by magnetic resonance imaging. Br J Radiol 1988;61:2–4.
18. Frija G, Schouman-Claeys E, Lacombe P, Bismuth V, Olivier J. A study of coronary artery bypass graft patency using MR imaging. J Comput Assist Tomogr 1989; 13:2.
19. White RD, Pflugfelder PW, Lipton MJ, Higgins CB. Coronary artery bypass grafts: evaluation of patency with cine MR imaging. Am J Roentgenol 1988;150:1271–74.
20. Aurigemma GP, Reichek N, Axel L, Schiebler M, Harris C, Kressel HY. Noninvasive determination of coronary artery bypass graft patency by cine magnetic resonance imaging. Circulation 1989;80:1595–602.
21. Galjee MA, van Rossum AC, Doesburg T, Hofman MB, Falke TH, Visser CA. Quantification of coronary artery bypass graft flow by magnetic resonance velocity mapping. Magn Reson Imaging 1996;14(5):485–93.
22. Hoodendoorn LI, Pattynama PMT, Buis B, Van der Geest RJ, Van Der Wall EE, DeRoos A. Noninvasive evaluation of aortocoronary bypass grafts with magnetic resonance flow mapping. Am J Cardiol 1995;75:845–48.
23. Vrachliotis TG, Bis KG, Aliabadi D, Shetty AN, Safian R, Simonetti O. Contrast enhanced breath-hold MR angiography for evaluating patency of coronary artery bypass grafts. Am J Roentgenol 1997;168:1073–80.
24. Galjee MA, van Rossum AC, Doesburg T, et al. Quantification of coronary artery bypass graft flow by magnetic resonance phase velocity mapping. Magn Reson Imag 1996;14(5):485–93.
25. Debatin JF, Strong JA, Sostman HD, et al. MR characterization of blood flow in native and grafted internal mammary arteries. J Magn Reson Imag 1993;3(3):443–50.

26. Sakuma H, Globits S, O'Sullivan M, et al. Breath-hold MR measurements of blood flow velocity in internal mammary arteries and coronary artery bypass grafts. J Magn Reson Imag 1996;6(1):219–22.

27. Kessler W, Achenbach S, Moshage W, et al. Usefulness of respiratory gated magnetic resonance coronary angiography in assessing narrowings > or = 50% in diameter in native coronary arteries and in aortocoronary bypass conduits. Am J Cardiol 1997;80(8):989–93.

28. Simonetti OP, Finn JP, White RD, et al. EKG-triggered breath-held gadolinium enhanced 3D MRA of the thoracic vasculature. *In*: Proceedings of the International Society for Magnetic Resonance in Medicine, vol. 2. New York: International Society for Magnetic Resonance in Medicine, 1996:703.

11
MRI of Coronary Artery Bypass Grafts

Bernd J. Wintersperger*

Coronary Artery Bypass Grafting

Coronary artery bypass grafting (CABG) is the most commonly performed revascularization procedure in patients suffering from multivessel ischemic heart disease (1). Although the first coronary artery revascularization had been performed using the internal mammary artery (IMA) (2), however, saphenous vein grafts were considered as first choice from beginning of routinely performed coronary artery bypass grafting (3), because of their higher flow volume compared with IMA grafts, their gross appearance, their easy harvesting, and their easy handling for coronary grafting. Venous grafts are still standard grafts for coronary bypass surgery and the graft of choice for emergency revascularization. The transfer into the high-pressure system, however, exposes the vein grafts to conditions for which they are not suitable, and most venous grafts develop atherosclerosis or occlude a few years after bypass surgery (4). One decade after surgery about 50% of venous bypass grafts are occluded, and those grafts that are still patent are mostly atherosclerotic (5–7). Arterial grafts using the IMA showed a significant higher patency rate in long-term studies than did venous grafts (5,6). Although clinical outcome is not improved by IMA grafting in the first postoperative year (8), the superior long-term patency rates of IMA grafts leads to improved long-term survival (9).

In early stages after coronary artery bypass grafting thrombosis is the main cause of graft occlusion, and in the first month after surgery up to 14% of grafts already failed due to thrombosis (8,10). Therefore follow-up examinations to determine bypass graft patency are necessary.

In patients with recurrent chest pain after bypass surgery, graft patency is routinely determined by X-ray angiography, which is still considered to be the gold standard in graft diagnostics. There are certain disadvantages of X-ray angiography, however, including invasiveness, high expenses, and X-ray burden. Although as a result of some decades of experience and technical improvements mortality of coronary angiography is only about 0.1% and the rate of complications about 3–4% (11), this technique is not useful for a frequently performed, routine-based bypass graft follow up. During years of improvement several noninvasive or minimally invasive cross-sectional techniques have become available for detection of CABG patency. Magnetic resonance imaging (MRI), in addition to helical computed tomography (CT) (12) and ultrafast CT (13), has the potential to visualize vessels in a noninvasive manner using special techniques for magnetic resonance angiography (MRA). MRI has the advantage to be a non- or minimally invasive method in combination with the absence of ionizing radiation and the use of a noniodinated contrast media in contrast to CT imaging.

MRA of Coronary Artery Bypass Grafts

The approaches to image and judge coronary bypass grafts are similar to those used in coronary MRA. Venous grafts, however, have a larger vessel diameter and a more limited mobility and displacement during rhythmic cardiac motion than native coronary arteries. Imaging of venous grafts, therefore, is easier to perform than coronary MRA. Imaging of IMA grafts is a little bit more tricky because of a diameter that is smaller than is the one of proximal major coronary vessels, which is why high spatial resolution techniques are necessary. MR bypass graft examinations have already been proposed as a useful screening procedure in assessment of graft patency (14,15). In combination with other cardiac examinations, such as analysis of cardiac function or morphology as well as coronary MRA or myocardial perfusion imaging, it is one step further to a comprehensive cardiac exam.

*Additional material can be found in Engelmann MG, Knez A, von Smekal A, et al. Non-invasive coronary bypass graft imaging after multivessel revascularisation. Int J Cardiol 2000;76(1):65–74.

Blood Flow–Based MRA Techniques

This will be a brief summary of noninvasive MRA techniques to explain fundamental aspects of coronary artery bypass graft imaging using MRA. Comprehensive literature is available to go into further details of MRA basics. Blood flow–based MRA techniques depict vessel territories with blood flow–related phenomena, such as flow void in spin-echo and flow-related enhancement or flow-induced phase shift in gradient echo techniques (16). Both effects can be combined with a two-dimensional (2-D) or three-dimensional (3-D) imaging technique; however, in regions with heavy motion, such as rhythmic respiratory or cardiac motion, these techniques often fail to visualize especially tiny vessel structures due to artifacts caused by long scanning times. In those regions respiratory gating in combination with EKG-triggering are useful to minimize respiratory and cardiac artifacts. Improvement of scanner and gradient systems as well as new imaging sequences enabled breathhold imaging that leads to superior image quality and the visualization of small moving vessels like the coronary arteries (17). These techniques can obtain 2-D data sets within a single breathhold period; however, 3-D data acquisition with blood flow–based MRA techniques is not possible today in a single breathhold.

Time-of-Flight MRA

Blood flow in spin-echo imaging leads to signal void within patent vascular structures. This is due to the sequence structure of spin-echo techniques. First a 90-degree RF pulse is used to swap the magnetization into the transversal plane, then a 180-degree pulse refocuses the dephasing spins within the transversal plane to measure a spin-echo signal. Spins in blood vessels moving out of the imaging plane or in this plane between these two RF pulses do not express any signal that leads to a "black blood" imaging of patent vessels. This effect is called the time-of-flight (TOF) effect and is one of the major basic effects of MRA.

In gradient-echo techniques with the use of a simplified RF pulse structure and de- and rephasing gradients, shorter repetition times are possible and the TOF effect shows a different vessel appearance. Stationary spins are exposed to many HF pulses within a short period of time and saturation occurs. Inflowing spins within patent vessels replace previously excited, saturated spins. During the next pulse repetition fresh magnetization within the imaging plane exists that leads to a vessel enhancement combined with background saturation. This is known as "bright blood" imaging (18). The maximum vessel enhancement is achieved at a flow velocity high enough to replace all previously exited spins within the imaging plane between two single RF excitations.

Phase-Contrast MRA

Special gradient-echo techniques based on phase effects are capable of flow direction and flow velocity determination (18,19). These techniques are equipped with special bipolar gradients additionally applied during MR measurements to induce phase differences between stationary and moving spins. Applying gradients in a special direction the lamor frequency of the spins becomes dependent on their exact position along the gradient axis. Thus, even though the gradient is switched on, spins accumulate different phase shifts according to their position. Stationary spins expressed to this gradient will be exactly refocused by the same gradient with just the opposite direction. Moving spins have a different behavior. As the spins move along between both gradient lobes their exact position within the magnet and therefore their lamor frequency changes, and the second gradient application cannot balance the phase shift of the first lobe, which results in a final phase shift of moving spins. At the end of this measurement, therefore, a final phase difference between moving and stationary spins will last. In combination with a second data set acquired with flow compensation images can be calculated that directly reflect flow velocity in the direction the velocity encoding gradient is applied. The resulting phase difference is proportional to the flow velocity. Exact flow velocity can be easily calculated by knowing the exact gradient strength.

Contrast-Enhanced MRA

Paramagnetic contrast media is known to shorten significantly the T1 values of tissues and blood. Based on this a new MRA technique has been implemented (20,21). This contrast-enhanced MRA technique, which relies on T1 shortening of blood within the vessels of interest by paramagnetic agents, enables much faster acquisitions of 3-D data sets (22). During first pass imaging after bolus injection bloods T1 value is reduced from about 900 ms to 50–100 ms. Ongoing advances in hardware with high-performance gradients lead to data acquisitions within a single breathhold period (23). Even with repetition times distinctly below 10 ms, no significant saturation of the blood and contrast agent mixture occurs. This technique is now established for examinations of the aorta and its major branches (22,24–27). With reduction of repetition times (TR) due to optimized gradient and sequence techniques acquisition time can be further reduced or spatial resolution increased. This fact is simply based on the calculation of 3-D data acquisition times (Formula 11.1):

$$T_{acqu} = Nex*Ph*Part*TR \qquad (11.1)$$

T_{acqu} = Time of data acquisition
Nex = Number of acquisitions
Ph = Number of phase-encoding steps
Part = Number of partitions
TR = Repetition time

Other strategies to reduce acquisition times further use partial Fourier scanning techniques that reduce the amount of phase-encoding steps. Based on the same formula scan time can be reduced without losing spatial resolution. The most important fact in using contrast-enhanced MRA is an adequate timing of the applied contrast media injection (Fig. 11.1). After using gadolin-

ium infusions with the first implemented sequence techniques with data acquisition times of more than a minute, in single breathhold acquisition a bolus injection is necessary to provide maximum enhancement within the vessels under investigation (Fig. 11.2). The injected paramagnetic agent, however, both enhances blood within the examined vessels as well as in adjacent vessels, such as

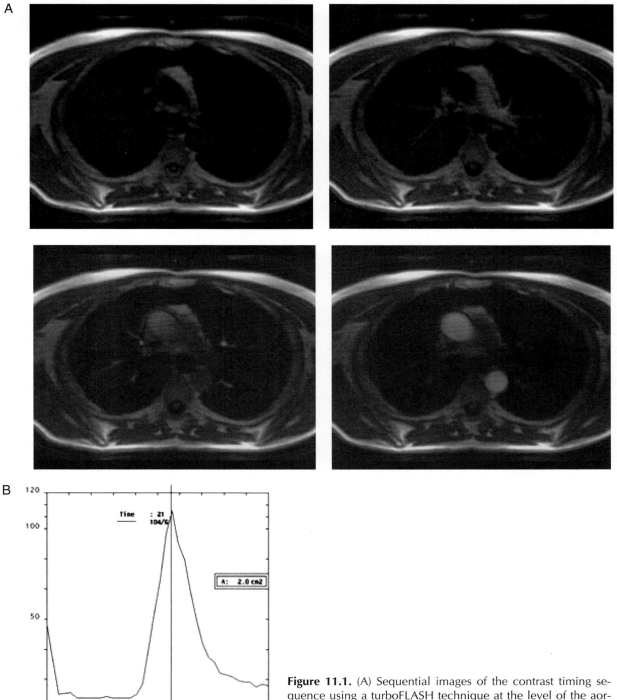

Figure 11.1. (A) Sequential images of the contrast timing sequence using a turboFLASH technique at the level of the aortic arch. (B) Time–intensity evaluation of the timing sequence showing the test bolus arrival.

A 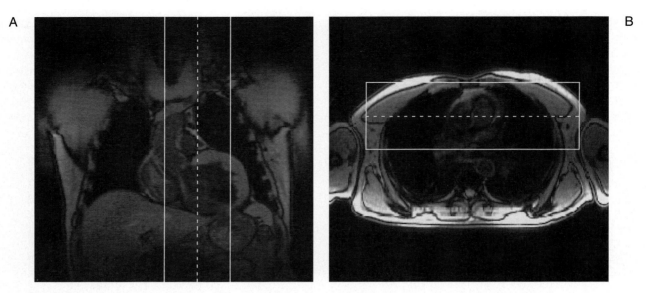 B

Figure 11.2. Positioning of the (A) sagittal and the (B) coronal slab for 3-D contrast-enhanced MRA of the bypass grafts.

venous structures, which may obscure interesting structures. For this reason timing of the contrast injection in relationship to the data acquisition is inalienable in order to maximize signal enhancement within the vessels of interest and to minimize enhancement within obscuring structures (28). This can be performed by automated detection of contrast arrival or by evaluation of individual contrast agent travel time in every patient (28,29).

Contrast behavior of MRI is dominated by the central lines of the MR raw data, the so-called k-space. Vessel enhancement can be maximized by timing the contrast bolus injection to occur within the acquisition of the central k-space lines with the low spatial frequency phase-encoding steps. Most sequence technologies acquire central k-space data during the middle of data acquisition. To cover this part of data acquisition with our paramagnetic agent this is the point of the data acquisition to which the contrast injection has to be addressed. Exact planning requires an automated bolus injection using an MR compatible power injector (Spectris™, Medrad, Pittsburgh, PA). Without automated contrast bolus detection, evaluation of individual contrast media transit time between the injection site and the vessels under investigation in every single patient can be performed using a sequential single slice turboFLASH technique with image updating of once a second (Fig. 11.1A). After time-intensity-analysis optimized scan delay time can be calculated (Fig. 11.1B). This can be easily performed with the known individual transit time and the duration of the data acquisition. There are slightly different calculation attempts to cover central data acquisition (Formulas 11.2 and 11.3), but both have been shown to be successful (28,30).

$$T_{delay} = T_{transit} - T_{acqu}/2 + 4s \text{ (Ref. 30)} \qquad (11.2)$$
T_{delay} = Delay between start of bolus injection and beginning of data acquisition in seconds
T_{acqu} = Time of data acquisition in seconds
$T_{transit}$ = Contrast travel time between injection site and vessel under investigation in seconds

$$T_{delay} = T_{1/2maxSI} - 40\%T_{acqu} \text{ (Ref. 28)} \qquad (11.3)$$
T_{delay} = Delay between start of bolus injection and beginning of data acquisition in seconds
T_{acqu} = Time of data acquisition in seconds
$T_{1/2maxSI}$ = Time to reach half of maximum SI in seconds

Comparison of Different Techniques

Blood Flow–Based MRA Techniques

After Herfkens et al. first had mentioned the visualization of coronary bypass grafts using spin-echo imaging in 1983 (31), several investigators designed studies for the assessment of CABG status using different MRA methods. The first efforts had been made using EKG-triggered T1-weighted spin-echo sequences. In spin-echo imaging patent CABGs appear as small circular structures with absence of luminal signal because blood moves rapidly through normal grafts (32).

Spin-echo techniques showed quite promising results with a correct judgment of bypass graft status in 73–90% (14,33–38). Although a specificity of 85% had been reported by Rubinstein and co-workers (34), other investigators calculated values of less than 80% that are not acceptable for a routine use of this technique (36,37).

Especially fast T1-weighted spin-echo imaging in a screening modality fashion with distinctly reduced scan times showed quite disappointing results with a specificity of only 56% (36). In addition, in early studies using spin-echo methods only venous grafts had been studied. Other investigators excluded existing IMA grafts from further data analysis due to obscuring artifacts. Limitations of spin-echo imaging are due to signal voids that arise from different factors: Metal artifacts may appear as patent grafts due to small signal voids, and in bypass grafting metallic hemostatic clips are commonly used. This especially affects IMA grafts along their course near the anterior chest wall and in addition to the small vessel size further complicates IMA graft judgment. With modern ultrafast T2 weighted half-Fourier acquired single-shot turbo spin-echo (HASTE) technique as used by Kalden and co-workers this limitation might have been overcome showing a sensitivity and specificity of 95% and 93% respectively (including IMA grafts) (53).

Gradient-recalled echo (GRE) imaging enables a much faster data acquisition and the spatial resolution or the temporal resolution can be improved. Cine MRI depicts laminar blood flow dynamically as bright signal, whereas flow abnormalities with turbulence and high-velocity flow are readily distinguishable due to signal voids (39,40). In contrast to conventional spin-echo imaging cine MRI obtains images throughout the whole cardiac cycle. Pulsatile graft flow can be viewed in an image movie loop (41). In 1988 White and co-workers discussed the potential advantages of cine MRI over conventional spin-echo techniques in terms of misinterpretation due to hemostatic clipping, air, or fibrosis (42). These problems of wrong judgment can be partially overcome by using gradient-echo techniques because patent grafts appear bright in gradient-echo imaging. In comparison to spin-echo techniques a better differentiation between graft flow and metal artifacts, air, and fibrosis is possible; however, gradient-echo sequences are more sensitive to susceptibility artifacts of metal clips that can obscure graft courses. Studies carried out to demonstrate the feasibility of GRE sequences showed improved specificity in comparison to spin-echo results with 86% (42) and even 100% (41). Aurigemma et al. could also demonstrate similar results in venous graft and IMA graft imaging (41).

As hardware and sequence technology improved in recent years, breathhold imaging became possible using GRE sequences, which tremendously pushed coronary MRI (17,43). Breathhold techniques can also be applied for CABG imaging, as shown in a study of von Smekal and co-workers at our institution (13). Although specificity reached 100%, the results in comparison to cine MRI were quite disappointing, with a sensitivity of 77% for saphenous vein grafts and only 53% for IMA

grafts (13) (Fig. 11.2). Another technique based on GRE sequences is capable of flow and flow velocity measurements based on modifications, as briefly mentioned earlier. This phase contrast (PC) MRI has been used by several investigators both to assess graft patency and to prove functional status of these grafts (44–46). The results of Galjee et al. showed in accordance to Hoogendoorn and co-workers that nonstenotic patent venous grafts show a biphasic flow pattern and comparable graft flow volumes. The latter study also pointed out that in stenotic grafts the biphasic flow pattern disappeared, which may be useful in the detection of graft malfunction (44). A biphasic flow velocity pattern has also been reported by other investigators using Doppler ultrasound (47). However all these MR studies excluded IMA grafts and only examined venous grafts because of their larger vessel diameter (Figs. 11.3). Debatin and co-workers reported on flow measurements of native and grafted internal mammary arteries and demonstrated flow curve and velocity differences (48) (Figs. 11.4A,B). Recent studies on IMA flow imaging confirmed these differences between native and grafted internal mammary arteries and showed good correlation in comparison to intraoperative flow measurements (49,50).

In general, 2-D gradient-echo techniques improved CABG imaging in comparison to spin-echo imaging, but there are still problems which have to be solved to establish these techniques in daily routine of CABG imaging. The most promising of these GRE techniques seems to be PC imaging with the ability to assess graft function in addition to patency.

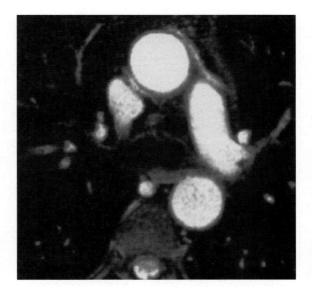

Figure 11.3. Patent IMA graft in a breathhold segmented 2-D FLASH sequence.

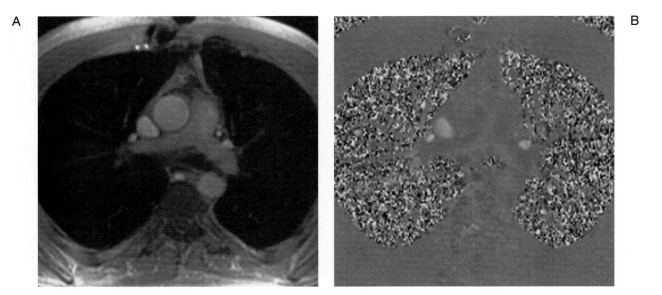

Figure 11.4. Phase-contrast (PC) technique showing a venous graft in the magnitude image (A) and the corresponding phase image (B).

Contrast-Enhanced MRA of CABG

Contrast-enhanced MRA has been shown to be a reliable method in assessment of venous and arterial CABG patency (51–53) (Figs. 11.5 to 11.9). Vrachliotis and coworkers used an EKG-triggered contrast-enhanced MRA technique and demonstrated a sensitivity in assessing graft patency of 97% (51). Our own investigations using contrast-enhanced MRA for venous and arterial coronary bypass grafts showed a sensitivity of 94%

and 95%, respectively (Table 11.1) (52,53). In contrast to Vrachliotis et al., however, we used a non-EKG-triggered technique that has the advantage of a distinctly higher spatial resolution. The specificity using a non-EKG-triggered technique was only 86% in comparison to the specificity using the EKG-triggered technique, which was 95% (51,52), but overall the results of these two studies are quite similar. In addition, contrast bolus timing might be easier to perform without triggering because of the known data acquisition time in

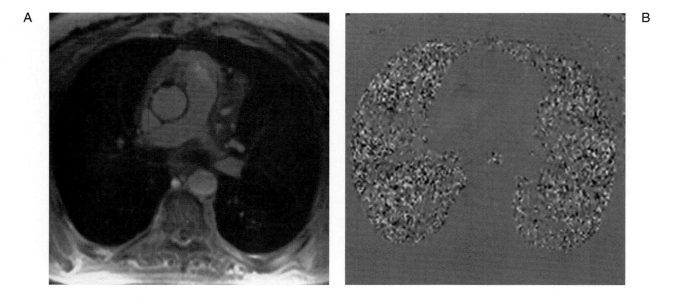

Figure 11.5. IMA graft in phase contrast MRA with the magnitude image on the left (A) and the phase image on the right (B).

A

B

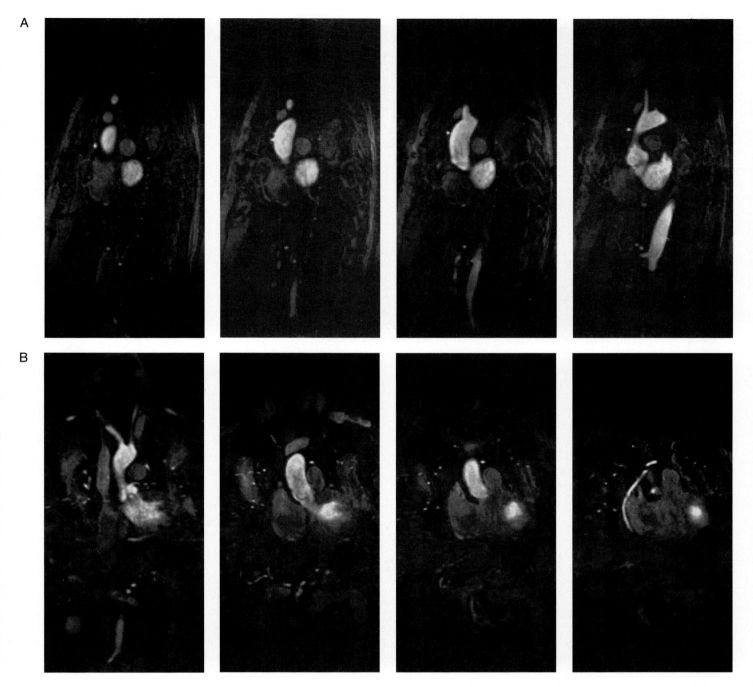

Figure 11.6. Source images of a sagittal and coronal data set showing origins of two venous grafts: one to the left anterior descending artery (LAD); the other one running down to its anastomosis with the right coronary artery (RCA).

comparison to a data acquisition time according to the patient's heart rate using EKG triggering. Using contrast-enhanced MRA, however, the distal anastomosis sites of the grafts at the level of the coronary arteries cannot be reliably identified and stenosis reliably judged because of image blurring as a result of imaging acquisition windows still too long to freeze cardiac mo-

tion and even EKG triggering does not improve visualization of these distal graft parts (51,53). These problems of visualization of distal graft anastomosis may be solved using coronary MRA techniques like 3-D navigator techniques that avoid cardiac and respiratory artifacts. Combinations of these techniques have been proposed to improve graft examinations and to get further

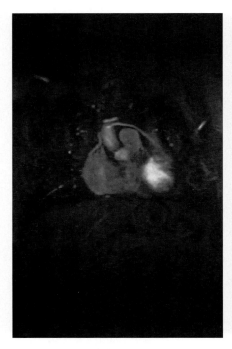
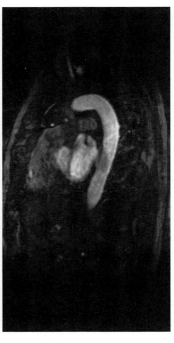

A   B

Figure 11.7. (A) Venous graft in a coronal data set with an additional origin of a second graft. (B) Maximum intensity projection (MIP) of the sagittal data set with the venous graft to the RCA.

information about the coronary artery anastomosis (54). In comparison to spin-echo or non-contrast-enhanced gradient echo techniques, metal hemostatic clips that are especially used in preparation of the internal mammary artery do not seem to severely influence patency judgment. This is mainly based on the fact that acquiring a three-dimensional data set allows to follow the graft courses in most parts.

Fractical Guide to CABG Imaging Using MRI

As shown previously contrast-enhanced MRA seems to be the most promising and reliable technique to examine and to visualize coronary bypass grafts in MRI. It is a quite simple and practical method to examine grafts that can be combined with routine cardiac MRI studies. However, a few fundamentals have to be considered to get high grade image quality. The following steps provide a guide to visualize CABG using contrast-enhanced MRA:

• Is the MR Examination Possible?
  Before every MRI examination potential contraindications have to be precluded. As cardiac patients often had undergone several interventional procedures intracoronary stents may be present. In addition, heart valve prostheses or other metal or ferromagnetic material can be found in elder cardiac patients. In any case of metallic implants, therefore, such as

prosthetic heart valves, coronary stents, or extracardiac implants it has to be proven if these devices are compatible to MRI without causing any risk to the patient. Modern implanted devices including heart valve prostheses, coronary stents, and joint prostheses are mostly suitable for MRI beside arising imaging artifacts, but a checkup is imperative and lists of MR compatibility are available (55). Although investigations are going on, however, cardiac pacemakers and defibrillators are still considered as strict contraindications for MRI.

• Patient preparation
  Informed consent of every patient is basically imperative. To improve image quality explanation of the examination to the patient is essential. Intravenous access is best provided by a 20-gauge vein catheter into an antecubital vein for a sufficient flow of 2 to 3ml/sec. In patients in whom CABG angiography is part of a comprehensive cardiac exam, EKG is also necessary, although it is not necessary for CABG angiography itself. Investigations that use small amounts of paramagnetic media like first-pass myocardial perfusion imaging should be performed prior to bypass MRA.

• Patient positioning in the magnet
  After preparation, patient positioning within the bore should center at approximately the third intercostal space in the magnetic field. The best signal-to-noise ratios can be achieved using phased-array body coils. Depending on the available coil

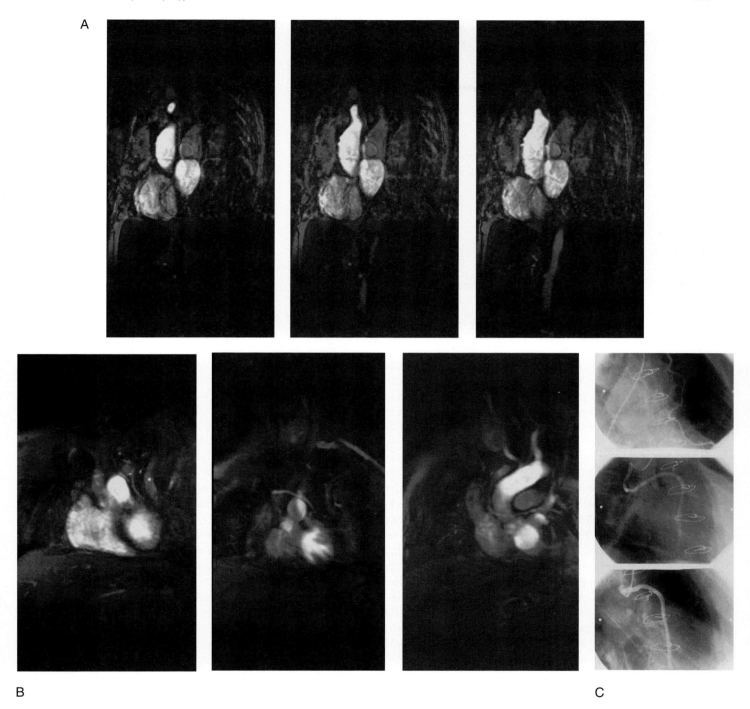

Figure 11.8. (A) Sagittal and coronal source images of a patient with two venous and one left IMA graft, all clearly patent in MRA. (B) Multiplanar reformats (MPR) of venous grafts to a branch of the LAD and one to the obtuse marginal branch of the left circumflex artery passing through the transversal pericardial sinus. (C) Corresponding X-ray angiogram indicating graft patency.

A
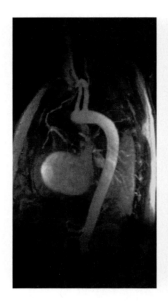
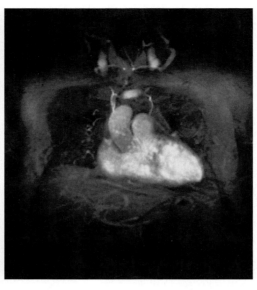
B **Figure 11.9.** MIPs of the sagittal (left side) and coronal (right side) data set with a patent left IMA graft.

technology the patient has to positioned in a prone but mostly in a supine position (using phased-array body coils). Scout views or localizers should be performed at the same respiratory level at which the MRA will be performed. Localizers in all three main plains are easily acquired using fast gradient-echo techniques in inspiration with a single breath-hold.

• Determination of contrast bolus transit time
The next step is one of the most important steps to provide an optimized enhancement within the ascending aorta, and the left internal mammary artery is the evaluation of the contrast agent transit time. Axial fast sequential turboFLASH techniques positioned at the level of the aortic arch with an update frequency of one frame per second can trace a small contrast bolus injection of 2–3 ml followed by a saline flush of about 20 ml (Fig. 11.1A). Simple time–intensity analysis can identify the signal peak that indicates the contrast bolus arrival (Fig. 11.1B). To ensure the detection of the signal peak a long scan of about 35 seconds is necessary. Without individual transit

time calculation, opacification of the aorta and the grafts may be insufficient (Fig. 11.10A,B).

• MRA Data Acquistion
After evaluation of a patient's individual contrast bolus transit time, the MRA data acquisition can be performed. We examine each patient in a sagittal and coronal data acquisition consecutively to ensure the imaging of all grafts, although information on graft number and insertion site is essential to provide maximum reliability. The use of a 512 matrix size with a minimum field-of-view of 500 mm allows a pixel size of 0.98 mm within the readout direction. Spatial resolution has also further improved recently (0.78mm) (Table 11.2). The 3-D slab in the sagittal acquisition should be positioned in a way to enclose a possible left IMA graft with its normal course to the left anterior descending (LAD) artery. With a slab thickness of about 100 mm the right margin of the ascending aorta will usually be covered. Sequence parameters should be adjusted to a patient's constitution, yielding an acquisition time of at most 30 seconds. Knowing the exact data-acquisition time, with the patient's contrast transit time, individual start delay can be easily calculated using the ways mentioned earlier. Coronal acquisition can be performed after sagittal data acquisition and image calculation in a similar way ensuring the coverage of the subclavian artery and the anterior chest wall (Fig. 11.10B). Remember to calculate a new start delay time when changing sequence parameters that affect the acquisition time. Using adequate sequence timing and MR-compatible power injectors, with 0.10–0.15 mmol/kg body weight gadopentetate dimeglumine for each angiography data acquisition, a sufficiently high image quality is obtained. Depending on the actual sequence technology and the data acquisition time a flow rate of 2–3

Table 11.1. MRA of CABG: results for different bypass graft types (52,53).

Graft Type	Sensitivity (%)	Specificity (%)	Pos. Predictive Value (%)
Venous Grafts	95	91	95
IMA[1]	94	67	94
Total	95	86	95

[1]IMA = internal mammary artery.
[2]*Note*: Excluding one false-positive IMA graft clearly patent in MRA but judged occluded in angiography leads to a specificity of 100% and 87%, respectively.

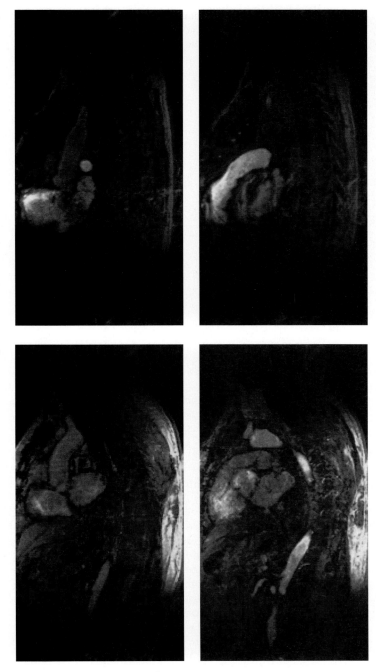

A

B

Figure 11.10. (A) Wrong timing of contrast bolus using hand injection with highest signal within the main pulmonary artery. The start delay between contrast injection and data acquisition has been too short. (B) Bad contrast in the pulmonary system and the aorta due to a start delay too long for this individual patent. This data acquisition has been made without previous transit time evaluation.

Table 11.2. Typical imaging parameters for MRA of CABG (52,53).

	MRI imaging parameters (3D-FLASH)
Repetition time (TR)	4.4/5.0 ms*
Echo time (TE)	1.8/2.0 ms*
Flip angle	40 degrees
Field-of-view (FOV)	500 mm
Matrix size	512†
Pixel size	0.98 × 1.40 mm (1.37) mm²
3-D slab thickness	96 mm

*Reduction to 70% in phase-encoding direction.
†Sequence version update.

ml/sec, followed by a saline flush, is sufficient. If all grafts are clearly depictable in the first data acquisition it is up to the investigator to end the graft angiography or go on with further aspects of comprehensive cardiac exams.

• Image postprocessing
  The acquired source images of the 3-D data sets can easily be used to calculate maximum intensity projections (MIP) or multiplanar reformats (MPR) (Fig. 11.11). In general, the source images and, in some cases, the MPR are the crucial image data to assess graft patency. A more reliable judgment is possible

A

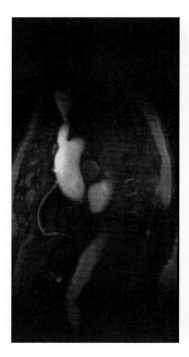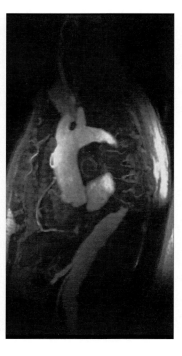

B **Figure 11.11.** Sagittal images of a patient with two venous grafts: Two aortic anastomosis sites are visible. By reviewing all the images it becomes clear that only one graft arises from the ascending aorta. The second (upper) graft is occluded and only a graft stump is visible.

by using both acquisition planes (sagittal and coronal).

References

1. Angelini GD, Newby AC. The future of saphenous vein as a coronary artery bypass conduit. Eur Heart J 1989; 10:273–80.
2. Olearchyk AS, Vasilli I. Kolesov. A pioneer of coronary revascularization by internal mammary-coronary artery grafting. J Thorac Cardiovasc Surg 1988;96:13–18.
3. Favoloro RG. Saphenous vein autograft replacement of severe segmental coronary artery occlusions: operative technique. Ann Thorac Surg 1968;5:334–39.
4. Grondin CM, Compean L, Lesperance J, Enjalbert M, Bourassa MG. Comparison of late changes in internal mammary artery and saphenous vein grafts in two consecutive series of patients 10 years after operation. Circulation 1984;70:208–12.
5. Barner HB, Standeven JW, Reese J. Twelve-year experience with internal mammary artery for coronary artery bypass. J Thorac Cardiovasc Surg 1985;90:668–75.
6. Lytle BW, Loop FD, Cosgrove DM, Ratliff NB, Easley K, Taylor PC. Long-term (5 to 12 years) serial studies of internal mammary artery and saphenous vein coronary bypass grafts. J Thorac Cardiovasc Surg 1985;89:248–58.
7. Grondin CM, Campeau L, Thornton JC, Engle JC, Cross FS, Schreiber H. Coronary artery bypass grafting with saphenous vein. Circulation 1989;79:I24–I29.
8. van der Meer J, Hillege HL, van Gilst WH, et al. A comparison of internal mammary artery and saphenous vein grafts after coronary artery bypass surgery: no difference in 1-year occlusion rates and clinical outcome. Circulation 1994;90:2367–74.
9. Cameron A, Davis KB, Green G, Schaff HV. Coronary bypass surgery with internal-thoracic-artery grafts—effects on survival over a 15-year period. N Engl J Med 1996; 334:216–19.
10. Sanz G, Pajaron A, Alegria E, et al. Prevention of early aortocoronary bypass occlusion by low-dose aspirin and dipyridamole. Grupo Espanol para el Seguimiento del Injerto Coronario (GESIC). Circulation 1990;82:765–73.
11. Wyman RM, Safian RD, Portway V, Skillman JJ, McKay RG, Baim DS. Current complications of diagnostic and therapeutic cardiac catheterization. J Am Coll Cardiol 1988;12:1400–6.
12. Engelmann MG, von Smekal A, Knez A, Kurzinger E, Huehns TY, Hofling B, et al. Accuracy of spiral computed tomography for identifying arterial and venous coronary graft patency. Am J Cardiol 1997;80:569–74.
13. von Smekal A, Knez A, Seelos KC, et al. A comparison of ultrafast computed tomography, magnetic resonance angiography and selective angiography for the detection of coronary bypass patency. Fortschr Röntgenstr 1997;166:185–91.
14. Jenkins JP, Love HG, Foster CJ, Isherwood I, Rowlands DJ. Detection of coronary artery bypass graft patency as assessed by magnetic resonance imaging. Br J Radiol 1988;61:2–4.
15. van Rossum AC, Galjee MA, Doesburg T, Hofman M, Valk J. The role of magnetic resonance in the evaluation of functional results after CABG/PTCA. Int J Card Imag 1993;1: 59–69.
16. Axel L. Blood flow effects in magnetic resonance imaging. Am J Radiol 1984;143:1157–66.
17. Edelman RR, Manning WJ, Burstein D, Paulin S. Coronary arteries: breath-hold MR angiography. Radiology 1991; 181:641–43.
18. Moran PR, Moran RA, Karstaedt N. Verification and evaluation of internal flow and motion: true magnetic resonance imaging by the phase gradient modulation method. Radiology 1985;154:433–41.
19. Dumoulin CL, Hart HR. Magnetic resonance angiography. Radiology 1986;161:717–20.

20. Prince MR, Yucel EK, Kaufman JA, Harrison DC, Geller SC. Dynamic gadolinium-enhanced three dimensional MR arteriography. J Magn Reson Imag 1993;3:877–81.

21. Prince MR. Gadolinium-enhanced MR aortography. Radiology 1994;191:155–64.

22. Prince MR, Narasimham DL, Jacoby WT, et al. Three-dimensional gadolinium-enhanced MR angiography of the thoracic aorta. Am J Roentgenol 1996;166:1387–97.

23. Shetty AN, Shirkhoda A, Bis KG, Alcantara A. Contrast-enhanced three-dimensional MR angiography in a single breath-hold: a novel technique. Am J Roentgenol 1995; 165:1290–92.

24. Holland GA, Dougherty L, Carpenter JP, et al. Breath-hold ultrafast three-dimensional gadolinium-enhanced MR angiography of the aorta and the renal and other visceral abdominal arteries. Am J Roentgenol 1996;166:971–81.

25. Snidow JJ, Johnson MS, Harris VJ, Trerotola SO. Three-dimensional gadolinium enhanced MR angiography for aortoiliac inflow assessment plus renal artery screening in a single breath-hold. Radiology 1996;198:725–32.

26. Siegelman ES, Gilfeather M, Holland GA, et al. Breath-hold ultrafast three-dimensional gadolinium-enhanced MR angiography of the renovascular system. Am J Roentgenol 1997;168:1035–40.

27. Carpenter JP, Holland GA, Golden MA, et al. Magnetic resonance angiography of the aortic arch. J Vasc Surg 1997;25:145–51.

28. Hany TF, McKinnon GC, Leung DA, Pfammatter T, Debatin JF. Optimization of contrast timing for breath-hold three-dimensional MR angiography. J Magn Reson Imag 1997;7:551–56.

29. Prince MR, Chenevert TL, Foo TK, Londy FJ, Ward JS, Maki JH. Contrast-enhanced abdominal MR angiography: optimization of imaging delay time by automating the detection of contrast material arrival in the aorta. Radiology 1997;203:109–14.

30. Kopka L, Vosshenrich R, Müller D, Fischer U, Rodenwaldt J, Grabbe E. Results of a contrast-medium supported 3D MR angiography in respiratory arrest following optimization of contrast medium bolus. Fortschr Röntgenstr 1997;166:290–95.

31. Herfkens RJ, Higgins CB, Hricak H, et al. Nuclear magnetic resonance imaging of the cardiovascular system: normal and pathologic findings. Radiology 1983;147:749–59.

32. van der Wall EE, Vliegen HW, de Roos A, Bruschke AV. Magnetic resonance imaging in coronary artery disease. Circulation 1995;92:2723–39.

33. White RD, Caputo GR, Mark AS, Modin GW, Higgins CB. Coronary artery bypass graft patency: noninvasive evaluation with MR imaging. Radiology 1987;164:681–86.

34. Rubinstein RI, Askenase AD, Thickman D, Feldman MS, Agarwal JB, Helfant RH. Magnetic resonance imaging to evaluate patency of aortocoronary bypass grafts. Circulation 1987;76:786–91.

35. Frija G, Schouman-Claeys E, Lacombe P, Bismuth V, Ollivier J-P. A study of coronary artery bypass graft patency using MR imaging. J Comput Assist Tomogr 1989;13:226–32.

36. Theissen P, Sechtem U, Langkamp S, Jungehulsing M, Hilger HH, Schicha H. Noninvasive assessment of aorto-coronary bypass using magnetic resonance tomography. Nuklearmedizin 1989;28:234–42.

37. Wicke K, Mühlberger V, Judmaier W, Moes N, zur Nedden D. The value of CT and MRT in assessing aortocoronary venous bypasses in comparison with coronary angiography. Fortschr Röntgenstr 1991;154:306–9.

38. Knoll P, Bonatti G, Pitscheider W, et al. The value of nuclear magnetic resonance tomography in evaluating the patency of aortocoronary bypass grafts. Z Kardiol 1994;83:439–45.

39. Sechtem U, Pflugfelder PW, White RD, et al. Cine MR imaging: potential for the evaluation of cardiovascular function. Am J Roentgenol 1987;18:239–46.

40. Schiebler M, Axel L, Reichek N, et al. Correlation of cine MR imaging with two-dimensional pulsed Doppler echocardiography in valvular insufficiency. J Comput Assist Tomogr 1987;11:627–32.

41. Aurigemma GP, Reichek N, Axel L, Schiebler M, Harris C, Kressel HY. Noninvasive determination of coronary artery bypass graft patency by cine magnetic resonance imaging. Circulation 1989;80:1595–602.

42. White RD, Pflugfelder PW, Lipton MJ, Higgins CB. Coronary artery bypass grafts: evaluation of patency with cine MR imaging. Am J Roentgenol 1988;150:1271–74.

43. Manning WJ, Li W, Edelman RR. A preliminary report comparing magnetic resonance coronary angiography with conventional angiography. N Engl J Med 1993;328:828–32.

44. Hoogendoorn LI, Pattynama PM, Buis B, van der Geest RJ, van der Wall EE, de Roos A. Noninvasive evaluation of aortocoronary bypass grafts with magnetic resonance flow mapping. Am J Cardiol 1995;75:845–48.

45. Galjee MA, van Rossum AC, Doesburg T, van Eenige MJ, Visser CA. Value of magnetic resonance imaging in assessing patency and function of coronary artery bypass grafts: an angiographically controlled study. Circulation 1996;93:660–66.

46. Galjee MA, van Rossum AC, Doesburg T, Hofman MB, Falke TH, Visser CA. Quantification of coronary artery bypass graft flow by magnetic resonance phase velocity mapping. Magn Reson Imag 1996;14:485–93.

47. Fusejima K, Takahara Y, Sudo Y, Murayama H, Masuda Y, Inagaki Y. Comparison of coronary hemodynamics in patients with internal mammary artery and saphenous vein coronary artery bypass grafts: a noninvasive approach using combined two-dimensional and Doppler echocardiography. J Am Coll Cardiol 1990;15:131–39.

48. Debatin JF, Strong JA, Sostman HD, et al. MR characterization of blood flow in native and grafted internal mammary arteries. J Magn Reson Imaging 1993;3:443–50.

49. Miller S, Scheule AM, Hahn U, et al. MR angiography and flow quantification of the internal mammary artery graft after minimally invasive direct coronary artery bypass. Am J Roentgenol 1999;172:1365–69.

50. Walpoth BH, Müller MF, Genyk I, et al. Evaluation of coronary bypass flow with color-Doppler and magnetic resonance imaging techniques: comparison with intraoperative flow measurements. Eur J Cardiothorac Surg 1999;15:795–802.

51. Vrachliotis TG, Bis KG, Aliabadi D, Shetty AN, Safian R, Simonetti O. Contrast-enhanced breath-hold MR angiography for evaluating patency of coronary artery bypass grafts. Am J Roentgenol 1997;168:1073–80.

52. Wintersperger BJ, Engelmann MG, von Smekal A, et al. Patency of coronary bypass grafts: assessment with breath-hold contrast-enhanced MR angiography—value of a non-electrocardiographically triggered technique. Radiology 1998;208:345–51.

53. Kalden P, Kreitner KF, Wittlinger T, et al. Assessment of coronary artery bypass grafts: value of different breath-hold MR imaging techniques. Am J Roentgenol 1999;172: 1359–64.

54. Parodi R, Sardanelli F, Molinari G, Caratti A, Zandrino F, Bruzzone F. Evaluation of coronary bypass graft patency with plain 3D navigator echo and breath-hold Gd-enhanced FISP MR angiography (abstr.). Radiology 1997; 205(P):153.

55. Shellock FG, Kanal E. Bioeffects and safety of MR procedures. *In*: Edelmann RR, Zladkin MB, Hesselink JR. Clinical Magnetic Resonance Imaging. Second ed. Philadelphia: W.B. Saunders Company, 1996;391–434.

12

Coronary Lesion Detection with Coronary MRA: When Will It Be Good Enough?

André J. Duerinckx

Introduction

The detection of coronary artery lesions by magnetic resonance (MR) is probably the most talked about and investigated future application of coronary magnetic resonance angiography (MRA). Interestingly enough, it is still the least mature and most experimental application. Coronary lesion detection represents the "holy grail" of cardiac magnetic resonance imaging (MRI) (1–5). From the beginning the hope was that coronary MRA could become a noninvasive screening tool for the detection of all (or most) coronary artery lesions. This is still our hope today, at least for proximal lesions in the main coronary arteries and their larger side branches. The fact that after 6 years of preclinical trials of coronary MRA techniques their sensitivity and specificity for coronary lesion detection still does not compare with traditional contrast coronary angiography (4,6–8) should not discourage us. There are many reasons why we have not yet seen "perfect" results, such as 99% sensitivity for detection of all coronary lesions.

First, the MRI technology and coronary MRA pulse sequences have changed and improved so quickly that few large preclinical trials were ever performed with any of them. Second, because the first- and second-generation coronary MRA techniques required great skills (see Chap. 15) or lesser skills, respectively, but much longer acquisition times (see Chaps. 16–19); few investigators were willing to take on the challenge. Third, many people wanted coronary MRA to perform like the established invasive gold standard, contrast X-ray coronary angiography, even though this was never the case for other noninvasive techniques (e.g., nuclear cardiology or exercise stress testing). There is a need to reassess unrealistic expectations about what coronary MRA should be able to do. Being able to detect 70–90% of all significant proximal coronary artery lesions is already a very worthwhile goal.

As this and later chapters will demonstrate we are almost getting to this point. It is not necessary for a noninvasive imaging technique for patients with ischemic heart disease to detect every single minor lesion in small coronary side branches. In addition, with the advent of the third-generation coronary MRA techniques (see Chaps. 20–21), improved postprocessing (see Chaps. 22–23), more interest from clinical users, the availability of new, dedicated "cardiac" MR scanners (see Chap. 3), and new MR blood pool agents (see Chaps. 24–25) (both indicating industry's interest in this issue), the use of coronary MRA in daily clinical practice will soon become reality. Coronary MRA for lesion detection is now available to clinical users, not just investigators at major academic centers or clinics. Coronary MRA will have an important role in the work up of patients with ischemic heart disease in the very near future.

Coronary Artery Lesion Detection by MRI: How Does It Differ from Other Vascular Territories?

The physiology of blood flow in coronary arteries is very different from the physiology of blood flow in large vessels (e.g., the carotid arteries and the abdominal aorta). In the coronary arteries flow velocities are lower than in other large vessels; there is less or no turbulent flow and there is potential for collateral blood flow. Normal coronary arteries and veins appear as high-signal linear structures on coronary MRA. Distal to a total occlusion vessels with no collateral flow have decreased signal intensity or background (fat-suppressed) signal intensity. Once in a while, however, a vessel shadow is visible, possibly corresponding to the wall of the occluded vessel. This could be misconstrued as representing reduced

A

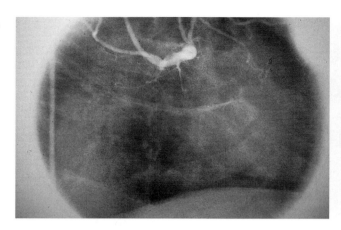

B

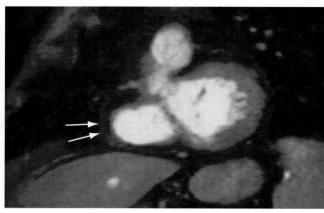

Figure 12.1. Total occlusion of the proximal RCA. (A) Conventional angiogram, left anterior oblique view. (B) Coronary MRA, the corresponding view, clearly shows the proximal RCA (long arrow). The middle and distal RCA are occluded. A low-signal-intensity band is seen on the MRA in the location of the occluded vessel. Also shown are: Ao = aortic root; PA = pulmonary artery; LV = left ventricle. (Reprinted with permission from Duerinckx (26).)

flow beyond a subtotal occlusion (Fig. 12.1). Reverse flow distal to a total occlusion cannot be distinguished from forward flow past a subtotal occlusion without determining direction of flow.

Figure 12.2 demonstrates a long hemodynamically significant proximal right coronary artery (RCA) lesion, as seen on both the conventional angiogram and on the coronary MRA. Figure 12.3 demonstrates another hemodynamically significant proximal left anterior descending (LAD) lesion, as seen on both the conventional angiogram and on the coronary MRA.

Discrete coronary lesions, both total and subtotal occlusions, may appear as either areas of signal void (9, 10), decreased flow signal (11), or vessel wall irregularity. It is thus very important to be aware of these important differences between coronary MRA and MRA of large vessels elsewhere in the body. In addition, be-

cause of collateral flow a total occlusion may have slow-moving fluid present in the vessel distal to the occlusion and show a normal vessel signal.

Diffuse diseased coronary arteries cannot be distinguished from small-caliber normal vessels by coronary MRA. A left dominant coronary system with a small-caliber RCA can simulate diffuse disease in the RCA, and vice versa. Women with small-caliber coronary vessels are also more difficult to study with coronary MRA.

Pioneering Work with First-Generation Coronary MRA: The 1992–1994 Period

A historical review of the initial reports on the use of coronary MRA for coronary artery lesion detection can be educational. It illustrates a typical cycle: The initial

A

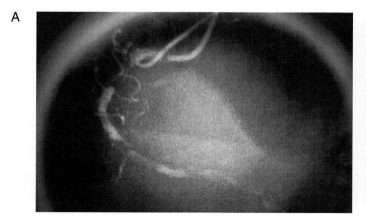

B

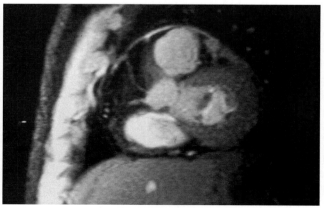

Figure 12.2. Long subtotal occlusion of the proximal RCA with additional distal lesions. (A) Conventional angiogram. (B) Coronary MRA clearly shows the segment of subtotal proximal occlusion. The more distal lesions are only faintly seen on the MRI. Also shown are: pericardial sac; Ao = ascending Aorta; P = pulmonary artery; LV = left ventricle; R = right chambers. (Reprinted with permission from Ref. 16; Radiology, RSNA, Inc.)

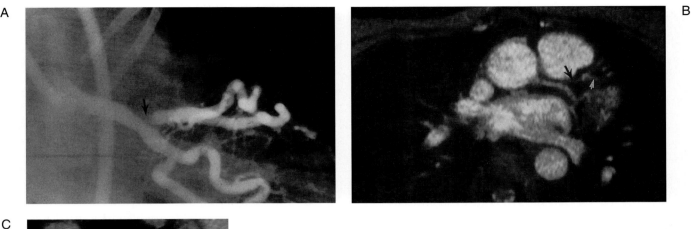

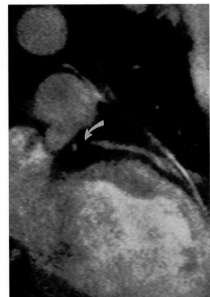

Figure 12.3. Subtotal occlusion of the proximal LAD. (A) Conventional angiogram, RAO caudal view showing a proximal LAD lesion (arrow). (B) Coronary MRA obtained in an oblique transaxial plane demonstrates the left main and LCx, with a signal void (black arrow) in the proximal LAD. Also noted are the more distal LAD and diagonal vessels (white arrow). (C) Coronary MRA obtained in a vertical two-chamber view which also shows the flow void area (curved arrow) in the proximal LAD. (Case provided by Dr. Warren Manning; reprinted with permission from Manning (48).)

enthusiasm of the first maybe overly positive and promising preclinical reports and then the more negative follow-up reports when other investigators try to duplicate the initial work. This seems to be a typical scenario encountered when new imaging technology or imaging applications are first implemented. Similar scenarios can be found in other areas of thoracic imaging, such as the use of CT angiography (CTA) for pulmonary embolism detection and the use of electron-beam computed tomography (EB-CT) for 3-D coronary artery visualization.

Work by Manning et al. Reported in 1993

Initial clinical testing of the first-generation coronary MRA technique was performed at the Beth-Israel Hospital in Boston and reported in a March 1993 issue of the *New England Journal of Medicine*. In this historical article, Manning et al. reported for the first time on the capability to detect coronary occlusion and stenosis using MRI in a series of 39 patients referred for elective coronary angiography (10). This article brought hope to the

field of cardiology and medicine that a noninvasive coronary imaging technique would soon become available. It created great interest by industry and MRI vendors for this new and extremely promising application of cardiac MRI. More than anything else it helped increase the research efforts in new uses of cardiac MR techniques. The national and international press became involved, and this report went beyond just the medical media.

In this first clinical study coronary MRA had a 90% sensitivity and a 92% specificity, as compared with conventional angiography, for correctly identifying individual vessels with $\geq$ 50% angiographic stenoses. The corresponding positive and negative predictive values were 0.85 and 0.95, respectively. The overall sensitivity and specificity for correctly classifying individual patients as having or not having serious coronary disease were 97% and 70%, respectively, with a corresponding positive and negative predictive value of 0.90 and 0.88, respectively. Lesion detection was highest in the LM. Coronary MRA showed the lowest sensitivity for lesion detection in LCx (71%) and the lowest specificity in the RCA (78%). In a follow-up study of 72 patients with 81 significant lesions in a total of 271 visualized coronary arteries (and 39% of patients without significant lesions), the sensitivity for an individual vessel with stenosis remained 90% (12).

Work by Duerinckx et al. Reported in 1994

Subsequent attempts by other investigators to reproduce these results based on blinded studies have not been as successful. Duerinckx et al. (13–15) were the first to report in December 1993 that the 90% sensitivity for lesion detection using first-generation coronary MRA was optimistic and could not be reproduced in a double-blinded prospective study. Their study was published in the December 1994 issue of *Radiology* (16). The publication of the article by Duerinckx et al. confirmed what several other investigators and industry people were starting to discover and had to admit. Although very promising, and in some patients spectacular, the images routinely produced with first-generation coronary MRA were not consistent enough to reproduce the results first reported by Manning et al. in the *New England Journal of Medicine*. This paper has historical importance because it set a more realistic tone for what first-generation coronary MRA can accomplish.

As can be expected great controversy erupted over these discrepancies in the performance of first-generation coronary MRA techniques (2,17,18). The original correspondence between Manning and Duerinckx was pub-lished in the June 1995 issue of *Radiology*. Duerinckx et al. were not alone in disagreeing with Manning et al. Indeed, during the 1994–1995 period the sensitivity for detection of significant ($\geq$ 50%) lesions in subsequent studies was varied: 36% based on an initial study by Post et al. of 14 patients, with 14 significant lesions (19); 33–75% based on a follow-up study by Post et al. of 35 patients with 35 stenoses (20); 63% average sensitivity (range: from 0% to 75%) based on a study by Duerinckx et al. of 20 patients with 27 proximal lesions (16); 65% based on an initial study by Pennell et al. of 17 patients with 23 lesions (9); 88% based on a follow-up study by Pennell et al. using a nonblinded analysis of 31 patients with 41 lesions (21); 83–100% in a study by Nitatori et al. in 50 patients (22); 56% in a study by Mohiaddin, Bogren, et al., in 16 heart transplant patients with 9 lesions (23). These results for lesion detection using the first-generation coronary MRA techniques in the 1994–1995 period are summarized in Figure 12.4.

Why the Discrepancy in Results Between Manning and Duerinckx?

The failure by other investigators to achieve a 90% sensitivity and 92% specificity for coronary lesion detection was not due to differences in techniques relating to relative poor temporal resolution, shorter echo times, or worse patient cooperation, unlike some statements to the contrary (7,17). Both Manning and Duerinckx used the same MR pulse sequences designed and provided by the same

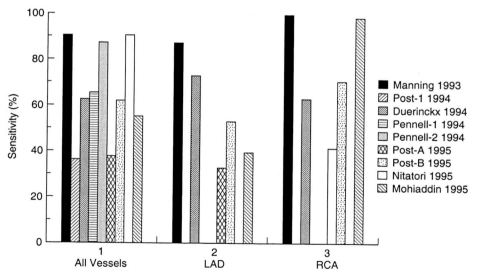

Figure 12.4. Plot of the sensitivities for detection of hemodynamically significant ($\geq$ 50%) coronary lesion as published in clinical studies: (1) all vessels; (2) LAD only; and (3) RCA only. The legend on the left lists the studies in the same sequence as the bars along the horizontal axis (from left to right). For two studies (Post et al., 1995, and Nitatori et al., 1995) the average of the sensitivities for detection of $\geq$ 50% lesions in the LAD and RCA was taken as the overall sensitivity. (Reprinted with permission from Duerinckx (26).)

company (Siemens Medical Systems, Inc, NJ). Both investigators took great care in patient preparation and prescan breathhold practice. In retrospect the discrepancy in results can most likely be explained by normal differences in human interpretation of a same set of MRI (24–26), as we will briefly explain. More detailed discussion of potential shortcomings of the first-generation coronary MRA techniques will be provided in a later chapter (Chap. 15). The most important key difference between the Manning and Duerinckx studies may well be the "human factor" (i.e., the level of confidence chosen by each investigator to call an anomaly on an MRI of a lesion).

An important practical problem with first-generation two-dimensional (2-D) coronary MRA is the potential for the overreading or underreading of coronary lesions. Because only one slice is viewed at a time, and spatial registration between slices is never guaranteed, it can be difficult to distinguish between out-of-plane vessel course and a lesion. This is compounded by the limited spatial and temporal resolution (typically 1 mm in-plane spatial and 80–100 msec temporal resolution). It is important for users of this technique to understand these interpretative difficulties. Many of these problems disappear with second- and third-generation coronary MRA techniques. Because of the great importance of such misinterpretatons, and to temper unrealistic expectations in users with lesser experience, we offer three challenging examples of missed lesions. Figure 12.5 shows a short mid–right coronary artery (RCA) lesion missed on coronary MRA that could easily have been misread as showing the lesion. The location and course of overlapping acute marginal branches causes partial voluming artifacts that simulate a lesion. Figure 12.6 demonstrates how a mid-RCA lesion is again missed; however, if sequential parallel images are not carefully analyzed (e.g., using a cine-loop display) one could erroneously conclude that there is a lesion present. Figure 12.7 illustrates another case of missed mid-RCA lesion. Here the lesion appears on a single right anterior oblique (RAO)-equivalent view, but is totally invisible on all other views. One has to adhere to strict radiological interpretation criteria, and call this a false negative; otherwise, one would have false-positive readings in almost 100% of normals.

There are several possible explanations for why a coronary lesion is not visualized by 2-D coronary MRA. These include spatial and temporal resolution, timing of the acquisition (within the cardiac cycle), irregular breathing and misregistration between breathholds, partial voluming of tortuous vessels and overlapping adjacent anatomical structures, reverse flow past an area of stenosis (collateral flow), and the unknown signal and contrast characteristics of vessel wall and plaque on coronary MRA sequences. We are planning several experiments to help clarify some of these problems (see later).

Methodology for Blind-Reading Used by Duerinckx et al. in Their 1994 Study

We will briefly detail the methodology used by Duerinckx et al. (16) in the blind comparison studies of elective cardiac catheterization with coronary angiography and 2-D coronary MRA because we believe that such methodology is essential to obtain valid clinical evaluations and to plan multicenter trials to compare techniques.

Twenty-one patients who underwent elective cardiac catheterization with coronary angiography were evaluated with 2-D coronary MRA. The MRI quality of each of the four segments of the proximal coronary artery tree (RCA, left main, LAD, and LCx) was graded from 0 to 5. If present, a ramus branch image quality grade was included in the LCx grading. The grading scale is shown in Table 12.1, and is based on the signal-to-noise, contrast-to-noise, and motion artifacts present in each image.

Confidence codes from 0 to 4 were assigned for lesion detection in each of the four proximal coronary segments. The confidence codes are given in Table 12.2, and are self-explanatory. A blinded prospective analysis of coronary lesion detection by MRI and conventional angiography was performed.

A receiver operating characteristic (ROC) analysis was also performed for lesion detection in coronary artery segments. For these receiver operating characteristic (ROC) analyses a degree of confidence decision task was used. Confidence codes from 0 to 4 were used to define four cutoffs at which sensitivity/specificity were calculated and ROC curves plotted for each of the four proximal coronary segments.

In the blinded prospective study by Duerinckx et al. of 21 patients studied with 2-D coronary MRA they were able to detect 62% of the hemodynamically significant ($\geq$ 50% reduction in diameter) coronary lesions in the RCA, and 72% in the left anterior descending (LAD) (16). Sensitivities and specificities were also derived for the different confidence levels. For example, the sensitivity for lesion detection in the RCA increases from 31% to 69% when the confidence level required is decreased from 4 to 1. For the LAD the sensitivity increases from 10% to 91% when the required confidence level drops from 4 to 1. The corresponding ROC curves for the RCA and LAD are shown in Figure 12.8. Included in this ROC curve are data from the studies by Manning et al. and Post et al. (10,20). The study by Post et al. provides a breakdown for LAD and RCA using two reading criteria that are equivalent to confidence levels as defined earlier: A = stenosis certainly present; and B = stenosis probably present (20). These ROC curves reflect both problems in image quality and problems with our ability to define coronary lesions on diagnostic valuable images.

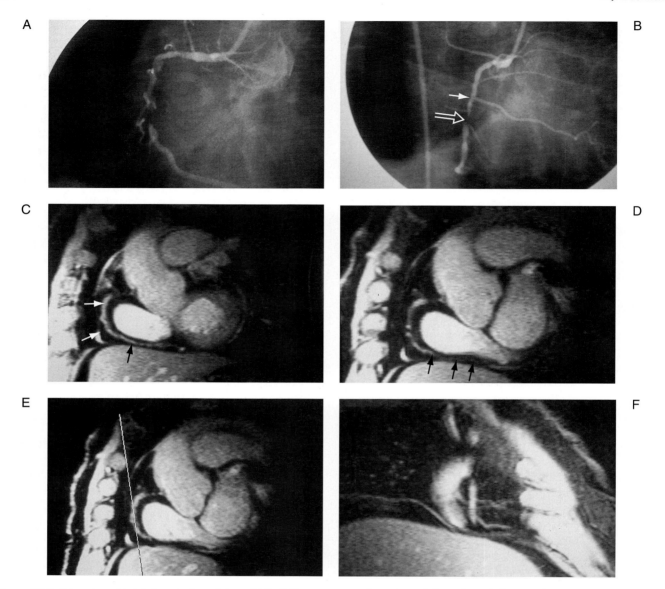

Figure 12.5. Discrete subtotal short lesion of the middle RCA not demonstrated on the coronary MRA, but erroneously suggested on a small subset of the MRI. (A) Conventional angiogram, LAO view. (B) Conventional angiogram, RAO view. The subtotal lesion is seen well on both projections. Also noted are two prominent acute marginal branches that originate just proximal (short arrow) and distal (open arrow) to the lesion. On the RAO view, a right atrial branch is also noted, which originates proximal to the discrete lesions. (C–E) Coronary MRA corresponding to the LAO view in four parallel imaging planes separated by a few millimeters. In the first plane (C), the proximal, middle, and portions of the distal RCA are shown (arrows). The origin of the RCA is located in a different plane and is not visible. There is no evidence of a discrete lesion in this plane. In the immediately adjacent plane (D), a similar appearance of the RCA is shown with a better visualization of the distal RCA (arrows). At the area of the short subtotal lesion, there is a slight bulge in the appearance of the mid-RCA. This corresponds to an overlap of the mid-RCA with two acute marginal branches. In (D) the appearance of the mid-RCA on the coronary MRA could erroneously sug-

gest detection of the subtotal short mid-RCA lesion. However, what is actually shown are cross-sections of the very tortuous proximal portions of the acute marginal branches as shown on the conventional angiogram (A, B). Using an LAO equivalent view of the mid-RCA as a localizer, an imaging plane was selected perpendicular to this view. (F) Coronary MRA corresponding to the RAO view taken at 90-degree angles from the images shown in (C–E). The acute marginal branches shown on the conventional angiogram (B) are clearly demonstrated. The visualized portion of the mid-RCA is located between the take-off of these two acute marginal branches and shows a slightly heterogeneous signal intensity but no clear evidence of a subtotal short lesion. This case illustrates how careful analysis of multiple adjacent parallel slices is needed to avoid under- or over-interpretation of lesions, and/or artifacts. In this particular case, the only evidence of a lesion can be seen on the RAO equivalent view and consists of a slight heterogeneity of MR signal at the location of the lesion. On the LAO equivalent views, however, there is no evidence of the lesion as shown in slice C and D. (Reprinted with permission from Duerinckx (26).)

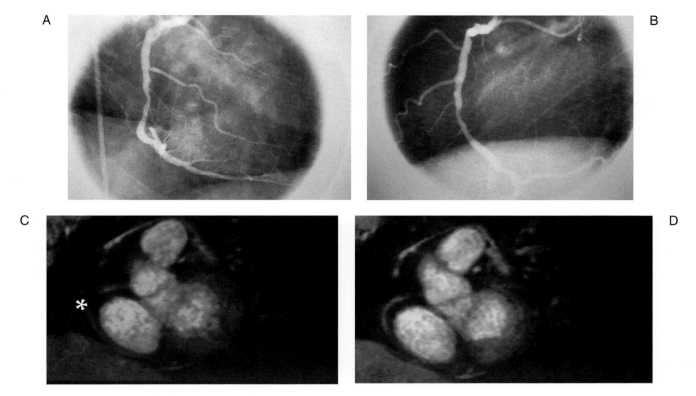

Figure 12.6. Discrete eccentric long stenosis in the mid-RCA not demonstrated on the coronary MRA. (A) Conventional angiogram, LAO view. (B) Conventional angiogram, RAO view. The discrete lesion in the RCA is best seen on the RAO view and to a lesser extent on the LAO view. (C,D) Coronary MRA corresponding to the LAO view in two parallel imaging planes located in the anterior atrioventricular groove are shown. In the first imaging plane (C), the proximal and middle RCA are shown. There is an appearance of flow void (asterisk) in the proximal RCA; however, in an adjacent plane (D), obtained just a few millimeters parallel to the original plane, there is clear continuity of the proximal into the mid-RCA illustrating continuity of RCA. (Reprinted with permission from Duerinckx (26).)

Lesion Detection Using First-, Second-, and Third-Generation Coronary MRA: The 1995–2000 Period

It was originally hoped that coronary MRA could become a noninvasive screening tool for the detection of coronary artery lesions. The results with first-generation coronary MRA in the 1993–1994 period were very promising but somewhat variable. The first-generation 2-D breathhold MRI technique (see also Chap. 15) was tested by several investigators on a total of approximately 224 patients and was able to detect significant coronary artery lesions (greater than 50% diameter narrowing) with a sensitivity ranging from 33% to 100% (see Table 12.3, top part). The reported sensitivity also varied depending upon the vessel examined, as shown in Figure 12.4. Because all the early studies were done with a surface coil positioned on the anterior chest wall, the more posteriorly located circumflex coronary artery was the more difficult one to visualize. More recent studies have used phased-array thoracic coils, with bet-

ter visualization of the circumflex coronary artery. The early 3-D techniques did not make a significant difference. The initial clinical results were very disappointing with a sensitivity of 0–38%, as shown in Table 12.3 (27,28). The second-generation 3-D coronary MRA trials came in 1994–1995 using navigator–pulse feedback (see also Chaps. 16–19). With the original implementation of these techniques a few investigators were able to demonstrate a sensitivity from 65% to 87% for lesion detection, as shown in Table 12.3 (28–30). Many modifications and improvements for this second-generation coronary MRA approach have since been proposed and implemented (see Chaps. 16–19). These improved second-generation coronary MRA show great promise. Even these improved navigator techniques, however, still require long acquisition times with all the inherent risks of erratic breathing or motion. Thus, we have the interest in developing newer techniques that allow multiple slice acquisition in one breathhold, referred to as the third-generation coronary MRA techniques. Only very preliminary clinical results are available for the third-generation coronary MRA techniques (31,32). The

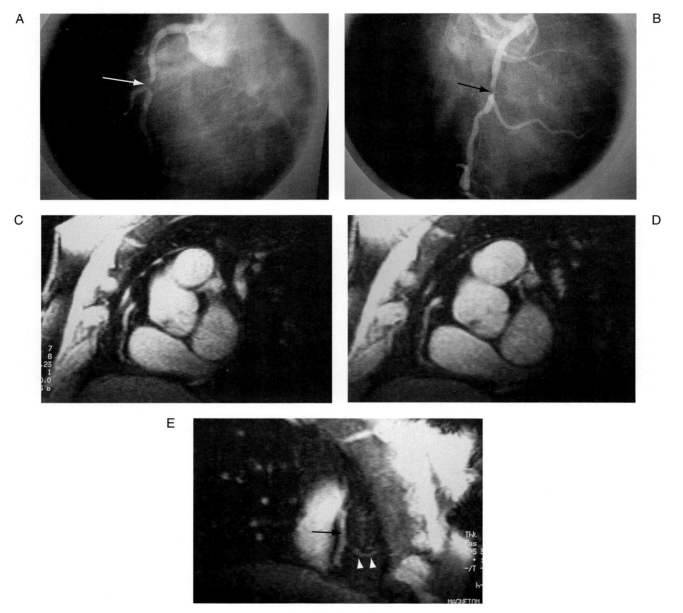

Figure 12.7. Short discrete lesion in the mid-RCA not demonstrated after careful review of all coronary MRA images, but with the potential of being overread as present on the MRA if all images are not analyzed. (A) Conventional angiogram, LAO view showing a short discrete lesion in the proximal RCA (arrow). (B) Conventional angiogram, RAO view showing the same short discrete lesion in the proximal RCA (arrow) with an acute marginal branch taking off just distal to the lesion (open arrow). (C,D) Coronary MRAs corresponding to the LAO view in two parallel imaging planes located in the anterior atrioventricular groove. On one of these images (C), an ill-defined region of decreased flow signal is seen that could erroneously be interpreted as representing the RCA lesion. On all other images (D) obtained in similar planes, however, the RCA appears without any evidence of lesion. (E) Coronary MRAs corresponding to the RAO view, showing the mid-RCA (arrow) and an acute marginal branch (arrowhead), as seen on the conventional angiogram (B). Again there is no evidence of lesions in the region of the RCA with a lesion. (Reprinted with permission from Duerinckx (26).)

Table 12.1. Image quality grading for MR coronary angiography images.

Description	Image quality grade
Not seen: severe artifact; could not be obtained	0
Very poor image quality	1
Poor image quality, insufficient to evaluate for lesions	2
Acceptable image quality (adequate to evaluate lesions)	3
Good image quality	4
Very good sharp images	5

From: Duerinckx AJ. Coronary MR angiography. *In*: Cardiac MR Imaging, Boxt LM, guest ed., *MRI Clin North Am* 1996;4(2):361–418; with permission.

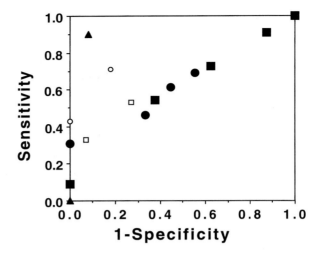

Figure 12.8. Receiver operating curve (ROC) for the detection of hemodynamically significant (≥ 50% diameter narrowing) coronary lesions in coronary arteries, based on data in three published clinical studies: (1) ● = RCA data and ■ = LAD data (Reprinted with permission from Duerinckx et al., 1994, (16).) (2) ○ = RCA data and □ = LAD data (Reprinted with permission from Post et al., 1995; (20).). (3) ▲ = all data (Reprinted with permission from Manning et al., (10).)

results of all these preclinical trials of the use of coronary MRA for coronary artery lesions detection are summarized in Table 12.3. After 6 years of preclinical trials of many different coronary MRA techniques, no technique has yet emerged as a clear winner that can provide a sensitivity and specificity for coronary lesion detection that compares with traditional contrast coronary angiography (4).

An important practical issue is the overreading or underreading of coronary lesions on 2-D coronary MRA. It is important for potential users of this technique to understand the interpretative difficulties with these techniques. There are several possible explanations for why a coronary lesion is not visualized by first-generation 2-D coronary MRA. These include spatial and temporal resolution, timing of the acquisition (within the cardiac cycle), irregular breathing and misregistration between breathholds, partial voluming of tortuous vessels and overlapping adjacent anatomical structures, reverse flow past an area of stenosis (collateral flow), and the unknown signal and contrast characteristics of vessel wall and plaque on coronary MRA sequences.

The performance of first-generation coronary MRA is still relatively time consuming and requires the pres-

Table 12.2. Response categories for ROC analysis for assessment of MR coronary angiography images.

Level of confidence of stenosis presence	Confidence code
Definitely absent	0
Probably absent	1
Uncertain either way	2
Probably present	3
Definitely present	4

From: Duerinckx AJ. Coronary MR angiography. *In*: Cardiac MR imaging, Boxt LM, guest ed., *MRI Clin North Am* 1996;4(2):361–418; with permission.

ence of a trained cardiac imager (25). With a moderate amount of training and practice, most radiologists and cardiologists should be able to perform these studies. Several excellent review articles have provided guidance for the time-efficient performance of these examinations (24,26,48,49).

Unresolved Issue: Will the Sensitivity for Lesion Detection Be Good Enough for Clinical Practice?

The most important limitation to the clinical implementation of coronary MRA is the great variation in the appearance of significant (≥ 50%) coronary lesions and the large number of image artifacts that can be misinterpreted as representing lesions (25). Although this has been best documented for first-generation 2-D coronary MRA techniques, preliminary evidence in normals seems to indicate that the problem may be worse with the initial implementations of the second-generation techniques using navigator pulses (45). In a study of normal volunteers imaged with a 3-D coronary MRA technique with navigator feedback, Stehling found that about 50% of the studies were of unacceptable quality, making interpretation of the images difficult or impossible.

It is obvious that the coronary MRA techniques available today have limitations when it comes to lesion detection. Clinical studies are needed to determine whether these techniques, with whatever limitation they have, would still have an impact on selecting clinical pathways for patient care and intervention. The ultimate

Table 12.3. Sensitivity and specificity for coronary lesion detection by coronary MRA: a literature survey (1993–2000).

	n	# les	Sensitivity	Specificity
First-generation techniques				
One slice; one breathhold				
Manning et al., 1993 (Ref. 10)	39	52*	90%	92%
Manning et al., 1994 (Ref. 12)	72	81	90%	
Duerinckx et al., 1993 (Ref. 13)	20	27	63%	n/a
Duerinckx et al., 1994 (Ref. 15)			(0% to	
& Duerinckx et al., Dec 1994 (Ref. 16)			75%)**	
Post et al., 1994 (Ref. 19)	14	14	36%	
Post et al., 1995 (Ref. 20)	35	35	33%-A **	
			75%-B **	
Pennell et al., 1994 (Ref. 9)	17	23	65%	
Pennell et al., 1995 (Ref. 21)	31	41	88% ***	
Nitatori et al., 1995 (Ref. 22)				
& Nitatori et al., 1995 (Ref. 33)	50	n/a	83% to 100%	
Pennell et al., 1996 (Ref. 34)	39	n/a	85 (75–100)	
Mohiaddin et al., 1996 (Ref. 35)				
& Mohiaddin et al., 1996 (Ref. 36)	16	9	56%	82%
Yoshino et al., Aug 1997 (Ref. 37)	36	31	83% LAD	98% LAD
			100% RCA	100% RCA
Post el al., March 1997 (Ref. 38)	35		53% LAD	73% LAD
			71% RCA	n/a RCA
Total number of patients = 224				
Transition from first- to				
second-generation				
Multislice acquisitions				
Post et al., 1994 (Ref. 27)	22	17	0%	
Post et al., 1996 (Ref. 28)	20	21	38%	95%
Second-generation techniques				
Navigator pulses; no breathholding				
Müller et al., 1996 (Ref. 30)	33	n/a	87%	97%
Müller et al., July 1997 (Ref. 39)	35	54	83%	94%
Kessler et al., Oct 1997 (Ref. 40)	73	43	65%	n/a
Woodard et al., (Ref. 29)	10	10	80%	
Woodard et al., April 1998 (Ref. 41)				
Huber et al., 1999 (Ref. 42)	20	53	73%	50%
		53+	79%	54%
Sandstede et al., 1999 (Ref. 43)	30	37	81%	89%
Van Geuns et al., 1999 (Ref. 44)	29	26	50%	91%
Sardanelli et al., 2000 (Ref. 45)	42	n/a	82%	89%
Second-generation techniques (3-D)				
Navigator pulses; no breathholding				
Prospective navigator approach				
Lethimmonier, 1999 (Ref. 46)	20	17	65%	93%
Total number of patients **** = 118				
Regenfus et al., 1999 (Ref. 47)	30	31	77	94
Third-generation techniques (3-D)				
Multiple slices; one breathhold				
Hu et al., April 1996 (Ref. 31)	23	27	63%	
van Geuns et al., April 2000 (Ref. 32)	13	9	66%	n/a

Results of clinical trials using coronary MRA (sensitivity and specificity), as compared with conventional angiography, to identify individual vessels with ≥ 50% angiographic stenoses. Results are expressed in percent (%), n = number of subjects; # les = number of lesions with significant disease; all results published as *peer-reviewed journal articles* are indicated in **BOLD** lettering.

*Number of vessels instead of lesions.

**Variable sensitivities depending upon detection threshold used to interpret images (see Duerinckx 1996, Ref. 26).

***Study interpretation not fully blinded.

****Total number of patients; this total does not reflect numbers reported at meetings in partial or preliminary oral or poster reports.

+sens. and spec. for subset of images with higher image quality.

Modified from: Duerinckx AJ. (Clinics) Coronary magnetic resonance angiography. *Radiol Clin North Am* 1999;37(2):273–318; and from Duerinckx AJ. Imaging of coronary artery disease—MR. *J Thorac Imaging* 2000;16(1):25–34; with permission.

clinical utility of a coronary MRA screening technique should be compared with the noninvasive alternatives, such as coronary calcium screening using electron-beam computed tomography (EB-CT) (51), EB-CT visualization of the coronary vessels (52,53), echocardiography, nuclear medicine studies, and even treadmill stress testing. None of the existing noninvasive techniques have a 100% sensitivity. Each technique has its own limitation, and the ultimate relative value of coronary MRA with respect to these techniques remains to be determined in future studies.

Another problem is that the expectations for coronary MRA were somewhat unrealistic to begin with. MRA in peripheral vessels and even in larger vessels, such as the carotid arteries, has well-known limitations and image artifacts (54). Nevertheless, MRA of the carotid arteries is well accepted and clinically used. It was unrealistic to expect that MRI techniques when applied to small vessels on the heart submitted to cardiac and respiratory motion would be able to perform any better than they can in relatively stationary vessels, such as the peripheral vasculature or the carotid arteries. In addition, one expects a very high sensitivity for lesion detection in the coronary territory, whereas a lesser sensitivity in the peripheral vasculature would be acceptable.

Lesion appearance and the presence of collateral flow also complicate image interpretation as described earlier. Discrete coronary lesions (total and subtotal occlusions) may appear as areas of signal void, decreased flow signal, or vessel wall irregularity (26). A subacute thrombus can mimic flowing blood (55). This is sometimes different from the more traditional appearance of lesions in larger vessels on MRA. In addition, because of collateral flow, a total occlusion may have slow-moving fluid present in a vessel distal to the occlusion and show a normal vessel flow signal. A correlate of this is the fact that the significance of a coronary lesion cannot be quantitated at the present time on coronary MRA. The typical spatial resolution is $1.5 \times 1 \times 4$ mm for coronary vessels measuring 2–4 mm in diameter. The problems with trying to measure luminal diameter narrowing for coronary MRA have been clearly outlined in two studies (34,56). Pennell et al. classified the degree of MR signal loss in the region of a known coronary artery lesion as severe or partial, and, additionally, noted when an irregular vessel outline was present. The main percentage of stenosis was significantly different for each type of signal loss, suggesting that visual assessment of signal loss can be a qualitative guide to stenotic severity. They also measured the relation between the proportion of magnetic resonance signal loss at the site of stenosis directly on the screen and the diameter stenosis assessed by X-ray angiography. There was a significant relation between stenosis severity and MR signal loss, although with a considerable scatter in individual measurements. They were never able to measure "lu-

minal diameter reduction." Shimamoto et al. (56) provided a detailed analysis of the use of spatial profile curves to better measure the diameter of coronary arteries on MR angiograms. This problem in quantitating the severity of stenosis was discussed early on by Duerinckx et al. (16) and Pennell et al. (34). Duerinckx et al. have suggested that this problem in quantitating the severity of stenosis can be circumvented by using "confidence levels" for the presence of significant disease and by using ROC analysis to interpret image data (16,26).

Is There a Gold Standard to Evaluate New Technologies?

A detailed protocol for the interpretation and reading of coronary MRA has been described by Duerinckx et al. and was briefly described in an earlier section. For each segment of vessel (for the visualized portion of the coronary anatomy), this protocol includes the following: (1) length and width of vessel, (2) grading of image quality, and (3) likelihood of presence of significant lesion or any (mild or moderate) disease (i.e., confidence levels for ROC analysis). This protocol, together with an estimate of intra- and interobserver variability in interpretation could form the basis for multicenter evaluations of any of these new coronary angiographic techniques. This preassumes the existence of a "gold" standard, however, to compare the new findings to. Does such a standard really exist? We will discuss the problems with the generally accepted standard of iodinated contrast-based angiography.

Presence or absence of coronary artery lesions is traditionally evaluated with coronary angiography. However, it has been well documented that there is great interobserver variability in the interpretation of coronary angiograms (57,58). Moreover, the assessment of significance of coronary stenosis based on interpretations of the coronary angiogram only is very questionable (59,60). We will briefly address both of these issues.

One older study by Zir et al. (58) from 1976 demonstrated that in only 65% of coronary angiograms did four observers agree about the significance of a stenosis (defined as greater than 50% of luminal narrowing) in the proximal or mid-left LAD. In this study four experienced coronary angiographers (two radiologists and two cardiologists) independently assessed the location and degree of coronary artery stenosis in 20 coronary angiograms and demonstrated the substantial degree of variability among four experienced coronary angiographers in the interpretation of coronary angiography. This was even more surprising in the sense that all four angiographers were from the same institutions and had frequently participated as a group in the interpretation of coronary angiograms. The 20 angiograms in their study included the typical spectrum of coronary angiographic findings with very few normal coronary arteries or single vessel disease.

The concept of what is a "gold" standard is constantly being reevaluated and questioned, and the problems of interobserver variability are not unique to the interpretation of coronary angiograms: They have also been reported in the interpretation of other vascular imaging studies (61–71). The reasons for the observed variability in coronary angiograms in the older studies like Zir et al. (58) can be related to: limited number of projections; partial visualization of the vessel segments with lesions; the quality of the coronary angiograms; differences in perception. Some of these problems no longer exist with the newer cardiac cathetherization laboratories; however, many important ones remain (62,63). One of the most important factors contributing to the variability was disagreement as to which portion of the vessel to use as a normal reference when calculating the percent coronary stenosis. Large portions of the vessels are frequently abnormal, making such determination difficult. There may be dilatation, lesions may be multiple, or lesions may be smooth or tapering. There are several approaches to reduce the error due to interobserver variability. One would be to combine independent readings. Another would be to use a consensus opinion based on joint reading of the coronary angiogram.

These difficulties in determining the level of stenosis of a coronary lesion could partially explain the problems with the poor correlation between coronary stenosis and functional significance of coronary lesion. The variations in cross-sectional shape of the lesions also accounts for some of the discrepancies. This well-known phenomenon can be solved by obtaining multiple projections of single lesions. In the case of a left main coronary artery or the proximal LAD, there are unfortunately often so many overlapping vessels that are difficult to separate even with several views.

One has to keep these discrepancies in interpretation of coronary angiographs in mind when designing and interpreting studies comparing new technologies, such as coronary MRA or EB-CT angiography with conventional coronary angiograms. If one preassumes that the conventional contrast-based coronary angiography is the gold standard, and does not take into account the great variability in interpretation, one may draw erroneous conclusions about the performance of either MR- or EB-CT–based coronary angiography. Thus, the results of prospective blind studies comparing both technologies should be interpreted with great caution. Each study should include a retrospective analysis of the data because in some instances coronary MRA or EB-CT angiography may provide additional information that is difficult to gain from a traditional conventional coronary angiogram with limited number of views of multiple superimposed vessels.

Coronary Lesion Detection by MRI in the Future

Coronary MRA technique development has been proceeding at a very fast pace. So fast, indeed, that most techniques never even have a chance of being evaluated by more than one or two investigators before everybody moves on to the next technique. Clinical users should not be disappointed by this or view this as an indication that these techniques are not working. As clearly demonstrated in Chapters 7–11, the first-generation coronary MRA techniques are more than adequate for a large number of specific clinical applications. They are even capable of detecting significant coronary lesions with 65–80% sensitivity in many centers. The early implementations of the second-generation coronary MRA techniques required long acquisition times, which explains their unpredictable behavior. When images were good, they were very good; however, equally often they were very bad and not interpretable. The improved second-generation coronary MRA techniques using navigator pulse feedback and adaptive prospective (or interactive) correction of slice position (72,73) or signal averaging (74) dramatically improve the reliability and image quality and thus increase the sensitivity of the technique. A multicenter trial has evaluated one implementation of the navigator-based coronary MRA techniques (75). The third-generation techniques, 3-D thin slab breathhold techniques, appear very promising and easy to use (see Chaps. 20–21). The advent of blood pool agents may also impact our capability to detect lesions better (see Chaps. 24–25) (76,77). Higher spatial resolution (down to 370 μm) may also help further delineate lesion severity (78). Hybrid techniques, as originally suggested by Wang et al., which combine the best of breathhold and navigator technology, are promising (79). Black-blood MR imaging may help better characterize coronary lesions (80–82). Direct MR imaging of the coronary vessel wall and plaque may also open new ways to characterize and detect lesion severity (83–86). We hope soon to have a useful array of complementary noninvasive MRA approaches to the evaluation of coronary lesions that will be easy to use and will provide reproducible results.

Acknowledgments: Images are partially reproduced from: Duerinckx AJ. Coronary MRA. *In*: Cardiac MR imaging, Boxt LM, guest ed.; *MRI Clin North Am* 1996;4(2): 361–418; with permission; and Duerinckx AJ. (Clinics) Coronary magnetic resonance angiography. *Radiol Clin North Am* 1999;37(2):273–318; with permission.

References

1. Caputo GC. Coronary arteries: potential for MR imaging (editorial). Radiology 1991;181(3):629–30.

2. Caputo RC. Coronary MR angiography: a clinical perspective (editorial). Radiology 1994;193(3):596–98.

3. Rogers LF. The heart of the matter: noninvasive coronary artery imaging (editorial). Am J Roentgenol 1998;170:841.

4. Dinsmore RE. Noninvasive coronary arteriography—here at last? [comment]. Circulation 1995;91(5):1607–8.

5. Goldsmith MF. Realizing potential of MR coronary angiography may ease patients' test load and diagnosis costs (editorial). JAMA 1994;271(4):256.

6. Duerinckx AJ. (Clinics) Coronary magnetic resonance angiography. Radiol Clin North Am 1999; March: (in press).

7. Danias PG, Edelman RR, Manning WJ. Coronary MR angiography. Cardiol Clin 1998;16(2):207–25.

8. Wielopolski PA, van Geuns RJ, de Feyter PJ, Oudkerk M. Coronary arteries. Eur Radiol 1998;8(6):873–85.

9. Pennell DJ, Bogren HG, Keegan J, Firmin DW, Underwood SR. Coronary artery stenosis: assessment by magnetic resonance imaging (abstr.). In: Book of Abstracts of the Eleventh Annual Scientific Meeting of the European Society for Magnetic Resonance in Medicine and Biology. Vienna, Austria, April 20–24, 1994:374.

10. Manning WJ, Li W, Edelman RR. A preliminary report comparing magnetic resonance coronary angiography with conventional angiography. N Engl J Med 1993;328:828–32.

11. Rogers WJ, Kramer CM, Simonetti OP, Reichek N. Quantification of human coronary stenoses by magnetic resonance angiography (abstr.). In: Printed Program of the Second Meeting of the Society of Magnetic Resonance (SMR), Vol. 1, p. 370. San Francisco, August 6–12, 1994; JMRI.

12. Manning WJ, Li W, Wielopolski P, Gaa J, Kannam JP, Edelman RR. Magnetic resonance coronary angiography: comparison with contrast angiography (abstr). In: Book of Abstracts and Proceedings of the Second Meeting of the the the Society of Magnetic Resonance (SMR). San Francisco, August 6–12, 1994; Vol. I: p. 368.

13. Duerinckx AJ, Urman M, Sinha U, Atkinson D, Simonetti O. Evaluation of gadolinium-enhanced MR coronary angiography (abstr.). In: Seventy-ninth Scientific Assembly and Annual Meeting of the Radiological Society of North America (RSNA). Chicago, Nov 28–Dec 3, 1993; Radiology 1993;189(P):278.

14. Duerinckx AJ, Urman MK, Atkinson DJ, Simonetti OP, Sinha U, Lewis B. Limitations of MR coronary angiography (abstr.). In: Printed Program of the First Meeting of the Society of Magnetic Resonance (SMR). Dallas, Texas, March 5–9, 1994; JMRI 1994;4:81.

15. Duerinckx AJ, Urman MK. Hemodynamically significant coronary artery lesions missed with MR coronary angiography (abstr.). In: Printed Program of the First Meeting of the Society of Magnetic Resonance (SMR). Dallas, Texas, March 5–9; 1994; J Magn Reson Imag 1994;4(P):80.

16. Duerinckx AJ, Urman M. Two-dimensional coronary MR angiography: analysis of initial clinical results. Radiology 1994;193:731–38.

17. Manning WJ, Edelman RR. Coronary MR angiography (letter-to-the-editor). Radiology 1995;195(3):875.

18. Duerinckx AJ. Coronary MR angiography (response-to-letter-to-the-editor). Radiology 1995;195(3):876.

19. Post JC, vanRossum AC, Hofman MBM, Valk J, Visser CA. Current limitations of two dimensional breathhold MR angiography in coronary artery disease (abstr.). In: Book of Abstracts and Proceedings of the Second Meeting of the the Society of Magnetic Resonance (SMR) (#508). San Francisco, August 7–12, 1994; Vol. I: 508.

20. Post JC, vanRossum AC, Hofman MBM, Valk J, Visser CA. Clinical utility of two dimensional breathhold MR angiography in coronary artery disease (abstr.). In: Book of Abstracts of the Third Meeting of the Society of Magnetic Resonance (SMR) and the Twelfth Annual Scientific Meeting of the European Society for Magnetic Resonance in Medicine and Biology (ESMRMB). Nice, France, August 20–25, 1995.

21. Pennell DJ, Bogren HG, Keegan J, Firmin DN, Underwood SR. Detection, localization and assessment of coronary artery stenosis by magnetic resonance imaging (abstr). In: Book of Abstracts and Proceedings of the Second Meeting of the the Society of Magnetic Resonance (SMR). San Francisco, August 6–12, 1994; Vol. I: 369.

22. Nitatori T, Hachiya J, Korenaga T, Hanaoka H, Yoshino, A. Clinical application of coronary MR angiography: studies on shortening of time for examination (abstr.). In: Book of Abstracts of the Third Meeting of the Society of Magnetic Resonance (SMR) and the Twelfth Annual Scientific Meeting of the European Society for Magnetic Resonance in Medicine and Biology (ESMRMB). Nice, France, August 20–25, 1995.

23. Mohiaddin RH, Bogren HG, Firmin DN, Keegan J. MR Angiography of the coronary arteries in heart transplants (abstr.). In: Book of Abstracts of Seventh International Workshop on Magnetic Resonance Angiography. Matsuyama, Japan; Oct 12–14, 1995.

24. Duerinckx AJ. Review: MR Angiography of the coronary arteries. Top Magn Reson Imag 1995;7(4):267–85.

25. Duerinckx AJ, Atkinson DP, Mintorovitch J, Simonetti OP, Urman MK. Two-dimensional coronary MR angiography: limitations and artifacts. Eur Radiol 1996;6(3):312–25.

26. Duerinckx AJ. Coronary MR angiography. In: Cardiac MR imaging, Boxt LM, guest ed. MRI Clin North Am 1996;4(2):361–418.

27. Post JC, vanRossum AC, Hofman MBM, Valk J, Visser CA. Respiratory-gated three dimensional MR angiography of coronary arteries and comparison with X-ray contrast angiography (abstr.). In: Book of Abstracts and Proceedings of the Second Meeting of the Society of Magnetic Resonance (SMR) (#509). San Francisco, August 7–12, 1994; Vol. I: 509.

28. Post JC, vanRossum AC, Hofman MB, Valk J, Visser CA. Three-dimensional repiratory-gated MR angiography of coronary arteries: comparison with conventional coronary angiography. Am J Roentgenol 1996;166(6):1399–1404.

29. Woodard PK, Li D, Dhawale P, et al. Identification of coronary artery stenosis with 3D retrospective respiratory gating (abstr.). In: Ninety-sixth Annual Meeting of the American Roentgen Ray Society, supplement to AJR. San Diego, May 5–10, 1996;166(3).

30. Müller MF, Fleisch M, Kroeker R. Coronary arteries: three-dimensional MR imaging with fat saturation and navigator echo (abstr.) Radiology 1996;201(P):274.

31. Hu BS, Meyer CH, Macovski A, Nishimura DG. Multislice spiral magnetic resonance coronary angiography

(abstr.). *In*: Book of Abstracts of the Fourth Meeting of the International Society of Magnetic Resonance in Medicine (ISMRM). New York, April 27–May 3, 1996; Vol. 1: 671.

32. van Geuns RJ, Wielopolski PA, de Bruin HG, et al. MR coronary angiography with breath-hold targeted volumes: preliminary clinical results. Radiology 2000;217(1):270–77.

33. Nitatori T, Hanaoka H, Yoshino A, et al. Clinical application of magnetic resonance angiography for coronary arteries: correlation with conventional angiography and evaluation of imaging time. Nippon Acta Radiol 1995;55:670–76.

34. Pennell DJ, Bogren HG, Keegan J, Firmin DN, Underwood SR. Assessment of coronary artery stenosis by magnetic resonance imaging. Heart 1996;75:127–33.

35. Mohiaddin RH, Bogren HG, Lazim F, et al. Magnetic resonance coronary angiography in heart transplant recipients (abstr.). *In*: Book of Abstracts of the Fourth Meeting of the International Society of Magnetic Resonance in Medicine (ISMRM). New York, April 27–May 3, 1996; Vol. 2: 671.

36. Mohiaddin RH, Bogren HG, Lazim F, et al. Magnetic resonance coronary angiography in heart transplant recipients. Cor Art Dis 1996;7(8):591–97.

37. Yoshino H, Nitatori T, Kachi E, et al. Directed proximal magnetic resonance coronary angiography compared with conventional contrast coronary angiography. Am J Cardiol 1997;80(4):514–18.

38. Post JC, van Rossum AC, Hofman MB, de Cock CC, Valk J, Visser CA. Clinical utility of two-dimensional magnetic resonance angiography in detecting coronary artery disease. Eur Heart J 1997;18(3):426–33.

39. Müller MF, Fleisch M, Kroeker R, Chatterjee T, Meier B, Vock P. Proximal coronary artery stenosis: three-dimensional MRI with fat saturation and navigator echo. J Magn Reson Imag 1997;7(4):644–51.

40. Kessler W, Achenbach S, Moshage W, et al. Usefulness of respiratory gated magnetic resonance coronary angiography in assessing narrowings >50% in diameter in native coronary arteries and in aortocoronary bypass conduits. Am J Cardiol 1997;80:989–93.

41. Woodard PK, Li D, Haacke EM, et al. Detection of coronary stenosis on source and projection images using three-dimensional MR angiography with retrospective respiratory gating: preliminary experience. Am J Roentgenol 1998;170:883–88.

42. Huber A, Nikolaou K, Ganschior P, Knez A, Stehling M, Reiser M. Navigator-echo-based respiratory gating for three-dimensional MR coronary angiography: results from healthy volunteers and patients with proximal coronary artery stenoses. Am J Roentgenol 1999;173(1):95–101.

43. Sandstede JJ, Pabst T, Beer M, et al. Three-dimensional MR coronary angiography using the navigator technique compared with conventional coronary angiography. Am J Roentgenol 1999;172(1):135–39.

44. van Geuns RJ, de Bruin HG, Rensing BJ, et al. Magnetic resonance imaging of the coronary arteries: clinical results from three-dimensional evaluation of a respiratory gated technique. Heart 1999;82(4):515–19.

45. Sardanelli F, Molinari G, Zandrino F, Balbi M. Three-dimensional, navigator-echo MR coronary angiography in detecting stenoses of the major epicardial vessels, with

conventional coronary angiography as the standard of reference [see comments]. Radiology 2000;214(3):808–14.

46. Lethimonnier F, Furber A, Morel O, et al. Three-dimensional coronary artery MR imaging using prospective real-time respiratory navigator and linear phase shift processing: comparison with conventional coronary angiography. Magn Reson Imag 1999;17(8):1111–20.

47. Regenfus M, Ropers D, Achenbach S, et al. Gadolinium enhanced 3D breathhold magnetic resonance angiography for detection of coronary artery stenosis in oblique projection angiograms (abstr). *In*: Book of Abstracts and Proceedings of the Seventh Meeting of the International Society of Magnetic Resonance in Medicine (ISMRM). Philadelphia, May 22–28:1999;1262.

48. Manning W, Edelman R. Magnetic resonance coronary angiography. Magn Reson Q 1993;9(3):131–51.

49. Pennell DJ, Keegan J, Firmin DN, Gatehouse PD, Underwood SR, Longmore DB. Magnetic resonance imaging of coronary arteries: technique and preliminary results. Br Heart J 1993;70(4):315–26.

50. Stehling M. Coronary arteries: experience with navigator echoes (abstr). *In*: Eighth International Workshop on Magnetic Resonance Angiography. Rome, Italy; Oct 16–19, 1996.

51. Wexler L, Brundage B, Crouse J, et al. Coronary artery calcification: pathophysiology, epidemiology, imaging methods, and clinical implications. A statement for health professionals from the American Heart Association Writing Group. Circulation 1996;94(5):1175–92.

52. Moshage WEL, Achenbach S, Seese B, Bachman K, Kirchgeorg M. Coronary artery stenosis: three-dimensional imaging with electrocardiographically triggered, contrast agent-enhanced, electron-beam CT. Radiology 1995;196(3):707–14.

53. Chernoff DM, Ritchie CJ, Higgins CB. Electron-beam CT coronary angiography: imaging characteristics in normal coronary arteries. Radiology 1996;201(P):274.

54. Patel MR, Klufas RA, Kim D, Edelman RE, Kent KC. MR angiography of the carotid bifurcation: artifacts and limitations. Am J Roentgenol 1994;162:1431–37.

55. Borelli C, Berthezene Y, Olteanu B, et al. Subacute coronary artery thrombus: MRI findings. JCAT 1997;21(6):962–64.

56. Shimamota R, Suzuki J-i, Nishikawa J-i, et al. Measuring the diameter of coronary arteries on MR angiograms using spatial profile curves. Am J Roentgenol 1998;170:889–93.

57. Galbraith JE, Murphy ML, Desoyza N. Coronary angiogram interpretation: interobserver variability. JAMA 1981;240:2053–59.

58. Zir LM, Miller SW, Dinsomore RE, et al. Interobserver variability in coronary angiography. Circulation 1976;53(4):627–23.

59. Marcus M, Skorton D, Johnson M, Collins S, Harrison D, Kerber R. Visual estimates of percent diameter coronary stenosis: "a battered gold standard." J Am Cell Cardiol 1988;11:882–85.

60. Nissen SE, Gurley JC. Assessment of the functional significance of coronary stenoses: is digital angiography the answer? (editorial comment). Circulation 1990;81(4):1431–35.

61. Karkow WS, Cranley JJ. Variations in interpretation of arterial stenosis. J Cardiovasc Surg 1989;30:826–32.

62. Feldman T, Laskey WK. Alchemy in the cath lab: creating a gold standard (editorial; comment). Catheter Cardiovasc Diag 1998;44(1):14–15.

63. Doriot PA, Dorsaz PA, Dorsaz L, Bodenmann JJ. Towards a gold standard for quantitative coronary arteriography. Phys Med Biol 1997;42(12):2449–62.

64. Rushing L, Joste N. The surgical pathology report: standardizing the "gold standard" (editorial). J Surg Oncol 1997;65(1):1–2.

65. Hastings MM, Andes S, Hsu A. The promises of autopsy: still the "gold standard" of quality? (abstr.) Abstr Book Assoc Health Serv Res 1997; 14(181).

66. Post JC, van Rossum AC, Bronzwaer JG, et al. Magnetic resonance angiography of anomalous coronary arteries: a new gold standard for delineating the proximal course? Circulation 1995;92(11):3163–71.

67. Hartnell GG, Hughes LA, Finn JP, Longmaid HE, III. Magnetic resonance angiography of the central chest veins: a new gold standard? Chest 1995;107(4):1053–57.

68. De Man F, De Scheerder I, Herregods MC, Piessens J, De Geest H. Role of intravascular ultrasound in coronary artery disease: a new gold standard? An overview. Acta Cardiol 1994;49(3):223–31.

69. Sacerdoti D, Gaiani S, Buonamico P, et al. Interobserver and interequipment variability of hepatic, splenic, and renal arterial Doppler resistance indices in normal subjects and patients with cirrhosis. J Hepatology 1997;27(6):986–92.

70. van Beek EJ, Bakker AJ, Reekers JA. Pulmonary embolism: interobserver agreement in the interpretation of conventional angiographic and DSA images in patients with non-diagnostic lung scan results. Radiology 1996;198(3):721–24.

71. Singh K, Bonaa KH, Solberg S, Sorlie DG, Bjork L. Intra- and interobserver variability in ultrasound measurements of abdominal aortic diameter: the Tromso Study. Eur J Vasc Endovasc Surg 1998;15(6):497–504.

72. Danias PG, McConnell MV, Khasgiwala VC, Chuang ML, Edelman RR, Manning WJ. Prospective navigator correction of image position for coronary. Radiology 1997; 203(3):733–36.

73. McConnell MV, Khasgiwala VC, Savord BJ, et al. Prospective adaptive navigator correction for breath-hold MR coronary angiography. Magn Reson Med 1997;37(1):148–52.

74. Oshinski JN, Hofland L, Mukundan S, Dixon WT, James WJ, Pettigrew RI. Two-dimensional MR coronary angiography without breath holding. Radiology 1996;201:737–43.

75. Botnar R, Stuber M, Manning WJ, Danias P, Kissinger K, et al. MR coronary artery multicenter study with the Boston Cookbook protocol (abstr.). In: Book of Abstracts of the First International Workshop on Coronary MR & CT Angiography. Lyon, France, Oct 1–3, 2000. Organized and published by the North American Society for Cardiac Imaging. Reprinted in: Int J Card Imag 2000;16(3):2200.

76. Hofman MB, Henson RE, Kovacs SJ, et al. Blood pool agent strongly improves 3D magnetic resonance coronary angiography using an inversion pre-pulse. Magn Reson Med 1999;41(2):360–67.

77. Johansson LO, Nolan NM, Taniuchi M, Fischer SE, Wickline SA, Lorenz CH. High resolution magnetic resonance coronary angiography of the entire heart using a new blood-pool agent, NC100150 injection: comparison with invasive X-ray angiography in pigs. J Cardiovasc Magn Reson 1999;2(1):139–44.

78. Stuber M, Botnar RM, Manning WJ. Towards X-ray angiography image resolution in coronary MRA (abstr.). In: Book of Abstracts of the First International Workshop on Coronary MR & CT Angiography. Lyon, France, Oct 1–3, 2000. Organized and published by the North American Society for Cardiac Imaging. Reprinted in: Int J Card Imag 2000;16(3):215.

79. Wang Y, Christy PS, Korosec FR, et al. Coronary MRI with a respiratory feedback monitor: the 2D imaging case. Magn Reson Med 1995;33(1):116–21.

80. Stuber M, Manning WJ. Black-blood coronary MRA (abstr.). In: Book of Abstracts of the First International Workshop on Coronary MR & CT Angiography. Lyon, France, Oct 1–3, 2000. Organized and published by the North American Society for Cardiac Imaging. Reprinted in: Int J Card Imag 2000;16(3)215.

81. Simonetti OP, Finn JP, White RD, Laub G, Henry DA. "Black blood" T2-weighted inversion-recovery MR imaging of the heart. Radiology 1996;199:49–57.

82. Steinman DA, Rutt BK. On the nature and reduction of plaque-mimicking flow artifacts in black blood MRI of the carotid bifurcation. Magn Reson Med 1998;39(4):635–41.

83. Luk-Pat GT, Gold GE, Olcott EW, Hu BS, Nishimura DG. High-resolution three-dimensional in vivo imaging of atherosclerotic plaque. Magn Reson Med 1999;42(4):762–71.

84. Shinnar M, Fallon JT, Wehrli S, et al. The diagnostic accuracy of ex vivo MRI for human atherosclerotic plaque characterization. Arterioscler Thromb Vasc Biol 1999;19(11):2756–61.

85. Zheng J, Finn JP, Li D. Contrast-enhanced MR coronary artery imaging on a porcine model: in vivo experience. (abstr.). In: Book of Abstracts of the First International Workshop on Coronary MR & CT Angiography. Lyon, France, Oct 1–3, 2000. Organized and published by the North American Society for Cardiac Imaging. Reprinted in: Int J Card Imag 2000;16(3):193.

86. de Bruin HG, vanGeuns RJM, Wielopolski PA, de Feyter PJ, Oudkerk M. Improvement of magnetic resonance imaging of the coronary arteries with a clinically available intravascular contrast agent (abstr.). In: Book of Abstracts of the First International Workshop on Coronary MR & CT Angiography. Lyon, France, Oct 1–3, 2000. Organized and published by the North American Society for Cardiac Imaging. Reprinted in: Int J Card Imag 2000;16(3):192–93.

13
Coronary Flow Measurements Using MRI

André J. Duerinckx

Introduction

Ischemic heart disease remains the leading cause of death in the United States. Much of the clinical care of patients with ischemic heart disease is still heavily based on the "gold standard" of visual interpretation of the coronary angiogram. Several studies, however, have seriously questioned the notion that this gold standard permits accurate assessment of the physiologic significance of coronary obstruction (1,2). In patients with multivessel coronary disease, visual estimates of angiographic percent stenosis correlate poorly with the direct measured physiologic significance of coronary lesions. This is particularly true for obstructions of intermediate severity. In patients with single vessel disease, however, vessel constriction as seen by coronary angiography correlates reasonably well with the physiological significance of obstruction. Clinical evaluations should add physiological information to the "gold standard" of visual interpretation of the coronary angiogram.

A similar conclusion can be drawn for coronary artery bypass grafts (CABGs). Evaluation of the functional status of CABGs is usually required in patients with grafts who have persistent or recurrent symptoms after surgery. From 10 to 30% of grafts are occluded 1–2 years after surgery; 45–55% are occluded by 10–12 years (3). The evaluation of postoperative flow capacity of CABG and native coronary arteries are equally important.

Coronary flow reserve is used to assess the capacity of a vessel to provide increased flow and to quantitate the functional importance of a stenosis. Coronary flow reserve is defined as the maximum flow under conditions of maximal vasodilatation divided by the resting flow. Changes in velocity (e.g., changes in peak diastolic velocity) in native coronary arteries or CABGs can be used to predict the functional significance of a lesion (4,5), plan interventional therapy (6), and predict postsurgical hemodynamics and/or complications (7,8).

Magnetic resonance imaging (MRI) can provide proximal *coronary artery anatomy* (9,10), and information about cardiac function (11), myocardial perfusion, and viability (12). MRI techniques have been used to quantitate *velocity, flow, and flow reserve* in native coronary arteries and CABG in humans (13–20) and in animals (21). The combination of coronary MRA of the proximal coronary arterial tree with MRI-derived information on coronary flow patterns and flow reserve could become a clinical alternative to the existing catheter-based techniques for the evaluation of ischemic heart disease (i.e., conventional coronary angiography and Doppler flow-wire studies).

Hemodynamics in Coronary Vessels

Hemodynamic data include velocity, velocity changes within a cardiac cycle (e.g., peak velocity during diastole), velocity profiles across a vessel (e.g., laminar flow), cross-sectional area, flow = velocity × cross-section, and flow reserve. The noninvasive measurement of any of these hemodynamic parameters can be difficult, and is subject to approximations. Nevertheless it is important to be able to predict the normal ranges of these parameters.

MR Quantification of Coronary Flow

Flow quantification in the cardiovascular system using MRI is well established (22). One category of MR techniques for flow quantification, called *velocity-encoded MRI* (also called "phase-contrast" MRI or cine PC-MRI), is based on the principle that flow across a magnetic field gradient induces a phase shift that is proportional to velocity. To measure the phase shift, pairs of images with different flow sensitivities are acquired and subtracted. Cine PC-MRI generates these pairs of images during several phases (typically 12–18) of the cardiac cycle. Each pair consists of a magnitude image, corresponding to a conventional cine MR image, and a phase image, which provides the velocity information. Traditional cine PC-MRI acquisitions typically take 3–6 minutes per two-dimensional (2-D) imaging plane with image pairs produced for each phase of the cardiac cycle.

There are several well-known problems with cine PC-MRI as discussed by Buonocore et al. (23). These are: (1) the zero-velocity background pixel value; (2) the size and shape of the vessel region-of-interest (ROI); (3) the maximum velocity encoded in diastole; and (4) the temporal resolution. For very small vessels the accuracy of flow estimates drops drastically unless there are at least 16 voxels to cover the cross-sectional area of the vessel lumen (24) or three voxels in a cross-sectional diameter (25). For portions of the cardiac cycle with low velocities, the noise levels due to background noise and intrinsic other noise can be overwhelming. The spatial resolution of these traditional PC-MRI sequences has been adequate for most clinical applications that deal with large vessels. The traditional PC-MRI techniques, as implemented by most commercial vendors, allow random orientations of the imaging plane and both in-plane and cross-plane velocity determination, i.e. these techniques allow one-dimensional (1-D) and full three-dimensional (3-D) velocity quantification. The appropriate selection of the Venc value (Venc = maximal velocity value that can be encoded), or the proper angulation of the plane to guarantee strict through-plane flow can easily be accommodated. Spatial resolution is not usually a problem in larger vessels. The only real remaining problems are the somewhat limited temporal resolution and the background noise.

Cine PC-MRI works well for large vessels and to quantitate blood flow through cardiac valves (22). Because of respiratory motion during the relatively long acquisition times (several minutes), cine PC MRI has been applied with only limited success in coronary bypass grafts (19,26), renal arteries (27,28), the coronary sinus (29), and the indirect estimate of coronary flow reserve in native coronary arteries (13).

Breathhold Velocity-Encoded Cine MRI

Flow quantification in small tortuous vessels subjected to significant physiological motion (e.g., coronary vessels and renal arteries) has required modifications of existing techniques. One of the more common variations relies on a breathhold k-space–segmented cine PC-MRI technique that provides quantitative flow measurements during a single breathhold acquisition (15,16,21,30). The acquisition of each velocity-encoded image pair is segmented over multiple heartbeats (R–R intervals), with each segment being acquired at a set time delay (TD) after the R-wave. The total segment duration per cardiac cycle (which corresponds to the temporal resolu-

Table 13.1. Protocol for segmented cine-PC coronary flow reserve quantification.

Step 1: Visualize the coronary vessel
Step 2: Select image planes for flow quantification
Step 3: Acquire velocity information
Step 4: Perform stress testing for coronary flow reserve
Step 5: Data analysis

From: Duerinckx AJ. Coronary MR angiography. *In*: Cardiac MR imaging, Boxt LM, guest ed. *MRI Clin North Am* 1996;4(2):361–418; with permission.

tion) is $2 \times n$ seg $\times$ TR, where n seg is the number of phase encodings per segment. To be able to acquire a velocity-encoded image pair within a single breathhold (16–20 heartbeats), the duration of each segment becomes a significant fraction of the cardiac cycle. It has been demonstrated that peak volume flow rates can be accurately measured using a segmented PC-MRI technique even when there is significant variation in flow rates over the duration of the segment by relying on the fact that the acquisition time in the low-order phase-encoding step determines the effective point of measurement (31).

A typical protocol for velocity and flow quantification using a breathhold segmented cine PC-MRI scheme would involve the steps described in Table 13.1.

This protocol will probably have to be slightly modified when breathhold PC MRI using segmented echoplanar (32) or spiral scanning (18) becomes routinely available.

Other Techniques

MR flow quantification techniques based on the time-of-flight (TOF) principle have also been modified for coronary artery applications, either using echo-planar imaging (17) or segmented gradient-recalled echo (GRE) pulse sequences (30).

Early Results in Animals and Humans (The 1993–1995 Period)

Only a handful of MRI-based coronary flow quantification studies were published in the 1993–1995 period (13,15,16,18,21). The findings from four of these five studies are summarized in Table 13.2. We will briefly comment on certain features of these published experimental MRI coronary flow studies.

Buonocore (13) measured global coronary flow reserve in healthy subjects and in patients indirectly by traditional phase-contrast MRI using a model that considers the antegrade and retrograde flows in the aorta during systole and diastole. Based on five healthy vol-

Table 13.2. Results of initial MR-based in vivo studies of coronary blood velocity and coronary flow reserve.

	Edelman et al., 1993 (15) Humans	Poncelet et al., 1993 (17) Humans	Clarke et al., 1995 (21) Animals	Keegan et al., 1994 (16) Humans
Through-plane imaging	yes	yes	yes	yes
Number of subjects	11 normals	10 normals	8 mongrel dogs LAD partial occlusion LCx normal	10 normals
Velocity ranges (Diastolic) at rest	Middiastole RCA; 9.9 ± 3.5 cm/sec LAD: 20.5 ± 5.2 cm/sec	Mean diastole LAD: 14 ± 3 cm/sec	Mean diastole LAD: 11.9 ± 5.1 cm/L LCx: 11.8 ± 5.2 cm/sec	3–29 cm/sec
Diastolic vel (stress)	>fourfold increase	LAD: 52% increase	LAD: 17.4 ± 10.8 cm/sec LCx: 21.5 ± 7.5 cm/sec	n/a
Cor flow reserve			LAD: 1.38 ± 0.31 LCx: 2.57 ± 0.92	
Type of stress	Adenosine	Isometric exercise	Adenosine	n/a
In-plane imaging	no	no	no	yes
Number of subjects				3
Velocity ranges (Diastolic)				n/a

Modified from: Duerinckx AJ. Coronary MR angiography. *In*: Cardiac MR imaging, Boxt LM, guest ed. *MRI Clin North Am* 1996;4(2):361–418; with permission.

unteers he measured a mean coronary artery flow of 252 mL/min ± 91. The flow could be measured with a standard error equal to 30% of the total coronary flow. Van Rossum et al. (29) similarly suggested a method to measure global coronary flow reserve from the coronary sinus flow patterns. The mean coronary sinus flow was 144 mL/min ± 62. There appears to be a major discrepancy between the two independent measurements. Moreover, global flow reserve is of limited usefulness.

The early breathhold k-space–segmented PC-MRI work reported by Edelman et al. (15) included coronary flow velocity measurements in 11 subjects (age range, 23–63 years), including eight healthy adult volunteers with no prior history of heart disease and three patients with angiographically normal coronary arteries. Physiological stimulation with intravenous adenosine was performed in four healthy adult volunteers (age range, 18–35 years). Venc was limited to 150 cm/sec with 96 × 256 acquisition matrix, with pixel dimensions 1.4 × 0.8 mm. The velocity measurements obtained in vivo were limited to middiastolic measurements. It was postulated that the MR velocities represented mean velocities, which for a laminar flow profile corresponds to half the peak velocity measured by Doppler ultrasound.

The early results reported by Keegan et al. (16) from the Royal Brompton National Heart and Lung Hospital in London were also limited to early diastolic velocity measurements, except for one normal volunteer in which the variation of flow velocity over the cardiac cycle was measured by repeating the procedure with varying TDs. Other parameters: Venc = 50 cm/sec; matrix 92–128 × 128; FOV 15–20 × 20 cm. They looked at in-plane as well as through-plane flow quantification.

Poncelet et al. (17), using a TOF echo-planer MRI approach measured the phasic flow pattern in the left anterior descending (LAD) and the coronary flow response to isometric exercise. Based on 11 subjects, the velocity varied in the range of 9–19 cm/sec in diastole and were all ≤5 cm/s in systole.

Clarke et al. (21) measured flow in eight mongrel dogs after creating a close chest model of partial LAD occlusion. Breathholding was obtained with the ventilator stopped. MRI parameters were: Venc = 138.4 cm/s; matrix: 160–220 × 256; FOV = 18–24 cm with pixel size range from 0.7 to 0.94 mm^2. Flow in the partially occluded LAD and normal circumflex (LCx) coronary arteries were measured using MRI and ultrasound (US). Measurements of absolute coronary flow and coronary flow reserve were highly correlated with US (r = 0.96 and 0.94, respectively). Flow reserve in the constricted LAD was significantly lower than that in the unconstricted LCx.

Breathhold Coronary MR Flow Measurements from 1995 to 2000

There has been a tremendous amount of scientific activity and interest in noninvasive MR-based flow quantification in coronary vessels. This is clearly shown by the large number of papers published and scientific presentations, starting with the Third Meeting of the Society of MR in Nice, France, August 20–25, 1995 (33–38) and continuing into 1998 (39–44), 1999 (45–49), 2000 and beyond. Multiple problems are unresolved and are currently being addressed: optimal sampling in k-space and k-space ordering; spatial resolution needed for accurate flow estimates; increased temporal resolution; dependence of flow accuracy on the number of cine frames (50); decreased noise levels; better background corrections. There is a need for clinical validation in larger groups of patients with correlation with Doppler ultrasound. The relative long breathholds required per image (30–40 seconds) and the total duration of the examination (1 hour or more) present tremendous challenges to clinical implementation.

Many investigators have used cine MRI variants of the first-generation coronary MRA techniques to measure coronary flow and flow reserve during a breathhold or sequential breathholds (51–60). A few have used navigator techniques (61) or spiral scanning (49). Other approaches have also been described, such as multibolus stimulated-echo imaging of coronary artery flow (62). Some investigators still question the validity of these techniques (63), although the majority would agree that we are getting very close to reproducible flow and flow reserve measurements.

Technical problems and basic physics limitations of the breathhold MR flow techniques have also received attention, such as: in-plane flow velocity quantification along the phase-encoding axis in MRI (64), k-space strategies (65), the effect of and correction for in-plane myocardial motion on estimates of coronary-volume flow rates (66), the small vessel size (25), the effect of cardiac and respiratory motion (67), accuracy estimates (24,63,68,69), the importance of the algorithm (phase-difference vs. complex-difference measurements) used (70), and vessel tortuosity (71).

A more detailed review of the principles and clinical applications of these techniques is provided in Chapter 14. Flow through coronary stents has also been measured or evaluated (41,45,72–74). Concepts are very relevant to the understanding of the importance of temporal resolution as discussed in the article by Hofman et al. on "Quantification of in-plane motion of the coronary arteries during the cardiac cycle: implications for acquisition window duration for MR flow quantification" (39), and we refer the reader to this excellent study.

Conclusions

The ability to measure blood flow is a major advantage of coronary MRA over coronary X-ray angiography. The clinical significance of determining coronary flow reserve and changes in velocity and flow in coronary vessels cannot be understated. Early work—before the advent of breathhold velocity-encoded cine MRI—has concentrated on flow measurements in mammary arteries because they are subjected to much less respiratory motion than the native vessels (19,26,75). Work using the breathhold velocity-encoded cine MRI has shown promising results (as described earlier) in native vessels (21,55,56,67), bypass grafts and mammary arteries (57).

These results are extremely encouraging and point us into the right direction. More basic and applied clinical work will be needed to validate these techniques. One can think of many theoretical reasons why none of the MRI-based techniques used to quantitate coronary flow should not work (39,43,66,76,77). Experimental evidence suggests that this may become a clinical tool in patients (40,42,78–82), in those with stents (83) and after bypass surgery (47,84,85) or interventions (86). First-generation (breathhold cine) and second-generation (navigator-based techniques) both appear to work well (48,87–88). Even color flow has been described (89). The techniques continue to be improved (90–91).

References

1. Marcus M, Skorton D, Johnson M, Collins S, Harrison D, Kerber R. Visual estimates of percent diameter coronary stenosis: "a battered gold standard." J Am Coll Cardiol 1988;11:882–85.
2. White C, Wright C, Doty D, et al. Does the visual interpretation of the coronary arteriogram predict the physiological significance of a coronary stenosis? N Engl J Med 1984;310:819–24.
3. Loop F. Progress in surgical treatment of coronary atherosclerosis (part I). Chest 1983;84:611–22.
4. Iliceto S, Marangelli V, Memmola C, Rizzon P. Transesophageal Doppler echocardiography evaluation of coronary blood flow velocity in baseline conditions and during dipyridamole-induced coronary vasodilation. Circulation 1991;83:61–69.
5. Iliceto S, Memmola C, Marangelli V, Caiato C, Rizzon P. Evaluation of coronary artery anatomy and physiology with the use of transesophageal echocardiography. Cor Art Dis 1992;3:357–63.
6. Deychak YA, Segal J, Reiner JS, Nachnani S. Doppler guide wire-derived coronary flow reserve distal to intermediate stenoses used in clinical decision making regarding interventional therapy. Am Heart J 1994;128(1):178–81.
7. Fusejima K, Takahara Y, Sudo Y, Murayama H, Masuda Y, Inagaki Y. Comparison of coronary hemodynamics in patients with internal mammary artery and saphenous vein coronary artery bypass grafts: a noninvasive approach using combined two-dimensional and Doppler echocardiography. J Am Coll Cardiol 1990;15(1):131–39.
8. Bandyk D, Galbraith T, Haasler G, Almassi H. Blood flow velocity of internal mammary artery and saphenous vein grafts to the coronary arteries. J Surg Res 1988;44:342–51.
9. Manning WJ, Li W, Edelman RR. A preliminary report comparing magnetic resonance coronary angiography with conventional angiography. N Engl J Med 1993;328:828–32.
10. Duerinckx AJ, Urman M. Two-dimensional coronary MR angiography: analysis of initial clinical results. Radiology 1994;193:731–38.
11. Blackwell GG, Pohost GM. The evolving role of MRI in the assessment of coronary artery disease. Am J Cardiol 1995;75(11):74D–78D.
12. Wilke N, Jerosch-Herold M, Stillman AE, et al. Concepts

of myocardial perfusion imaging in magnetic resonance imaging. Magn Reson Q 1994;10(4):249–86.

13. Buonocore MK. Estimation of total coronary artery flow using measurements of flow in the ascending aorta. Magn Reson Med 1994;32(5):602–11.

14. Bogren HG, Buonocore MH. Measurement of coronary flow reserve by magnetic resonance velocity mapping in the aorta. Lancet 1993;342(8876):899–900.

15. Edelman RR, Manning WJ, Gervino E, Li W. Flow velocity quantification in human coronary arteries with fast breath-hold MR angiography. J Magn Reson Imag 1993; 3(5):699–703.

16. Keegan J, Firmin D, Gatehouse P, Longmore D. The application of breath hold phase velocity mapping techniques to the measurement of coronary artery blood flow velocity: phantom data and initial in vivo results. Magn Reson Med 1994;31:526–36.

17. Poncelet BP, Weisskoff RM, Vedeen VJ, Brady TJ, Kantor H. Time of flight quantification of coronary flow with echo-planar MRI. Magn Reson Med 1993;30(4):447–57.

18. Gatehouse PD, Firmin DN, Longmore DB. Real time blood flow imaging by spiral scan phase velocity mapping. Magn Reson Med 1994;31:504–12.

19. Debatin JR, Strong JA, Sostman HD, et al. MR characterization of blood flow in native and grafted internal mammary arteries. J Magn Reson Imag 1993;3(3):443–51.

20. Burstein D. MR imaging of coronary artery flow in isolated and in vivo hearts. J Magn Reson Imag 1991;1:337–46.

21. Clarke GD, Eckels R, Chaney C, et al. Measurement of absolute epicardial coronary artery flow and flow reserve with breathhold cine phase-contrast magnetic resonance imaging. Circulation 1995;91(10):2627–34.

22. Mostbeck GH, Caputo GR, Higgins CB. MR measurements of blood flow in the cardiovascular system. Am J Roentgenol 1992;159:453–61.

23. Buonocore M, Bogren H. Factors influencing the accuracy and precision of velocity-encoded phase imaging. Magn Reson Med 1992;26:141–54.

24. Tang C, Blatter DD, Parker DL. Accuracy of phase-contrast flow measurements in the presence of partial-volume effects. J Magn Reson Imag 1993;3(3):377–87.

25. Hofman MBM, Visser FC, vanRossum AC, Vink GQM, Sprenger M, Westerhof N. In vivo validation of magnetic resonance blood volume flow measurements with limited spatial resolution in small vessels. Magn Reson Med 1995; 33(6):778–84.

26. Duerinckx AJ. Coronary hemodynamics in patients with artery bypass grafts using phase contrast MRI (abstr.). In: Sixteenth Annual Meeting of Society for Cardiac Angiography and Interventions. San Antonio, May 18–22, 1993.

27. Debatin JF, Ting RH, Wegmüller H, et al. Renal artery blood flow: quantification with phase-contrast MR imaging with and without breathholding. Radiology 1994;190: 371–78.

28. Thompson C, Cortsen M, Söndergaard L, Heriksen O, Stählberg F. A segmented k-space velocity mapping protocol for quantification of renal artery blood flow during breath-holding. J Magn Reson Imag 1995;5(4):393–402.

29. vanRossum AC, Visser FC, Hofman MBM, Galjee MA, Westerhof N, Valk J. Global left ventricular perfusion: non-invasive measurement with cine MR imaging and phase

velocity mapping of coronary venous outflow. Radiology 1992;182:685–91.

30. Chien D, Laub G, Simonetti O, Anderson CM. Time-resolved velocity quantification of pulsatile flow: segmented k-space bolus tagging in a single breathhold (abstr.). In: Proceedings of the First Meeting of the Society of Magnetic Resonance (SMRM). Dallas, March 5–9, 1994; J Magn Reson Imag 1994;4(P) Work-in-Progress Supplement: S27.

31. Polzin JA, Korosec FR, Alley MT, Grist TM, Mistretta CA. Peak flow measurements using a segmented 2-D phase-contrast acquisition (poster #989) (abstr.). In: Printed Program of the Second Meeting of the Society of Magnetic Resonance (SMR). San Francisco, August 6–12, 1994.

32. Wielopolski PA, Manning WJ, Edelman RE. Single breath-hold volumetric imaging of the heart using magnetization-prepared 3-dimensional segmented echo-planar imaging. J Magn Reson Imag 1995;5(4):403–9.

33. Sakuma H, Sebastian G, O'Sullivan M, et al. Measurement of phasic coronary blood flow velocity and vasodilator coronary flow reserve in man using breathhold velocity-encoded cine MR imaging (abstr.). In: Book of Abstracts of the Third Meeting of the Society of Magnetic Resonance (SMR) and the Twelfth Annual Scientific Meeting of the European Society for Magnetic Resonance in Medicine and Biology (ESMRMB). Nice, France, August 20–25, 1995.

34. Grist TM, Polzin JA, Bianco JA, et al. Measurement of absolute coronary flow and flow reserve using phase-contrast MRI techniques (abstr.). In: Book of Abstracts of the Third Meeting of the Society of Magnetic Resonance (SMR) and the Twelfth Annual Scientific Meeting of the European Society for Magnetic Resonance in Medicine and Biology (ESMRMB). Nice, France, August 20–25, 1995.

35. Davis CP, Hauser M, Göhde SC, et al. Measurement of coronary flow with segmented k-space phase contrast MRI pre- and post-dipyridamole (abstr.). In: Book of Abstracts of the Third Meeting of the Society of Magnetic Resonance (SMR) and the Twelfth Annual Scientific Meeting of the European Society for Magnetic Resonance in Medicine and Biology (ESMRMB). Nice, France, August 20–25, 1995.

36. vonSmekal A, Knetz A, Seelos KC, et al. Assessment of coronary bypass graft patency: comparison of coronary arteriography, ultrafast-CT and MR-angiography (abstr.). In: Book of Abstracts of the Third Meeting of the Society of Magnetic Resonance (SMR) and the Twelfth Annual Scientific Meeting of the European Society for Magnetic Resonance in Medicine and Biology (ESMRMB). Vol. 1, p. 14. Nice, France, August 20–25, 1995.

37. Sakuma H, Sebastian G, O'Sullivan M, et al. Flow velocity measurements in native internal mammary arteries and coronary artery bypass grafts with breathhold velocity-encoded cine MR imaging (abstr.). In: Book of Abstracts of the Third Meeting of the Society of Magnetic Resonance (SMR) and the Twelfth Annual Scientific Meeting of the European Society for Magnetic Resonance in Medicine and Biology (ESMRMB). Nice, France, August 20–25, 1995.

38. Li D, Kaushikkar S, Haacke M, Dhawale P. Coronary artery flow quantification using segmented phase contrast sequence with retrospective respiratory gating (abstr.). In: Book of Abstracts of the Third Meeting of the Society of Magnetic Resonance (SMR) and the Twelfth Annual Sci-

entific Meeting of the European Society for Magnetic Resonance in Medicine and Biology (ESMRMB). Nice, France, August 20–25, 1995.

39. Hofman MB, Wickline SA, Lorenz CH. Quantification of in-plane motion of the coronary arteries during the cardiac cycle: implications for acquisition window duration for MR flow quantification. J Magn Reson Imag 1998; 8(3):568–76.

40. Kessler W, Moshage W, Galland A, et al. Assessment of coronary blood flow in humans using phase difference MR imaging. Comparison with intracoronary Doppler flow measurement. Int J Card Imag 1998;14(3):179–86; discussion 187–89.

41. Nagel E, Hug J, Bunger S, et al. Coronary flow measurements for evaluation of patients after stent implantation. Magma 1998;6(2–3):184–85.

42. Voigtlander T. Coronary artery and bypass flow measurement—basic methodology and current status. Magma 1998;6(2–3):96–97.

43. Wedding KL, Grist TM, Folts JD, et al. Coronary flow and flow reserve in canines using MR phase difference and complex difference processing. Magn Reson Med 1998; 40(5):656–65.

44. Buonocore MH. Visualizing blood flow patterns using streamlines, arrows, and particle paths. Magn Reson Med 1998;40(2):210–26.

45. Klein C, Hug J, Bünger S, et al. Determination of coronary blood flow velocity after stent implantation (abstr.). In: Society for Cardiovascular Magnetic Resonance, Second Meeting, January 22–24, 1999. Atlanta, 1999:52.

46. Voigtländer T, Kreitner K-F, Wittlinger T, Scharhag J, Abegunewardene N, Meyer J. MR measurements of flow reserve in coronary grafts (abstr.). In: Society for Cardiovascular Magnetic Resonance, Second Meeting, January 22–24, 1999. Atlanta, 1999:53.

47. Schreiber WG, Voigtländer T, Kreitner K-F, et al. Measurement of flow reserve in coronary bypass grafts (abstr.). In: Book of Abstracts and Proceedings of the Seventh Meeting of the International Society of Magnetic Resonance in Medicine (ISMRM). Philadelphia, May 22–28, 1999. 1999;Vol. 1.

48. Doornbos J, Langerak SE, Kunz P, et al. Coronary artery bypass graft MR flow measurements: high temporal resolution and respiratory compensation (abstr.). In: Book of Abstracts and Proceedings of the Seventh Meeting of the International Society of Magnetic Resonance in Medicine (ISMRM). Philadelphia, May 22–28, 1999. 1999;Vol. 1.

49. Keegan J, Gatehouse PD, Yang GZ, Firmin DN. Interleaved spiral cine coronary artery velocity mapping (abstr.). In: Book of Abstracts and Proceedings of the Seventh Meeting of the International Society of Magnetic Resonance in Medicine (ISMRM). Philadelphia, May 22–28, 1999. 1999;Vol. 1.

50. Clarke GD, Hundley WG, McColl RW, et al. Velocity-encoded, phase-difference cine MRI measurements of coronary artery flow: dependence of flow accuracy on the number of cine frames. J Magn Reson Imag 1996;6(5): 733–42.

51. Davis CP, Liu PF, Hauser M, Gohde SC, von Schulthess GK, Debatin JF. Coronary flow and coronary flow reserve measurements in humans with breath-held magnetic res-

onance phase contrast velocity mapping. Magn Reson Med 1997;37(4):537–44.

52. Globits S, Sakuma H, Shimakawa A, Foo TF, Higgins CB. Measurement of coronary blood flow velocity during handgrip exercise using breath-hold velocity encoded cine magnetic resonance imaging. Am J Cardiol 1997;79: 234–37.

53. Grist TM, Polzin JA, Bianco JA, Foo TK, Bernstein MA, Mistretta CM. Measurement of coronary blood flow and flow reserve using magnetic resonance imaging. Cardiology 1997;88(1):80–89.

54. Harada M, Taoka Y, Nishitani H, Nomura M. [The measurement of the coronary flow by the phase contrast method (cine PC, Fastcard PC)]. Nippon Rinsho. Jap J Clin Med 1997;55(7):1828–32.

55. Hundley WG, R A Lange GCC, B M Meshack JP, C Landau, et al. Assessment of coronary arterial flow and flow reserve in humans with magnetic resonance imaging. Circulation 1996;93:1502–8.

56. Sakuma H, Blake LM, Amidon TM, et al. Coronary flow reserve: noninvasive measurement in humans with breath-hold velocity-encoded cine MR imaging. Radiology 1996;198:745–50.

57. Sakuma H, Globits S, O'Sullivan M, et al. Breath-hold MR measurements of blood flow velocity in internal mammary arteries and coronary artery bypass grafts. J Magn Reson Imag 1996;6(1):219–22.

58. Sakuma H, Saeed M, Takeda K, et al. Quantification of coronary artery volume flow rate using fast velocity-encoded cine MR imaging. Am J Roentgenol 1997;168(5): 1363–67.

59. Sakuma H, Takeda K, Nakagawa T. [Assessment of coronary flow reserve using fast phase contrast cine MR imaging]. Nippon Rinsho. Jap J Clin Med 1997;55(7):1833–38.

60. van Rossum AC, Galjee MA, Post JC, Visser CA. A practical approach to MRI of coronary artery bypass graft patency and flow. Int J Card Imag 1997;13(3):199–204.

61. Post JC, Hofman MBM, Piek JJ, Galjee MA, vanRossum AC, Visser CA. Flow assessment in the right coronary artery: navigator-echo-based respiratory-gated MR measurements vs intravascular Doppler guidewire measurements (abstr.). In: Book of Abstracts and Proceedings of the Fifth Meeting of the International Society of Magnetic Resonance in Medicine (ISMRM). Vancouver, B.C., Canada, April 12–18, 1997; Vol. 1: 446.

62. Chao H, Burstein D. Multibolus stimulated echo imaging of coronary artery flow. J Magn Reson Imag 1997;7(3): 603–5.

63. Nitz WR, Kessler W, Stingl D, Moshage W, Laub G. Can we trust breathhold MR velocity measurements of coronary blood flow? (abstr.). Radiology 1996;201(P):166.

64. Duerk JL, Pattany PM. In-plane flow velocity quantification along the phase encoding axis in MRI. Magn Reson Imag 1988;6:321–33.

65. Franck A, Selby K, vanTyen R, Nordell B, Saloner D. Cardiac-gated MR angiography of pulsatile flow: k-space strategies. J Magn Reson Imag 1995;5:297–307.

66. Frayne R, Polzin JA, Mazaheri Y, Grist TM, Mistretta CA. Effect of and correction for in-plane myocardial motion on estimates of coronary-volume flow rates. J Magn Reson Imag 1997;7(5):815–28.

67. Hofman MBM, vanRossum AC, Sprenger M, Westerhof N. Assessment of flow in the right human coronary artery by magnetic resonance phase contrast velocity measurements: effects of cardiac and respiratory motion. Magn Reson Med 1996;35:521–31.

68. Li H, Clarke GD, NessAiver M, Liu H, Peshock R. Magnetic resonance imaging k-space segmentation using phase-encoding groups: the accuracy of quantitative measurements of pulsatile flow. Med Phys 1995;22(4):391–99.

69. Strauss WL, Tsuruda JS, Richards TL. Accuracy of MR phase contrast velocity measurements for unsteady flow. J Magn Reson Imag 1995;5(4):428–32.

70. Polzin JA, Korosec FR, Wedding KL, et al. Effects of through-plane myocardial motion on phase-difference and complex-difference measurements of absolute coronary artery flow. J Magn Reson Med 1996;6(1):113–23.

71. vanTyen R, Saloner D, Jou LD, Berger S. MR imaging of flow through tortuous vessels: a numerical simulation. Magn Reson Imag 1994;31:184–195.

72. Duerinckx AJ, Atkinson D, Hurwitz R, Mintorovitch J, Whitney W. Coronary MR angiography after coronary stent placement (case report). Am J Roentgenol 1995; 165(3):662–64.

73. Duerinckx AJ, Atkinson D, Hurwitz R. Assessment of coronary artery patency after stent placement using magnetic resonance angiography. J Magn Reson Med 1998;8: 896–902.

74. DeCobelli F, Guidetti D, Vanzulli A, Mellone R, Chierchia S, Del Maschio A. Magnetic resonance angiography of coronary arteries: assessment in patients with coronary stenosis and control after stent positioning. Radiol Med 1998;95(1–2):54–61.

75. Debatin J, Strong J, Negro-Vilar R, Sostman H, Pelc N, Herfkens R. MR characterization of blood flow in native and grafted internal mammary arteries (abstr.). In: Proceedings of the RSNA Seventy-eighth Scientific Assembly and Annual Meeting. Chicago: 1992;185(P):102.

76. Duerinckx AJ, Atkinson DP. Coronary MR angiography during peak-systole: work-in-progress. J Magn Reson Imag 1997;7(6):979–86.

77. Marcus JT, Smeenk HG, Kuijer JP, Van der Geest RJ, Heethaar RM, Van Rossum AC. Flow profiles in the left anterior descending and the right coronary artery assessed by MR velocity quantification: effects of through-plane and in-plane motion of the heart. J Comput Assist Tomogr 1999;23(4):567–76.

78. Firmin D. Report from the June 28–30, 1999 ISMRM Workshop on Flow and Motion: how it relates to coronary MRA. (abstr.) In: Book of Abstracts of the First International Workshop on Coronary MR & CT Angiography. Lyon, France, Oct 1–3, 2000. Organized and published by the North American Society for Cardiac Imaging. Reprinted in: International Journal of Cardiac Imaging. 2000.

79. Sakuma H, Kawada N, Takeda K, Higgins CB. MR measurement of coronary blood flow. J Magn Reson Imag 1999;10(5):728–33.

80. Hundley WG, Hillis LD, Hamilton CA, et al. Assessment of coronary arterial restenosis with phase-contrast magnetic resonance imaging measurements of coronary flow reserve. Circulation 2000;101(20):2375–81.

81. Lund GK, Sakuma H, Higgins CB. Coronary flow reserve: assessment by magnetic resonance imaging. Rays 1999; 24(1):119–30.

82. Amano Y, Hayashi H, Ishihara M, Kumazaki T. Coronary flow reserve estimated with fast cine phase-contrast magnetic resonance imaging in 4 patients with syndrome X: technical note. Can Assoc Radiol J 1999;50(5):298–300.

83. Lethimonnier F, Bouligand B, Thouveny F, et al. Error assessment due to coronary stents in flow-encoded phase contrast MR angiography: a phantom study. J Magn Reson Imag 1999;10(5):899–902.

84. Miller S, Scheule AM, Hahn U, et al. MR angiography and flow quantification of the internal mammary artery graft after minimally invasive direct coronary artery bypass. Am J Roentgenol 1999;172(5):1365–69.

85. Walpoth BH, Muller MF, Genyk I, et al. Evaluation of coronary bypass flow with color-Doppler and magnetic resonance imaging techniques: comparison with intraoperative flow measurements. Eur J Cardiothorac Surg 1999; 15(6):795–802.

86. Rutishauser W. The Denolin Lecture 1998. Towards measurement of coronary blood flow in patients and its alteration by interventions. Eur Heart J 1999;20(15):1076–83.

87. Keegan J, Gatehouse PD, Yang GZ, Firmin DN. Navigator-echo controlled interleaved spiral phase velocity mapping of coronary artery blood flow (abstr). In: Book of Abstracts of the First International Workshop on Coronary MR & CT Angiography. Lyon, France, Oct 1–3, 2000. Organized and published by the North American Society for Cardiac Imaging. Reprinted in: Int J Card Imag 2000;16.

88. Nagel E, Bornstedt A, Hug J, Schnackenburg B, Wellnhofer E, Fleck E. Noninvasive determination of coronary blood flow velocity with magnetic resonance imaging: comparison of breath-hold and navigator techniques with intravascular ultrasound. Magn Reson Med 1999;41(3): 544–49.

89. Nayak KS, Pauly JM, Kerr AB, Hu BS, Nishimura DG. Real-time color flow MRI. Magn Reson Med 2000;43(2): 251–58.

90. Langerak SE, Kunz P, Vliegen HW, Lamb HJ, Jukema JW, van der Wall EE, de Roos A. Improved MR flow mapping in coronary artery bypass grafts during adenosine-induced stress. Radiology 2001;218(2):540–47.

91. Book of Abstracts of the Second Workshop on Coronary MR & CT Angiography, Sept 29–Oct 2, 2001, Chicago. Organized and published by the North American Society for Cardiac Imaging. Reprinted in the Int J Card Imag 2001; (17):5.

14
Coronary Flow Reserve

Hugo G. Bogren and Michael H. Buonocore

Coronary artery flow reserve is the ratio of maximum coronary blood flow induced by ischemia or pharmacological stimulation to resting flow and is based on the original data from animal experiments (1). The experiments indicated that approximately 50% stenosis is required to reduce the coronary flow reserve (Fig. 14.1). This finding forms the basis for our clinical judgment that a stenosis of 50% or more is physiologically significant and therefore, under certain circumstances, should be bypassed or balloon dilated. The data were based on experiments in 12 healthy dogs and were extrapolated to human beings with atherosclerosis. Furthermore, the weight of the dogs varied between 17 and 40 kilos, and no normalization for body weight was performed. The measurements were made with an electromagnetic flow meter in the left circumflex artery. The flow in that artery may have varied somewhat individually, but not as much as three times because all dogs are left dominant. The resting and maximum flow in milliliters per minute per gram cardiac muscle therefore probably varied significantly (Fig. 14.2A,B). Note in Figure 14.2 that the same degree of stenosis (e.g., 70%) results in different flows in different individuals. Nevertheless, coronary flow reserve became the gold standard and a 50% stenosis came to be considered significant.

Later data and experiments by the same and other authors have cast some doubt on the validity of flow reserve as it was first defined as a gold standard (2–5). The coronary flow reserve varies with heart rate and blood pressure. True coronary flow reserve in a vessel can only be known if the flow at rest and at maximum dilatation of the coronary artery are both known. One would think that maximum exercise would give maximum dilatation of the vessel, but such is evidently not the case because the flow reserve increases if Dipyridamol is given after maximum exercise (4–7). Furthermore, flow reserve is spatially heterogeneous. The regional coronary flow reserve, defined as the ratio of maximum to resting flow in dog experiments, ranged from 1.75 to 21.9 in a study by Austin et al. (8). This wide range of values suggests that regional coronary flow reserve is of questionable value. Global flow reserve as an absolute measure also has limited value because the coronary flow appears to vary by a factor of 2–3 (9). Global or regional flow reserve may only have relevance as a measure of deterioration or improvement for example by intervention.

The gold standard for measurement of significance of coronary artery stenosis is percent reduction of its diameter or area that can be visually estimated or measured with calipers or via computer. All three of these methods involve judgment and error by the operator. Even if we were able to measure the stenosis and regional flow reserve correctly, we would still not be able to correct for possible collateral flow (10).

Global flow reserve may have value as an indicator of impaired coronary flow due to atherosclerosis or of improved flow after coronary artery intervention. It is likely that only measurements of flow expressed in milliliters per minute per gram heart muscle is valid in evaluating ischemia in an individual case. Percent stenosis, whether determined by computerized methods or manually and coronary flow reserve measurements with ultrasound magnetic resonance (MR) or other techniques may have limited value in the individual case other than as a relative measure.

Nevertheless, coronary artery flow reserve appears to be the best measurement we have at the present time, but it must be used with caution. The MR method has the potential to evaluate the arterial wall and measure flow as well as flow reserve that would be superior to all other previous methods, invasive or noninvasive.

Attempts to measure coronary flow reserve have been made by invasive methods [e.g., digital selective coronary arteriography (11–13) and Doppler tip catheters (14–16)]. Positron emission tomography has been used to measure coronary artery flow reserve (17–20), perhaps more accurately than other methods as advocated by Gold (19). Positron emission tomography, however, is expensive and not readily available. It is still predominantly a research technique that continues to give us new insights into coronary flow

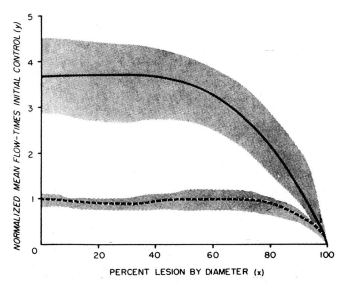

Figure 14.1. Flow and flow reserve in the left circumflex artery in dogs versus percent constriction. (Reprinted from American Journal of Cardiology, volume number 33, Gould et al., Physiologic basis for assessing critical coronary stenosis, pages 87–94, copyright 1974, with permission from Excerpta Media, Inc.)

and flow reserve (20,21). The only method that is used occasionally but seldom in clinical practice is the Doppler flow meter, which may be available in cardiac catheterization laboratories. It is used as a complement to coronary angiography in doubtful cases. Its application is based on the assumption that the coronary blood flow velocity is proportional to blood flow (14). This is not always true because the velocity may increase in a stenosis reflecting reduced flow rather than increased flow. Area measurements are also uncertain especially because the catheter itself gives a relative obstruction in the examined vessel especially in a diseased vessel.

Global Coronary Artery Flow Reserve Measurements with MRI Blood Flow Into the Coronary Arteries

Blood flow in the coronary arteries is predominantly diastolic because the intramyocardial pressure is equal to or higher than the aortic and coronary pressure (22). Only the left atrial branches of the left anterior descending (LAD) and perhaps the sinus node artery, if it originates in the left circumflex artery, may have significant systolic flow. The right coronary artery (RCA) has more systolic flow than does the left because it supplies the low pressure right ventricle and atrium; however, it also supplies some high pressure left ventricle in the posterior lateral branches and the posterior descending branch. In infarcted myocardium the intramyocardial pressure may be lower and it is likely that the little blood flow that there is to the infarct may take place in systole as well as diastole. The septal vessels have retrograde flow in systole (23) and there is also some systolic retrograde flow in the LAD. Ideally, one should measure the coronary flow all through the cardiac cycle, but a reasonable compromise is to measure it only in diastole when there is also less motion of the vessels.

The coronary circulation is unique, since it is dependent on retrograde flow in the aorta and how it is provided (9,24,25). A small amount of blood flows into the coronary arteries in systole especially into the right coronary artery (Fig. 14.3A,B). In mid- to late-systole blood turns around clockwise in the ascending aorta and returns in a well-defined posterior lateral channel towards the left coronary sinus. Immediately above the left coronary sinus blood crosses over to the right coronary sinus. Some blood also reverses in the distal part of the aortic arch (26). The reverse flow amounts to approxi-

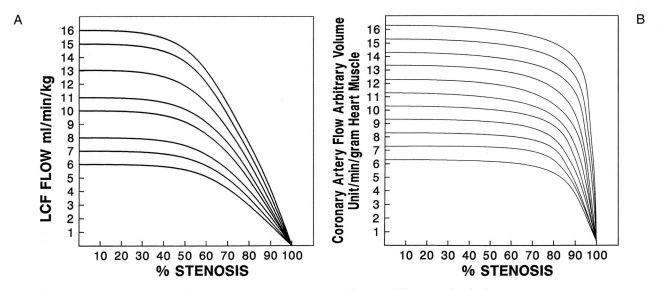

Figure 14.2. Resting (A) and maximum (B) coronary artery flow in different individuals versus percent stenosis.

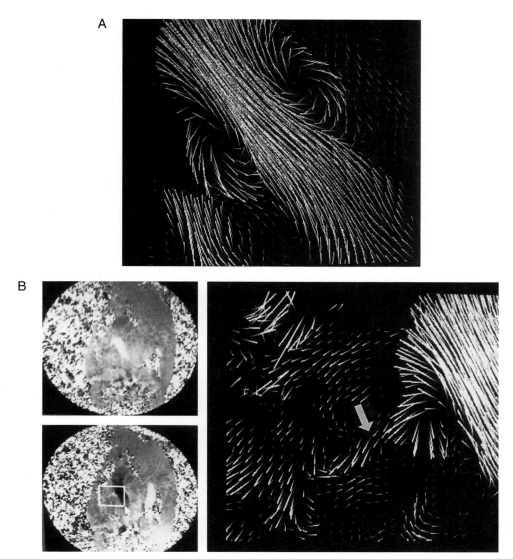

Figure 14.3. Systolic vortices in the coronary sinuses (A) leading to flow into the right coronary artery (arrow in B). Velocity maps are seen to the left in B and vector maps in A and to the right in B in an oblique coronal plane equivalent to a left anterior oblique projection. In the velocity maps black represents velocity up the image in vertical encoding in the lower image and to the right in the upper image with horizontal encoding. White represents motion down the image and to the left, respectively. The velocity maps are displayed for orientation and are from early systole, when the flow directions are best seen.

mately 1–1.5 L/min, out of which 200–300 ml flow into the coronary arteries. The remainder turns forward again in or above the sinuses and is part of the antegrade flow during diastole, most of which goes to the brain (25). In patients with atherosclerosis the blood flow patterns in the ascending aorta are more irregular and unpredictable (26).

Measurement of Coronary Artery Flow Reserve in the Ascending Aorta

It is possible to measure global diastolic coronary flow and flow reserve by measuring ante and retrograde flows in the ascending aorta:

Coronary Artery Flow
= Retrograde Aortic Flow in Systole and Diastole
− Antegrade Aortic Flow in Diastole

with some adjustments (see later). An example of velocity mapping in the mid-ascending aorta, where such measurements may be and were performed by Bogren and Buonocore (24), is seen in Figure 14.4. A diagram of the flow measurements is seen in Figure 14.5. Velocity mapping has an accuracy of 5–10% in the ascending aorta (27) that is sufficient to measure, for example, cardiac output that is dependent predominantly on systolic very high volume flow. The measurements of smaller flows in diastole that are used to compute coronary

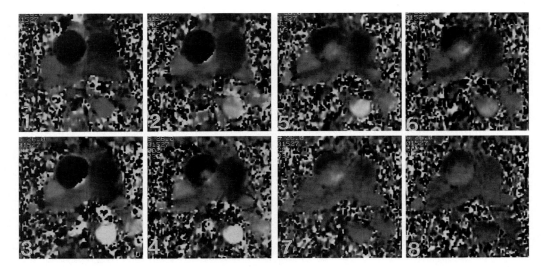

Figure 14.4. Axial velocity maps in the ascending and descending aorta at the level of the pulmonary artery bifurcation seen from below. Black denotes velocities away from the viewer (towards the head), white towards the viewer (towards the feet). The first image (top left) was obtained in early systole, 32 msec after the R-wave. The interval between images is 66 msec. Late diastolic images are not included. R–R-interval = 1277 msec. Note the retrograde flow in late systole and diastole. (*From*: Flow measurements in the aorta and major arteries with MR velocity mapping. Bogren et al., *J Magn Reson Imag* 1994. Reprinted by permission of Wiley-Liss, Inc., a subsidiary of John Wiley & Sons, Inc.)

artery flow have large errors at velocity encoding of 150–200 cm/sec (i.e., error is 5–10% of 200), as was used in most of the study by Bogren and Buonocore (24). Accuracy increases if encoding can be done at 30 cm/sec in diastole (the error is then 5–10% of 30), which was also used with improved results (24).

Bogren and Buonocore (24) performed measurements before and after intravenous Dipyridamol 0.57 mg/kg. The studies were performed using a General Electric Signa scanner (1.5 T), Milwaukee, with phase-contrast velocity mapping [Repetition times (TR) 25 msec, TE 7.4 msec, flip angle 30 degrees, field-of-view (FOV) 40 cm]. Voxel size was 1.5 × 3 × 5 mm and the temporary resolution 50 msec. Velocity encoding was set at 200 cm/sec or 200 in systole and 30 in diastole. The acquisition time was approximately 30 minutes for the pre- and 15 minutes for the post-Dipyridamol study in a slice through the mid-ascending aorta that was performed immediately after the 4-minute-long infusion of Dipyridamol. The study was performed in combination with Cardiolite (technicium-99m 2-metoxy isobutyl isonitrile, Dupont Pharma) myocardial perfusion scans. One-directional through-plane velocity mapping was performed in an axial slice of the mid-ascending aorta at the level of the pulmonary artery bifurcation (Fig. 14.4). The retrograde flow, in systole and diastole minus the antegrade flow during diastole, equals the coronary diastolic flow adjusted for the change in volume of the ascending aorta below the slice of measurement between systole and diastole (caused by compliance) (see Fig. 14.5A).

Because coronary flow reserve is the difference in coronary flow, pre- and post-Dipyridamol, its estimate is insensitive to known errors in magnetic resonance velocity mapping (Fig. 14.5A,B). These errors influence the accuracy and precision of absolute estimates of coronary artery flow, but not the before and after difference. For example, systematic errors in the zero velocity (background) pixel value should be the same pre- and post-Dipyridamol and should not influence the flow reserve estimate (Fig. 14.6). Another error arises because the ascending aorta is elastic and its volume decreases during diastole, which may contribute to diastolic coronary artery flow and may not be detected by velocity mapping in the mid-ascending slice. The overall volume change between systole and diastole was assumed to be unaffected by Dipyridamol. The other possible sources of errors, such as recirculation before aortic valve closure, were also assumed to be the same before and after Dipyridamol.

In eight normal subjects and in four patients with possible ischemic heart disease but with normal perfusion scans, the mean coronary flow reserve was 269 ml/min. Coronary flow reserve was zero in seven patients with coronary artery disease.

Although true coronary flow before and after Dipyridamol could not be reliably measured, it was shown that MR velocity mapping could be used to measure coronary flow reserve indirectly. This was the first noninvasive measurement of coronary flow reserve preceding transesophageal Doppler echocardiography (15,16). The method has not had much clinical demand because only global flow reserve can be measured. In the individual case it is considered more important to find out whether there is ischemic heart disease due to coronary artery stenosis and a decreased regional flow reserve. The global flow reserve would be of interest as a screening method for coronary artery disease or, perhaps, as a measure of successful or failed coronary artery bypass grafting or angioplasty.

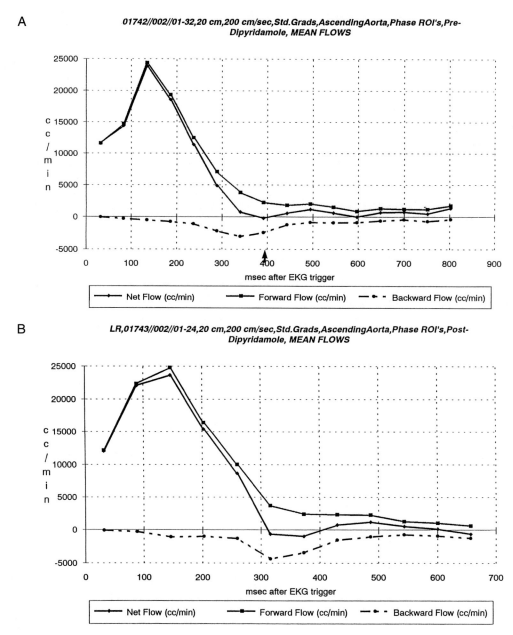

Figure 14.5. Plot of blood flow in the mid-ascending aorta averaged from 256 heartbeats before (A) and after Dipyridamol (B). The flow was 227 ml/min before and 667 ml/min after Dipyrimadol.

We have subsequently studied blood flow patterns in the ascending aorta and found very irregular flows in patients with ascending aortic aneurysms and severe coronary artery disease, as well as in asymptomatic individuals above the age of 70 (26,28). Due to these highly irregular flows and vortex formations, it may be difficult to measure coronary flow reserves in patients with severely abnormal ascending aortas.

Another attempt to measure total coronary flow and flow reserve was made by Buonocore (29) who measured flow in the ascending aorta below and above the origin of the right and left coronary arteries. The standard error was 90 cc/min. No flow reserve measure-

ments were performed, but they are feasible and may be accurate despite the large error in total flow measurements.

Measurement of Coronary Flow Reserve in the Coronary Arteries

The long acquisition times in traditional phase-contrast velocity mapping and in other traditional sequences (e.g., T1, which is used for localization of the coronary arteries) has put time constraints on flow reserve measurements. Flow reserve after exercise has not been pos-

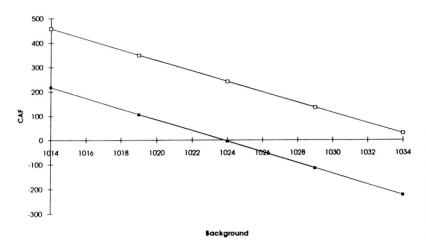

Figure 14.6. Coronary artery flow. Background denotes zero flow. Coronary artery flow reserve is 247 ml/min at all background levels. Filled in squares = pre- and open squares = post-Dipyridamol. (*From*: Measurement of coronary artery flow reserve using magnetic resonance velocity mapping in the aorta. Bogren and Buonocore, Lancet 1993;341:891. Reprinted with permission by The Lancet Ltd.)

sible. Pharmacological stress has to be continuous for a long time if adenosine is used or is somewhat uncertain in effect when Dipyridamol is used because the maximum effect may be limited in time. If MR flow data could be acquired within a few heartbeats the maximum effect of stress would be more readily detectable.

The development of breathhold velocity-encoded cine magnetic resonance imaging (MRI) by Edelman et al. (30) opened up new possibilities for timely coronary artery flow and flow reserve measurements (see Fig. 4 in Ref. 30). Edelman (30) developed an imaging sequence called turboFLASH (fast low angle shot) on a 1.5 T Siemens (Erlangen, Germany) Scanner for imaging coronary and other arteries, and modified the sequence for phase-contrast applications. Similar sequences were developed and used for flow measurements by Keegan et al. (31), Clarke et al. (32), and Sakuma et al. (33). Other fast-imaging techniques (e.g., echo-planar and spiral imaging) have also been adopted for flow or velocity measurements in the coronary arteries (34–36). In segmented turboFLASH technique developed by Edelman (30), data is acquired from the central *k*-space only, so that data from eight or even more lines/cardiac cycle can be obtained hereby reducing the acquisition time from 128 to 16 or fewer heartbeats. The acquisition can be made during one breathhold. For further details about the techniques see the physics part of this chapter or Pearlman and Edelman (37). Only one phase–cardiac cycle could initially be acquired, but with improving and stronger gradients three to four phases/cycle (32) or even nine (33) or more (37). Most studies have involved only velocity measurements, but attempts to measure total flow and flow reserve have been made (32). It is obvious that there is a great advantage to include as many phases as possible in the cardiac cycle and that measurements at a single time point in the cardiac cycle for each breathhold data acquisition has limitations since the peak flow or peak velocity may not have been sampled. Echo-planar methods hold great

promise (36), but they are still not very well explored (34,36). Spiral imaging may hold the most promise (35), but it is even less explored. After rapid development of stronger and faster gradients, echo-planar and spiral imaging could very well dominate the field, but as of today, all serious attempts to measure coronary flow and flow reserve have been made using segmented *k*-space techniques of the turboFLASH type, with only one exception (36). In the remainder of this chapter we will therefore analyze the results from use of these turboFLASH or turboFLASH-like sequences.

Edelman et al. (30) were the pioneers and showed the possibility of measuring blood flow velocity at one point in the cardiac cycle before and after pharmacologic stress induced by intravenous adenosine. They showed that the velocities at one point in time increased from 9.9 cm/sec ± 3.5 to 20.5 cm/sec ± 5.2 in the right coronary artery after adenosine, a four-fold increase. Normal subjects therefore demonstrated a physiologic response to pharmacologic stimulation of a magnitude consistent with earlier experience from, for example, ultrasound (14–16). No patients were studied. The acquisition was made in diastole 350–600 msec after the R wave. Peak velocity may not have been recorded, but the response to adenosine appeared adequate.

Keegan et al. (31) presented a similar study measuring velocities at one point of time at a time in each heartbeat in diastole (see Fig. 6 in Ref. 31). In one patient up to 14 points in the cardiac cycle were acquired, showing a typical biphasic RCA flow with almost equal amounts of flow in systole and diastole while the diastolic flow dominated in the LAD and the left circumflex artery (see Fig. 9 in Ref. 31). Absolute flow could not be measured, only velocities due to the smallness of the coronary arteries and the relatively large size of the pixels (1.6 × 1.6 mm).

Keegan et al. calibrated their method extensively in a phantom. They found increasing velocities in arterial stenosis and thought that the velocity increase could be used in the future to evaluate the severity of a coronary artery stenosis. Keegan et al. did not perform any stress measurements, but their methodology is open to such measurements. They worked with a modified 1.5 T Picker (Cleveland, Ohio) scanner.

Clarke et al. (32) measured flow and flow reserve in eight dogs before and after adenosine using a similar breathhold cine-phase contrast sequence. They acquired four to six frames/cardiac cycle with a segmented k-space sequence called phase-encode grouping (PEG) (SCOPEG) on a 1.5 vista, HPQ MRI scanner (Picker International, Cleveland). They found very close agreement between the results from perivascular ultrasound flow meters and MR measurements. Their pixel size was less than 1×1 mm. The measurements were made in the left circumflex and the left anterior descending branches of the left coronary artery (Fig. 14.7). The flow reserve in the left circumflex was 2.57 ± 0.92, in the LAD 1.38 ± 0.31, and there was a very close correlation with the ultrasound measurements. The total flow in the left coronary artery, however, which is a very dominant artery in dogs who have very small RCAs, was approximately 90 ml/min. The mean weight of the dogs was 36.6 kg and the average mongrel dog has 4 g heart mass/kg body weight. The flow in milligrams per minute per gram heart muscle amounted to 0.63, which appears low because normal coronary artery flow is approximately 1 ml/min/g heart muscle.

There are several possible errors in their measurements (e.g., that the dogs were anesthetized and that the blood pressure during adenosine was 58 systolic and 36 diastolic). Autoregulation is not in force during adenosine medication and we know from dog experiments that the nonautoregulated coronary artery flow decreases below a pressure of 60 mmHg (38). These factors may have influenced the total flow and flow reserve measurements. The results, however, suggest that there is high accuracy in the MR measurements because they were very similar to the ultrasound measurements, although both may be incorrect as measurements of normal absolute blood flow in the coronary arteries. Hundley et al. (39) of the same group thereafter investigated 12 patients with chest pain using the same technique with similar results. Their average LAD flow was 18–163 ml/min (mean 49), and only 2 of their 12 patients had significant (>50%) stenosis. Their flow volumes are unrealistic whereas the flow reserves again make sense. The through-plane motion was evaluated by measuring the frame-to-frame displacement of landmarks on the myocardium near the arteries. They therefore measured velocity in the arteries compared to the arterial wall and not necessarily velocity in space and therefore not true volumes.

Keegan et al. (31) chose to calibrate and correct their velocities against a large stationary uniform body phantom at the end of each in vivo study. Their velocities may therefore represent true velocities more accurately, but even this is unknown at the present time. Their velocities were smaller than the others. Sakuma et al. (33) chose to calibrate and correct their method against the surrounding myocardium, and they measured blood velocity compared with the vascular wall. They performed a two-part study, one published in 1996 (33) and one appearing in abstract form only (40). The study was published later in Japanese with abstract in English (41). Their full sequence employed for breathhold flow

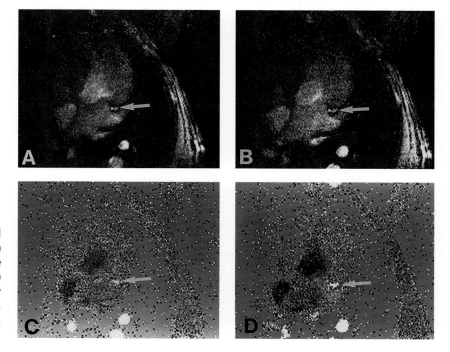

Figure 14.7. Arrows indicate cross-sectional views of the left circumflex artery (LCx) in (A) a baseline magnitude image, (B) a magnitude image acquired during adenosine infusion, (C) a baseline velocity image, and (D) a velocity image obtained during adenosine infusion. (Reproduced with permission from Clark et al., (32) and *Circulation*, 1995.)

measurements was a phase-contrast fast gradient echo sequence with resonance frequency phase spoiling (Fast Card-PC, GE Medical Systems, Milwaukee). They measured flow velocity in mid-LAD in eight healthy young volunteers (33) and in 10 patients with LAD stenosis (40). Up to nine frames/cardiac cycle were acquired. The velocities were corrected by subtracting the myocardial velocities. They used view sharing processing and their effective temporal resolution was 64 msec. Data were acquired during 24 heartbeats in suspended, shallow inspiration. They used Dipyridamol 0.56 mg/kg of body weight injected over 4 minutes and measured immediately afterward (see Fig. 2 in Ref. 33). Coronary flow reserve was calculated as the ratio of hyperemic to baseline coronary blood flow velocity. The volume flow was not calculated because of the small diameter of the LAD in relation to the spatial resolution of the images. Their study has the advantage of multiple phase acquisition in one breathhold compared to one acquisition/breathhold which is difficult to reproduce when collecting more data. The flow reserve based on their velocity data was significantly higher in the normal volunteers than in the patients (Fig. 14.8). An interesting finding was that in five of the ten patients with less than 75% stenosis some flow reserve was preserved while none was preserved in the five who had more than 75% lesions.

Davis et al. (42) measured coronary flow reserve in normal subjects and found the flow reserve to be 5.0 ± 2.6 (median 4.15). They did not state how they calibrated their velocities, and the accuracy of their absolute measurements of a flow of 38 ± 11 ml/min in the LAD is uncertain. Kawada et al. have later measured coronary flow reserve in the coronary sinus compared with the

flow reserve in the coronary arteries with good correlation (43). Absolute flows in milliliters per minute was not measured. The same group (44) measured absolute myocardial flow and vasodilator flow reserve in patients with hypertrophic cardiomyopathy. They found that the flow in milliliters per minute per gram heart muscle was significantly lower in hypertrophic hearts who also had lower flow reserve. The data are only in abstract form, and it is unknown how they calculated zero velocity.

Hundley et al. (45) measured coronary flow and flow reserve in proximal middle or distal LAD at rest and after intravenous adenosine using breathhold technique. The measurements correlated well with similar measures using intracoronary Doppler flow wires. A review of MR measurements of coronary blood flow has been published by Sakuma (46):

> Calculation of zero velocity is absolutely crucial for volume flow measurements in the coronary arteries (47). The FOV is too small to include stationary structures, and large errors in absolute flow volumes occur if the effects of through-plane myocardial motion is not corrected for. The myocardial motion is largest in peak systole (10 cm/sec) and is larger during stress than rest so that flow reserve measurements may become uncertain as well (48, 49).

The only published clinical study using echo-planar imaging is by Poncelet et al. (36). They used a time of flight (TOF) model with echo-planar imaging to derive coronary flow velocities from wash in curves free of cardiac wall motion contamination. They used short axis studies as all the others with through-plane velocity measurements. Ten to 20 singular or multislice images were acquired within a single breathhold. Flow velocity was measured in the proximal LAD at rest and during isometric exercise. The data demonstrated the known phasic pattern of the LAD with systolic velocities of five cm/sec and diastolic of fourteen. During isometric exercise the LAD flow velocities increased to an average of 52 cm/sec in eight out of nine subjects. The TOF echo-planar imaging method therefore appears as useful as the turboFlash-segmented k-space sequences. None of them, however, appears to be useful for absolute flow measurements.

In summary, it appears that we can now measure something equivalent to flow reserve in individual coronary arteries with MR phase-contrast velocity mapping, but not absolute flow due to insufficient spatial resolution (approximately 1 × 1 mm) and lack of zero velocity accuracy. Peak velocity and total flow volume may have different peak periods at stress. In large vessels the accuracy of phase-contrast velocity and flow measurements is 5–10%, but it is much larger in very small vessels like coronary arteries, maybe 50–100%. The velocity encoding should be kept at the minimum to keep

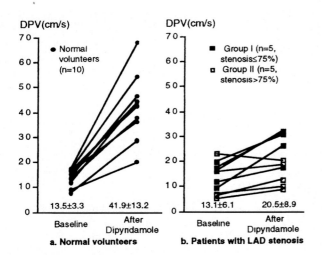

Figure 14.8. Diastolic peak velocity (DPV) in the baseline state and after Dipyridamole injection. (Reprinted with permission from Proceedings of the International Society for Magnetic Resonance in Medicine Fourth Scientific Meeting and Exhibition. New York, April 27–May 3, 1996,1:672. (40).)

errors low. As high flow encoding as 150 cm/sec has been used in coronary arteries, which gives a large error and should be avoided because the maximum velocities appear to be in the region of 50 cm/sec.

The value of flow reserve in itself is not quite clear. The flow reserve varies regionally and flow reserve measurement in one branch may be of limited value due to this variation and the uncertainty of collateral flow. We may have to measure flow reserve in the LAD, the left circumflex, and the RCA to obtain an overall evaluation of flow reserve. The global flow reserve may after all be more important than the regional. It is likely, though, that flow measurements in the three main branches would be superior to measurement in the aorta in a clinical case of coronary artery stenosis. The global flow reserve measurement may be of value as a screening method for coronary artery disease or as a measure of success or failure of therapy, but it has to be much simplified to be practical.

The competing methods include the intravascular Doppler method, which has the disadvantage of being invasive and may only be useful in connection with cardiac catheterization. It increases radiation exposure to patients who, after cardiac cath and balloon angioplasty, already have obtained high radiation doses. The transesophageal echocardiography method is invasive, or at least semi-invasive, and requires general anesthesia in some instances.

Myocardial scintigraphy with radioisotopes and exercise or pharmacologic stress may show ischemia better than any other method and thereby the functional severity of a stenosis. Myocardial perfusion studies with MR are being developed (50) and have been extended to measurements of regional myocardial flow reserve in experimental animals and a few patients with apparent success by one frontier research group (49). MR coronary angiography and MR flow reserve measurements are also being developed, but they are not clinically useful yet. With ingenuity and rapid technological development, however, the MR station may be the future for the diagnosis of ischemic heart disease with capabilities to perform angiography, measure flow and flow reserve, and myocardial perfusion.

Coronary Flow Reserve: Technical Aspects

General Principles of Flow Measurement by Phase Contrast

Phase-contrast cine MRI velocity measurement requires that at least two independent images are acquired (51). By manipulating the magnetic field gradient pulses to set the first moment equal to zero, one image is "motion-compensated" in that no dephasing of the echo

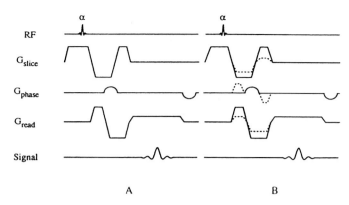

Figure 14.9. Phase-contrast gradient echo pulse sequence for acquisition of a "motion-compensated" and "velocity-encoded" pulse sequence. (A) Gradient pulses in which the first moments are equal to zero at the echo, producing a "motion-compensated" image. (B) For acquisition of an image that is "velocity encoded" in one direction, a second data set is acquired with the gradient waveform along that direction changed from the solid line to the dashed line. Gradient pulse shapes are set by the desired velocity selectivity. (Reprinted with permission from Pelc et al. (51).)

signal due to first-order motion occurs. By manipulating the magnetic field gradient pulses to set the first moment equal to specific value, the second image is "velocity encoded" for a predetermined range of velocities (Fig. 14.9). The difference in the phases of the two complex MRI signals arising from moving spins is directly proportional to the spins' velocity. Phase differences proportional only to velocity may also be derived from subtraction of data encoded to different nonzero velocities, neither motion-compensated. The VENC value is defined as the velocity that generates a 180-degree phase difference. In quantitative phase-contrast MRI velocity images, the spatial distribution of the signal phase, which is distinct from the more commonly used signal amplitude, is displayed. This velocity image is composed of the pixel-by-pixel differences between the motion-compensated and velocity-encoded phase images. Pixels containing blood with velocity VENC are displayed as maximal white or black, depending on flow direction. Motion-compensated and velocity-encoded data acquisitions could be done separately in time, but they are usually interleaved to reduce view-to-view misregistration artifacts (52). Accurate velocity maps also require the application of correction algorithms to remove residual background phase error in the subtraction image (53,54).

Phase-contrast sequences employ gradient waveforms for encoding the velocity in the phase of the blood spin. Velocity-encoding gradients are typically applied in the slice select direction. For each k-space view, positive and negative velocity-encoding data (encoding typically 100–200 cm/sec), or velocity-encoded and flow-compensated data, are acquired as sequential pairs. Eight or more lines of k-space data are typically collected in each R–R interval. The true temporal resolution, defined as the data acquisition window over which motion is averaged, was typically 128 msec, and is generally expressed as $m \times n \times TR$, where m is the number of flow-encoding directions in each k-space line, n is the number of lines collected per segment, and TR is the repetition time.

Evolution of Pulse Sequences for Coronary Flow Reserve

Non-breathhold Techniques

Bogren and Buonocore (24) first measured coronary flow reserve using flow measurements in the ascending aorta. Compelling reasons for choosing aorta flow measurements include: (1) Relative lack of motion of the aorta compared to the coronary arteries. (2) Improved accuracy of low flow measurements (with appropriate reduction in encoding value, over large cross-sectional area (i.e., the aorta) relative to higher velocity measurement across a smaller cross-sectional area (i.e., the coronary vessel). Asynchronously (retrospectively) gated velocity-encoded phase imaging using a velocity-encoded cine pulse sequence (GE Medical Systems) was

used (Fig. 14.10) with TR: 33 ms, TE: 9 ms, Flip: 30 degrees, slice thickness: 5 mm, FOV: 40 cm, matrix: 128 × 256, NEX: 2, VENC: 200 cm/s, Flow Comp On, and sequential phase encode ordering. Velocity data was obtained in an axial slice at the level of the pulmonary artery bifurcation, with velocity encoding perpendicular to the slice plane. Velocity images were constructed by subtracting the phase angles of a velocity-encoded phase image from a nonencoded reference image. Encoded and nonencoded raw data was acquired in alternate TR intervals, giving a temporal resolution of 66 msec. Linear interpolation of the encoded and nonencoded data is used to create new data at specified time points for reconstruction of images.

Original Segmented k-Space Technique

Atkinson and Edelman were first to implement a breath-hold MRA technique for depicting the coronary arteries and for potentially quantifying flow velocities (55,56). This imaging and flow quantification method is based on an approach called segmented turboFLASH (fast low-angle shot). Data acquisition, in which a gradient-echo pulse sequence that is synchronized with the cardiac cycle, is divided into multiple portions of k-space (segments) (Fig. 14.11). For angiography without flow quan-

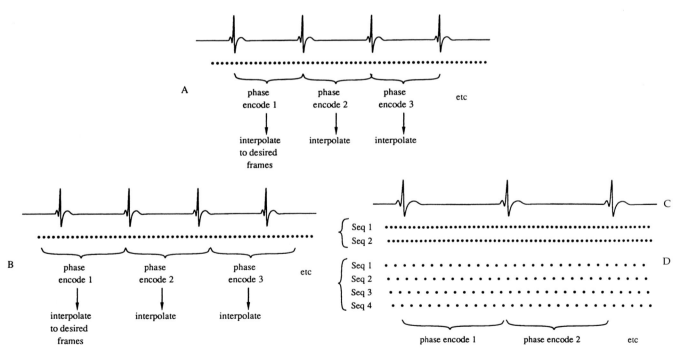

Figure 14.10. (A) Retrospectively gated cine pulse sequence with sequential phase-encode ordering. Each cardiac cycle is associated with a single phase-encode step. The phase-encode step is incremented with each EKG trigger. Acquired data is interpolated to the desired "cardiac frames," typically defined at equally spaced time points within the average cardiac cycle. (B) Single slice acquisitions with different velocity encodings are interleaved within each cardiac cycle. Acquisitions in the same cycle have the same spatial phase encoding, but alternating velocity encoding. Spatial phase encoding is incremented with each new cardiac cycle. (C) Interleaving of two different velocity encodings for imaging velocity in one direction. (D) Interleaving of four different velocity encodings for imaging all three directions of velocity. Different velocity encodings include the "motion-compensated" case in which there is 0 cm/sec velocity encoding. (Reprinted with permission from Pelc et al. (51).)

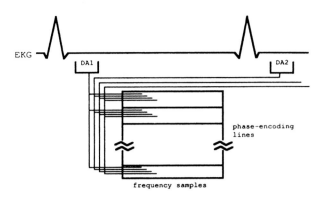

Figure 14.11. Association of EKG triggering and k-space demonstrates the process of segmented data acquisition. Two of 16 segments, denoted DA1 and DA2, are shown. Each segment has a short acquisition window (e.g., 50 ms), within which eight distinct k-space lines (with eight different phase-encode steps) are acquired for a single image. Within each segment, every sixteenth line of k-space is acquired. Thus, the first segment (DA1) acquires lines 1, 17, 33, 49, 65, 81, 97, and 113, and DA2 acquires 2, 18, 34, and so on. The acquisition shown is for production of one image at one distinct phase of the cardiac cycle (frame). Depending on heart rate and variability, data for production of up to 20 frames might be acquired. (Reprinted with permission from Atkinson and Edelman (55).)

tification, the duration of each segment was brief (50 ms) to reduce blurring related to cardiac motion. The acquisition was completed within a single breathhold to eliminate respiratory artifacts. The final image was reconstructed from a data set that is a composite of all the segments acquired within the breathhold. For the phase-contrast modification of this approach, two segmented

turboFLASH images were acquired in a single breath-hold (Fig. 14.12). The data for a rephased and a dephased image are acquired on alternate heartbeats. In the first R–R interval, every twelfth k-space line is acquired with rephasing section select gradients. In the second R–R interval, the same lines are acquired by using partially dephasing section select gradients. This pattern is continued until all 96 phase-encoding steps have been applied for both the rephased and dephased images. The section select, however, is performed using a three-lobed, velocity-compensated waveform insensitive to flow, and a bilobed waveform resulting in a measurable shift in the phase of the MR signal of flowing blood.

The main advantage of the segmented acquisition developed by Edelman was the ability to use breathholding to reduce respiratory motion artifacts. Breathholding can typically be implemented by having the subject take a deep breath in and breath out, then suspend breathing in shallow inspiration. Imaging data can be acquired for 12 or more heartbeats, depending on patient capability. The turboFLASH sequence for coronary flow measurement is rapid and noninvasive. Using the fat-suppressed segmented turboFLASH sequence, coronary arteries are identified in most subjects (57), and provide the necessary anatomical image requisite to flow velocity measurement.

Improvements in the Original Segmented Sequence
The segmented k-space sequences used today for the majority of coronary flow reserve measurements are based on the original technique developed by Edelman. They employ k-segmentation that allows the acquisition of several phase-encoding steps for each cine frame in

Figure 14.12. Pulse sequence diagram for interleaved, segmented turboFLASH imaging and phase-contrast velocity measurement. Data for a rephased and a dephased image are acquired on alternate heartbeats. In the first R–R interval, every twelfth k-space line (i.e., 1, 13, 25, etc.) is acquired with rephasing (i.e., motion-compensated) section-selection gradients. In the second R–R interval, the same lines are acquired using partially dephasing (i.e., velocity-encoded) section-selection gradients. Every twelfth k-space line starting with the second (i.e., 2, 14, 26, etc.) are acquired with rephasing and dephasing gradients in the third and fourth R–R intervals. This pattern is continued until all (e.g., 96) phase-encoding steps have been applied for both rephased and dephased images. (*From*: Flow velocity quantification in human coronary arteries with fast, breath-hold MR angiography. Edelman et al., *J Magn Reson Imag*, copyright 1993. Reprinted by permission of Wiley-Liss, Inc., a subsidiary of John Wiley & Sons., Inc.)

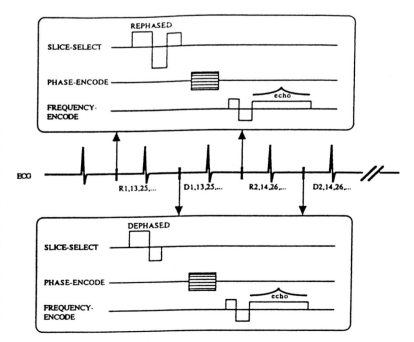

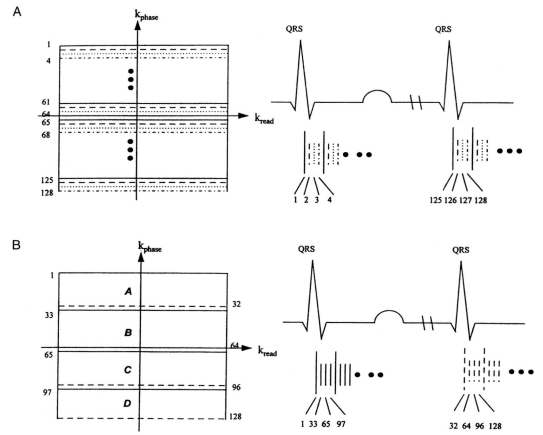

Figure 14.13. Depiction of "sequential" and "interleaved" (also called "simple") segmented phase-encode grouping methods with a phase-encode grouping (PEG) size of 4. (A) In the sequential method, four adjacent lines of *k*-space are acquired in each heartbeat for each cardiac frame, starting at 1. Subsequent heartbeats acquire four adjacent lines in numerical sequence (i.e., starting at 5, 9, 13, etc.). In this scenario, the two central lines (e.g., numbers 64 and 65) are acquired with the greatest possible temporal difference (64 at the end of the frame, 65 at the beginning). (B) In the interleaved method [originally proposed by Atkinson (41)] *k*-space is divided into four segments. Within each heartbeat one line from each segment is acquired in each cardiac frame. The two central lines are acquired at adjacent time points within the frame, and image ghosting due to variations across the cardiac frame are reduced compared with the sequential method. The sequential method, however, reduces image ghosting due to trigger-to-trigger variations. Additional useful variations of *k*-space acquisition ordering have been developed; in particular, the acquisition of symmetrically placed *k*-space lines at the same time point within the frame is an important feature of the SCOPEG technique. (Reprinted with permission from Li et al. (64).)

a single heartbeat. The principal difference in the new techniques are the options with respect to the temporal order in which different phase-encoding steps are acquired, and the routine acquisition of greater number of cardiac frames (e.g., Fig. 14.13). Data is acquired in groups of *k*-space lines referred to as phase-encode groupings (PEGS), among other names. Ultrashort repetition times (TR) are used to acquire multiple phase-encoding steps for each cardiac frame for each R–R interval. A complete cardiac cine with four to eight frames (instead of one acquired in the original implementation of the phase-contrast technique) can be easily obtained during a single breathhold.

Fat saturation is generally utilized because the coronary vessels are surrounded by fat and local contrast is improved by reducing this signal. There is disagreement, however, over whether fat saturation is necessary for adequate visualization and flow measurements. There are time penalties associated with implementation of the pulse, and disruption of steady-state conditions in retrospectively gated cine acquisitions. Hundley (53) did not use fat saturation because in-plane spatial presaturation pulses were used to suppress signal from tissue in the slice. Flowing blood appeared bright and of different contrast relative to stationary tissue with this technique.

Flow Reserve Using EPI
Echo-planar imaging (EPI) is a unique tool that provides images in 60 ms (58), effectively freezing heart motion.

Detection and quantification of flow of the left anterior descending (LAD) coronary artery has been demonstrated in healthy volunteers using gradient-echo EPI. In the first application of EPI to coronary flow and flow reserve measurement (59,60), flow velocity was derived by modeling the TOF effects of a laminar flow wash-in through a slice, as described by Wehrli (61). A gated, flow-compensated, gradient-echo EPI pulse sequence (GE Signa 1.5T retrofitted by Advanced NMR Inc., TE = 29 ms, alpha = 90, slice = 10 mm, FOV = 20 × 40 cm, pixel 1.5 × 3.0 mm, 75% partial k-space and fat suppression) was used for short axis studies of the heart. Images were collected during a 4–20-second breath-hold.

In the TOF technique, two 90-degree RF pulses are applied: The first saturates a large slab (3 cm); the second excites the imaging slice (1 cm) within it. By including a presaturation slab larger than the imaging slice, the effects of through-plane displacement of the coronary vessel during the cardiac cycle are reduced (62). The slice excitation pulse timing is fixed to a particular cardiac gate delay, and the interval between the 2 pulses, T_{sat}, is progressively lengthened backward in time from this fixed gate delay. A series of 20 images is collected, increasing T_{sat} by 10 ms at each heartbeat. The signal intensity change due to blood wash-in through the slice as a function of T_{sat} was measured. Reference signal intensity was obtained using the first three images of the series collected without presaturation. Maximum flow velocity, V_{max}, is then derived from fitting the wash-in curve to the model. Assuming laminar flow, $V_{max} = 2 \langle V \rangle$, where $\langle V \rangle$ is the mean flow velocity. On 11 subjects, EPI determined the peak mean flow velocity in diastole and the mean flow velocity in systole: $\langle Vd \rangle$ ranged from 9 to 19 cm/s (peak $\langle Vd \rangle$ = 14 ± 3 cm/s) in diastole and $\langle Vs \rangle$ were all ≤4 cm/s in systole. Repeating measurements for several delays demonstrated good reproducibility (sigma = 1.2 cm/s). While EPI imaging has been used more extensively, spiral imaging (63) offers comparable imaging times and should also have major impact.

Special Attributes of Newer Segmented Techniques

The optimized k-space segmentation used by Clarke et al. (32) involving symmetrical, centrally ordered PEGs, referred to as SCOPEG (Fig. 14.14) (54,64). Heartbeat-to-heartbeat misregistration of the data is minimized with this technique by acquiring the data in the central portion of k-space (low spatial frequencies) at the same time period in the cardiac cycle for successive heartbeats. This characteristic of data acquisition was not provided in the original segmented k-space method. Eddy currents can be a problem with any

rapid imaging sequence that uses rapid pulsing of the gradients. In the SCOPEG technique, these are minimized by using phase-encoding gradient pulses temporally arranged so that a positive gradient pulse is always followed by a negative pulse. To provide a smooth and symmetrical modulation of the gradient pulses, the positive and negative regions of k space are sampled separately, resulting in a data set that is symmetrically ordered about the zeroth phase-encoding step. This segmentation scheme reduces the incidence of ghosting and eddy current effects while also minimizing the blurring due to motion between low spatial frequency phase-encode steps.

Pulse sequences that use cine retrospective acquisition (33,48) also provide images at multiple temporal phases during a single breathhold period (Fig. 14.15). Uniform repetition time and constant resonance frequency excitation was implemented to maintain spins at a dynamic equilibrium, which decreased artifacts and, very importantly, allowed acquisition of data immediately before and after the electrocardiographic R-wave trigger. Acquisition during diastole had not been possible with previous techniques. In addition, by maintaining the steady state, these sequences eliminated the increased signal intensity typical in the first few temporal images that results from the longer T1 recovery period—the so-called lightning flash artifact. The view acquisition order in these sequences is sequential or centric rather than interleaved, and images show fewer artifacts because low spatial frequency k-space lines are acquired within a single R–R interval, reducing effects of beat-to-beat variability. Images obtained with sequential ordering have better edge definition because adjacent spatial frequency data are acquired close in time.

View-sharing reconstruction was implemented with velocity encoding (Fig. 14.16) to improve effective temporal resolution by shifting a virtual acquisition window by half the original temporal resolution, thereby providing better sampling for diastolic peak flow velocity (33,48). Images at intermediate temporal phases were generated by using the last $n/2$ views in each segment of one temporal phase image with the first $n/2$ views in each segment of the succeeding temporal phase, where n is the number of views per segment. If m temporal phase images were originally obtained with velocity-encoded cine MRI, this method increases the number of temporal phase images to $2m - 1$. The true temporal resolution, that is the time necessary to acquire data for all n views within a segment, is unchanged (128 ms); however, the effective temporal resolution (i.e., the temporal separation between images), is halved (64 ms). Magnitude and phase cine images with 7–13 temporal phases for an average cardiac cycle were reconstructed from the data acquired within a single breathhold period.

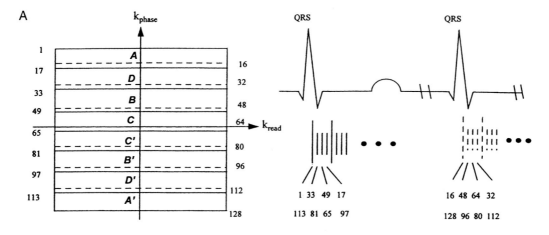

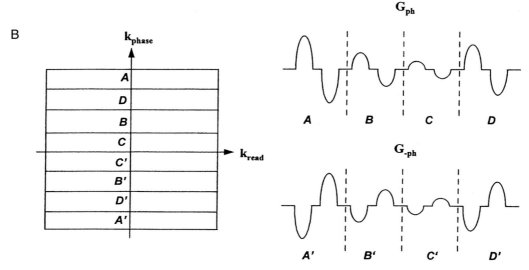

Figure 14.14. Depiction of the SCOPEG method for a single cardiac frame, showing acquisition of central *k*-space lines at the same time point within the frame. (A) For a phase-encode grouping (PEG) size of 4, *k*-space is divided into eight segments. One line from segment A, B, C, or D in the top half of *k*-space, *or* A′, B′, C′, or D′ in the bottom half of *k*-space, is acquired in each heartbeat. Top and bottom halves of *k*-space are acquired separately; however, lines from segments A and A′ (1–16 and 113–128 in figure), B and B′ (33–48 and 81–96), C and C′ (49–80, which are the central lines of *k*-space), and from D and D′ (17–32 and 97–112) are acquired at the same (first, second, third, or fourth, respectively) time points within the frame. (B) Each phase-encoding pulse is paired with a rewinding pulse. The top and bottom halves of *k*-space are sampled separately, so that a positive gradient pulse is always followed by a negative pulse (e.g., negative rewinding pulse is never followed by a negative encoding pulse that would be required for the bottom half of *k*-space), which provides more reliable transitions and less phase distortions due to eddy currents within each phase-encoding group. (Reprinted with permission from Li et al. (64).)

Special Hardware for Coronary Flow Measurement

Most studies have been performed at 1.5 T using systems with conventional gradients (10 mT/m, 500 μsec rise time). High-speed gradients, however, can result in 50–100% increase in the number of frames per cardiac cycle that can be acquired (32). In these studies, standard imagers (e.g., the 1.5 T Vista HPQ MRI system) have been fitted with prototype high-performance gradient coils (e.g., 65). These gradient coils can provide 15 mT/m or more with reduced rise times of 300 μsec or less. Quad-

rature and phased-array surface radiofrequency coils have been used to improve signal-to-noise ratio (SNR) and image depth compared with standard linear surface coils. They have been used in both the supine or prone position. Receive-only quadrature surface coils (20 cm/25 cm) designed for spine imaging have also been used (32).

Testing of Flow Measurement Accuracy and Precision

Quantitative evaluation of the segmented sequences in phantom studies has yielded good results; however,

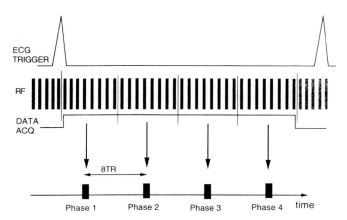

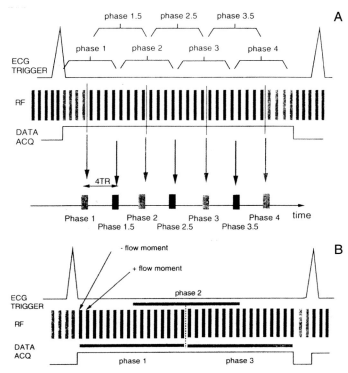

Figure 14.15. Diagram shows the radiofrequency excitation that is temporally uniform (interval TR between pulses) and continuous throughout the scan, combined with so-called prospectively gated acquisition in which data is obtained immediately after the EKG trigger. Note that this gating scheme is equivalent to previously defined *retrospective* acquisition in the standard cine acquisition (41), except that data is not interpolated across the EKG trigger. Eight views acquired in succession are grouped into a segment to generate data for an image at a particular cardiac phase (i.e., frame). This organization is depicted by the vertical lines and arrows. With RF excitation at uniform TR, the steady-state magnetization is maintained, and the first view is closer to the R wave because dummy excitations that would be needed to create the steady state are not necessary. (Reprinted with permission from Foo TKF, Bernstein MA, Aisen AM, Hernandez RJ, Collick BD, Bernstein T. Improved ejection fraction and flow velocity estimates using view sharing and uniform TR excitation with fast cardiac techniques. Radiology 1995;195:471–78.)

Figure 14.16. (A) View sharing using the data acquisition as presented in Figure 14.15; however, views from adjacent segments are now grouped to generate intermediate (half-integer) segments centered at time points midway between those of the original segments. This is equivalent to shifting the acquisition window for a segment by four TR intervals. Although the effective temporal resolution is increased to four TR intervals, motion in each image (corresponding to a particular cardiac phase) is still averaged over eight TR intervals. Hence, the true temporal resolution is not improved; rather, the cardiac cycle motion will be smoother in the resulting time sequence of images. Given m frames in the original, view sharing will nearly double the number of frames to $2m - 1$. (B) Diagram shows the modification of the acquisition for velocity encoding (VENC) in a single direction with eight views per segment. The number of velocity-encoded frames decreases by a factor of two (to $m/2$), whereas view sharing increases the number of such frames to $m/2 - 1$. The diagram depicts plus and minus velocity encoding as sequential pairs, but compensated, velocity encoding is also compatible. (Reprinted with permission from Foo TKF, Bernstein MA, Aisen AM, Hernandez RJ, Collick BD, Bernstein T. Improved ejection fraction and flow velocity estimates using view sharing and uniform TR excitation with fast cardiac techniques. *Radiology* 1995;195:471–78.)

phantom studies that accurately mimic the motion and small size of the coronary vessel have not yet been performed. Using the velocity-encoded turboFLASH sequence, Edelman et al. (56) found excellent correlation ($r = 0.99$, $p = 0.0001$) between MR and volume displacement flow measurements using a steady flow phantom. Velocity measurements and laser Doppler methods obtained in a pulsatile flow phantom, and those obtained in volunteers in the abdominal aorta, also correlated well. There was also good agreement between flow measurements from breathhold-segmented sequences and standard velocity-encoded cine sequences.

The most thorough verification of flow measurements with fat-suppressed segmented k-space sequences, using phantoms, has been carried out by Keegan et al. (66). Flow measurement accuracy and precision was evaluated using two encoding strategies. In the first, a nonvelocity-sensitized reference image and an image sensitized to 25 cm/sec were obtained in a single acquisition. In the second, two velocity-sensitized images, both to 50 cm/sec, but in the opposite sense, were obtained in a single acquisition, giving a combined sensitivity equal to the first strategy. Phase encoding was performed in PEGs of four per cardiac cycle, resulting in

data acquisition over 32 heartbeats or less. The segmented sequence velocity measurements were compared with those obtained from conventional velocity-encoded acquisition.

Significant differences in performance were found using the two encoding strategies. Small beat to beat flow variations and relatively higher velocity sensitivity of the velocity-sensitized image in the first (25–0) sequence resulted in the sensitized magnitude image having considerably more artifacts than the nonvelocity-sensitized reference image obtained in the same acquisition. In the second (50–50) sequence, the artifacts were less. The study concluded that distributing the encoding across the two sequences was preferred for coronary artery imaging. Increasing the phase-encoding grouping size from 1 to 4 did not appreciably change the flow measured in the pulsatile flow phantom, thus validating higher grouping size. Maximum and mean velocities measured at 34% and 57% stenoses were consistent with theoretical predictions of velocity increase.

The absolute accuracy of the flow measurements in coronary arteries in vivo has not been demonstrated. In lieu of a gold standard, some investigators have evaluated interstudy reproducibility of coronary flow velocity measurements in humans by performing the velocity-encoded scan twice, with separate breathholds, in the baseline state prior to dipyridamole administration (33). Reproducibility is sufficient to detect differences due to pharmacological stress in flow reserve measurements reliably.

Sequence Parameters and Data Acquisition

In Edelman's original implementation, gradients waveforms were calibrated for unambiguous flow velocity measurements up to 150 cm/sec. Minimum TR and TE of the imager is used to get the highest duty cycle, and an acquisition matrix of 96×256 to 224×256 is typically used, resulting in pixel dimensions of 0.8–2 mm in each direction [e.g., 1.4×0.8 mm (56)]. Four images were produced at each cardiac phase, consisting of magnitude and phase reconstructions of each of the two encodings. In modern implementations, four to six phases (more if view sharing is employed) of the cardiac cycle are obtained in a single breathhold. The flow-insensitive magnitude image best showed vessel anatomy, whereas subtraction of the flow insensitive and flow-sensitive phase images produced a phase difference image in which the phase shift was proportional to flow velocity along the section select direction. Image subtraction was necessary to eliminate background phase shifts unrelated to blood flow.

In human studies using the SCOPEG technique, velocity compensation and encoded acquisitions were acquired with a PEG size of 3–7 to yield four to five frames per cardiac cycle. With 7-mm slice thickness, 256×256 or 256 to 224 matrix, FOV of 21 to 23 cm, flip angle of 40 degrees, repetition time of 19.5 ms, and echo time of 11 ms. The total number of views was limited to keep the duration of the breathhold at 15–25 seconds. In animal studies using the SCOPEG technique (32), the MRI image parameters were TR = 19.1 ms, TE = 11 ms, 40-degree flip angle, slice thickness 7 mm. FOV 18–24 cm (depending on orientation and animal size) corresponding to a pixel size range of 0.7 to 0.94 mm² with

phase-encoded aspect ratios ranging from 160:256 to 220:256, and PE grouping sizes of two to three. Each cine set of four to six images was acquired during a 30- to 40-second breathhold. The longer breathhold and higher resolution imaging were possible in dog studies, but are probably not achievable in human subjects.

Double oblique thick sections perpendicular to the LAD artery, 16 ms repetition time, and 9 ms echo time, 96 phase encoding steps, 24×18 cm FOV, 256×192 reconstructed image matrix, and 32 kHz receiver bandwidth were used with the Fast Card segmented breathhold sequence (33). This sequence (65) employed resonance frequency phase spoiling, permitting slightly improved TR. High receiver bandwidth permitted significantly shorter TE. The phase-encoding direction was chosen so ghosting from ventricular chamber blood would not overlap the coronary vessel.

Protocols for Locating the Vessels

All studies have utilized pilot scans in order to localize the coronary vessels both in space and time. Because of the errors associated with measurements of flow in vessels that are obliquely oriented to the slice, special care was taken to set up slices exactly transverse to the vessels at the point in time of interest.

In original studies by Edelman (56), coronary artery localization images were acquired over 16–20 heartbeats during a single breathhold. Localization sequences were EKG gated, with single-image acquisition during diastole. Oblique views were then acquired along the long axis of each proximal coronary artery. Double oblique sections perpendicular to the long axis of the vessel of interest were then obtained to visualize the vessel in cross-section.

Most studies imaged human subjects in the supine position using EKG monitoring for cardiac triggering, a respiratory bellows to monitor the breathholds and provide respiratory gating, and an anterior surface coil. Scans were done to image the artery in short axis, tangential, and longitudinal planes. These scout images were acquired with the same sequences as used for velocity measurement, incorporating breathhold, gradient echo with first moment compensation (no velocity encoding), and frequency fat suppression, with shortest possible TR (e.g., 20 ms) and TE (e.g., 9.4 ms) and 4–6 PEG size. In subjects showing a signal void in the vessel of interest proximally (indicating a potential arterial stenosis), cross-sectional images using similar scan parameters were obtained distal to the area of dropout (53). FOV was then decreased to 21–23 cm to decrease pixel sizes (to 0.82–1.00 mm) and thereby reduce intravoxel dephasing. In-plane presaturation pulses were applied at the first frame of each cardiac cycle to remove unwanted signals.

Because the LAD artery has a tortuous course, it was typical to choose the imaging plane among three to five consecutive cardiac short axis planes, such that the orientation of the LAD artery was closest to perpendicular (33). The imaging plane on which the LAD artery was depicted as a small round vessel, and where the adjacent imaging plane showed the LAD artery at a similar location, was chosen. To allow for the positional variation of the arteries over the cardiac cycle, some investigators performed an additional pilot scan at each gating delay at which velocity mapping was to be performed (66).

Clarke et al. (32) used the sagittal view in dog studies, and continued if necessary with oblique orientations, to obtain a series of high-resolution cine images with the LAD and LCx in the image plane. Breathhold MRI pilot images were then obtained with the ventilator stopped to determine the position of the LCx and LAD that would occur during a breathhold. A perpendicular view of the vessel was then acquired to confirm that the section was straight and adequate for the slice thickness of the anticipated flow measurement and that there was no excessive through-plane motion. Through-plane motion was evaluated by measuring the frame-to-frame displacement of landmarks on the myocardium near the arteries that were visible on the initial cine scout images.

Data Analysis

The major concerns in extracting velocity and flow measurements from the coronary arteries are typically (1) correctly tracking the position of the coronary vessel on the individual frames through the cardiac cycle, (2) drawing an region of interest (ROI) that extracts velocity data that accurately represents the intraluminal velocity and is not contaminated by partial volume effects, and (3) finding a region of the image that can be assumed to be not moving to serve as a zero-velocity phase reference value. The magnitude images are first displayed in a cine loop and the position and shape of the artery are noted. To make identification of the vessel as easy as possible, the lumen cross-sectional area is determined from the magnitude images, and is typically chosen from the magnitude image in which the vessel appears to be largest and brightest from flow signal enhancement. Previous studies have demonstrated that mean variation in coronary vessel size is 3% from beat to beat and is 6% from systole to diastole, suggesting that beat to beat and phasic changes in coronary arterial diameter could not be measured at typical MRI spatial resolutions (67). Thus, ROI size and shape are usually kept constant, whereas the location of the ROI is changed from frame to frame to move with the vessel on the magnitude images. The ROI is then automatically placed at the identical position on the associated velocity image for measurement of the mean velocity in the vessel. A relatively large region of interest (30–50 pixels) is then placed on tissue adjacent to the artery for each cardiac phase, and mean velocity in the artery is adjusted using the mean velocity in the surrounding tissue as baseline. The flow during each phase of the cardiac cycle is then calculated from the product of the mean velocity in the ROI and the ROI area. The average coronary flow in mL/min is estimated as the mean of the calculated flow values for the entire set of images across the cardiac cycle. Coronary flow reserve is calculated as the ratio of hyperemic to baseline coronary blood flow. Flow velocities in each coronary artery should be measured independently by two or more observers.

In some investigations (33), the volume flow was not calculated, because the small diameter of the LAD artery in relation to the spatial resolution of the images was thought to make the accuracy of this measurement questionable. Moreover, the contrast of the LAD arterial edge in the basal and dipyridamole vasodilation states varied because of the increased signal intensity in the artery associated with increased flow velocity. Because flow measurements are very sensitive to edge effects in small vessels, comparisons were thought to be inaccurate. These investigators used only the measured velocities to estimate coronary flow reserve, thus avoiding these errors associated with calculation of flow. Peak diastolic flow velocities in the baseline state and after dipyridamole administration were identified and measured with time–velocity curves through the cardiac cycle. Coronary flow reserve was then calculated as the ratio of hyperemic to baseline peak coronary blood velocity. Data were expressed as the mean plus or minus the standard deviation, except where noted. The peak diastolic flows were compared with a paired Student t-test. Interstudy and interobserver variabilities were calculated as the absolute difference between the two measurements divided by the mean of the two measurements.

Common Limitations of MRI Coronary Flow Reserve Measurement

Several limitations are commonly presented regarding the use of MRI for coronary artery flow measurement.

Complex Geometry and Motion of Coronary Arteries
The most common limitation is that the coronary arteries exhibit complex curvature and are moving; therefore, it is exceedingly difficult to obtain true transverse slice orientations that provide the most accurate flow measurements. Phase-contrast velocity measurements with the vessel in the plane of the images, studied by Kraft et al. (67) and others, suffer from partial volume effects due to static tissue on either side of the vessel that cause severe phase errors. These studies conclude that small vessels, such as the coronary arteries, must be imaged transversely.

Cardiac contraction generates two different components of motion in the coronary arteries, through-plane and in-plane. The effect of through-plane motion and of the offset error in phase is handled, in principle, by subtracting the velocity in the tissue surrounding the coronary artery (33). Large in-plane motion may blur the coronary artery during data acquisition in velocity-encoded cine MRI. The LAD artery generally has peak flow velocity in the diastolic phase, and no blurring of the artery was observed in diastole; however, the RCA may demonstrate peak velocity in the systolic phase, and, therefore, flow reserve measurement of the RCA necessitates flow measurements throughout the cardiac cycle. Measurement of flow velocity over the entire cardiac cycle necessitates use of better temporal resolution (<64 ms typically used) or of a novel method to correct for coronary arterial motion (68).

Breathhold Requirement

Another common limitation is the length of the breathhold period. Patients with known myocardial infarction have been able to hold their breaths repeatedly for as long as 30 seconds (32). Many patients, however, do not have this capability, especially those with pulmonary disease. The length of the breathhold can be reduced by decreasing TR using a very-high-performance gradient system, and by reducing the number of frames obtained per cardiac cycle. Reducing the number of frames is not advisable because coronary vessels are much easier to see in a cine loop presentation with high temporal resolution, in which magnitude and velocity images are projected side by side to visualize the cyclic motion and flow-related signal changes. Even with a breathholding protocol, investigators have reported problems with inadequate compliance or patient movement during a breathhold in real-time cardiac imaging (69). It is clear that technology advances should be utilized to make the breathholding durations as short as possible.

Requirement for Diastolic Measurements

In studies using prospective EKG gating (32,53), raw data cannot be taken during the last 30–80 msec in diastole. For this portion of the cardiac cycle, flow is typically estimated as equal to flow observed in the last imaged frame. This may be a poor assumption. The degree to which flow reserve estimates are affected by the technique should be investigated because retrospective gating with acquisition over the entire cycle might be strongly preferred for this reason. One advantage of using peak velocity for coronary flow reserve estimation is that it is not important to obtain the flow curve over the entire cardiac cycle, provided that the missing frames do not contain the peak velocity (33).

Optimal Time for Acquiring the Velocity Measurement

Coronary artery flow is biphasic, so it is difficult to be certain that acquisitions are being performed during peak flow. Keegan et al. observed that changing the gating delay by as little as 100 msec may result in the maximum velocities measured being reduced from 15 cm/sec to 5 cm/sec (64). Based on these and previous measurements, the optimum time for velocity mapping appears to be in early diastole, when coronary flow has achieved its second peak and the motion of the heart is relatively low.

Flow Volume Versus Peak Velocity

There is disagreement over whether the spatial resolution is sufficient to measure coronary flow reserve based on flow, or whether it should be based on relative peak blood velocities. The accuracy of flow volume measurement with phase-contrast MRI has been shown for large vessels in several studies (69–71) in which a sufficient number of image pixels were included in the vessels. For small vessels, however, such as a coronary artery, the effects of partial volume averaging along the endothelial border of the artery can be significant and may dictate alternate, complex-difference analysis techniques (72,48). Typical in-plane spatial resolution of approximately 1×1 mm may not be sufficient to quantify volume flow accurately (73). Many researchers have assumed that in-plane spatial resolution is *not* sufficient (33,56) for accurate flow measurements. In these studies, flow reserve is instead based on relative *peak velocity*. The use of peak velocity will result in incorrect values for coronary flow reserve if the shape of the flow versus the time curve and diameter of the coronary artery change significantly under stress (33).

Clarke (32) provided submillimeter in-plane resolution, and accurate transverse positioning of the slice, to claim that flow measurements were within the theoretical specifications necessary for 10% accuracy. Tang et al. (74) demonstrated in phantoms that the error in measured volume flow rate will be < 10% if the ratio between in-plane pixel dimension and vessel radius is >0.5. The spatial resolution of the images obtained in Clarke's study were at the margin of the preceding criterion, about 3 pixels in diameter. Tang et al. also noted that the error observed in conditions of laminar flow is much less than that seen in plug flow. It is likely that laminar flow predominates within the coronary arteries, making the errors somewhat less.

Baseline Phase Offset Correction

A known error of velocity measurement with phase-contrast MRI is phase-offset caused by imperfection in the magnetic field gradient, due mainly to eddy currents (75). Because the offset varies slowly with spatial location, this error can be corrected by measuring the offset in the surrounding stationary tissue. Because the coronary arteries and their surrounding tissue undergo considerable motion due to cardiac contraction, however, this offset can be used only to determine relative velocity, and has inherently more error due to motion artifacts. The absolute flow velocity in coronary arteries measured with MRI may consequently have greater error relative to flow measurements in static tissue. Insufficient tissue for baseline measurements has been reported as a serious problem. Small FOV, together with fat suppression and the use of a surface coil, in studies by Keegan (31) resulted in there being insufficient stationary material in the resulting images for performing phase-offset corrections. To overcome this, phase data was acquired from a large uniform body phantom in the same orientations as the in vivo acquisitions, and used to determine a baseline correction. The similarity of phase data created by the human body versus a large phantom was not confirmed, and it is possible that the phantom phase variations were more severe. It is not known whether a single calibration scan could be performed and then applied to all subjects without calibration for each subject.

References

1. Gould KL, Lipscomb K, Hamilton GW. Physiologic basis for assessing critical coronary stenosis. Instantaneous flow response and regional distribution during coronary hyperemia as measures of coronary flow reserve. Am J Cardiol 1974;33:87–94.
2. Gould KL, Kirkeeide RL, Buchi M. Coronary flow reserve as a physiologic measure of stenosis severity. J Am Coll Cardiol 1990;15(2):459–74.
3. Klocke FJ. Measurements of coronary flow reserve: defining pathophysiology versus making decisions about patient care. Circulation 1987;76(6):1183–89.
4. Hoffman JIE. A critical view of coronary reserve. Circulation 1987;75(Suppl. I):I-6–I-11.
5. Collins P. Editorial: coronary flow reserve. Br Heart J 1993;69:279–81.
6. Rossen JD, Winniford MD. Effect of increases in heart rate and arterial pressure on coronary flow reserve in humans. J Am Coll Cardiol 1993;21(2):343–48.
7. Barnard RJ, Duncan HW, Livesay JJ, Buckberg GD. Coronary vasodilatory reserve and flow distribution during near maximal exercise in dogs. J Appl Physiol 1979;43:988–92.
8. Austin Jr RE, Aldea GS, Coggins DL, Flynn AE, Hoffman JIE. Profound spatial heterogeneity of coronary reserve. Discordance between patterns of resting and maximal myocardial blood flow. Circ Res 1990;67(2):319–31.
9. Bogren HG, Mohiaddin RH, Klipstein RK, Firmin DN, Underwood SR, Rees SR, et al. The function of the aorta in ischemic heart disease: a magnetic resonance and angiographic study of aortic compliance and blood flow patterns. Am Heart J 1989;118(2):234–47.
10. Legrand V, Mancini GBJ, Bates ER, Hodgson JM, Gross MD, Vogel RA. Comparative study of coronary flow reserve, coronary anatomy and results of radionuclide exercise tests in patients with coronary artery disease. J Am Coll Cardiol 1986;8(5):1022–32.
11. Vogel RA, Bates ER, O'Neill WW, Aueron FM, Meier B, Gruentzig AR. Coronary flow reserve measured during cardiac catheterization. Arch Intern Med 1984;144:1773–76.
12. Vogel RA. The radiographic assessment of coronary blood flow parameters. Circulation 1985;72:460–65.
13. Nissen SE, Elion JL, Booth DC, Evans J, DeMaria AN. Value and limitations of computer analysis of digital subtraction angiography in the assessment of coronary flow reserve. Circulation 1986;73:562–71.
14. Wilson RF, Laughlin DE, Ackell PH, et al. Transluminal subselective measurement of coronary artery blood flow velocity and vasodilator reserve in man. Circulation 1985;72:82–92.
15. Stoddard MF, Prince CR, Morris GT. Coronary flow reserve assessment by dobutamine transesophageal Doppler echocardiography. J Am Coll Cardiol 1995;25(2):325–32.
16. Redberg RF, Sobol Y, Chou TM, Malloy M, Kumar S, Botvinick E, et al. Adenosine-induced coronary vasodilation during transesophageal Doppler echocardiography: rapid and safe measurement of coronary flow reserve ratio can predict significant left anterior descending coronary stenosis. Circulation 1995;92(2):190–96, 215.
17. Kirkeeide R, Gould KL, Parsel L. Assessment of coronary stenoses by myocardial imaging during coronary vasodilation. VII. Validation of coronary flow reserve as a single integrated measure of stenosis severity accounting for all its geometric dimensions. J Am Coll Cardiol 1986;7:103–13.
18. Gould KL, Goldstein RA, Mullani NA, et al. Noninvasive assessment of coronary stenoses by myocardial perfusion imaging during pharmacologic coronary vasodilation. VIII. Clinical feasibility of positron cardiac imaging without a cyclotron using generator-produced rubidium-82. J Am Coll Cardiol 1986;7:775–89.
19. Gould KL, Ornish D, Scherwitz L, Brown S, Edens RP, Hess MJ, et al. Changes in myocardial perfusion abnormalities by positron emission tomography after long-term, intense risk factor modification. JAMA 1995;274(11):894–901.
20. Di Carli M, Czernin J, Hoh CK, Gerbaudo VH, Brunken RC, Huang SC, et al. Relation among stenosis severity, myocardial blood flow, and flow reserve in patients with coronary artery disease. Circulation 1995;91(7):1944–51.
21. Uren NG, Melin JA, De Bruyne B, Winjns W, Baudhuin T, Camici PG. Relation between myocardial blood flow and the severity of coronary artery stenosis. N Engl J Med 1994;330(25):1782–88.
22. Westerhof N. Physiological hypotheses—intramyocardial pressure: a new concept, suggestions for measurement. Basic Reson Cardiol 1990;85(2):105–19.
23. Hoffmann JIE, Spaan JA. Pressure flow relation in coronary circulation. Physiol Rev 1990;70:347.
24. Bogren HG, Buonocore MH. Measurement of coronary artery flow reserve using magnetic resonance velocity mapping in the aorta. Lancet 1993;341:899–900.
25. Bogren HG, Buonocore MH. Blood flow measurements in the aorta and major arteries with MR velocity mapping. J Magn Reson Imag 1994;4(2):119–30.
26. Bogren HG, Mohiaddin RH, Jimenez-Borreguero LJ, Kilner PJ, Yang GZ, Firmin DN. Blood flow patterns in the thoracic aorta studied with three-directional magnetic resonance velocity mapping: the effects of age and coronary artery disease. J Magn Reson Imag 1997;784–93.
27. Bogren HG, Klipstein RH, Firmin DN, Mohiaddin RH,

Underwood SR. Quantitation of antegrade and retrograde blood flow in the human aorta by magnetic resonance velocity mapping. Am Heart J 1989;117:1214–22.

28. Bogren HG, Mohiaddin RH, Yang GZ, Kilner PJ, Firmin DN. Magnetic resonance velocity vector mapping of blood flow in thoracic aortic aneurysms and grafts. J Thor Cardiol Surg 1995;110:704–14.

29. Buonocore MH. Estimation of total coronary artery flow using measurements of flow in the ascending aorta. Magn Reson Med 1994;32:602–11.

30. Edelman RR, Manning WJ, Gervino E, Li W. Flow velocity quantification in human coronary arteries with fast, breath-hold MR angiography. J Magn Reson Imag 1993; 3:699–703.

31. Keegan J, Firmin D, Gatehouse P, Longmore D. The application of breath hold phase velocity mapping techniques to the measurement of coronary artery blood flow velocity: phantom data and initial in vivo results. Magn Reson Med 1994;31:1–11.

32. Clarke GD, Eckels R, Chaney C, Smith D, Dittrich J, Hundley WG, NessAiver M, et al. Measurement of absolute epicardial coronary artery flow and flow reserve with breath-hold cine phase-contrast magnetic resonance imaging. Circulation 1995;91(10):2627–34.

33. Sakuma H, Blake LM, Amidon TM, O'Sullivan M, Szolar DH, Furber AP, et al. Coronary flow reserve: noninvasive measurement of humans with breath-hold velocity-encoded cine MR imaging. Radiology 1996;198:745–50.

34. Firmin DN, Klipstein RH, Hounsfield GL, Paley MP, Longmore DB. Echo-planar high-resolution flow velocity mapping. Magn Reson Med 1989;12(3):316–27.

35. Gatehouse PD, Firmin DN, Hughes RL, Collins S, Longmore DB. Phase contrast velocity mapping by spiral scanning. Society of Magnetic Resonance in Medicine Book of Abstracts 1992;1:216.

36. Poncelet BP, Weisskoff RM, Wedeen VJ, Brady TJ, Kantor H. Time of flight quantification of coronary flow with echo-planar MRI. Magn Reson Med 1993;30(4):447–57.

37. Pearlman JD, Edelman RR. Ultrafast magnetic resonance imaging. Segmented turboflash, echo-planar, and real-time nuclear magnetic resonance. Radiol Clin North Am 1994;32(3):593–612.

38. Mosher P, Ross J, McFate PA, Shaw RF. Control of coronary blood flow by an autoregulatory mechanism. Circ Res 1964;14:250–59.

39. Hundley WG, Hillis LD, Hamilton CA, et al. Assessment of coronary arterial restenosis with phase-contrast magnetic resonance imaging measurements of coronary flow reserve. Circulation 2000;101(20):2375–81.

40. Sakuma H, Shibata M, Isaka N, Nakano T, Takeda K, Nakagawa T, et al. MR measurement of coronary flow reserve in patients with coronary artery stenosis. Proc Int Soc Magn Reson Med 1996;1:672.

41. Sakuma H, Takeda K, Nakagawa T. Assessment of coronary flow reserve using fast phase contrast cine MR imaging. Nippon Rinsho. Jap J Clin Med 1997;55(7):1833–38.

42. Davis CP, Liu PF, Hauser M, Göhde SC, von Schulthess GK, Debatin JF. Coronary flow and coronary flow reserve measurements in humans with breath-held magnetic resonance phase contrast velocity mapping. Magn Reson Med 1997;37:537–44.

43. Kawada N, Sakuma H, Matsumura K, Takeda K, Yamakado T, Nakano T. MR measurement of coronary flow reserve (CFR): correlation between CFR measured in the coronary sinus and CFR measured in the coronary artery. MAGMA Suppl. Vol. V (11), June 1997, Book of Abstracts, ESMRMB '97 p. 38 abstract 119.

44. Kawada N, Sakuma H, Takeda K, Nakagawa T, Yamakado T, Nakano T, et al. MR assessment of absolute myocardial blood flow and vasodilator flow reserve in patients with hypertrophic cardiomyopathy. Proceedings of the International Society for Magnetic Resonance in Medicine, Fifth Scientific Meeting and Exhibition, Vancouver, B.C., 1997, Vol. 1.

45. Hundley WG, Hamilton CA, Clarke GD, Hillis LD, Herrington DM, Lange RA, et al. Visualization and functional assessment of proximal and middle left anterior descending coronary stenoses in humans with magnetic resonance imaging. Circulation 1999;99:3248–54.

46. Sakuma H, Kawada N, Takeda K, Higgins CB. MR measurement of coronary blood flow. J Magn Reson Imag 1999;10(5):728–33.

47. Polzin JA, Korosec FR, Wedding KL, Grist TM, Frayne R, Peters DC, et al. Effects of through-plane myocardial motion of phase-difference and complex-difference measurements of absolute coronary artery flow. J Magn Reson Imag 6(1):113–123.

48. Grist TM, Polzin JA, Bianco JA, Foo TKF, Bernstein MA, Mistretta CM. Measurement of coronary blood flow and flow reserve using magnetic resonance imaging. Cardiology 1997;88:80–89.

49. Wilke N, Jerosch-Herold M, Wang Y, Huang Y, Christensen BV, Stillman AE, et al. Myocardial perfusion reserve: assessment with multisection, quantitative, first-pass MR imaging. Radiology 1997;204:373–84.

50. Wilke N, Jerosch-Herold M, Stillman AE, Kroll K, Tsekos N, Merkle H, et al. Concepts of myocardial perfusion imaging in magnetic resonance imaging. Magn Reson Q, 1994;10(4):249–86.

51. Pelc NJ, Herfkens RJ, Shimakawa A, Enzmann DR. Phase contrast cine magnetic resonance imaging. Magn Reson Q 1991;7:229–54.

52. Sprikzer CE, Pelc NJ, Lee JN, Evans AJ, Sostman HD, Riederer SJ. Rapid MR imaging of blood flow with a phase sensitive limited flip angle gradient recalled pulse sequence: preliminary experience. Radiology 1990;176: 255–62.

53. Hundley WG, Li HF, Hillis LD, Meshack BM, Lange RA, Willard JE, et al. Quantitation of cardiac output with velocity encoded phase difference magnetic resonance imaging. Am J Cardiol 1995;75:1250–1255.

54. NessAiver M. Breath hold cines using phase encode groupings. In: Pohost GM, ed. Cardiovascular Applications of Magnetic Resonance. Mount Kisco, NY: Futura Publishing, 1993, 33–145.

55. Atkinson DJ, Edelman RR. Cineangiography of the heart in a single breath hold with a segmented turbo FLASH sequence. Radiology 1991;178:357–60.

56. Edelman RR, Manning WJ, Burnstein D, Paulin S. Coronary arteries: breath hold MR angiography. Radiology 1991;181:641–3.

57. Manning WJ, Boyle N, Li W, Edelman RR. Fat suppressed

breath hold magnetic resonance coronary angiography. Circulation 1992;87:94–104.

58. Stehling MK, Turner R, Mansfield P. Echo planar imaging: magnetic resonance imaging in a fraction of a second. Science 1991;254:43–50.

59. Poncelet B, Weisskoff RM, Wedeen VJ, Brady TJ, Kantor H. Measurement of coronary flow using time-of-flight echo planar MRI. Proc SMRM 1993;1:217.

60. Poncelet B, Zervos J, Weisskoff RM, Wedeen VJ, Brady TJ, Kantor H. Measurement of coronary flow reserve with time-of-flight EPI in normal and diseased LAD coronary. Proc Soc Magn Reson 1994;1:374.

61. Wehrli FW, Shimakawa A, Gullberg GT, MacFall JR. Time-of-flight MR flow imaging: selective saturation recovery with gradient refocusing. Radiology 1986;160(3):781–85.

62. Poncelet B, Kantor H. Weisskoff RM, Holmvang F, Brady TJ, Wedeen VJ. Proc Soc Magn Reson Med 1992;(2):604.

63. Pike GB, Meyer CH, Brosnan TJ, Pelc NJ. Magnetic resonance velocity imaging using a fast spiral phase contrast sequence. Magn Reson Med 1994;32(4):476–83.

64. Li H, Clarke GD, NessAvier M, Liu H, Peshock R. Magnetic resonance imaging k-space segmentation using phase-encoding groups: the accuracy of quantitative measurements of pulsatile flow. Med Phys 1995;22(4):391–99.

65. Morich MA. MRI self-shielded gradient coils. US Patent 5,296,810, assigned 1994.

66. Keegan J, Firmin DN, Gatehouse PD, Longmore DB. The study of coronary artery flood flow using breath hold phase velocity mapping techniques. Proc SMRM 1993;1:223.

67. Tomoike H, Ootsubo H, Sakai K, Kikuchyi Y, Nakamura M. Continuous measurement of coronary artery diameter in situ. Am J Physiol 1981;240:1173–79.

68. Scheidegger MB, Hess OM, Boesiger P. Assessment of coronary flow over the cardiac cycle and diastolic to systolic flow ratio with correction for vessel. Proc SMR 1994:498.

69. Maiser SE, Maier D, Boesiger P, Moser UT, Vieli A. Human abdominal aorta: comparative measurements of blood flow with MR imaging and multigated Doppler US. Radiology 1989;171:487–92.

70. Pelc LR, Pelc NJ, Rayhill SC, et al. Arterial and venous blood flow: noninvasive quantifications with MR imaging. Radiology 1992;185:809–12.

71. Mostbeck GH, Caputo GR, Higgins CB. MR measurement of blood flow in the cardiovascular system. Am J Roentgenol 1992;159:453–61.

72. Polzin JA, Alley MT, Korosec FR, Grist TM, Wang Y, Mistretta CA. A complex-difference phase-contrast technique for measurement of volume flow rates. J Magn Reson Imag 1995;5(2):129–37.

73. Wolf RL, Ehman RL, Riederer SJ, Rossman PJ. Analysis of systemic and random error in MR volumetric flow measurements. Magn Reson Med 1993;30:82–91.

74. Tang C, Blatter DD, Parker DL. Accuracy of phase contrast flow measurements in the presence of partial volume effects. Magn Reson Med 1993;3:387–85.

75. Hofman MBM, van Rossum AC, Sprenger M, Westerhof N. Assessment of flow in the right human coronary artery by magnetic resonance phase contrast velocity measurement. In: Hofman M, ed. Blood Flow Measurement by Magnetic Resonance Imaging. Utrecht, The Netherlands: Hofman, 1994.

15
First-Generation Coronary MRA Techniques

André J. Duerinckx

Introduction and Overview

First-generation coronary magnetic resonance angiography (MRA) techniques can be simplistically described as the "one-breathhold one image" technique, or the 2-D breathhold technique. There are, however, many different implementations. For example, the temporal resolution of these techniques is quite variable depending upon the geometry of k-space traversal (rectangular or spiral). We will summarize some of the more important features in this chapter, and refer the reader to other chapters for technique description (Chap. 3), history (Chap. 4), and clinical applications (Chaps. 5, 7–10).

We will start by reiterating some of the history discussed in Chapter 4. The history of first-generation coronary MRA started, at least in the published literature, in February 1991 with the article where Atkinson and Edelman (1) described a new EKG-triggered k-space segmented pulse sequence for cardiac imaging. This was followed in December 1991 by a second article by Edelman et al. (2) that described its application to coronary artery magnetic resonance imaging (MRI). EKG-triggered k-space segmented techniques allow a significant reduction of the total acquisition time for two-dimensional (2-D) imaging such that images can be acquired within a single breathhold (1,2). These techniques are now referred to as the "first-generation coronary MRA techniques." They are available on most commercial MRI scanners. The concept of k-space segmentation is widely used in other MRI applications (3). This same technique has since been shown to also work with nonrectangular k-space sampling schemes (e.g., spiral scanning) (4). Spiral coronary MRA has some advantages over the traditional approach, but is not yet routinely available on most commercial MRI scanners.

There are, however, several problems with these first-generation techniques. First, although adequate for 2-D coronary MRA, breathholding cannot easily be extended to three-dimensional (3-D) acquisitions (5,6). Second, the duration of the total examination can be long because of the need to acquire many sequential 2-D images, each requiring one breathhold. Thus, inconsistent breathholding and image misregistration problems can happen (7). Third, the technique requires a significant amount of user experience, skill, and familiarity with the cardiac and coronary anatomy to produce good results. With some training and practice, most technologists, radiologists, and/or cardiologists can learn how to perform these studies (7–9) (see also Chap. 5). It has also been demonstrated that the first-generation techniques can provide relatively good image quality for cardiac imaging, and even coronary imaging, in patients who cannot cooperate with breathholding commands by relying on signal averaging (10). Hands-on cardiac MRI courses have been organized to teach these coronary MRA techniques. One such 2-day cardiac MRI seminar was offered in Leuven, Belgium, October 3–4, 1997 (11). Several of the images shown in Chapter 5 of this book were acquired during this 1997 European course, using participants of the course as volunteers. We hope that this book and such courses will help teach these techniques to many more users. Initial clinical results with these techniques have been very promising with the sensitivity for significant coronary lesion detection ranging from 56 to 100% (12–20). Initial clinical results have also been very successful in imaging bypass grafts, coronary stents (21, 22), and coronary artery variants, such as anomalous origin or proximal course of the coronary vessels (23–26) or aneurysms as in Kawasaki disease (27,28).

Principles of Pulse Sequence Design and k-Space Segmentation for First-Generation Coronary MRA

Temporal Resolution

Image sharpness of coronary MRA is greatly influenced by cardiac motion and temporal resolution. Coronary

MRA requires the avoidance of motion (cardiac and respiratory motion) and compensation for pulsatile blood flow, all of which degrade the image quality by causing ghosting and image blurring.

Cardiac Motion

EKG-triggering synchronizes data acquisition to the cardiac cycle, and allows a better depiction of the heart and surrounding structures. The heart shows a highly variable motion pattern, most pronounced during systole and early diastole, but nearly absent during mid- and late diastole (29,30). Because coronary flow decreases from early to late diastole, middiastole appears to be optimally suited for coronary MRA.

k-Space segmentation is a new concept used to improve the temporal resolution of fast EKG-triggered MRI (31). For example, for conventional cardiac-triggered SE imaging and a typical 144×256 matrix, one would need 144 heartbeats (2 minutes, 24 seconds) to get one or multiple images (i.e., multiple respiratory cycles). For conventional nontriggered GRE imaging with one-shot acquisition and a typical 144×256 matrix with a TR = 13 ms, one would need a 1872 msec acquisition to obtain one image, which is approximately two heartbeats (i.e., multiple cardiac cycles). k-Space segmentation refers to the acquisition of small groups of phase-encoding lines, [i.e., phase-encoding groups (PEGs) or segments of k-space, during each heartbeat]. For the same 144×256 matrix and 9 phase acquisitions per segment (PEG = 9), one would only need $144/9 = 16$ heartbeats for a full image acquisition, much less than the 144 heartbeats for traditional SE (Fig. 15.1). This "segmented" acquisition scheme thus decreases the total image acquisition time when compared with conventional cardiac SE, but it is still insensitive to most cardiac motion. The segment of nine phase steps (PEG = 9) is acquired over a 117-msec period, which is much less than the 1872 msec per image for a similar traditional nontriggered one-shot gradient-recalled echo (GRE).

Although a 117-ms PEG duration (i.e., the duration of a k-space segment acquisition per heartbeat used in the early implementations of 2-D breathhold techniques) may seem long for cardiac motion, the center of k-space is actually acquired in much less time, with an effective temporal resolution of 30–40 ms (32). The "effective" temporal resolution of 20–30 msec, as opposed to the "nominal" temporal resolution of 70–120 msec, should be used when calculating vessel motion. Thus, assuming that the coronary vessel tracks the cardiac chamber motion, and using the data from Karwatowski et al (33) (see previous discussion on cardiac motion), during a 20-msec window the coronary vessel would move 1.6 mm in peak-diastole but only 0.2 mm in middiastole. In addition, better coil designs and faster gradients have improved the time duration of each PEG, thus ultimately improving the temporal resolution.

Respiratory Motion

Because a PEG only contains a small portion of the total number of phase encodings needed to obtain an ac-

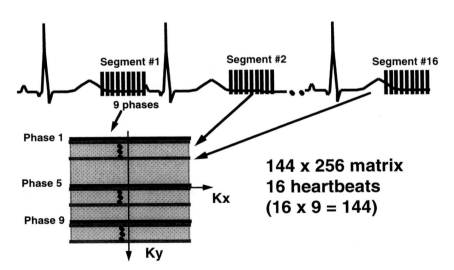

Figure 15.1. Pulse-sequence timing for the 2-D coronary MRA technique using k-space segmented breathhold ultrafast GRE and a 144×256 matrix with PEG = 9. At the top is shown the electrocardiogram signal (EKG signal) used to trigger the MR pulse sequence. The horizontal axis (time-axis) is not shown to scale. The timing of the data acquisition in middiastole for 3 of 16 segments (covering PEG = 9 phase-encoding steps each) is shown. Preceding the nine-phase acquisition within each heartbeat is an additional pulse (not shown) needed to suppress the signal from fat surrounding the coronary arteries. At the bottom is shown how k-space data are acquired: the nine phase acquisitions in each segment cover k-space (ky) sequentially. Each new segment adds nine more phase steps, until $16 \times 9 = 144$ phase steps are acquired in 16 heartbeats. (*From:* Duerinckx AJ. Coronary MR angiography. *In:* Cardiac MR imaging, Boxt LM, guest ed. *MRI Clin North Am* 1996;4(2):361–418; with permission.)

ceptable image, image acquisition over multiple heart-beats is needed. Breathholding and/or respiratory compensation/feedback schemes thus come into play.

For first- and third-generation coronary MRA techniques using breathholding, the corresponding breath-hold period varies between 12 and 25 seconds, depending on the heart rate and the number of phase-encoding steps (i.e., the number of k-space lines) acquired during each heartbeat. It should be noted that the duration of breathholding, even though it is only 12–20 seconds, can be exhausting for sick patients because of the need for repeated breathholds at 1-minute intervals for up to 1 hour. Because the heart moves considerably during respiratory motion (see also Table 15.1), image data have to be acquired during the same phase of each respiratory cycle (34). At most institutions, imaging is done at end-expiration, following a shallow or deep inspiration. Experience has shown that end-expiration breathholding is easier and more consistent (35).

Spatial Resolution

Temporal resolution, as described earlier, is a key factor which determines the size of the acquisition matrix for a breathhold scan. For a given field-of-view (FOV), this then determines the spatial resolution. The spatial resolution and signal to noise in coronary MRA can be further improved by either switching to nonbreathhold techniques (thus eliminating the time constraints) or by using better coil designs and faster gradients. Because of the increased signal-to-noise ratio, one can then decrease the FOV and increase the spatial resolution with a fixed data acquisition matrix (e.g., 144×256). Initial 2-D coronary MRA techniques required prone patient positioning with the arms pulled up along the head for a typical in-plane spatial resolution of 1–2 mm. This can be uncomfortable for patients with shoulder pain or recent coronary bypass surgery. Even healthy volunteers experienced some discomfort with this position after a long study.

Phased-array thoracic surface coils now allow coronary artery MRA in the supine position (36–38). Better and faster gradients have improved the spatial resolution via larger matrix sizes for equivalent repetition times (TR).

Small vessel detail may be obscured in these scans by slight cardiac motion and limited flow-to-background contrast. Spatial resolution for human in vivo work of 0.5 mm has been reported (39). Microscopic imaging of small distal coronary vessels with higher spatial resolution in the isolated rat heart (40) and imaging of smaller vessels in cadaveric human hearts (41) have been successfully performed.

Blood-to-Background Noise Contrast Ratio

Coronary MRA requires enhancement of the signal from moving (arterial) blood in the coronary arteries, while the signal from the surrounding stationary tissue and venous blood in the coronary veins has to be suppressed as much as possible. The signal from flowing blood-to-background noise ratio can be increased by inflow enhancement (modify the MR pulse sequence), by the use of paramagnetic contrast agents (MR contrast agents) which enhance the magnetic relaxation in the blood pool (42,43), and by suppression of signal from surrounding fat (2), muscle, and coronary veins (44,45).

Coronary arteries are usually embedded in fat, which has high signal intensity on T1-weighted images. Suppression of the high signal from fat offers improved coronary vessel detection with MRA. This technique is called "fat-saturation" and is essential in coronary MRA to suppress the signal from the peri- and epicardial fat.

A magnetization-prepared T2-contrast technique (T2-prep) takes advantage of the differences in T2 for muscle, arterial and venous blood to suppress signal from muscle and fat (44, 45). It is a robust technique that can be used with spiral scanning.

Magnetization transfer contrast (MTC) is another technique used to suppress the signal from certain types of stationary tissue. This technique has been used by Li et al. (46) to suppress the signal from the myocardium and could potentially be used to visualize coronary arteries embedded in the myocardium (e.g., myocardial bridges). Although promising, its clinical utility for coronary MRA and cardiac imaging is unproven at the present time (46).

The MR contrast agents now in clinical use are extracellular agents and they rapidly diffuse from the blood pool into the extracellular compartment (47). They do not, therefore, provide a long enough duration of signal enhancement of the blood signal. Newer blood pool contrast agents, manufactured by the binding of Gadolinium to macromolecules (e.g., albumin, dextran, polylysine) prolong the effect of signal changes in the blood pool considerably (48–50). Experimental use of these intravascular contrast agents has shown a significant and persistent increase of the blood signal intensity. The use of these intravascular contrast agents, therefore, might allow a better visualization of coronary vessels and a more accurate detection of coronary artery disease (42,43,51–53).

Optimization of the flip angle series used during a segmented acquisition can also change the relative T1 and T2* contrast in these ultrafast coronary MR angiographic sequences (43,54,55). This is a well-known concept in conventional 3-D time-of-flight MRA. Variable flip angles have improved image quality for the 2-D coronary MRA techniques, and also helped improve 3-D techniques with retrospective respiratory gating.

Timing of Data Acquisition Within Each Heart Cycle

Because of the complex pattern of cardiac motion and the biphasic flow patterns in the coronary vessels, it would appear that middiastole offers the best compromise when imaging coronary vessels (56,57). Flow in the left coronary system is maximal during early diastole. In the right coronary system, however, it can peak during late systole. Thus coronary MRA acquisitions performed during middiastole may not be optimal to visualize the period of maximal flow in the right coronary system.

There has been great interest in measuring velocity and flow in the proximal coronary arteries using newly developed breathhold MR flow quantification techniques that are variants of these first-generation coronary MRA techniques (58–62). One of the requirements for MR quantification of flow reserve is to be able to visualize the proximal portions of the coronary arteries throughout the cardiac cycle. It has also been suggested that cine displays of the coronary arteries can help facilitate the distinction between arteries and veins based on the early diastolic increased flow in the arteries (63). Implicit in this is the assumption that good-quality images can be obtained during all phases of the cardiac cycle. This goes against a commonly held belief that coronary MRA can only be performed during mid-diastole (8,12).

Because of this uncertainty about the optimal timing, several studies were undertaken to investigate this (29,64,65). In the study by Duerinckx et al. (64) coronary MRA was successfully performed in all cases in systole and diastole in 14 coronary vessels. In 8 of 14 vessels (57%) there was no visible coronary MRA image degradation when comparing peak-systolic with middiastolic images. In 4 of 14 vessels (29%) there was mild MR image degradation. There was significant MR image degradation in only one case (7%). In one case (7%) there was mild image improvement during systole. The width and length of the visualized coronary vessels did not significantly change from diastole to systole. Although the study confirms that it is possible to visualize large portions of the proximal coronary tree throughout the cardiac cycle, it does not necessarily imply that velocity and flow measurements throughout the cardiac cycle will be available with any coronary MRA sequence and in all patients.

Direction of Flow in a Vessel

Two-dimensional coronary MRA techniques visualize enhancement with in-plane and through-plane flow. This is a problem clinically as arteries and veins have similar appearances. As will be explained later (see the section on limitations) it occasionally becomes important to know the direction of flow to be able to distinguish between vein or artery. In addition, distal to a significant lesion the direction of flow is needed to distinguish between a lesion with forward flow and a total lesion with reversed flow due to collateral blood supply.

The conventional application of an upstream saturation pulse [e.g., with 2-D time of flight (TOF)] may not distinguish between the two, or determine the direction of flow. A T2-preparation pulse can be used to eliminate signal from venous blood, but is not widely used (44). Several alternative techniques have been developed. Segmented k-space alternatives of the bolus tracking techniques can help, but this requires a rather wide area to be visible (66). Another technique is to use temporal cine loops, and to take advantage of the fact that flow peaks at different points of the cardiac cycle in arteries and veins (63).

Typical 2-D Coronary MRAs

Typical 2-D coronary MRA is shown in Chapter 1, with additional typical images shown in Chapter 5. In most volunteers and a significant number of patients who can cooperate with breathholding commands, large portions of the proximal coronary arterial tree can be imaged.

Coronary MRA studies done mostly in normal volunteers (6,67–71) and several studies done in patients only (13,72) have measured the length of the coronary arteries typically visualized with the coronary MRA technique. The findings from the early 1993–1995 studies are summarized in Table 15.1. For comparison we have included data from a transesophageal study (TEE) of proximal coronary artery lesions (73) (see also later discussion). The difference in measured lengths between the different studies may be explained by a different approach to the selection of imaging planes.

Flow in the diagonal branches of the left anterior descending (LAD) was visible in 80% of the subjects in a study by Manning et al. (67). In a study of 15 patients by Duerinckx et al., however, the branch vessels were seldom visualized except for the acute marginal and diagonal branches. Moreover, the proximal circumflex artery was poorly visualized due to the use of a surface coil and prone positioning (69).

As stated earlier (see Chap. 2) the frequency of significant lesions in the left circumflex artery (LCx) is relatively low. Because of this lesion distribution pattern 2-D coronary MRA, even with its poor visualization of the LCx, may still be a valuable noninvasive screening tool for coronary artery disease.

Artifacts and Limitations of 2-D Breathhold Coronary MRA

The most important limitation of today's coronary MRA is the great variation in the appearance of significant (>50%) coronary lesions and the large number of image artifacts that can be misinterpreted as representing lesions. It can be very tempting to interpret an artifac-

Table 15.1. Comparison of the length of coronary arteries visualized by first-generation coronary MRA in the 1993–1995 period.

	n	RCA	LM	LAD	LCX
2-D: Manning et al., 1993 (Ref. 67)	25	58 (24–122)	10 (8–14)	44 (28–93)	25 (9–42)
2-D: Pennell et al., 1993 (Ref. 68)	26	53.7 ± 27.9	10.4 ± 5.2	46.7 ± 22.8	26.3 ± 17.5
2-D: Duerinckx et al., 1994 (Ref. 13)	21	65 ± 23	12 ± 3	53 ± 19	19 ± 12
2-D: Sakuma et al., 1994 (Ref. 70)	18	65 ± 23	n/a	62 ± 10	23 ± 11
2-D: Duerinckx et al., 1994 (Ref. 69)	15	78.4	13.9	54.9	14.7
2-D: Hofman et al., 1995* (Ref. 71)	10	55 ± 11	8 ± 2	42 ± 14	16 ± 12
3-D: Li et al.** (Ref. 46)	?	3 to 7**	n/a	5 to 50**	5 to 50**
3-D: Paschal et al.* (Ref. 6)	7	34 (12–50)	5 (4–14)	24 (5–47)	24 (8–64)
3-D: Hofman et al., 1995* (Ref. 71)	10	37 ± 14	7 ± 3	37 ± 9	11 ± 12
3-D gated: Hofman et al., 1995* (Ref. 71)	10	46 ± 10	8 ± 4	37 ± 11	17 ± 14
2-D: Post et al. (Ref. 72)	35	89 ± 32	9 ± 4	62 ± 16	21 ± 9
TEE: Samdarshi et al., 1992 (Ref. 73)	111	7 ± 2	9.3 ± 1	8.2 ± 8	6.7 ± 9

From: Duerinckx AJ. Coronary MR angiography. *In*: Cardiac MR imaging, Boxt LM, guest ed. *MRI Clin North Am* 1996;4(2):361–418; with permission.
Results are expressed in millimeters, and, depending on the study, as: mean ± standard deviation or mean (range: min–max). *n* = number of subjects; RCA = right coronary artery; LM = left main stem artery; LAD = left anterior descending artery; LCx = left circumflex artery. *Not all vessels could be visualized in each subject; **range reflects the most frequently measured lengths, not the full range.

tual change in the signal intensity of flow in a vessel as representing a lesion, especially if the artifact just happens to be located in the vicinity of the real lesion. Such erroneous overinterpretation of artifacts as lesions will increase the sensitivity for lesion detection, as will be explained and illustrated in the next section. If done consistently, it would unfortunately also significantly reduce the specificity of the technique, thus ultimately reducing its clinical impact. Issues relating to "lesion" appearance on MR will be discussed in the next section. The discussion here will be limited to general artifacts and limitations as seen in healthy normal volunteers without coronary lesions.

Due to increasing interest in exploring and defining the ultimate clinical roles of the commercially available first-generation 2-D breathhold coronary MRA techniques (8,13,74–76), Duerinckx et al. undertook a study of the artifacts and limitations of 2-D coronary MRA (7,69). A similar study was undertaken by Lentschig et al. (77).

The purpose of the study by Duerinckx et al (7,69) was to describe and illustrate: (1) artifacts due to data and image acquisition problems that cause reduced image quality and limit the number of high-quality images per study, and (2) limitations due to problems in the interpretation of 2-D coronary MRA images. The first category pertains to those sets of problems that influence the acquisition of a good image and overall study. The second category itemizes problems that may cause a misinterpretation of a technically adequate exam.

Problems were divided into two areas: data acquisition (artifacts) and image interpretation (limitations).

"Artifacts" refer to the consequences of data acquisition problems that preclude the gathering of good-quality images at the desired anatomic locations. These items can cause image degradation, poor image quality, and diminish the number of high-quality images available for the clinical study. In some cases, these can be overcome during the examination by readjustment of the systems or better patient cooperation. Examples of these problems are: intermittent difficulty with breathholding (blurring), image reconstruction artifacts (ghosting, ringing, and blurring), poor cardiac triggering (ghosting) and poor fat-suppression (decreased flow contrast-to-background).

"Limitations" refer to the fact that there will sometimes be ambiguity in the interpretation of images. This is partially due to the artifacts described earlier, but there are additional causes. The inherent 2-D nature of the image acquisition requires the examination of serial images because the complex anatomy is often only demonstrated in successive sections. Complete but inconsistent breathholding or patient motion will cause misregistration. The fact that veins, arteries, and pericardial sac contents all have similar signal intensity can also cause misinterpretation of anatomical structures. Some of these problems of interpretation are inherent in the 2-D nature of the technique. Examples of these are potential misinterpretation of vessel continuity due to slice misregistration, misidentification of adjacent vein and artery, confusion between superimposed anatomical structures (e.g., pericardium) and the coronary artery, confusion between a vessel and the upper pericardial recess area, and susceptibility artifacts caused by sternal wires, surgical clips, or coronary stents.

Duerinckx et al. quantitated the frequency of occurrence of these problems (see Table 15.2) and recommended possible methods to overcome artifacts and deal with limitations.

We will discuss three frequently encountered limitations in more detail.

Irregular Breathholding

Under ideal circumstances (i.e., with perfectly consistent breathholding throughout the study) analysis of a sufficient number of sequential serial images in more than one plane would clarify the cardiac and coronary anatomy. Coronary vessels can unfortunately sometimes be very tortuous with multiple branches and overlapping venous structures. This presents a problem clinically in that the typical 50-minute examination is not adequate to obtain a sufficient image data in orthogonal planes to follow each vessel.

The initial reports on 2-D coronary MRA suggested that proximal portions of a tortuous coronary artery can easily and reliably be imaged with a stack of parallel overlapping slices (12). It was assumed that successive sections would demonstrate the anatomy of the coronary arteries and that serial images could be examined using either film or cine display (video loops). The irreproducibility of breathholding in many patients unfortunately undermines the reliability of this technique.

Third-generation (3-D breathhold) coronary MRA techniques, such as the experimental segmented 3-D breathhold echoplanar techniques (78–83), offer the promise to avoid these misregistration problems; however, they either expand the scan times to a longer scan period and/or require expensive instrument upgrades.

Veins Versus Arteries
Superposition of a venous and arterial structure in the same 2-D image may cause interpretation difficulties or artifactual lesions.

Left Main Coronary Artery
Usually the entire left main coronary artery can be imaged; however, not all portions of the left main coronary artery are equally visualized. The origin of the left main artery is often not clearly seen and blends in with surrounding tissues on the oblique axial images. A slightly oblique coronal plane along the left atrioventricular groove is sometimes a better imaging plane for the origin of the left main.

Hybrid Techniques: Nonbreathhold Approaches to 2-D Coronary MRA

Inconsistency in breathholding for 2-D techniques can be avoided with real-time or retrospective navigator pulses (84–86), thus effectively turning these "breathhold" 2-D techniques into nonbreathhold techniques. The use of navigator pulses allows for nonbreathhold acquisitions by tracking diaphragmatic motion (84,87,88). The concept of navigator pulses has been used for thoracic and abdominal imaging (89). Whether or not these nonbreathhold 2-D coronary MRI will be as diagnostic as the breathhold images is unresolved.

Table 15.2. Frequency of artifacts and limitations with 2-D breathhold coronary MRA.

Artifacts	Description	Frequency (%)
	1. Intermittent difficulty with breathholding	40
	2. Ghosting	22
	3. Ringing	19
	4. Blurring	22
	5. Poor fat-suppression	19
Limitations	1. Misregistration due to inconsistent breathholding*	37
	2. Difficulty distinguishing arteries from veins*	37
	3. Overlapping structures	26
	4. Poor visualization of the left main artery*	59

Based on a study in 27 subjects by Duerinckx et al.; Ref. 7.
*For further discussion see text; for others refer to Ref. 7.
From: Duerinckx AJ. Coronary MR angiography. *In*: Cardiac MR Imaging, L M Boxt, Guest Editor; *MRI Clin North Am* 1996;4(2):361–418; with permission.

Cardiac and Thoracic MRI Using First-Generation Coronary MRA Techniques

The use of *k*-space segmentation has had a dramatic effect upon thoracic and cardiac MRI in general (3,31,90–92). It has generated a whole new set of breathhold cardiac MR pulse sequences (93–96).

Other Technique Variants and Improvements

Improvements in MR hardware will allow faster imaging. Higher resolution imaging using interleaved spirals (4,97), SMASH or SENSE (98,99) has been implemented

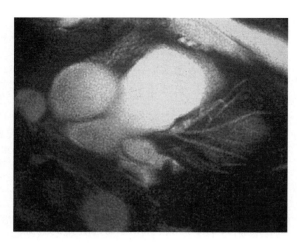

Figure 15.2. Spiral coronary MR angiogram of the left coronary system. Multiple side-branches are shown. (Courtesy of Meyer et al., Standford University.)

on a limited number of scanners (These concepts are explained in more detail in Chapters 2, 4, and 16). For example spiral *k*-space traversal does provide better spatial resolution and allows routine visualization of coronary side branches, as shown in Figure 15.2 (4,100). Other variants include real-time imaging (101–103).

Black-blood imaging offers an interesting alternative to bright-blood imaging of coronary vessels (104–106). Bright-blood coronary MRA may not sufficiently suppress the signal coming from the coronary vessel walls, thrombus, and plaque. Artifactual narrowing of focal stenosis has also been reported. Metallic implants as frequently present in patients post–cardiac surgery are a further limitation. This has prompted the development of black-blood techniques, which combine a dual-inversion prepulse and a turbo spin-echo sequence for black-blood coronary MRA. Examples of this are the half-Fourier acquired single-shot turbo spin echo (HASTE) technique (Siemens terminology), also referred to as a half-Fourier turbo spin-echo technique (HF-TSE, Philips) or a single-shot fast spin echo technique (Single-Shot FSE, General Electric) (107,108). Stuber et al. (104) have shown that extensive portions including higher-order branches of the left and right coronary system could be visualized with a high contrast between the coronary blood pool and the surrounding tissue. They also found a good agreement with X-ray coronary angiography and artifacts originating from metallic implants could successfully be minimized.

Other variants of the first-generation techniques rely on the pulse sequences developed for real-time cardiac MRI (101,102). Deshpande et al. (109) have described 2-D and 3-D MR coronary artery imaging using magnetization-prepared EKG-triggered TrueFISP. TrueFISP is Siemens terminology, also called balanced FFE (BFFE) by Philips or single-shot free processing (SSFP) by General Electric. TrueFISP is a fast imaging approach that gives rise to high signal-to-noise ratio and T1/T2-weighted contrast because it maintains the transverse magnetization within each TR that contributes to the signal intensity. The major problem with TrueFISP has been off-resonance artifacts due to field inhomogeneities. These effects can be minimized by using short TRs with a high-performance gradient system. As a result, TrueFISP has dramatically improved blood signal and contrast over conventional FLASH in cardiac cine imaging. Deshpande et al. (109) investigated the utility of TrueFISP for 3-D coronary artery imaging, but this technique could also be used for real-time 2-D coronary imaging. More information on this promising thin-slab 3-D approach will be provided in Chapter 20.

As discussed in Chapter 2, we have gained a much better understanding of cardiac and coronary artery motion within a caridac cycle (110–112). It has been suggested that the motion of the heart within a cardiac cycle should first be assessed to pick the best temporal window for imaging, which may vary from patient to patient, as opposed to picking a set time frame during diastole (Wang, personal communication). Nevertheless, successful performance of coronary MRA during portions of the cardiac cycle other than mid- to late diastole has been also demonstrated by Duerinckx et al. (30). This can partially be explained by findings from studies on changes in cardiac motion during the cardiac cycle (29,34).

Today we also have a better understanding of what breathholding means. There is indeed diaphragmatic motion during a breathhold, and it appears to be different for end-inspiration and end-inspiration breathholds (35,112,113). This may lead to real-time adaptive motion correction schemes during each heartbeat within a single breathhold (114).

The Use of Contrast Agents

Limited work on the use of extracellular contrast agents with the first-generation techniques has been performed (42,43). Two to three times the 0.1 mole/kg dose seems to be needed in order to see a signal increase with these somewhat proton-weighted pulse sequences. With dynamic bolus injection and bolus timing the results appear to improve (105).

The availability of blood-pool agents may dramatically change our potential to take advantage of the added MR contrast: they remain in the blood long enough to allow multiple 2-D or 3-D slab acquisitions (116–118). When using today's blood-pool agents with 2-D breathhold techniques, however, a low dose of contrast is needed due to the short T2 values, which would otherwise decrease signal intensity for many commercial breathhold 2-D coronary MRA sequences.

The Future

Both first- and second-generation coronary MRA techniques are universally available on commercial MRI scanners and have a proven clinical track record. Nevertheless, first-generation 2-D coronary MRA techniques will remain very important in the future, as there is more clinical experience with these techniques, and they provide quicker feedback than 3-D navigator techniques (119–120). The new hybrid versions of the breathhold 2-D techniques rely on navigators that are used to eliminate inconsistencies between breathholds, opening the door for much higher spatial resolution. Spiral 2-D imaging also offers improved spatial resolution.

Coronary lesion detection is still problematic, but progress is being made. Vessel wall imaging and plaque characterization using 2-D techniques are possible (121). A combination of the best of first-, second-, and third-generation coronary MRA principles may lead to a hybrid acquisition mode for 2-D or very thin 3-D slab acquisitions, acquired during sequential breathholds, but with superior spatial and temporal resolution and adequate coverage to image large portions of the coronary arteries. For these hybrid applications the use of contrast agents will probably be very helpful. Real-time imaging will decrease the study duration by making it easier to find the best imaging planes.

References

1. Atkinson D, Edelman R. Cineangiography of the heart in a single breathhold with a segmented TurboFLASH sequence. Radiology 1991;178:359–62.
2. Edelman R, Manning W, Burstein D, Paulin S. Coronary arteries: breath-hold MR angiography. Radiology 1991;181(3):641–43.
3. Mezrich R. A perspective on k-space. Radiology 1995;195:297–315.
4. Meyer CH, Hu BS, Nishimura DG, Macovski A. Fast spiral coronary artery imaging. Magn Reson Med 1992;28(2):401–6.
5. Paschal C, Haacke E, Adler L, Finelli DA. Magnetic resonance coronary artery imaging. Cardiovasc Intervent Radiol 1992;15:23–31.
6. Paschal CB, Haacke EM, Adler LP. Three-dimensional MR imaging of the coronary arteries: preliminary clinical experience. J Magn Reson Imag 1993;3(3):491–501.
7. Duerinckx AJ, Atkinson DP, Mintorovitch J, Simonetti OP, Urman MK. Two-dimensional coronary MR angiography: limitations and artifacts. Eur Radiol 1996;6(3):312–25.
8. Duerinckx AJ. Review: MR angiography of the coronary arteries. Top Magn Reson Imag 1995;7(4):267–85.
9. Duerinckx AJ. Coronary MR angiography. In: Cardiac MR imaging, Boxt LM, guest ed. MRI Clin North Am 1996;4(2):361–418.
10. Duerinckx AJ, Lewis BS, Louie HW, Urman MK. MRI of pseudoaneurysm of a brachial venous coronary bypass graft. Catheter Cardiovasc Diag 1996;37:281–86.
11. Duerinckx AJ. Coronary arteries: how do I image them? In: Bogaert J, Duerinckx AJ, Rademakers F, eds. Magnetic Resonance of the Heart and Great Vessels: Clinical Applications. Berlin: Springer-Verlag, 1999:223–43.
12. Manning WJ, Li W, Edelman RR. A preliminary report comparing magnetic resonance coronary angiography with conventional angiography. N Engl J Med 1993;328:828–32.
13. Duerinckx AJ, Urman M. Two-dimensional coronary MR angiography: analysis of initial clinical results. Radiology 1994;193:731–38.
14. Pennell DJ, Bogren HG, Keegan J, Firmin DW, Underwood SR. Coronary artery stenosis: assessment by magnetic resonance imaging (abstr.). In: Book of Abstracts of the Eleventh Annual Scientific Meeting of the European Society for Magnetic Resonance in Medicine and Biology. Vienna, April 20–24, 1994:374.
15. Pennell DJ, Bogren HG, Keegan J, Firmin DN, Underwood SR. Detection, localization and assessment of coronary artery stenosis by magnetic resonance imaging (abstr.). In: Book of Abstracts and Proceedings of the Second Meeting of the the Society of Magnetic Resonance (SMR). San Francisco, August 6–12, 1994; Vol. I:369.
16. Mohiaddin RH, Bogren HG, Lazim F, et al. Magnetic resonance coronary angiography in heart transplant recipients. Cor Art Dis 1996;7(8):591–97.
17. Nitatori T, Hanaoka H, Yoshino A, Tominaga M, et al. Clinical application of magnetic resonance angiography for coronary arteries: correlation with conventional angiography and evaluation of imaging time. Nippon Acta Radiol 1995;55:670–76.
18. Post JC, van Rossum AC, Hofman MB, de Cock CC, Valk J, Visser CA. Clinical utility of two-dimensional magnetic resonance angiography in detecting coronary artery disease. Eur Heart J 1997;18(3):426–33.
19. Yoshino H, Nitatori T, Kachi E, et al. Directed proximal magnetic resonance coronary angiography compared with conventional contrast coronary angiography. Am J Cardiol 1997;80(4):514–18.
20. Duerinckx AJ. MRI of coronary arteries. Int J Card Imag 1997;13(3):191–97.
21. Duerinckx AJ, Atkinson D, Hurwitz R, Mintorovitch J, Whitney W. Coronary MR angiography after coronary stent placement (case report). Am J Roentgenol 1995;165(3):662–64.
22. Duerinckx AJ, Atkinson D, Hurwitz R. Assessment of coronary artery patency after stent placement using magnetic resonance angiography. J Magn Reson Med 1998;8:896–902.
23. Post JC, vanRossum AC, Bronzwaer JGF, et al. Magnetic resonance angiography of anomalous coronary arteries: a new gold standard for delineating the proximal course? Circulation 1995;92:3163–71.
24. McConnell MV, Ganz P, Selwyn AP, Li W, Edelman RR, Manning WJ. Identification of anomalous coronary arteries and their anatomic course by magnetic resonance coronary angiography. Circulation 1995;92:3158–62.
25. Manning WJ, Li W, Cohen SI, Johnson RG, Edelman RR. Improved definition of anomalous left coronary artery by magnetic resonance coronary angiography. Am Heart J 1995;130(3 Pt. 1):615–17.

26. Duerinckx AJ, Bogaert J, Jiang H, Lewis BS. Anomalous origin of the left coronary artery: diagnosis by coronary MR angiography (case report). Am J Roentgenol 1995; 164:1095–97.

27. Duerinckx AJ, Takahashi M. Coronary MR angiography in Kawasaki disease (abstr.). Radiology 1996;201(P): 274.

28. Duerinckx AJ, Troutman B, Allada V, Kim D. Coronary MR angiography in Kawasaki disease: a case report. Am J Roentgenol 1997;168:114–16.

29. Sodickson DK, Chuang ML, Khasgiwala VC, Manning WJ. In-plane motion of the left and right coronary arteries durign the cardiac cycle (abstr.). In: Book of Abstracts and Proceedings of the Fifth Meeting of the International Society of Magnetic Resonance in Medicine (ISMRM). Vancouver, B.C., April 12–18, 1997; Vol. 2: 910.

30. Duerinckx AJ, Atkinson DP. Coronary MR angiography during peak-systole: work-in-progress. J Magn Reson Imag 1997;7(6):979–86.

31. Pearlman JD, Edelman RE. Ultrafast magnetic resonance imaging: segmented TurboFLASH, echo-planar, and real-time nuclear magnetic resonance. Radiol Clin North Am 1994;32(3):593–612.

32. Matsuda T, Yamada H, Kida M, Sasayama S. Is 300 msec too long for cardiac MR imaging? Feasibility study demonstrating changes in left ventricular cross-sectional area with use of single-shot TurboFLASH imaging. Radiology 1994;190:353–62.

33. Karwatowski SP, Mohiaddin RH, Yang GZ, Firmin DN, StJohnSutton M, Underwood SR. Regional myocardial velocity image by magnetic resonance in patients with ischaemic heart disease. Br Heart J 1994;72(4):332–38.

34. Wang Y, Riederer SJ, Ehman RL. Respiratory motion of the heart: kinematics and implications for the spatial resolution in coronary imaging. Magn Reson Med 1995; 33(5):713–19.

35. Holland A, Goldfarb JW, Barentsz JO, Edelman RR. Diaphragm motion during suspended breathing: implications for MR imaging of the heart (abstr.). In: Proceedings of the Sixth Scientific Meeting of the International Society for Magnetic Resonance in Medicine (ISMRM), April 18–24, 1998. Sydney, Australia, 1998; Vol. 1: 276.

36. Hatabu H, Gefter WB, Listerud J, et al. Pulmonary MR angiography utilizing phased-array surface coils. JCAT 1992;16(3):410–17.

37. Constantinides CD, Westgate CR, O'Dell WG, Zerhouni EA, McVeigh ER. A phased array coil for human cardiac imaging. Magn Reson Med 1995; July; 34(1):92–98.

38. Fayad ZA, Connick TJ, Axel L. An improved quadrature or phased-array coil for MR cardiac imaging. Magn Reson Med 1995;34(2):186–93.

39. Meyer CH, Sachs TS, Hu BS, Macovski A, Nishimura DG. High resolution spiral coronary angiography. (abstr.). In: Book of Abstracts of the Third Meeting of the Society of Magnetic Resonance (SMR) and the Twelfth Annual Scientific Meeting of the European Society for Magnetic Resonance in Medicine and Biology (ESMRMB). Nice, France, August 20–25, 1995.

40. Bauer WR, Hiller K-H, Roder F, et al. Investigation of coronary vessels in microscopic dimensions by two- and three-dimensional NMR microscopic imaging in the isolated rat heart. Circulation 1995;92:968–77.

41. Gates ARC, Huang CL-H, Crowley JJ, et al. Magnetic resonance imaging planes for the 3-dimensional characterization of human coronary arteries. J Anat 1994;185: 335–46.

42. Stillman AE, Wilke N, Li D, Haacke EM, McLachlan SJ. MRA of renal and coronary arteries using an intravascular contrast agent (#944) (abstr.). In: Printed program of the second meeting of the Society of Magnetic Resonance (SMR). San Francisco, August 6–12, 1994.

43. Duerinckx AJ, Urman M, Sinha U, Atkinson D, Simonetti O. Evaluation of gadolinium-enhanced MR coronary angiography (abstr.). In: Seventy-ninth Scientific Assembly and Annual Meeting of the Radiological Society of North America (RSNA). Chicago, November 28–December 3, 1993; Radiology 1993;189(P):278.

44. Brittain JH, Hu BS, Wright GA, Meyer CH, Macovski A, Nishimura DG. Coronary angiography with magnetization-prepared T2 contrast. Magn Reson Med 1995; May;33(5):689–96.

45. Brittain JH, Hu BS, Wright GA, Meyer CH, Macovski A, Nishimura DG. Multislice coronary angiography with muscle and venous suppression (#367) (abstr.). In: Printed Program of the Second Meeting of the Society of Magnetic Resonance (SMR). San Francisco, August 7–12, 1994.

46. Li D, Paschal CB, Haacke EM, Adler LP. Coronary arteries: three-dimensional MR imaging with fat saturation and magnetization transfer contrast. Radiology 1993;187: 401–6.

47. Saeed M, Wendland MF, Higgins CB. Contrast media for MR imaging of the heart (review). J Magn Reson Imag 1994;4:269–79.

48. Marchal G, Bosmans H, VanHecke P, et al. MR angiography with gadopentetate dimeglumine-polylysine: evaluation in rabbits. Am J Roentgenol 1990;155:407–11.

49. Adam G, Neuerburg J, Spüntrup E, Mühler A, Scherer K, Günther RW. Gd-DTPA-Cascade-Polymer: potential blood pool contrast agent for MR imaging. J Magn Reson Imag 1994;4:462–66.

50. Bogdanov AA, Weissleder R, Frank HW, et al. A new macromolecule as a contrast agent for MR angiography: preparation, properties, and animal studies. Radiology 1994;187(3):701–6.

51. Taylor AM, Panting JR, Gatehouse PD, et al. Safety and preliminary findings with an intravascular contrast agent, NC100150 for MR coronary angiography (abstr.). In: Proceedings of the Sixth Scientific Meeting of the International Society for Magnetic Resonance in Medicine (ISMRM), April 18–24, 1998 (paper #18). Sydney, Australia, 1998; Vol. 1: 18.

52. Stuber M, Botnar RM, McConnell MV, et al. Coronary artery imaging with the intravascular contrast agent MS-325 (abstr.). In: Proceedings of the Sixth Scientific Meeting of the International Society for Magnetic Resonance in Medicine (ISMRM), April 18–24, 1998 (paper #316). Sydney, Australia, 1998; Vol. 1: 316.

53. Li D, Dolan RP, Walovitch RC, Lauffer RB. Three-dimensional MRI of coronary arteries using an intravas-

cular contrast agent. Magn Reson Med 1998;39(6):1014–18.

54. Simonetti O, Cadena G, Laub G. Strategies for improving contrast in Coronary MR angiography (abstr.). *In*: Proceedings of the RSNA Seventy-eighth Scientific Assembly and Annual Meeting. Chicago, November 28–December 4, 1992;185(P):103.

55. Li D, Kaushikkar S, Woodard P, Dhawale P, Haacke EM. Three-dimensional MRI of Coronary Arteries (abstr.). *In*: Book of Abstracts of Seventh International Workshop on Magnetic Resonance Angiography. Matsuyama, Japan; October 12–14, 1995.

56. Duerinckx AJ. Coronary MR angiography (response-to-letter-to-the-editor). Radiology 1995;195(3):876.

57. Manning WJ, Edelman RR. Coronary MR angiography (letter-to-the-editor). Radiology 1995;195(3):875.

58. Edelman RR, Manning WJ, Gervino E, Li W. Flow velocity quantification in human coronary arteries with fast, breath-hold MR angiography. J Magn Reson Imag 1993;3(5):699–703.

59. Gatehouse PD, Firmin DN, Longmore DB. Real time blood flow imaging by spiral scan phase velocity mapping. Magn Reson Med 1994;31:504–12.

60. Keegan J, Firmin D, Gatehouse P, Longmore D. The application of breath hold phase velocity mapping techniques to the measurement of coronary artery blood flow velocity: phantom data and initial in vivo results. Magn Reson Med 1994;31:526–36.

61. Buonocore MK. Estimation of total coronary artery flow using measurements of flow in the ascending aorta. Magn Reson Med 1994;32(5):602–11.

62. Clarke GD, Eckels R, Chaney C, et al. Measurement of absolute epicardial coronary artery flow and flow reserve with breathhold cine phase-contrast magnetic resonance imaging. Circulation 1995;91(10):2627–34.

63. Hundley WG, Clarke GD, Landau C, et al. Noninvasive determination of infarct artery patency by cine magnetic resonance angiography. Circulation 1995;91:1347–53.

64. Duerinckx AJ, Atkinson D. Coronary MR angiography during peak-systole (abstr.). *In*: Book of Abstracts of the Third Meeting of the Society of Magnetic Resonance (SMR) and the Twelfth Annual Scientific Meeting of the European Society for Magnetic Resonance in Medicine and Biology (ESMRMB), Vol. 3, p. 1396. Nice, France, August 20–25, 1995.

65. Hofman MB, Wickline SA, Lorenz CH. Quantification of in-plane motion of the coronary arteries during the cardiac cycle: implications for acquisition window duration for MR flow quantification. J Magn Reson Imag 1998;8(3):568–76.

66. Chien D, Laub G, Simonetti O, Anderson CM. Time-resolved velocity quantification of pulsatile flow: segmented *k*-space bolus tagging in a single breath hold (abstr.). *In*: Proceedings of the First Meeting of the Society of Magnetic Resonance (SMRM). Works in Progress Suppl. Dallas, March 5–9, 1994; J Magn Reson Imag 1994; 4 (P) Work-in-Progress Supplement: S27.

67. Manning WJ, Li W, Boyle NG, Edelman RE. Fat-suppressed breath-hold magnetic resonance coronary angiography. Circulation 1993;87:94–104.

68. Pennell DJ, Keegan J, Firmin DN, Gatehouse PD, Underwood SR, Longmore DB. Magnetic resonance imaging of coronary arteries: technique and preliminary results. Br Heart J 1993;70(4):315–26.

69. Duerinckx AJ, Urman MK, Atkinson DJ, Simonetti OP, Sinha U, Lewis B. Limitations of MR coronary angiography (abstr.). *In*: Printed Program of the First Meeting of the Society of Magnetic Resonance (SMR). Dallas, March 5–9, 1994; J Magn Reson Imag 1994;4:81.

70. Sakuma H, Caputo GR, Steffens JC, et al. Breath-hold MR cine angiography of coronary arteries in healthy volunteers: value of multiangle oblique imaging planes. Am J Roentgenol 1994;163(3):533–37.

71. Hofman MBM, Paschal CB, Li D, Haacke M, vanRossum AC, Sprenger M. MRI of coronary arteries: 2D breath-hold vs 3D respiratory-gated acquisition. JCAT 1995; 19(1):56–62.

72. Post JC, vanRossum AC, Hofman MBM, Valk J, Visser. CA. Clinical utility of two dimensional breathhold MR angiography in coronary artery disease (abstr.). *In*: Book of Abstracts of the Third Meeting of the Society of Magnetic Resonance (SMR) and the Twelfth Annual Scientific Meeting of the European Society for Magnetic Resonance in Medicine and Biology (ESMRMB). Nice, France, August 20–25, 1995.

73. Samdarshi T, Nanda N, Gatewood R, et al. Usefulness and limitations of transesophageal echocardiography in the assessment of proximal coronary artery stenosis. J Am Coll Cardiol 1992;19:572–80.

74. Manning WJ, Li W, Wielopolski P, Gaa J, Kannam JP, Edelman RR. Magnetic resonance coronary angiography: comparison with contrast angiography (abstr.). *In*: Book of Abstracts and Proceedings of the Second Meeting of the the Society of Magnetic Resonance (SMR). San Francisco, August 6–12, 1994; Vol. I: p. 368.

75. Manning W, Edelman R. Magnetic resonance coronary angiography. Magn Reson Q 1993;9(3):131–51.

76. Bogaert J, Duerinckx AJ, Baert AL. Coronary MR angiography: a review. Journal Belge de Radiologie / Belgisch Tijdschrift voor Radiologie. 1994;77:255–61.

77. Lentschig MG, Brinkmann A, Reimer P, Tombach B, Rummeney EJ. Two-dimensional breath-hold coronary MR angiography: diagnostic value and limitations (abstr.). *In*: 1997 Scientific Program of the 83rd Scientific Assembly and Annual Meeting of the Radiological Society of North America (RSNA). Chicago, November 30–December 5, 1997. Radiology; 1997;205(P):153.

78. McKinnon GC. Ultrafast interleaved gradient-echo-planar imaging on a standard scanner. Magn Reson Med 1993;30:609–16.

79. Wielopolski PA, Scharf JG, Edelman RR. Multislice coronary angiography within a single breath hold (abstr.). *In*: Printed Program of the First Meeting of the Society of Magnetic Resonance (SMRM). Dallas, March 5–9, 1994; J Magn Reson Imag 1994;4(P):80.

80. Wielopolski PA, Manning WJ, Edelman RE. Single breath-hold volumetric imaging of the heart using magnetization-prepared 3-dimensional segmented echo-planar imaging. J Magn Reson Imag 1995; 5(4):403–9.

81. Wielopolski PA, vanGeuns RJM, deFeyter PJ, Oudkerk M. VCATS (volume coronary arteriography using targeted

scans), MR coronary angiography using breath-hold volume targeted acquistions (abstr.). *In*: Proceedings of the Sixth Scientific Meeting of the International Society for Magnetic Resonance in Medicine (ISMRM), April 18–24, 1998 (paper #14). Sydney, Australia, 1998.

82. Wielopolski PA, van Geuns RJ, de Feyter PJ, Oudkerk M. Coronary arteries. Eur Radiol 1998;8(6):873–85.

83. Wielopolski P, vanGeuns RJ, deFeyter PJ, Oudkerk M. Breath-hold coronary MR angiography with volume targeted imaging. Radiology 1998;209:209–20.

84. Sachs TS, Meyer CH, Hu BS, Kohli J, Nishimura DG, Macovski A. Real-time motion detection in spiral MRI using navigators. Magn Reson Med 1994;32(5):639–45.

85. Sachs TS, Meyer CH, Irazzabal P, Hu BS, Nishimura DG, Macovski A. The diminishing variance algorithm for real-time reduction of motion artifacts in MRI. Magn Reson Med 1995;34:412–22.

86. McConnell MV, Khasgiwala VC, Savord BJ, et al. Prospective adaptive navigator correction for breath-hold MR coronary angiography. Magn Reson Med 1997;37(1):148–52.

87. Wang Y, Christy PS, Korosec FR, et al. Coronary MRI with a respiratory feedback monitor: the 2D imaging case. Magn Reson Med 1995;33(1):116–21.

88. Brittain JH, Sachs TS, Hu BS, Nishimura DG. Non-breathheld 2DFT coronary angiography (abstr.). *In*: Book of Abstracts of the Third Meeting of the Society of Magnetic Resonance (SMR) and the Twelfth Annual Scientific Meeting of the European Society for Magnetic Resonance in Medicine and Biology (ESMRMB). Nice, France, August 20–25, 1995.

89. Butts K, Riederer SJ, Ehman RL. The effect of respiration on the contrast and sharpness of liver lesions on MRI. Magn Reson Med 1995;33:1–7.

90. Hernandez RJ, Aisen AM, Foo TKF, Beekman RH. Thoracic cardiovascular anomalies in children: evaluation with a fast gradient-recalled-echo sequence with cardiac-triggered segmented acquisition. Radiology 1993;188:775–80.

91. Bluemke DA, Boxerman JL, Mosher T, Lima JA. Segmented *k*-space cine breath-hold cardiovascular MR imaging: part 2. Evaluation of aortic vasculopathy. Am J Roentgenol 1997;169(2):401–7.

92. Bluemke DA, Boxerman JL, Atalar E, McVeigh ER. Segmented *k*-space cine breath-hold cardiovascular MR imaging: part 1, principles and technique. Am J Roentgenol 1997;169(2):395–400.

93. Reeder SB, McVeigh ER. Tag contrast in breathhold CINE cardiac MRI. Magn Reson Med 1994;31(5):521–25.

94. Sakuma H, Fujita N, Foo TK, et al. Evaluation of the left ventricular volume and mass with breathhold cine MR imaging. Radiology 1993;188:377–80.

95. Sakuma H, Globitis S, Shimakawa A, Bernstein MA, Higgins CB. Breathhold coronary flow measurements with a cine phase-contrast technique (#375) (abstr.). *In*: Printed Program of the Second Meeting of the Society of Magnetic Resonance (SMR). San Francisco, August 6–12, 1994.

96. Simonetti OP, Laub G, Finn JP. Breathhold T2-weighted imaging of the heart (#1499) (abstr.). *In*: Printed Program of the Second Meeting of the Society of Magnetic Resonance (SMR). San Francisco, August 6–12, 1994.

97. Liao J-R, Sommer G, Herfkens RJ, Pelc NJ. Cine spiral imaging. Magn Reson Med 1995;34(3):490–93.

98. Sodickson DK, Manning WJ. Simultaneous acquisition of spatial harmonics (SMASH): fast imaging with radiofrequency coil arrays. Magn Reson Med 1997;38(4):591–603.

99. Jakob PM, Griswold MA, Edelman RR, Manning WJ, Sodickson DK. Cardiac imaging with SMASH (abstr.). *In*: Proceedings of the Sixth Scientific Meeting of the International Society for Magnetic Resonance in Medicine (ISMRM), April 18–24, 1998 (paper #16). Sydney, Australia, 1998.

100. Meyer C, Hu B, Nishimura D, Macovski A. Fast spiral coronary artery imaging (abstr.). *In*: Proceedings of the Eleventh Annual Scientific Meeting of the Society of Magnetic Resonance Imaging (SMRM). Berlin, Germany, August 8–14, 1992; 211.

101. Hardy CJ. Real-time cardiovascular MR imaging. *In*: Reiber JHC, vanderWall EE, eds. What's New in Cardiovascular Imaging? Dordrecht: Kluwer Academic Publishers, 1998: 207–19.

102. Hardy CJ, Darrow RD, Pauly JM, et al. Interactive coronary MRI. Magn Reson Med 1998;40(1):105–11.

103. Sodickson DK, Stuber M, Botnar RM, Kissinger KV, Manning WJ. SMASH real-time cardiac imaging at echocardiographic frame rates. (abstr.). *In*: Book of Abstracts and Proceedings of the Seventh Meeting of the International Society of Magnetic Resonance in Medicine (ISMRM). Philadelphia, May 22–28, 1999, Vol. 1.

104. Stuber M, Manning WJ. Black-blood coronary MRA (abstr). *In*: Book of Abstracts of the First International Workshop on Coronary MR & CT Angiography. Lyon, France, Oct 1–3, 2000. Organized and published by the North American Society for Cardiac Imaging. Reprinted in: Int J Card Imag 2000;16.

105. Simonetti OP, Finn JP, White RD, Laub G, Henry DA. "Black blood" T2-weighted inversion-recovery MR imaging of the heart. Radiology 1996;199:49–57.

106. Jara H, Barish MA. Black-blood MR angiography: techniques and clinical applications. Magn Reson Imag Clin North Am 1999;7(2):303–17.

107. Regan F. Clinical applications of half-Fourier (HASTE) MR sequences in abdominal imaging. Magn Reson Imag Clin North Am 1999;7(2):275–88.

108. Wittlinger T, Voigtlander T, Grauvogel K, et al. Noninvasive evaluation of coronary bypass grafts by magnetic resonance imaging: comparison of the Haste and Fisp-3-D sequences with the conventional coronary angiography. Z Kardiol 2000;89(1):7–14.

109. Deshpande V, Gerhard Laub, Orlando Simonetti, et al. 3D MR coronary artery imaging using magnetization-prepared TrueFISP (abstr.). *In*: Book of Abstracts of the First International Workshop on Coronary MR & CT Angiography. Lyon, France, Oct. 1–3, 2000. Organized and published by the North American Society for Cardiac Imaging. Reprinted in: Int J Card Imag 2000; 16.

110. Wang Y, Vidan E, Bergman GW. Cardiac motion of coronary arteries: variability in the rest period and implications for coronary MR angiography. Radiology 1999;213(3):751–8.

111. Wang Y, Vidan E, Bergman GW. Characteristics of cardiac motion of coronary arteries (abstr.). *In*: Book of Abstracts of the First International Workshop on Coronary MR & CT Angiography. Lyon, France, Oct. 1–3, 2000. Organized and published by the North American Society for Cardiac Imaging. Reprinted in: Int J Card Imag 2000;16.

112. Firmin D. Report from the June 28–30, 1999 ISMRM Workshop on Flow and Motion: how it relates to coronary MRA. (abstr.). *In*: Book of Abstracts of the First International Workshop on Coronary MR & CT Angiography. Lyon, France, Oct. 1–3, 2000. Organized and published by the North American Society for Cardiac Imaging. Reprinted in: Int J Card Imag 2000;16.

113. Holland AE, Goldfarb JW, Edelman RR. Diaphragmatic and cardiac motion during suspended breathing: preliminary experience and implications for breath-hold MR imaging. Radiology 1998;209(2):483–9.

114. McGee KP, Felmlee JP, Manduca A, Riederer SJ, Ehman RL. Rapid autocorrection using prescan navigator echoes. Magn Reson Med 2000;43(4):583–88.

115. Ho VB, Foo TKF, Arai AE, Wolff SD. Gadolinium-enhanced two-dimensional coronary MR angiography using an automated contrast bolus detection algorithm (MR smartprep) (abstr.). *In*: Proceedings of the Sixth Scientific Meeting of the International Society for Magnetic Resonance in Medicine (ISMRM), April 18–24, 1998 (paper #19). Sydney, 1998 (in press).

116. Hofman MB, Henson RE, Kovacs SJ, et al. Blood pool agent strongly improves 3D magnetic resonance coronary angiography using an inversion pre-pulse. Magn Reson Med 1999;41(2):360–67.

117. Johansson LO, Nolan NM, Taniuchi M, Fischer SE, Wickline SA, Lorenz CH. High resolution magnetic resonance coronary angiography of the entire heart using a new blood-pool agent, NC100150 injection: comparison with invasive X-ray angiography in pigs. J Cardiovasc Magn Reson 1999;2(1):139–44.

118. Taylor AM, Panting JR, Keegan J, et al. Safety and preliminary findings with the intravascular contrast agent NC100150 injection for MR coronary angiography. J Magn Reson Imag 1999;9(2):220–27.

119. Duerinckx AJ. Coronary MR angiography. Radiol Clin North Am 1999;37(2):273–318.

120. Wielopolski PA, van Geuns RJ, de Feyter PJ, Oudkerk M. Coronary arteries. Eur Radiol 2000;10(1):12–35.

121. Meyer CH, Hu BS, Macovski A, Nishimura DG. Coronary vessel wall imaging (abstr.). *In*: Proceedings of the Sixth Scientific Meeting of the International Society for Magnetic Resonance in Medicine (ISMRM), April 18–24, 1998 (paper #15). Sydney, 1998; Vol 1: 15.

16
Second-Generation Coronary MRA Techniques

André J. Duerinckx

Introduction and Overview

Second-generation coronary magnetic resonance angiography (MRA) techniques can be simplistically described as the "multiple images during free breathing" techniques using navigator echo feedback for respiratory motion. In general, no breathholding is required. There is not a single second-generation technique, but a whole class of variants and improved versions. There are even more differences in implementations between commercial vendors and academic institutions with these techniques than there are with the first-generation techniques. Nobody yet knows what the best "modification" of the basic navigator technique will be (1–6). This is an active area of fascinating and promising ongoing research.

We will summarize some of the more important features of these techniques in this chapter, and refer the reader to other chapters for technique description (Chap. 3), history (Chap. 4), clinical applications (Chap. 6), and technical considerations (Chaps. 17–19).

Soon after the development of the first-generation single breathhold coronary MRA techniques there was also an interest in extending them to three-dimensional (3-D) imaging. Three-dimensional imaging offers the advantages of higher signal-to-noise ratio, shorter echo times, more isotropic pixel resolution, and the ability to examine the data set with a multiplanar reformatting technique. The initial attempts at using signal averaging (without breathholding) for 3-D coronary imaging did not produce very good results (7–10). Another 3-D coronary MRA technique, developed by Scheidegger at al., used a brief coached breathholding strategy that only required a 1-second breathhold in every 4 seconds (with the respiratory cycle typically lasting four heartbeats) (11–15) (see also Chap. 23). The results were very good and have inspired others to continue in this direction. Scheidegger et al. were the first to use sophisticated 3-D imaging display technology. This and other pioneering work on 3-D coronary magnetic resonance

imaging (MRI) formed the basis for the development of the second-generation coronary MRA techniques and has been reviewed in detail elsewhere (16).

The second-generation 3-D techniques for coronary MRA require less training to perform, can provide higher spatial resolution, and are very promising. These techniques are referred to as the "navigator" techniques. They allow higher-resolution two-dimensional (2-D) and low or high-resolution 3-D data acquisitions. These techniques were first described in 1993–1994 (6,17), but because the initial proposed implementations had severe shortcomings they underwent many improvements (1,3). The initial implementations of these second-generation techniques are still available on some commercial MR scanners and use visual feedback (17–20) or retrospective respiratory gating (21–25) to compensate for respiratory motion. They rely upon a navigator pulse to determine motion of the diaphragm (breathing motion). By either providing feedback to the patient (as to when to hold his/her breath) for repeated breathholds, or by feeding information back to the MRI computer, respiratory motion and/or inconsistency in repeated breathholding are eliminated. This allows more time to acquire image data (as one is not limited to a single breathhold), and thus allows for acquisition of 3-D data sets (6,26) or higher-resolution 2-D data sets (3,27). The technique can also be used with a spiral data acquisition scheme (22). The navigator pulse most often determines the motion of the diaphragm, but in some implementations it directly monitors the motion of portions of the left ventricular wall.

For the repeated breathholding versions, inconsistent breathholding is no longer a problem because the patient receives feedback as to when to stop breathing. For the nonbreathhold versions, the regularity of the breathing pattern during the long scan acquisition (sometimes up to 15 minutes) is important. It has been recommended that the navigator echo (NE) window be placed around end-expiratory position, that subjects should not sleep, and that scan efficiency should be monitored and, if needed, the NE window needs to be repositioned (5). Because of these and similar recommendations many adaptations and improvements to this navigator scheme have been made to improve its efficacy, including adaptive windowing (to correct for upward creep of the diaphragm in the supine position after 15–20 minutes) and the use of three orthogonal navigator echoes (to minimize motion in all three directions) (1,3,5,28). Once implemented, this technique requires less expertise and training because a 3-D transaxial slab covering the top of the heart and aortic root can be acquired and images can be analyzed later. In this sense it is very similar to electron-beam computed tomography (EB-CT) acquisitions for coronary calcium determination.

There are some problems with the second-generation coronary MRA technique found on some of the commercial MRI scanners. First, each acquisition takes much longer than it did with first-generation techniques (up to 12–15 minutes in some cases vs. a single 10–15-second breathhold) before the first images are generated. Second, it has been recognized that the initial implementation of the navigator techniques sometimes did not work in up to 50% of normal volunteers (for a variety of unknown reasons) (29), can be very noisy, and is very much a function of the regularity and type of breathing pattern. Navigator pulse correction techniques have also been used with the first-generation coronary MRA techniques to avoid slice misregistration between breathholding (2,3,30). These are the hybrid, first-generation techniques alluded to in Chapter 15. The navigator techniques have also been used to acquire small volume scan acquisitions (thin 3-D slabs) oriented along the right coronary artery (RCA) (4). The initial clinical results with a 3-D navigator technique have shown sensitivities for coronary artery lesion detection from 65 to 87% (31–33).

We will now review some of the early history leading to today's better understanding of these techniques

Early Three-Dimensional "Repeated Breathholding" Techniques

Typical 3-D acquisitions are too long to perform with breathholding; however, several schemes have been tested to help patients perform consistent repeated breathholds for a time period long enough to complete the 3-D data set acquisition.

One such modification of nonbreathhold 3-D coronary MRA techniques (described in next subsection) has incorporated visual feedback, derived from a navigator echo, to facilitate consistent repeated periods of breathholding (20). The 3-D acquisition in effect becomes a "breathhold" acquisition, but with much improved consistency. The patient alternates between "breathing"

and "breathhold" states. This technique was implemented on a 1.5 Tesla Signa scanner (General Electric, Milwaukee). Typical scan parameters were: TR = 9.9 ms, 32 slices, and a 256 × 128 matrix with 2-mm slice thickness. Each breathhold consisted of 10 heartbeats, with data acquisition disabled during the first two heartbeats to prepare spin equilibrium, and then segmental acquisition of 16 phases per heartbeat during 8 heartbeats. This amounted to 16 × 8 (or 32 × 4) views per breathhold. The total of 128 × 32 views needed was thus acquired in 32 breathholds typical with a total scan time of 10 minutes. The feedback system was able to reduce the variation of diastolic heart position to less than 2 mm. A drawback of this technique is the need for patient cooperation; however, with the respiratory feedback the patient can control the pace of data acquisition.

Another group of investigators introduced a breathholding strategy that only required a 1-second breathhold in every 4 seconds (with the respiratory cycle typically lasting 4 heartbeats) (11,12). A set of cross-sectional images, typically 30 slices, was acquired in approximately 10 minutes and 3-D renderings of the coronary arteries were produced from these (Fig. 16.1). Imaging started in late systole and proceeded throughout the entire diastolic period, thus covering a much longer portion of the cardiac cycle than the other techniques. Due to the cardiac motion occurring throughout each relatively long acquisition window (600 msec), however, there is an "S" shape deformity to the end of the visualized coronary vessels. The technique was implemented on a 1.5 Tesla S15/ACS Gyroscan (Philips Medical Systems, Best, The Netherlands). This group has obtained excellent results in patients with coronary lesions studied before and after angioplasty (13,14). The 3-D image rendering routine used produced images very similar to the ones obtained more recently with EB-CT.

Pulse Sequence Developments Prior to Today's "Free-Breathing" 3-D Coronary MRA

Inconsistency in breathholding with first-generation 2-D coronary MRA techniques is a well-known problem. Technical developments made to resolve this problem paralleled those made to develop the 3-D techniques. The use of real-time or retrospective navigator pulses (22,24) can help avoid this problem, but effectively turns these "breathhold" 2-D techniques into "FREE-BREATHING" (nonbreathhold) techniques. The use of navigator pulses allows acquisitions during free breathing by tracking diaphragmatic motion (18,22,34). The concept of navigator pulses has been used for thoracic and abdominal imaging (35). Whether or not these nonbreathhold 2-D coronary MRI will be as diagnostic as the breathhold images is unresolved.

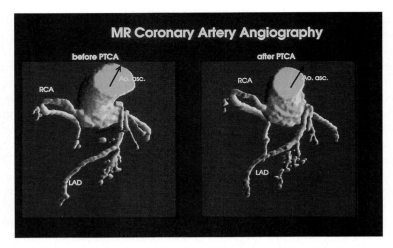

Figure 16.1. Three-dimensional reconstruction of the coronary vessels of a 53-year-old patient with a severe lesion in the proximal left anterior descending (LAD). A 3-D image stack was obtained by acquiring individual image data during consecutive 2–2.5-second periods of apnea at the end of normal exhalations, repeated approximately every 4 seconds. One to two cardiac cycles at the end of each exhalation were used for data acquisition. (Left) Image acquired 1 day prior to the treatment of the lesion with PTCA; the proximal LAD lesion (long arrow) is clearly demonstrated. The lesion is rendered as a short interruption, due to signal loss within the stenosis. (Right) Image acquired 1 day after PTCA. The dilated vessel segment is now open. Also shown are the: right coronary artery (RCA), left circumflex artery (LCx), and aortic root. (Case provided by M.B. Scheidegger, MD; reprinted with permission from Scheidegger (14); Springer-Verlag.)

The early 3-D coronary MRA techniques relied on either averaging during one or more respiratory cycles or pseudo-respiratory gating in patients with a regular breathing pattern (7–9,36,37). A typical 3-D pulse sequence is shown in Figure 16.2.

An early 3-D coronary MRA protocol developed by Paschal et al. (8) used subtraction to suppress fat. Imaging parameters were: a 128×256 matrix with 16 partitions; 2–3-mm slice thickness; TR = 11.1 msec; up to four averages to reduce respiratory motion artifacts. First, all the section-encoding (kz) lines were acquired, which took TR $\times$ 16 = 178 msec per cardiac cycle. This was repeated four times for each in-plane phase-encoding (ky), thus requiring $128 \times 4 = 512$ heartbeats, or (for a heart rate of 60 beats/second) approximately 8 minutes and 32 seconds per 3-D data set. This 3-D data set acquisition was repeated with and without a magnetization preparation pulse to reproduce the best nulling of blood signal. The two 3-D data sets were then subtracted to remove fat and most of the myocardium. This 3-D technique relying on four averages during a respiratory cycle produced adequate images in normal volunteers and in a small number of patients.

Newer improved versions of the 3-D technique included fat saturation and magnetization transfer contrast without the need for subtraction (9,37). They also used thinner slices, allowing better multiplanar reconstructions. Typical imaging parameters were: a 128×256 matrix with 31 partitions; TR = 8.4 msec, TE = 2.9 msec, with a flip angle of 10 degrees, and an effective slice thickness of 2.1 mm. All 31 kz phase-encoding steps were obtained within one cardiac cycle, resulting in a

time window of 260 msec. Six interleaved acquisitions per ky step were obtained to cover the respiratory cycle. This technique was compared to a 2-D breathhold using a 140×256 matrix, with TR = 12.6 msec and TE =

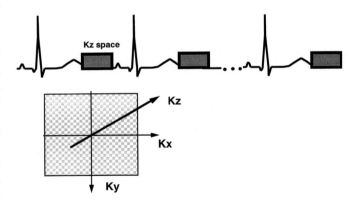

Figure 16.2. Pulse sequence timing for a 3-D coronary MRA technique using k-space segmented non-breathhold ultrafast gradient-recalled echo (GRE) with a $144 \times 256 \times 16$ matrix. At the top is shown the electrocardiogram signal (EKG signal) used to trigger the MR pulse sequence. The horizontal axis (time-axis) is not shown to scale. The timing of the data acquisition for one of 144 segments (covering 16 kz encoding steps) is shown in mid-diastole. Preceding the segment acquisition within each heartbeat is an additional pulse (not shown) needed to suppress the signal from fat surrounding the coronary arteries. At the bottom is a representation of the way k-space data are being acquired: each segments acquires 16 kz data points, repeated 144 times for the 144 ky steps (in 144 heartbeats) until all data are acquired. If averaging over a respiratory cycle is used, one typically repeats this 4 to 6 times. (Reprinted with permission from Duerinckx (16).)

7.0 msec, variable flip angle, seven phase-encodings per segment, and a 4-mm slice thickness, with an acquisition window of 88 msec per cardiac cycle. The image quality was somewhat better for images obtained by 2-D breathholding in 83% of the vessels, probably due to less blurring by remnant respiratory motion and higher inflow contrast (9). The 3-D acquisition, however, is less operator dependent, faster, and less strenuous for patients.

Wang et al. showed that the blurring differences between nonbreathhold 3-D and breathhold 2-D images are mainly caused by respiration because coronary displacement caused by cardiac motion during the somewhat longer diastolic acquisition window is negligible (38) (see also earlier discussion). This explains the strong emphasis on techniques that compensate for respiratory motion by using either feedback devices (20) or real-time and retrospective respiratory gating.

More recently the use of navigator pulses has allowed to transform these sequences into "repeated breath-hold" acquisitions with visual feedback, or nonbreath-hold sequences with real-time or retrospective respiratory gating (9,25,39). Even during early attempts, the introduction of retrospective respiratory gating improved the image quality in 76% of the 3-D images (9). Since then, using improvements in the retrospective respiratory gating technique, Li et al. and others have obtained very impressive clinical images of coronary arteries in volunteers and patients (25,39,40). In addition to the use of retrospective respiratory gating, their 3-D MR pulse sequence parameters were highly optimized as follows: the acquisition window was reduced from 260 msec to 120 msec (by reducing the number of partitions from 32 to 16 and slightly reducing the TR from 8.4 to 8 msec); a variable flip angle (20 to 90 degrees) was used in the 3-D partition encoding direction. Improvements in MRI equipment, such as the ability to use a faster gradient rise time of 600 sec from 0 to 25 mT/m on the new 1.5 Tesla VISION MR imager (Siemens Medical Systems, Inc., Iselin, NJ) and other scanners also allowed additional improvements in signal bandwidth and resolution.

The Free-Breathing 3-D Coronary MRA Since Year 2000

Commercial implementations of highly sophisticated and improved versions of the navigator echo guided free-breathing 3-D coronary MRA are now available. Manning et al. (41) with support from Philips Medical Systems have organized an MR coronary artery multicenter study with the Boston Cookbook protocol using the latest navigator-based technology. Prospective adaptive navigator motion correction will probably replace the older retrospective motion correction schemes

(see also Chaps. 17–19). 3-D MRA techniques have several advantages: favorable signal-to-noise ratios (SNR), the acquisition of thin contiguous sections and the ability to postprocess/reformat the data set. When compared to 2-D techniques they also have a lower contrast between coronary blood and myocardium. This disadvantage of 3-D can be overcome by using contrast agents or prepulses (23).

T2 preparation prepulses (T2-prep) allow suppression of tissues with short T2 relaxation times, e.g. cardiac muscle (T2 = 50 m/sec), cardiac veins with deoxygenated blood (20% O_2 saturation, T2 = 35 m/sec), and epicardial fat. Tissues with long T2 relaxation times e.g., arterial blood (T2 = 250 m/sec), are minimally influenced. The contrast-to-noise between arterial blood and myocardium can be adjusted by varying parameters in the pulse sequence.

Botnar et al. (42) showed that the use of a T2prep pulse resulted in significant increase in contrast-to-noise and improved coronary edge definition. Reduction of the acquisition windows from 120 to 60 m/sec (improved temporal resolution) allowed for only a small improvement in vessel definition, at the expense of a doubled scan time. For this study Botnar et al. (42) used a T2prep pulse, a cranial-caudal oriented 2-D selective navigator through the basal LV with prospective slice correction and a 3-mm gating window, and a frequency-selective fat-suppressed pulse to suppress signal from epicardial fat preceding the imaging acquisition. The field of view (FOV) was 360 × 305 mm with an image matrix of 512 × 304 (in plane resolution of 0.7 × 1.0 mm). The 3-D slab had 10 slices with a 3-m slice thickness, interpolated to 20 slices with a 1.5-m thickness. Each 3-D volume slice was acquired during data collection over 38 consecutive acquisition windows (or "shots") by use of a centric k-space ordering scheme with a TR = 7.4 m/sec and TE = 2.5 m/sec. Acquisition windows of 120 m/sec (16 echoes/shot) and 60 m/sec (8 echoes/shot) were compared. All data were acquired at middiastole. At a heart rate of 60 beats per minute, with 16 echoes/shot and with a (theoretical) scan efficiency of 100%, this would require an acquisition duration of 19 heartbeats per slice, or 190 heartbeats (3.2 minutes) per 3-D volume. Scan efficiency is defined as the number of shots accepted (within the navigator window) divided by the total number of heartbeats used for completing the scan. The actual total imaging time for each acquisition of 10 slices (interpolated to 20 slices) varied from 10 to 20 minutes depending on heart rate and navigator efficiency. To cover a large heart multiple such acquisitions would be needed.

This typical 10- to 20-minute duration for one 3-D slab navigator acquisition can present a real problem. Respiratory patterns vary during such a long period of free-breathing and can be quite different for normal volunteers and patients (5,43). Thus faster implementation of the 3-D techniques have been developed to overcome this problem. One such implementation allows 3-D volume data acquisitions in less than 5 minutes with a slight worsening in spatial resolution (44). Botnar et al. (44) used a navigator-gated and corrected EKG triggered ultra-fast 3-D interleaved gradient echo planar imaging sequence (TFE-EPI) to acquire a 3-D slab, consisting of 20 slices with a reconstructed slice thickness of 1.5 mm with free-breathing. The diastolic TFE-EPI acquisition block was preceded by a T2prep prepulse, a diaphragmatic navigator pulse, and a fat suppression prepulse. With a TR of 19 ms and an effective TE of 5.4 ms, the duration of the data acquisition window was 38 ms. The in-plane spatial resolution was 1.0–1.3 mm × 1.5–1.9 mm. As will be described later (see Chap. 20) this can be taken even further using a HYBRID technique of volume splitting using prospective real-time navigator technology (45). Using this approach, Stuber et al. acquired a 9-cm thick volume with in-plane resolution of 1.2 × 2.2 mm, which can be acquired during five breathholds of 15 second duration each (45).

Another approach to reducing the excessive measurement times associated with large volume acquisitions is the use of double-oblique free-breathing high resolution 3-D coronary MRA (46). By planning the 3-D volume sets along the major axis of the coronary vessels successful submillimeter coronary MRA was possible within reasonable time frames, with the scanning time per double-oblique high resolution 3-D scan less than 16 minutes. This is very similar to the image slice and 3-D thin-slab position selection described in Chapter 5 for first- and third-generation coronary MRA (47–51).

Other unresolved problems remain. The ratio of cardiac motion to diaphragmatic motion is greatly variable from person to person, thus making it difficult to use a universal correction factor when using navigator echoes to measure motion of the diaphragm only (52). Several investigators have looked at navigator echo triggering off a cardiac structure (53). Stuber et al. (53) compared images acquired with the navigator localized at the right hemidiaphragm and at the left ventricle. The diaphragmatic navigator was found to be superior for vessel delineation of middle to distal portions of the coronary arteries. It has also been observed that the chest wall motion and the diaphragmatic motion are not always synchronized. Because of this Stuber (54) has conducted

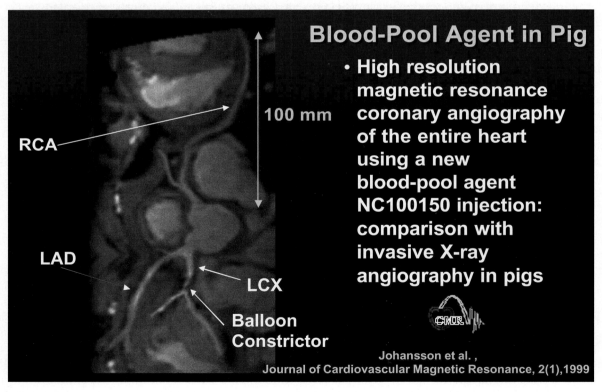

Figure 16.3. Coronary MRA (curved reformat) in a pig with an externally placed balloon constrictor on the left circumflex artery. Images were obtained with NC100150 injection, 5 mg Fe/kg body weight (Nycomed Amersham Imaging) using a 3-D spoiled gradient echo sequence with fat suppression and a flip angle sweep optimized to maintain constant maximum signal in the blood (TR/TE 6.7/2.3 msec). A 2-D RF selective navigator placed on the diaphragm was used for motion compensation. Images were obtained on a 1.5T Gyroscan NT, PT 6000 (Philips Medical Systems, The Netherlands). Resolution was 0.9 × 0.9 × 0.9 mm³, and the acquisition window per cardiac cycle was 55 msec. (Images are courtesy of Lars Johansson, Nycomed, Oslo, Norway and Christine Lorenz, Siemens Medical Center, London, UK; Images acquired while both were working at Center for Cardiovascular MR, Barnes-Jewish Hospital at Washington University Medical Center, St. Louis, MO.)

a study to show that prone positioning may be superior in free-breathing 3-D coronary MRA in patients. If this is significant (and it probably will be for some patients) then we may have to return to the what we did during the early days (the 1993–1995 period) with first-generation coronary MRA when all patients were studied in the less comfortable prone position.

Higher resolution imaging has become possible, with spatial in-plane resolution down to 390 micrometers (55). Such high-resolution MRI can also be used to image the coronary vessel wall and plaque (56,57). There are other ways to further improve spatial and temporal resolution, such as SMASH imaging or SENSE, which are new MRI techniques that can be used to multiply the speed of existing imaging sequences (58–63). SMASH operates by using an array of radiofrequency (RF) detection coils to perform some of the spatial encoding normally accomplished with magnetic field gradients. The speed of the SMASH technique results from appropriate combinations of coil array RF signals in which multiple lines of image data are gathered simultaneously, rather than one after another.

Preclinical and clinical work with navigator techniques has been quite impressive. Several studies for coronary lesion detection using retrospective navigator gating reported good results, as described in Chapter 12 (64–66). Examples of recently published coronary MRA using these retrospective navigator gated techniques are shown in Figure 16.3. Much better results are expected from techniques using prospective and adaptive gating, such as used by Manning et al. (41) for the MR coronary artery multicenter study with the Boston Cookbook protocol. Motion adaptive gating techniques are still being refined (67).

The Use of Contrast Agents

Lorenz et al. have reviewed the use of MR contrast agents for coronary MRA for a special December 1999 cardiac MRI issue of the *Journal of Magnetic Resonance in Medicine* (68). We will only briefly reference some of the publications in this field, as this is an embryonic but promising topic.

Limited work on the use of gadolinium contrast agents with the first-generation techniques has been done (69–73). The use of contrast agents with the third-generation coronary MRA techniques (see Chaps. 20, 24–25) seems more promising and is easier to implement (74–77). Some very promising early work with the second-generation techniques has also been performed, however, in animals and humans (78–83).

Keyhole Imaging

Scanning efficiency can be further increased by using the concept of keyhole imaging. Jhooti et al. (84) have proposed the use of centrically ordered acquisitions in which the central portion of the *k*-space is collected with a small respiratory gating window (like 1 mm), while the data for the outer portions of *k*-space are scanned with increasing gating windows (from 3 to 5 to 7 mm). Another such approach is the 3-D zonal EPI coronary MRA, described by Yang et al. (85). Both approaches claim increases in scanning efficiency, without significant image degradation.

The Future

The second-generation coronary MRA sequences have a great future. Today they allow the highest spatial resolution with a user-friendly MR scanning technique. Commercial implementations exist, with Philips Medical Systems being the first to offer its customers a great reliable implementation of navigator-echo-based coronary MRA since 1999. At the time of this writing, preliminary data from the MR coronary artery multicenter study with the Boston Cookbook protocol appear very promising (41). Many investigators are actively working on further improving these techniques. A more detailed description of second-generation technique design and variants is provided in Chapters 17 to 19.

References

1. Danias PG, McConnell MV, Khasgiwala VC, Chuang ML, Edelman RR, Manning WJ. Prospective navigator correction of image position for coronary. Radiology 1997; 203(3): 733–36.
2. McConnell MV, Khasgiwala VC, Savord BJ, et al. Comparison of respiratory suppression methods and navigator locations for MR coronary angiography. Am J Roentgenol 1997;168(5):1369–75.
3. McConnell MV, Khasgiwala VC, Savord BJ, et al. Prospective adaptive navigator correction for breath-hold MR coronary angiography. Magn Reson Med 1997;37(1):148–52.
4. Oshinski JN, Dixon WT, Pettigrew RI. Magnetic resonance coronary angiography with navigator echo gated real-time slice following. The International J Card Imag 1998;14(3):191–99.
5. Taylor AM, Jhooti P, Wiesmann F, Keegan J, Firmin DN, Pennell DJ. MR navigator-echo monitoring of temporal changes in diaphragm position: implications for MR coronary angiography. J Magn Reson Imag 1997;7(4):629–36.
6. Wang Y, Rossman PJ, Grimm RC, Riederer SJ, Ehman RL. Navigator-echo-based real-time respiratory gating and triggering for reduction of respiration effects in three-dimensional coronary MR angiography. Radiology 1996; 198:55–60.
7. Paschal C, Haacke E, Adler L, Finelli DA. Magnetic resonance coronary artery imaging. Cardiovasc Intervent Radiol 1992;15:23–31.
8. Paschal CB, Haacke EM, Adler LP. Three-dimensional MR imaging of the coronary arteries: preliminary clinical experience. J Magn Reson Imag 1993;3(3):491–501.
9. Hofman MBM, Paschal CB, Li D, Haacke M, vanRossum AC, Sprenger M. MRI of coronary arteries: 2-D breath-hold

vs. 3-D respiratory-gated acquisition. J Comput Assist To-mogr 1995;19(1):56–62.

10. Li D, Kaushikkar S, Haacke EM, et al. Coronary arteries: three-dimensional MR imaging with retrospective respiratory gating (technical development and instrumentation). Radiology 1996;201:857–63.

11. Scheidegger M, deGraaf R, Doyle M, Vermeulen J, vanDijk P, Pohost G. Coronary artery MR imaging during multiple brief (1 sec) expiratory breathholds (abstr.). In: Proceedings of the Eleventh Annual Scientific Meeting of the Society of Magnetic Resonance Imaging (SMRM). Berlin, August 8–14, 1992:602.

12. Doyle M, Scheidegger MB, DeGraaf RG, Vermeulen J, Pohost GM. Coronary artery imaging in multiple 1-sec breath holds. Magn Reson Imag 1993;11:3–6.

13. Scheidegger MB, Müller R, Boesiger P. Magnetic resonance angiography: methods and its applications to the coronary arteries. Technol Health Care 1994;2:255–65.

14. Scheidegger MB, Boesiger P. Coronary MR imaging. In: Lanzer P, Rösch J, ed. Vascular Diagnosis. Berlin: Springer-Verlag, 1994: 415–420.

15. Scheidegger MB, Stuber M, Boesiger P, Hess OM. Coronary artery imaging by magnetic resonance. Herz 1996; 21(2):90–96.

16. Duerinckx AJ. Coronary MR angiography. In: Cardiac MR imaging, Boxt LM, guest ed. MRI Clin North Am 1996; 4(2):361–418.

17. Liu YL, Rossman PJ, Grimm RC, Debbins JP, Ehman RL, Riederer SJ. Comparison of two breath-hold feedback techniques for reproducible breath holds in MRI (abstr.). In: Printed Program of the First Meeting of the Society of Magnetic Resonance (SMR). Dallas, Texas, March 5–9, 1994; J Magn Reson Imag 1994;4(P):61.

18. Wang Y, Christy PS, Korosec FR, et al. Coronary MRI with a respiratory feedback monitor: the 2D imaging case. Magn Reson Med 1995;33(1):116–21.

19. Liu YL, Riederer SJ, Rossman PJ, Grimm RG, Debbins JF, Ehman RL. A monitoring, feedback, and triggering system for reproducible breath-hold MR imaging. Magn Reson Med 1993;30:507–11.

20. Wang Y, Grimm RC, Rossman PJ, Debbins JP, Riederer SJ, Ehman RL. 3D coronary MR angiography in multiple breath-holds using a respiratory feedback monitor. Magn Reson Med 1995;34(1):11–16.

21. Brittain JH, Hu BS, Wright GA, Meyer CH, Macovski A, Nishimura DG. Multislice coronary angiography with muscle and venous suppression (#367) (abstr.). In: Printed Program of the Second Meeting of the Society of Magnetic Resonance (SMR). San Francisco, August 7–12, 1994.

22. Sachs TS, Meyer CH, Hu BS, Kohli J, Nishimura DG, Macovski A. Real-time motion detection in spiral MRI using navigators. Magn Reson Med 1994;32(5):639–45.

23. Brittain JH, Hu BS, Wright GA, Meyer CH, Macovski A, Nishimura DG. Coronary angiography with magnetization-prepared T2 contrast. Magn Reson Med 1995;33(5): 689–96.

24. Sachs TS, Meyer CH, Irazzabal P, Hu BS, Nishimura DG, Macovski A. The diminishing variance algorithm for real-time reduction of motion artifacts in MRI. Magn Reson Med 1995;34:412–22.

25. Li D, Kaushikkar S, Woodard P, Dhawale P, Haacke EM.

Three-dimensional MRI of coronary arteries (abstr.). In: Book of Abstracts of Seventh International Workshop on Magnetic Resonance Angiography. Matsuyama, Japan, October 12–14, 1995.

26. Fu Z, Wang Y, Grimm RC, et al. Orbital navigator echoes for motion measurement in magnetic resonance imaging. Magn Reson Med 1995;34(5):746–53.

27. Oshinski JN, Hofland L, Dixon WT, Parks WJ, Pettigrew RI. Magnetic resonance coronary angiography without breathholding using navigator echoes (abstr.). In: Book of Abstracts of the Fourth Meeting of the International Society of Magnetic Resonance in Medicine (ISMRM). New York, April 27–May 3, 1996; Vol. 1: 449.

28. Taylor AM, Jhooti P, Firmin DN, Pennell DJ. Automated monitoring of diaphragm end-expiratory position for real-time navigator echo MR coronary angiography (abstr.). In: Proceedings of the Sixth Scientific Meeting of the International Society for Magnetic Resonance in Medicine (ISMRM), April 18–24, 1998 (paper #21). Sydney, Australia, 1998; Vol. 1: 21.

29. Stehling M. Coronary arteries: experience with navigator echoes. (abstr.). In: Eighth International Workshop on Magnetic Resonance Angiography. Rome, Italy, October 16–19, 1996.

30. Oshinski JN, Hofland L, Mukundan S, Dixon WT, James WJ, Pettigrew RI. Two-dimensional MR coronary angiography without breath holding. Radiology 1996;201:737–43.

31. Müller MF, Fleisch M, Kroeker R, Chatterjee T, Meier B, Vock P. Proximal coronary artery stenosis: three-dimensional MRI with fat saturation and navigator echo. J Magn Reson Imag 1997;7(4):644–51.

32. Kessler W, Achenbach S, Moshage W, et al. Usefulness of respiratory gated magnetic resonance coronary angiography in assessing narrowings >50% in diameter in native coronary arteries and in aortocoronary bypass conduits. Am J Cardiol 1997;80:989–93.

33. Achenbach S, Kessler W, Moshage WE, et al. Visualization of the coronary arteries in three-dimensional reconstructions using respiratory gated magnetic resonance imaging. Cor Art Dis 1997;8(7):441–48.

34. Brittain JH, Sachs TS, Hu BS, Nishimura. DG. Nonbreath-held 2DFT coronary angiography (abstr.). In: Book of Abstracts of the Third Meeting of the Society of Magnetic Resonance (SMR) and the Twelfth Annual Scientific Meeting of the European Society for Magnetic Resonance in Medicine and Biology (ESMRMB). Nice, France, August 20–25, 1995.

35. Butts K, Riederer SJ, Ehman RL. The effect of respiration on the contrast and sharpness of liver lesions on MRI. Magn Reson Med 1995;33:1–7.

36. Paschal C, Haacke E, Adler L, Lin W, Shetty A, Altidi R. High resolution 3-D cardiac imaging (abstr.). In: Proceedings of the Ninth Annual Meeting of the Society of Magnetic Resonance in Medicine (SMRM). Berkeley, California, 1990: 278.

37. Li D, Paschal CB, Haacke EM, Adler LP. Coronary arteries: three-dimensional MR imaging with fat saturation and magnetization transfer contrast. Radiology 1993;187:401–6.

38. Wang Y, Grist TM, Korosec FR, et al. Respiratory blur in 3D coronary MR imaging. Magn Reson Med 1995;April; 33(4):541–48.

39. Haacke EM, Li D, Kaushikkar S. Cardiac MR imaging: principles and techniques. Top Magn Reson Imag 1995; 7(4):200–17.

40. Woodard PK, Li D, Haacke EM, et al. Detection of coronary stenosis on source and projection images using three-dimensional MR angiography with retrospective respiratory gating: preliminary experience. Am J Roentgenol 1998;170:883–88.

41. Manning WJ, Danias P, Kissinger K, Stuber M, Botnar R, et al. MR coronary artery multi-center study with the Boston Cookbook protocol (abstr.). In: Book of Abstracts of the First International Workshop on Coronary MR & CT Angiography. Lyon, France, Oct. 1–3, 2000. Organized and published by the North American Society for Cardiac Imaging. Reprinted in: Int J Card Imag 2000;16.

42. Botnar RM, Stuber M, Danias PG, Kissinger KV, Manning WJ. Improved coronary artery definition with T2-weighted, free-breathing, three-dimensional coronary MRA. Circulation 1999;99(24):3139–48.

43. Taylor AM, Keegan J, Jhooti P, Gatehouse PD, Firmin DN, Pennell DJ. Differences between normal subjects and patients with coronary artery disease for three different MR coronary angiography respiratory suppression techniques. J Magn Reson Imag 1999;9(6):786–93.

44. Botnar RM, Stuber M, Danias PG, Kissinger KV, Manning WJ. A fast 3D approach for coronary MRA. J Magn Reson Imag 1999;10(5):821–25.

45. Stuber M, Botnar RM, Danias PG, Kissinger KV, Manning WJ. Breathhold three-dimensional coronary magnetic resonance angiography using real-time navigator technology. J Cardiovasc Magn Reson 1999;1(3):233–38.

46. Stuber M, Botnar RM, Danias PG, et al. Double-oblique free-breathing high resolution three-dimensional coronary magnetic resonance angiography. J Am Coll Cardiol 1999; 34(2):524–31.

47. Duerinckx AJ. Review: MR angiography of the coronary arteries. Topics Magn Reson Imag 1995;7(4):267–85.

48. Duerinckx AJ, Urman M. Optimal imaging planes for MR coronary angiography. (abstr.). In: Book of Abstracts of the Eleventh Annual Scientific Meeting of the European Society for Magnetic Resonance in Medicine and Biology. Vienna, Austria, April 20–24, 1994;83.

49. Duerinckx AJ. Coronary arteries: how do I image them? In: Bogaert J, Duerinckx AJ, Rademakers F, ed. Magnetic Resonance of the Heart and Great Vessels: Clinical Applications. New York: Springer-Verlag, 2000:223–43.

50. Wielopolski P, vanGeuns RJ, deFeyter PJ, Oudkerk M. Breath-hold coronary MR angiography with volume targeted imaging. Radiology 1998;209:209–20.

51. Wielopolski PA, van Geuns RJ, de Feyter PJ, Oudkerk M. Coronary arteries. Eur Radiol 2000;10(1):12–35.

52. Danias PG, Stuber M, Botnar RM, Kissinger KV, Edelman RR, Manning WJ. Relationship between motion of coronary arteries and diaphragm during free breathing: lessons from real-time MR imaging. Am J Roentgenol 1999;172(4):1061–65.

53. Stuber M, Botnar RM, Danias PG, Kissinger KV, Manning WJ. Submillimeter three-dimensional coronary MR angiography with real-time navigator correction: comparison of navigator locations. Radiology 1999;212(2):579–87.

54. Stuber M. Superiority of prone position in free-breathing 3D coronary MRA in patients with coronary disease. (abstr.). In: Program Book of the Society for Cardiovascular Magnetic Resonance, Third Meeting. Atlanta, Georgia, January 21–23, 2000:2000;13.

55. Stuber M, Botnar RM, Manning WJ. Towards X-ray angiography image resolution in coronary MRA (abstr.). In: Book of Abstracts of the First International Workshop on Coronary MR & CT Angiography. Lyon, France, Oct. 1–3, 2000. Organized and published by the North American Society for Cardiac Imaging. Reprinted in: Int J Card Imag 2000;16.

56. Botnar RM, Matthias Stuber, Kraig V Kissinger, Manning WJ. Real-time navigator gated and corrected coronary vessel wall imaging (abstr.). In: Cardiovascular Imaging 1999. The Twenty-seventh Annual Meeting of the North American Society for Cardiac Imaging (NASCI), Nov. 6, 1999. Atlanta, Georgia: 1999.

57. Botnar RM, Stuber M, Kissinger KV, Manning WJ. In vivo imaging of coronary artery wall in humans using navigator and free-breathing (abstr.). In: Book of Abstracts and Proceedings of the Eighth Meeting of the International Society of Magnetic Resonance in Medicine (ISMRM 2000 Proceedings Available on CD-ROM). Denver, Colorado, April 1–7:2000.

58. Sodickson DK, Griswold MA, Jakob PM, Edelman RR, Manning WJ. Signal-to-noise ratio and signal-to-noise efficiency in SMASH imaging. Magn Reson Med 1999;41(5): 1009–22.

59. Sodickson DK, Stuber M, Botnar RM, Kissinger KV, Manning WJ. SMASH real-time cardiac imaging at echocardiographic frame rates. (abstr.). In: Book of Abstracts and Proceedings of the Seventh Meeting of the International Society of Magnetic Resonance in Medicine (ISMRM). Philadelphia, Pennsylvania, May 22–28, 1999.

60. Sodickson DK, Griswold MA, Jakob PM. SMASH imaging. Magn Reson Imag Clin North Am 1999;7(2):237–54, vii–viii.

61. Griswold MA, Jakob PM, Chen Q, et al. Resolution enhancement in single-shot imaging using simultaneous acquisition of spatial harmonics (SMASH). Magn Reson Med 1999;41(6):1236–45.

62. Pruessmann KP, Weiger M, Scheidegger MB, Boesiger P. SENSE: sensitivity encoding for fast MRI. Magn Reson Med 1999;42(5):952–62.

63. Weiger M, Pruessmann KP, Boesiger P. High performance cardiac real-time imaging using SENSE (abstr.). In: Book of Abstracts and Proceedings of the Seventh Meeting of the International Society of Magnetic Resonance in Medicine (ISMRM). Philadelphia, Pennsylvania, May 22–23, 1999:1999.

64. Huber A, Nikolaou K, Gonschior P, Knez A, Stehling M, Reiser M. Navigator echo-based respiratory gating for three-dimensional MR coronary angiography: results from healthy volunteers and patients with proximal coronary artery stenoses. Am J Roentgenol 1999;173(1):95–101.

65. Sandstede JJ, Pabst T, Beer M, et al. Three-dimensional MR coronary angiography using the navigator technique compared with conventional coronary angiography. Am J Roentgenol 1999;172(1):135–39.

66. Sardanelli F, Molinari G, Zandrino F, Balbi M. Three-dimensional, navigator-echo MR coronary angiography in

detecting stenoses of the major epicardial vessels, with conventional coronary angiography as the standard of reference [see comments]. Radiology 2000;214(3):808–14.

67. Nagel E, Bornstedt A, Schnackenburg B, Hug J, Oswald H, Fleck E. Optimization of realtime adaptive navigator correction for 3D magnetic resonance coronary angiography. Magn Reson Med 1999;42(2):408–11.

68. Lorenz CH, Johansson LO. Contrast-enhanced coronary MRA. J Magn Reson Imag 1999;10(5):703–8.

69. Duerinckx AJ, Urman M, Sinha U, Atkinson D, Simonetti O. Evaluation of gadolinium-enhanced MR coronary angiography (abstr.). In: Seventy-ninth Scientific Assembly and Annual Meeting of the Radiological Society of North America (RSNA). Chicago, November 28–December 3, 1993; Radiology 1993;189(P):278.

70. Stillman AE, Wilke N, Li D, Haacke EM, McLachlan SJ. MRA of renal and coronary arteries using an intravascular contrast agent (#944) (abstr.). In: Printed Program of the Second Meeting of the Society of Magnetic Resonance (SMR). San Francisco, August 6–12, 1994.

71. Saeed M, Wendland MF, Engelbrecht M, Sakuma H, Higgins CB. Contrast-enhanced magnetic resonance angiography in the coronary and peripheral arteries. Acad Radiol 1998;17 Vol. 5, Suppl. 1: S108–S12.

72. Ho VB, Foo TKF, Arai AE, Wolff SD. Gadolinium-enhanced two-dimensional coronary MR angiography using an automated contrast bolus detection algorithm (MR smartprep) (abstr.). In: Proceedings of the Sixth Scientific Meeting of the International Society for Magnetic Resonance in Medicine (ISMRM), April 18–24, 1998 (paper #19). Sydney, Australia, 1998.

73. Taylor AM, Panting JR, Keegan J, et al. Safety and preliminary findings with the intravascular contrast agent NC100150 injection for MR coronary angiography. J Magn Reson Imag 1999;9(2):220–27.

74. Goldfarb JW, Edelman RR. Coronary arteries: breath-hold, gadolinium-enhanced, three-dimensional MR angiography. Radiology 1998;206(3):830–34.

75. deBruin HG, vanGeuns RJM, Wielopolski PA, deFeyter PJ, Oudkerk M. Improvement of magnetic resonance imaging of the coronary arteries with a clinically available intravascular contrast agent (abstr.). In: Book of Abstracts of the First International Workshop on Coronary MR & CT Angiography. Lyon, France, Oct. 1–3, 2000. Organized and published by the North American Society for Cardiac Imaging. Reprinted in: Int J Card Imag 2000;16.

76. Kessler W, Laub G, Achenbach S, Ropers D, Moshage W, Daniel WG. Coronary arteries: MR angiography with fast contrast-enhanced three-dimensional breath-hold imaging—initial experience. Radiology 1999;210(2):566–72.

77. Kruger DG, Busse RF, Johnston DL, Ritman EL, Ehman RL, Riederer SJ. Contrast-enhanced 3D MR breathhold imaging of porcine coronary arteries using fluoroscopic localization and bolus triggering. Magn Reson Med 1999; 42(6):1159–65.

78. Li D, Dolan RP, Walovitch RC, Lauffer RB. Three-dimensional MRI of coronary arteries using an intravascular contrast agent. Magn Reson Med 1998;39(6):1014–18.

79. Li D, Zheng J, Weinmann H-J, et al. Comparison of intravascular and extravascular contrast agents in coronary artery imaging. (abstr.). In: Proceedings of the Sixth Scientific Meeting of the International Society for Magnetic Resonance in Medicine (ISMRM), April 18–24, 1998 (paper #17). Sydney, Australia, 1998: Vol. 1: 17.

80. Stuber M, Botnar RM, McConnell MV, et al. Coronary artery imaging with the intravascular contrast agent MS-325. (abstr.). In: Proceedings of the Sixth Scientific Meeting of the International Society for Magnetic Resonance in Medicine (ISMRM), April 18–24, 1998 (paper #316). Sydney, Australia, 1998: Vol. 1: 316.

81. Sakuma H, Goto M, Nomura Y, Kato N, Takeda K. Higgins CB. Three-dimensional coronary magnetic resonance angiography with injection of extracellular contrast medium. Invest Radiol 1999;34(8):503–8.

82. Stuber M, Botnar RM, Danias PG, et al. Contrast agent-enhanced, free-breathing, three-dimensional coronary magnetic resonance angiography. J Magn Reson Imag 1999;10(5):790–99.

83. Zheng J, Bae KT, Woodard PK, Haacke EM, Li D. Efficacy of slow infusion of gadolinium contrast agent in three-dimensional MR coronary artery imaging. J Magn Reson Imag 1999;10(5):800–5.

84. Jhooti P, Keegan J, Gatehouse PD, et al. 3D coronary artery imaging with phase reordering for improved scan efficiency. Magn Reson Med 1999;41(3):555–62.

85. Yang GZ, Burger P, Gatehouse PD, Firmin DN. Locally focused 3D coronary imaging using volume-selective RF excitation. Magn Reson Med 1999;41(1):171–78.

17
Motion Reduction Techniques for Coronary MRA

Yi Wang

Introduction

Significant progress has been made in coronary magnetic resonance angiography (MRA) (1–16). Motion reduction techniques have contributed significantly to this progress (1,2,9–16). Motion of the heart consists of cardiac contraction and respiration. For effective reduction of the effects of cardiac contraction, coronary data acquisition is enabled only during a brief diastolic period (~100 msec) of the cardiac cycle when the cardiac contraction is minimum and coronary arterial flow is maximum. Many cardiac cycles are accordingly required to complete acquisition of the coronary tree, and respiration occurred during data acquisition is the major factor limiting image quality.

The challenge to reduce respiration effects in magnetic resonance imaging (MRI) is that respiration cannot be modeled or predicted accurately. Breathholding has been a popular method used to reduce respiration effects. Multiple breathholds are typically required to acquire the whole coronary tree with sufficient spatial resolution and signal-to-noise ratio. Misregistration between different breathholds may limit diagnostic accuracy (7,10).

A systematic and effective approach to reduce respiration effects in coronary MRA as well as in other areas of MRI affected by motion is the navigator-based motion reduction method: Motion is monitored using navigator echoes and data acquisition is modified accordingly. This concept was introduced in the early 1950s for correcting the distorting effects of the Earth's atmosphere in ground-based astronomical imaging, where the angular resolution is limited by the atmospheric turbulence deforming the image on a millisecond time scale, not by the size of the primary mirrors of telescopes (17). Adaptive optical systems consisting of natural or artificial guide stars, wavefront sensors, and real-time phase-delay corrections have significantly improved image resolution (18).

Spatial resolution of coronary MRA is similarly limited by physiological motion, not by the capability of the MRI system to sample high spatial frequency information. Navigator-based motion gating and correction techniques were separately introduced in MRI in the late 1980s to reduce motion effects (19,20). Navigator-based motion correction techniques are currently used widely to correct undesired motion effects in diffusion imaging (21–24), neuro-fMRI (26–28), body MRA (29–32), and spectroscopy (33). The initial results from our group and others vindicate the effectiveness of these navigator-based methods for reducing motion effects in coronary MRA (9–16). These navigator methods will very likely play a significant role in future development of coronary MRA.

This chapter will attempt to review systematically navigator-based motion reduction techniques for coronary MRA: (1) kinematics and imaging effects of respiration; (2) navigator echo techniques for monitoring motion; and (3) motion reduction techniques for coronary MRA.

Kinematics of Respiration and Imaging Effects of Respiration

Kinematics of Respiration

The effects of respiration on cardiac position can be measured by imaging the diastolic heart at various positions of tidal respiration with a breathhold magnetization prepared segmented fast gradient echo technique (34). The cranial–caudal (superior–inferior, SI) motion of the heart due to respiration is the dominant component of motion. The SI motion range is six to eight times that of the anterior–posterior (AP) motion (Fig. 17.1b). The SI motion of the heart is linearly correlated to the SI motion of the diaphragm (Fig. 17.1). Motion variation across the heart is three times smaller than the motion at the inferior margin. The respiratory motion of the heart is primarily a monotonic linear translation within the tidal breathing range.

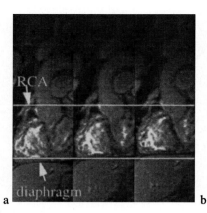

anatomy	coordinate	range(mm)	SI/AP
heart IM	SI	18.1 ± 9.1	10.3 ±9.1
AM	AP	2.4 ± 1.5	
apex	SI	16.0 ±7.1	10.6 ±7.7
	AP	3.0 ± 2.8	
RCA root	SI	10.5 ± 4.8	6.2 ±3.6
	AP	2.3 ± 1.4	
LAD	SI	13.1 ± 4.1	8.2 ± 4.1
	AP	2.0 ± 0.7	

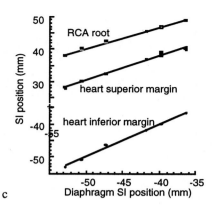

Figure 17.1. Respiration kinematics. (a) An RCA section of the heart at three different respiration levels: inspiration (left), middle, and expiration (right). (b) Comparison of SI versus AP displacements over 10 subjects: SI/AP ~ 10. Notation for the table: IM = inferior margin, AM = anterior margin, mean ± standard deviation. (c) Linear regression between the SI positions of cardiac landmarks and the diaphragm at different respiration levels.

The respiratory motion ranges measured in this kinematics manner are in agreement with those measured with other real-time techniques such as real-time MR line scan (35), ultrasound (36), cineangiography, and nuclear medicine (37).

Respiratory Motion Effects on Imaging

Respiratory kinematics define the physical environment for developing motion reduction techniques for reducing respiration effects in coronary MRA. Effects of respiration in MRI can be sorted as ghosting (structure repetition) and blurring (loss of image sharpness or resolution). The dominant effects of respiration in 3-D coronary MRA is blurring: The achievable minimal full width at half maximum (FWHM) of coronary vessels is 3–4 m under tidal breathing (8). These motion effects significantly limit the depiction of coronary arteries.

The motion range is an important determinant for the degree of motion blurring in MRI (8,34). Because the SI motion is the dominant component of respiration (Fig. 17.1b), the effects of respiratory motion in coronary MRA can be decomposed into the first order effects (o(1)) due to the principal SI displacement, and the second-order effects (o(ϵ), $\epsilon \sim$ SI/AP $\sim$ 0.1) due to AP and right-left (RL) displacements, dilation (D), rotation (R), phase effects of stationary inhomogeneous background susceptibility (S), and cardiac twisting contraction (T):

$$\text{Motion Effects} = o(1)[\text{ SI }]$$
$$+ o(\epsilon) \ [\text{AP} + \text{RL} + \text{D} + \text{R} + \text{S} + \text{T}]. \quad (17.1)$$

Navigator Echo Techniques for Monitoring Motion

Because respiration cannot be modeled accurately, effective reduction of respiration effects in MRI requires monitoring of respiration. Beltlike devices have been used widely to monitor respiration in MRI for respiratory-gating and phase-ordering schemes (38–41). Measurements of the circumference of the trunk are unfortunately only loosely and indirectly related to the actual motion of visceral structures in the abdomen and thorax. The respiratory motion of most structures near the diaphragm is predominantly in the SI direction (34–37). The use of navigator echoes that are processed in real-time provides a direct method for monitoring such motion (19,20,42). Navigator-based methods have been shown to be applicable to respiratory-gating techniques (12,29,31,42).

Pencil-Beam Navigator Echo

Spin-echo (SE) techniques have been used initially to acquire navigator echoes. SE navigator echo acquisitions, however, may alter the magnetization of the object being monitored, which is not desirable for fast image acquisition. Gradient-recalled echo (GRE) techniques are more suitable for monitoring purposes (43–46) because a small flip angle can be used, which only causes small perturbation to the magnetization. For the purpose of reducing the first-order motion effects, navigator pulse based on 2-D radiofrequency (RF) excitation can be used to acquire a longitudinal cylinder of tissue through the left-posterior part of the diaphragm (Fig. 17.2). The superior-inferior (SI) respiratory motion of the heart is estimated from the SI motion of the diaphragm. This beam navigator provides good detection of the change in the SI position of the diaphragm because the principally anterior-posterior (AP) oriented motion of the chest wall and the upper abdominal wall is excluded from the beam navigator region. (*Note*: Square beams of tissue can also be acquired using SE navigator echoes with perpendicular slice selection gradients for the 90 and 180 RF pulses.)

Figure 17.2. Acquisition of the beam navigator echo. The navigator echo is acquired from a longitudinal cylinder of tissue through the left-posterior part of the diaphragm (Fig. 17.1a), using a 2-D excitation pulse (Fig. 17.1b).

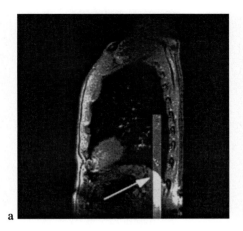

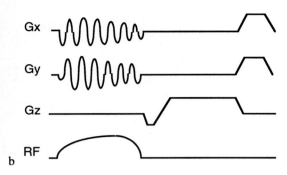

Least Squares Algorithm for Motion Detection

Algorithms to extract motion information reliably from navigator echoes are crucial to motion reduction techniques. Three algorithms have been reported for processing motion information from the navigator echo signals: edge-detection (46,47), correlation (20,42), and least-squares (48)–based methods. The edge-detection algorithm selects one edge of a navigator profile as the reference feature for determination of movement. When there is no well-defined edge in the navigator profile, the algorithm cannot be implemented to extract motion information reliably. The correlation algorithm computes the correlation between a shifted current navigator echo and a reference echo. The displacement is determined by locating the shift position that gives the maximum correlation. The least squares algorithm computes the variance for a shifted current navigator echo with respect to a reference echo and determines the displacement by locating the shift position that gives the minimum variance. The minimum variance used by the least squares algorithm corresponds to the maximum likelihood estimation of the match between the shifted current navigator echo and the reference echo (49).

The accuracy of the motion detection can be affected by noise and profile deformation of the navigator echoes. Noise always exists within the MR signal. A motion estimation algorithm should minimize noise propagation. In addition to a global displacement of the mass center of a structure in the image physiologic motion can cause local change in the structure itself (profile deformation). This, too, can cause error in the estimation of the global displacement of the structure. Studies using computer simulation and in vivo imaging experiments demonstrated that the least squares algorithm is more resistant to the effects of noise and motion-induced profile-deformation than the correlation algorithm and that the least squares algorithm provides motion information with error < 0.5 pixel in practice (50) (Fig. 17.3).

Orbital Navigator Echo

For reducing the second order motion effects, it is necessary to detect rotation in addition to translation in all directions. Orbital navigator echoes can be used to achieve this goal (51). Data points in an orbital navigator echo describe a circle in 2-D k-space and permit simultaneous measurement of in-plane rotation and translation (Fig. 17.4a). An object $f(x)$ after in-plane motion is

$$f'(x) = f(R(x - t)), \qquad (17.2)$$

where R is the orthogonal rotation matrix and t is the translation vector. The corresponding representation of the motion effect (Eq. 17.2) in the Fourier space ($F(k) = \int dx\, f(x) \cdot e^{ikx}$) is

$$F'(k) = e^{ikt} \cdot F(Rk). \qquad (17.3)$$

Figure 17.3. Algorithms for extracting motion information from navigator echoes. Errors in both the correlation (corr) and least squares (ls) algorithms versus (a) signal-to-noise ratios (SNR) and (b) signal-to-deformation ratios (SDR) indicate that least square algorithm is more accurate than correlation. Noise and deformation encountered in practice are indicated by the gray areas.

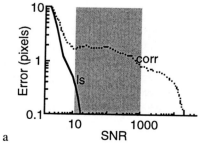

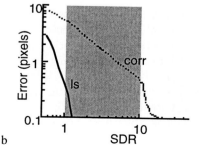

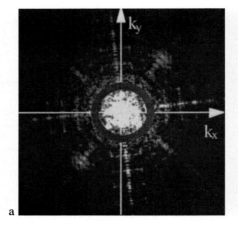 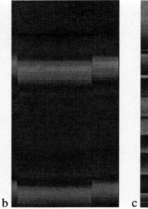 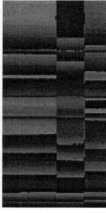

Figure 17.4. Orbital navigator echo. (a) Navigator orbit in *k*-space (gray circle). (b) Magnitude records of orbital navigator echoes acquired from a resolution phantom that was rotated three times during scanning. The horizontal axis is time. The vertical axis is the azimuth angle (0, 2p) of the navigator orbit in *k*-space. The rotation angle is the profile shift in the navigator record. (c) Phase records of orbital navigator echoes acquired from a resolution phantom that was displaced twice during scanning. The displacement can be derived from the phase changes in the record.

Based on Eq. 17.3, rotation can be determined from the shift in the magnitude profile of the orbital echo with respect to a reference orbital echo using a least squares algorithm (Fig. 17.4b), and displacements can be calculated from the phase difference between the current echo and a rotated reference echo (Fig. 17.4c):

$$\Delta\Psi(\theta) = kt = k_\rho(t_x \cos\theta + t_y \sin\theta),$$

$$t_x = \frac{1}{\pi k_\rho}\int_0^{2\pi}\Delta\Psi(\theta)\cos\theta d\theta,$$

$$t_y = \frac{1}{\pi k_\rho}\int_0^{2\pi}\Delta\Psi(\theta)\sin\theta d\theta. \quad (17.4)$$

Orbital navigator echoes, therefore, can be used to measure simultaneously both rotation and translation components of motion.

Motion Reduction Techniques for Coronary MRA

Real-Time versus Postprocessing

The general strategy to reduce motion effects is to modify data acquisition using motion information derived from navigator echoes. Data acquisition can be modified in real-time (prospectively) or postprocessing (retrospectively). Real-time modification requires use of real-time communication and processing hardware (12). Postprocessing is typically performed on data acquired with a fixed scan time or signal averages (15). Real-time and postprocessing techniques can be combined together to address different components of motion.

The effectiveness of motion reduction can be mea-sured by the range of residual motion. In real-time modification of data acquisition, the residual motion range can be controlled effectively by the targeted specification at the price of scan time. In postprocessing modification of data acquisition, there is no mechanism to control the residual motion range and data points may be missing or containing large motion effects (11,13,15,51). Modifying data acquisition in real-time is accordingly more effective than in real-time modification.

Triggering, Gating, and Correction

The commonly used modifications on data acquisition are triggering, gating, and correction. In triggering, data acquisition is enabled or data is accepted for a fixed duration when a motion parameter rises to a reference level (Fig. 17.5a). EKG triggering and respiratory bellow triggering are the commonly used triggering techniques. The widely used breathholding can be considered as a triggering technique (12,46). Triggering can reduce the motion range, but its effectiveness is limited because motion occurring during data acquisition will contaminate images (Fig. 17.5a). Two reference levels are used in gating (Fig. 17.5b). Data acquisition is enabled or data is accepted only when the motion parameter is within the range specified by the two reference levels (12,29,38,39,42). Gating is accordingly more effective than triggering (at the price of scan time). In correction, a model relating motion parameters and image effects (e.g., Eq. 17.3) is used to correct the image effects corresponding to the measured motion (20). Correction can further reduce the residual motion within the gating window (52).

Up to now, all efforts have been in reducing the dom-

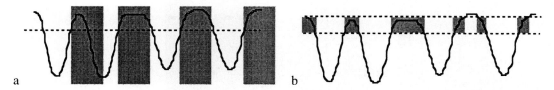

Figure 17.5. (a) Triggering and (b) gating. Gray areas represent data accepted or data acquisition enabled.

inant first-order motion effects in Eq. 17.1 in coronary MRA. We will review a variety of techniques to achieve this goal: (1) multiple breathhold acquisition using a real-time respiratory feedback monitor, (2) real-time navigator-gated acquisition, and (3) adaptive correction for residual motion in gated acquisition.

Multiple Breathhold Acquisition Using Real-Time Respiratory Feedback Monitor

It typically takes multiple breathholds to complete acquisition of a coronary tree with adequate spatial resolution and signal-to-noise ratio. Consistency in the breathholding position (i.e., returning the heart to the same position at each breathhold) is necessary to prevent image artifacts. Without any feedback signal to aid breathholding, the position of the coronary arteries may vary as much as 8 mm among different breathholds (Fig. 17.6). A navigator echo signal from the diaphragm can be used to reduce the variation in the coronary position among different breathholds to about 1 mm (9,10,46). Multiple breathhold acquisitions using a respiratory feedback monitor can provide significant reduction in motion effects (Fig. 17.7).

Real-Time Navigator-Gated Acquisition

Breathholding can be difficult for patients to perform. Failures to suspend respiration during data acquisition degrade breathhold images. Real-time navigator gating overcomes these limitations by monitoring motion during data acquisition and accepting data only when motion is at the desired level (12,42). Figure 17.8a illustrates one implementation of real-time navigator gating in

coronary MRA (12). The pencil-beam navigator echoes are acquired immediately before and after the image data readout train in every cardiac cycle. The SI positions of the diaphragm were extracted from the two navigator echoes in real-time (< 5 msec) to control data acquisition: When both positions are within the gating window, image data collected between the navigator echoes are accepted and image data acquisition is advanced to the next segment of k-space. Image data are otherwise rejected and the same segment of k-space is reacquired in the next heartbeat. Such an implementation rejects data if motion occurs during the image data acquisition period. Such a real-time navigator gating (at a gating window of 3 mm SI range of the diaphragm) provides significant reduction of respiration effects (Figs. 17.8b vs. 17.8c).

Adaptive Correction of Residual Motion Effects in Real-Time Navigator-Gated Acquisition

Effective real-time navigator gating requires a narrow gating window, but this implies undesirable increase in scan time. To shorten scan time, one method is to use modified respiration with brief pauses at the gating window and respiratory feedback (bottom of Fig. 17.8a). This method, however, required active participation from patients, which might be difficult for certain patients. A more promising approach is to use a wide gating window to increase the data acceptance rate (thus reduce scan time) and to correct the residual displacements within the wide gating window (Fig. 17.9):

$$F_c(k) = F(k) \cdot \exp\left[-ik \cdot t\right] \qquad (17.5)$$

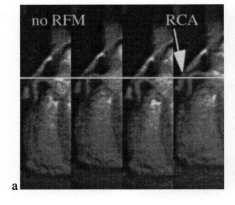
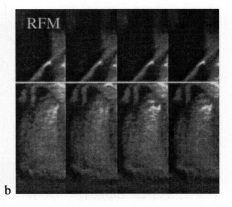

Figure 17.6. Respiratory feedback monitor (RFM). The range of variation in the SI position of the right coronary artery (RCA) imaged in four different breathholds is reduced from 5.6 mm in (a) without using RFM to approximately zero in (b) using RFM.

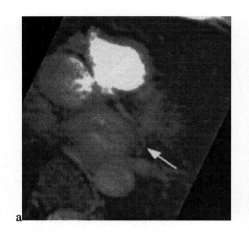
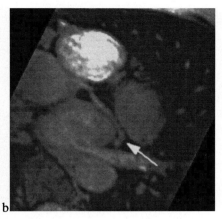

Figure 17.7. Navigator-echo-guided multiple breathhold 3-D acquisition. Image blurring is substantially reduced from (a) two-signal averaged under tidal breathing to (b) multiple breathhold 3-D acquisition. Images were reformatted to show the proximal Cx (arrows).

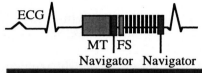

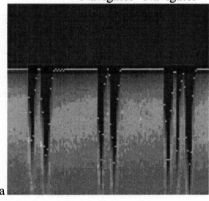
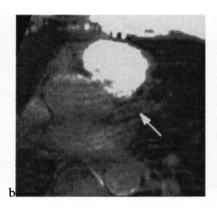
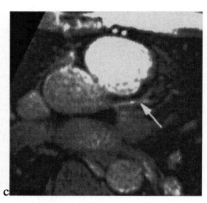

Figure 17.8. Real-time navigator gating. (a, top) Two navigator echoes are acquired before and after the readout train in each heartbeat. (a, bottom) Record of pencil-beam navigator echoes acquired through the diaphragm (Fig. 17.3). The horizontal axis is time, and upward is the superior direction (to the lung). If the diaphragm positions from both navigator echoes (shown as white dots near the diaphragm edge) are within the gating window (indicated as the dark band), image data are accepted and acquisition is advanced; otherwise, image data are rejected and reacquired in the next heartbeat. Respiration here is modified with a brief pause in the gating window (near normal end-expiration) to shorten the scan time. Motion effects (ghosting and blurring) are substantially reduced from (b) acquired continuously under tidal breathing to (c) real-time navigator gated. Images are reformatted to show the proximal left anterior descending (LAD) (arrows).

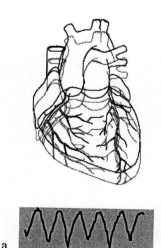
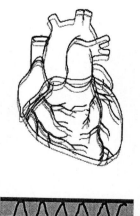
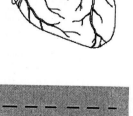

Figure 17.9. (a) The full range of quiet breathing. (b) The range of residual motion (light band) in image data acquired with real-time gating, where motion effects in image data can be approximately described by Eq. (17.2). (c) Image sharpness improvement by adaptive correction of residual motion in the gating window.

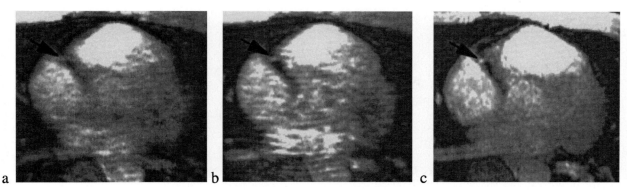

a   b   c

Figure 17.10. Adaptive motion correction (AMC). The sharpness of the RCA (arrow) is substantially increased from (a) acquisition using 8.4-mm gating window to (b) same acquisition processed with AMC at a scaling factor of 0.4, and become comparable to (c) acquired with a 3-mm gating window. Images are axial sections at same location from 3-D image set. Note AMC also introduced chest wall ghosting, which does not interfere depiction of the RCA here.

Adaptive correction for the first-order motion effects in Eq. (17.1) caused by the dominant SI displacement t_{SI} was implemented (52). It was found that such a combination of real-time navigation gating and adaptive motion correction can reduce motion effects without the need for extensive patient cooperation and without an undesirable increase in scan time (Fig. 17.10).

Summary and Discussion

Motion reduction techniques for coronary MRA are summarized in Fig. 17.11, according to their effectiveness, scan time, and patient compliance. For reference, the residual motion range ($\sim$ 10 mm) in acquisitions without motion reduction (nmr in Fig. 17.11) and in acquisitions with two signal averages (2sa in Fig. 17.11) are indicated. The size of a coronary artery stenosis ($\sim$ 1 mm) is also depicted, which is the spatial resolution goal of coronary MRA using our proposed motion reduction techniques (proposed mrt in Fig. 17.11).

- Multiple breathhold acquisitions (bh & bh+fb in Fig. 17.11) are very demanding on patients and require respiratory feedback to minimize breathhold inconsistency.
- Real-time navigator-gated acquisitions at a narrow gating window (gn & gn+fb in Fig. 17.11) might undesirably prolong scan time. Use of respiratory feedback reduces scan time but requires active participation from patients.
- Real-time navigator-gated acquisitions at a wide gating window (gw & gw+amc1 in Fig. 17.11) window and adaptive motion correction provides the shortest scan time and highest patient compliance. The first-order motion effects (Eq. 17.1), however, remain in all these techniques.
- Further development of motion reduction techniques is required for coronary MRA in order to reduce the residual motion to a range comparable with the size of coronary stenosis (future mrt in Fig. 17.11), which would be adequate for depiction stenosis. This might require more effective reduction of the first-order

Figure 17.11. Motion reduction techniques and their scan time, patient compliance, and residual motion range within image data (black bar height). Notation: ·nmr: no motion reduction; 2sa: two signal averaging; gw: gating with a wide window; amc1: first order AMC; mrt: motion reduction techniques; gn: gating with a narrow window; fb: feedback; bh: breathhold. Techniques in the middle of the graph (bh, bh+fb, gn+fb, gw, gw+amc1) have approximately the same scan time as that of two signal averaging (2sa).

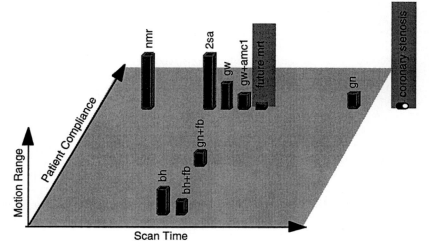

effects and correction of the second-order motion effects in Eq. (17.1).

References

1. Edelman RR, Manning WJ, Burstein D, Paulin S. Coronary arteries: breath-hold MR angiography. Radiology 1991; 181:641–43.
2. Meyer CH, Hu BS, Nishimura DG, Macovski A. Fast spiral coronary artery imaging. Magn Reson Med 1992;28: 202–13.
3. Li D, Paschal CB, Haacke EM, Adler LP. Coronary arteries: three-dimensional MR imaging with fat saturation and magnetization transfer contrast. Radiology 1993;187:401–6.
4. Manning WJ, Li W, Edelman RR. A preliminary report comparing magnetic resonance coronary angiography with conventional angiography. N Engl J Med 1993;328:828–32.
5. Pennell DJ, Keegan J, Firmin DN, Gatehouse PD, Underwood SR, Longmore DB. Magnetic resonance imaging of coronary arteries: technique and preliminary results. Br Heart J 1993;70(4):315–26.
6. Paschal CB, Haacke EM, Adler LP. 3D MRI of the coronary arteries: preliminary clinical experience. J Magn Reson Imag 1993;3:491–500.
7. Duerinckx AJ, Urman MK. Two-dimensional coronary MR angiography: analysis of initial clinical results. Radiology 1994;193:731–38.
8. Wang Y, Grist TM, Korosec FR, Christy PS, Alley MT, Polzin JA, et al. Respiratory motion blurring in 3D coronary MR imaging. Magn Reson Med 1995;33:541–48.
9. Wang Y, Christy PS, Korosec FR, Alley MT, Grist TM, Polzin JA, et al. Coronary MRI with a respiratory feedback monitor: the 2D case. Magn Reson Med 1995;33:116–21.
10. Wang Y, Grimm RC, Rossman PJ, Debbins JP, Riederer SJ, Ehman RL. Coronary MR angiography in multiple breath-holds using a respiratory feedback monitor. Magn Reson Med 1995;34:11–16.
11. Hofman MBM, Paschal CB, Li D, Haacke EM, van Rossum AC, Sprenger M. MRI of coronary arteries, 2D breath-hold vs 3D respiratory gated acquisition. J Comput Assist Tomogr 1995;19:56–62.
12. Wang Y, Rossman PJ, Grimm RC, Riederer SJ, Ehman RL. Navigator-echo-based real-time respiratory gating and triggering for reduction of respiration effects in three-dimensional coronary MR angiography. Radiology 1996; 198:55–60.
13. Post JC, van Rossum AC, Hofman MBM, Valk J, Visser CA. Three-dimensional respiratory-gated MR angiography of coronary arteries: comparison with conventional coronary angiography. Am J Roentgenol 1996;166:1399–404.
14. Oshinski JN, Hofland L, Mukundan S, Dixon WT, Parks WJ, Pettigrew RI. Two-dimensional coronary MR angiography without breath-holding. Radiology 1996;201:737–44.
15. Li D, Kaushikkar S, Haacke EM, Woodard PK, Dhawale PJ, Kroeker RM, et al. Coronary arteries: three-dimensional MR imaging with retrospective respiratory gating. Radiology 1996;201:857–63.
16. McConnell MV, Khasgiwala VC, Savord BJ, Chen MH, Chuang ML, Edelman RR, Manning WJ. Prospective adaptive navigator correction for breath-hold MR coronary angiography. Magn Reson Med 1997;37:148–52.
17. Babcock HW. The possibility of compensating astronomical seeing. Publ Astron Soc Pac 1953;65:229.
18. Thompson LA. Adaptive optics in astronomy. Phys Today 1994;27(12):24–31.
19. Hinks RS. Monitored echo gating (mega) for the reduction of motion artifacts. Proceedings of the Sixth Meeting of the Society of Magnetic Resonance Imaging, 1988:48.
20. Ehman RL, Felmlee JP. Adaptive technique for high-definition MRI of moving structures. Radiology 1989;173: 255–63.
21. Anderson AW, Gore JC. Analysis and correction of motion artifacts in diffusion weighted imaging. Magn Reson Med 1994;32:379–387.
22. Ordidge RJ, Helpern JA, et al. Correction of motional artifacts in diffusion-weighted MR images using navigator echoes. Magn Reson Imag 1994;12:455–60.
23. de Crespigny A, Marks M, et al. Navigated diffusion imaging of normal and ischemic human brain. Magn Reson Med 1995;33:720–28.
24. Butts K, de Crespingy A, et al. Diffusion-weighted interleaved echo-planer imaging with a pair of orthogonal navigator echoes. Magn Reson Med 1996;35:763–70.
26. Hu X, Kim S. Reduction of signal fluctuation in functional MRI using navigator echoes. Magn Reson Med 1994;31: 495–503.
27. Jiang A, Kennedy D, et al. Motion detection and correction in functional MRI. Proceedings of the Second Meeting of the Society of Magnetic Resonance Imaging, 1994: 351.
28. Lee CC, Grimm RC, et al. Real-time adaptive motion correction in fMRI. Proceedings of the Fourth Meeting of International Society of Magnetic Resonance in Medicine, 1996:342.
29. Sachs TS, Meyer CH, Irarrazabal P, Hu BS, Nishimura DG, Macovski A. The diminishing variance algorithm for real-time reduction of motion artifacts in MRI. Magn Reson Med 1995;34:412–22.
30. Wilman AH, Riederer SJ, Grimm RC, Rossman PJ, Wang Y, King BF, et al. Multiple breathhold 3D TOF MR angiography of the renal arteries. Magn Reson Med 1996; 35:426–34.
31. Wang Y, Rossman PJ, Grimm RC, Wilman AH, Riederer SJ, Ehman RL. 3D MR angiography of pulmonary arteries using real-time navigator gating and magnetization preparation. Magn Reson Med 1996;36:579–87.
32. Schmidt MA, Yang GZ, et al. Lung MRI with real-time navigation and feedback. Proceedings of the Fourth Meeting of International Society of Magnetic Resonance in Medicine, 1996:17.
33. Tyszka JM, Silverman JM. Navigated short echo time ^{1}H MRS of moving objects. Proceedings of the Fourth Meeting of International Society of Magnetic Resonance in Medicine, 1996:375.
34. Wang Y, Riederer SJ, Ehman RL. Respiratory motion of the heart: kinematics and the implications for the spatial resolution of coronary MR imaging. Magn Reson Med 1995;33:713–19.
35. Korin HW, Ehman RL, Riederer SJ, Felmlee JP, Grimm RC. Respiratory kinematics of the upper abdominal organs: a quantitative study. Magn Reson Med 1992;23:172–78.
36. Suramo I, Paivansalo M, Myllyla V. Cranio-caudal move-

ments of the liver, pancreas and kidneys in respiration. Acta Radiol Diagn 1984;25:129–31.

37. Harauz G, Bronskill MJ. Comparison of the liver's respiratory motion in supine and upright positions: concise communication. J Nucl Med 1979;20:733–35.

38. Runge VM, Clanton JA, Partain CL, James AE. Respiratory gating in magnetic resonance imaging at 0.5 Tesla. Radiology 1984;151:521–23.

39. Ehman RL, McNamara MT, Pallack M, Hricak H, Higgins CB. Magnetic resonance imaging with respiratory gating: techniques and advantages. Am J Roentgenol 1984;143:1175–82.

40. Bailes DR, Gilderdale DJ, Bydder GM, Collins AG, Firmin DN. Respiratory ordered phase encoding (ROPE): a method of reducing respiratory motion artifacts in MR imaging. J Comput Assist Tomogr 1985;9:835–38.

41. MacFall JR, Dahlke J. Respiratory triggering circuit and application to 3D pulmonary angiography and abdominal fast spin echo MR imaging. In: Proceedings of the Society of Magnetic Resonance in Medicine, Twelfth Annual Meeting, New York, 1993:574.

42. Sachs TS, Meyer CH, Hu BS, Kohli J, Nishimura DG, Macovski A. Real-time motion detection in spiral MRI using navigators. Magn Reson Med 1994;32:639–45.

43. Pauly J, Le Roux P, Nishimura D, Macovski A. Parameter relations for the Shinnar-Le Roux selective excitation pulse design algorithm. IEEE Trans Med Imag 1991;10:53–65.

44. Pauly J, Nishimura D, Macovski A. A k-space analysis of small-tip-angle excitation. J Magn Reson 1989;81:43–56.

45. Hardy CJ, Cline HE. Broadband nuclear magnetic resonance pulses with two-dimensional spatial selectivity. J Appl Phys 1989;66:1513–16.

46. Liu Y, Riederer SJ, Rossman PJ, Grimm RC, Debbins JP, Ehman RL. A monitoring, feedback, and triggering system for reproducible breath-hold MR imaging. Magn Reson Med 1993;30:507–11.

47. Felmlee JP, Ehman RL, Riederer SJ, Korin HW. Adaptive motion compensation in MR imaging without use of navigator echoes. Radiology 1991;179:139–42.

48. Felmlee JP, Korin HW, Ehman RL, Riederer SJ. Adaptive motion correction of high-resolution spine images with navigator echoes (abstr.). Radiology 1991;181(P): 237.

49. Bronshtein IN, Semendyayev KA. Handbook of Mathematics, Third Edition. New York: Van Nostrand Reinhold, 1985:635.

50. Wang Y, Grimm RC, Riederer SJ, Ehman RL. Algorithms to extract motion information from navigator echoes. Magn Reson Med 1996;36:117–23.

51. Fu ZW, Wang Y, Grimm RC, Rossman PJ, Felmlee JP, Riederer SJ, et al. Orbital navigator echoes for motion measurements in MRI. Magn Reson Med 1995;34:746–53.

52. Wang Y, Riederer SJ, Ehman RL. Adaptive motion correction for real-time navigator gated coronary MR angiography. Proceedings of the Fourth Meeting of International Society of Magnetic Resonance in Medicine, 1996:175.

18

Coronary MRA Techniques Without Breathholding

Debiao Li, Mark B.M. Hofman, Christine H. Lorenz, and E. Mark Haacke

Introduction

Noninvasive visualization of coronary arteries using magnetic resonance imaging (MRI) is a challenging task. A number of factors have hindered its progress, including the motion of the heart during cardiac and respiratory cycles, the highly tortuous course and the small size of coronary arteries, and the adjacency of coronary arteries to epicardial fatty tissues, atrial appendages, coronary veins, and major blood pools. The spatial displacement of coronary arteries during each heartbeat and respiratory cycle is on the order of several centimeters. The proximal coronary arteries have calibers in the range of 2–4 mm and rarely exceed 5 mm in normal humans (1,2). Distal portions of coronary arteries and branch vessels are even smaller. As a result, the visualization of coronary arteries requires elimination or significant reduction of motion effects during cardiac and respiratory cycles and high-resolution volumetric coverage of the region of interest. Because of the technical difficulties (both in hardware and software) of achieving these capabilities, early efforts of visualizing coronary arteries using conventional spin-echo (SE) and gradient-recalled echo (GRE) cine techniques have had only marginal success (3–7).

A major limiting factor in the visualization of coronary arteries using MRI is image degradation from motion of the heart and coronary arteries. Motion artifacts include image ghosts, blurs, and signal loss. The sources of motion that affect heart and coronary arteries include bulk translations secondary to respiratory motion, motion due to contraction and relaxation of the heart muscle, and spurious patient motion. To reduce the effect of heart motion during the cardiac cycle, the execution of the imaging sequence is synchronized with the heartbeat by emitting a trigger signal from the R-wave of the electrocardiographic (EKG) signal. Certain delay time from the trigger signal is allowed to ensure that data are collected during middiastole, when heart has the least motion. This effectively freezes the heart motion, provided that the heart returns to the same position for each heartbeat, and the data acquisition window is short compared with the duration of diastole.

A major breakthrough in coronary MRI came with the ability to acquire a segment of the k-space data (a few phase-encoding lines or a spiral interleave), rather than a single phase-encoding line, within each heartbeat (8–10). Segmented data acquisition permitted a two-dimensional (2-D) gradient-echo image to be acquired within a single breathhold, eliminating the respiratory motion effects. Another important technical advancement was improved magnetic field homogeneity, which permits the consistent suppression of signals from epicardial fat that surrounds proximal portions of coronary arteries and their major branches (1,8,11). Fatty tissue has a shorter T1 than muscle and blood, and tends to have a much larger signal than blood in coronary arteries with a T1-weighted gradient-echo sequence. With adequate fat saturation and the ability to collect images within a single breathhold, proximal portions of coronary arteries have consistently been visualized in cooperative healthy subjects.

Initial clinical trials with the 2-D segmented technique have been promising (12–14); however, several problems exist with 2-D imaging that decreased its clinical utility. First, only one slice was collected within a single breathhold on conventional imaging systems. Since the coronary arteries are highly tortuous, multiple breathholds are needed to cover a vessel. Misregistration of slices caused by inconsistent breathhold positions may make image interpretation difficult. Second, experience is needed for the operator to set up the 2-D image plane orientation because the long axis of the vessel needs to be in the image plane, making the 2-D technique somewhat operator dependent. Finally, many patients may have difficulty holding their breath with adequate duration and consistency to enable collection of images of diagnostic value. Modifications to the 2-D imaging approach have been made in both data acquisition and image processing (15–17) in an attempt to overcome these problems; however, limitations remain.

Three-dimensional (3-D) data acquisition methods have also been used to image coronary arteries (2,11,18–35). In principle, 3-D imaging can overcome many of the problems associated with 2-D methods. The advantages of 3-D imaging include the acquisition of thin and contiguous slices so that image processing can be performed, a high signal-to-noise ratio, and less operator dependence compared with 2-D imaging because the orientation of the imaging volume is less critical and can be just orthogonal. For multislice 2-D imaging, the acquisition time of each separate slice fits in a single breathhold period. For conventional 3-D gradient-echo imaging, there is one total acquisition time for the whole volume which is relatively long, and it is not feasible for patients to hold their breath during the entire acquisition. Although a 3-D segmented echo-planar data acquisition can be collected with a single breathhold (27), this approach requires special hardware that is still not available at most clinical sites. Furthermore, the clinical utility of these 3-D echo-planar imaging of coronary arteries remains to be determined because of its relatively low signal-to-noise ratio and resolution.

There is a strong need, therefore, for alternatives to the breathhold approach to reduce respiratory motion effects for visualizing coronary arteries. These alternatives are necessary for a 3-D acquisition to be collected with relatively high resolution. In addition, it is desirable to eliminate the need for breathhold even for 2-D imaging, avoiding the problem of misregistration between adjacent slices that may exist in breathhold imaging. Nonbreathhold approaches will also remove the limit on imaging time, allowing for the acquisition of high-resolution images, and make coronary MRI more patient friendly.

In this chapter, we will review commonly used methods of compensating respiratory motion effects without breathholding and show applications of these techniques for MRI of coronary arteries. A retrospective respiratory gating approach in conjunction with 3-D imaging will then be discussed in greater detail.

Different Approaches of Respiratory Motion Compensation Without Breathhold

Motion Artifacts

In MRI there are more motion artifacts than just blurring of the moving object itself. This is due to the fact that in MRI the raw data in k-space is the Fourier trans-

form of the image. After data collection, the actual image is obtained by performing the inverse Fourier transform to the raw data. This process dictates that the object to be imaged needs to remain constant during the entire imaging process. If this condition is not satisfied (i.e., if the structure to be imaged changes position from the time that one part of k-space is acquired to the time that another part of k-space is acquired) this structure will not be reconstructed correctly, and image artifacts will occur. For periodic physiological motion (e.g., heartbeat and respiration) the image artifacts include image blurs as expected. They also appear as image ghosts, which are periodic replicas of the moving anatomical structures superimposed on nonmoving structures. In 2-D and 3-D Fourier transform imaging, the frequency encoding is obtained quickly compared with physiological motion (heartbeat and respiration); therefore, no obvious motion artifacts will occur in this direction. In the remaining directions, however, where phase encoding is performed, this ghosting artifact will occur when the object moves during data acquisition.

Techniques that compensate for respiratory motion can be separated into two groups. In the first group, techniques such as respiratory-ordered phase encoding and pseudogating will remove or reduce the effect of ghosting, but will not remove image blur, or loss of resolution. In the second group, the respiratory-gating techniques limit both ghosting and blurring. Respiratory gating techniques, therefore, are of greater importance and will be discussed more thoroughly.

Respiratory-Ordered Phase Encoding

Ghosting artifacts are caused by the periodicity of tissue motion. These artifacts can be eliminated by destroying the periodicity of motion in data collection. This can be accomplished by ordering the acquisition of phase-encoding lines to match the amplitude of the respiratory motion. This method is referred to as respiratory-ordered phase encoding (ROPE) (36,37). If the moving structure is not within the region of interest and the goal is to remove the interference of the ghosts with the stationary tissue, or if a simple loss of resolution in the moving structure is acceptable, the ROPE technique will help improve image quality.

Because the ROPE technique does not remove image blur caused by respiratory motion of coronary arteries, this technique itself is not sufficient for motion reduction in MR coronary angiography. The same basic principle, however, is used to limit ghosting effects induced by cardiac motion when multiple phase-encoding steps are collected within one cardiac cycle. These phase-encoding steps are arranged such that the periodic variations of phase in k-space are eliminated in a technique referred to as the segmented k-space acquisition (8,9, 38,39).

Pseudorespiratory Gating and Signal Averaging

A pseudogating approach (40) has also been used to remove ghosting artifacts. The principle of pseudogating is that each phase-encoding step is repeated N times consecutively during the period of motion and data are averaged to eliminate periodicity. No motion signal is needed here. If the motion is strictly periodic, then the resultant image will be a sum of N images, with each collected at a different time of the motion cycle. The image will be blurred, resulting in a loss of resolution in regions of motion. Nevertheless, there will be no replicas of moving objects in the image and the stationary tissue will be reconstructed correctly, with a $\sqrt{N}$ gain in signal-to-noise (SNR) ratio over a single data acquisition (e.g., with the ROPE technique). On the other hand, the imaging time is also prolonged by a factor of N.

In practice, a subject's respiration may not be consistent. Nevertheless, data averaging is still effective in eliminating major ghosting artifacts. For coronary artery imaging using a 3-D gradient-echo sequence (11), the 3-D partition encoding loop corresponding to each in-plane phase-encoding step is collected during one cardiac cycle. If the collection of each in-plane phase-encoding step is repeated four to five times consecutively within a single breathing cycle (approximately four to five heartbeats), data averaging will then eliminate most image ghosts of cardiac structures that would otherwise blur the depiction of coronary arteries.

Examples of coronary artery visualization with pseudorespiratory gating are shown in Figures 18.1 and 18.2. The coronary arteries have been consistently visualized using a 3-D gradient-echo sequence with this technique (11,19,20). In an anecdotal case, a significant stenosis in the proximal left anterior descending (LAD) coronary artery was detected (Fig. 18.3). The vessel boundary blur, however, limited the utility of the technique for consistently detecting coronary artery stenoses. Nevertheless, these initial results provided important initial evidence that it is feasible to visualize coronary arteries consistently using a 3-D technique without breathhold. This technique was found useful in visualizing complicated anatomical structures in the thorax and in detecting congenital heart diseases and great vessel diseases (21).

Techniques for Respiratory Gating

Basic Principles of Respiratory Gating

Similar to EKG-triggering where data acquisition is synchronized to the heartbeat, respiratory signal can also

A

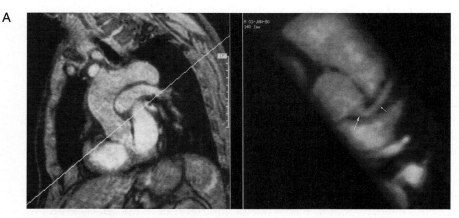

B

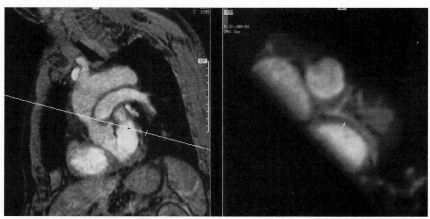

Figure 18.1. Coronary artery depiction with a 3-D gradient-echo sequence using signal averaging (pseudogating) to reduce ghosting artifacts caused by respiratory motion. The images on the left side of both (A) and (B) are individual partition images of a 3-D data set. The images on the right were created by multiplanar reconstruction (MPR) depicting the left main (long arrow in A), left anterior descending (short arrow in A), and the left circumflex (arrow in B) coronary arteries. The original data set was collected by averaging four signals. No apparent image ghosts are visible in the images; however, the delineation of the coronary arteries are blurred. (Reprinted with permission from Li et al. (11).)

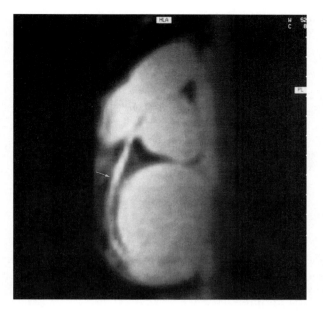

Figure 18.2. An MPR image generated from a 3-D data set acquired with the same sequence as in Figure 18.1. The right coronary artery (RCA) (arrow) is clearly visualized; however, image blur remains.

be used to control the timing of data acquisition or to select data used for image reconstruction. The basic principle of respiratory gating is that data are used for image reconstruction only when the respiration falls within a certain range, the gate window, as illustrated in Figure 18.4. Respiratory gating, therefore, will lengthen the total imaging time because effectively no data are collected during the remaining part of the respiratory cycle. In general, motion artifacts are reduced more with a narrower gate window, but this also results in longer imaging time. Thus, it is important to collect

data around the most consistent respiratory position. This position is usually at the relaxed state at the end of expiration. In principle, if the heart returns to exactly the same position during each respiratory cycle, the respiration can be frozen and reconstructed images will be free of respiration effects.

In the next few sections, methods to obtain the respiratory signal will first be introduced. Different methods of setting the gate window, both prospectively and retrospectively, will be discussed.

Techniques to Obtain a Respiratory Signal

Abdominal Belt

The reference for the respiratory motion was initially obtained by placing a belt containing a displacement transducer around the upper abdomen (41,42). The anterior–posterior (AP) displacement of the abdomen is hereby determined. The disadvantage of this technique is that the belt does not give the absolute displacement value of the respiratory motion in the superior–inferior (SI) direction. In addition, there are variations in the correlation between the abdominal respiratory motion and the actual motion of coronary arteries.

Navigator Echoes

A more direct and absolute measurement of the respiration-induced motion can be obtained by the use of navigator echoes. This technique was first developed to monitor respiratory motion to improve abdominal MRI (43–45), and was later successfully applied for respiratory gating of MR coronary artery imaging (2,28,31, 46–49). The motion of the diaphragm in the SI direction is typically tracked, assuming that the SI motion of the diaphragm is synchronized to that of the heart (and coronary artery) caused by respiration.

A

B

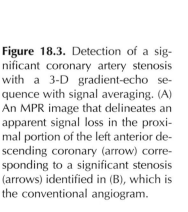

Figure 18.3. Detection of a significant coronary artery stenosis with a 3-D gradient-echo sequence with signal averaging. (A) An MPR image that delineates an apparent signal loss in the proximal portion of the left anterior descending coronary (arrow) corresponding to a significant stenosis (arrows) identified in (B), which is the conventional angiogram.

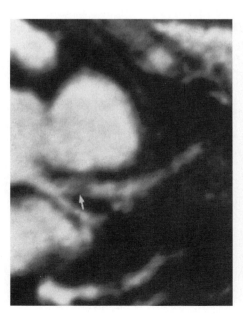

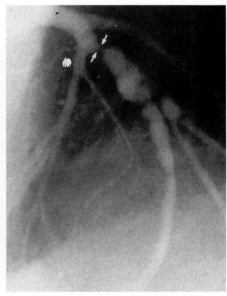

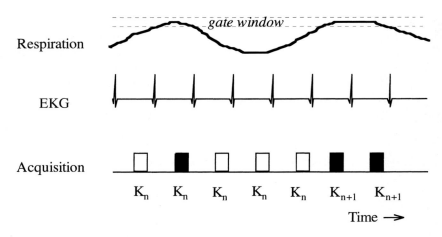

Figure 18.4. Schematic diagram of respiratory gating. The dotted lines in the respiratory signal show the position of the gate window. Only data obtained when the respiratory signal is within the gate window are used for image reconstruction (shown as black boxes). The phase encoding is updated every five cardiac cycles. Data are collected during diastole of each cardiac cycle through EKG-triggering.

With the navigator echo technique, the MR signal of a beam is measured, using frequency encoding along the long axis of the beam. After data acquisition, a one-dimensional Fourier transform is performed, and a one-dimensional image along the beam is created. When this beam is placed over a structure that moves during respiration along the direction of the beam, this motion can be measured by tracking a marker in the beam (typically the boundary between high and low signal intensities). These navigator echoes should have a spatial resolution of 1 mm or less in order to detect the motion of the heart with adequate resolution. These one-dimensional images can be obtained within 10–20 msec, thereby showing real-time information of the respiratory motion. There are two methods to obtain such a beam for a navigator image: the spin echo method or the 2-D selective excitation method.

The first method to obtain a navigator echo is by applying a pair of 90- and 180-degree pulses at an angle such that a spin echo is formed in the intersection of the two pulses with frequency encoding and data readout in the SI direction (43,50). The advantage of this method is the relative simple implementation. The disadvantage is that the high excitation flip angles used will result in magnetization saturation of the entire two slices within

the object. The 90- and 180-degree pulses could saturate the blood magnetization and reduce the coronary artery signal if they cut across the heart. This interference limits the flexibility in positioning the navigator echo beam.

A more flexible way of implementing the navigator echo is using a 2-D selective excitation pulse (51,52). By modulating both the RF pulse shape and gradients, only the signal within a pencil beam is excited. This allows the use of lower excitation angles and a greater flexibility in positioning the beam without interfering with coronary artery signal.

The next question is where to place this navigator beam in order to obtain the best motion signal for respiratory gating. From motion studies of the heart, it is found that the major component of respiratory motion is in SI direction (53). Most studies up to now have used the dome of the diaphragm to detect the craniocaudal motion. Figure 18.5 illustrates the placement of 90- and 180-degree pulses to measure the displacement of the diaphragm during respiration. Here, the sharp interface between liver and lung results is a clear edge on the navigator echo image (Fig. 18.6).

The use of diaphragmatic displacement for respiratory gating is based on the assumption that the motion detected from the navigator echo is correlated to that of

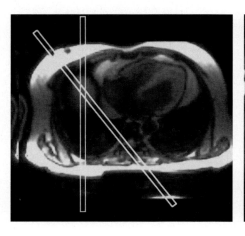

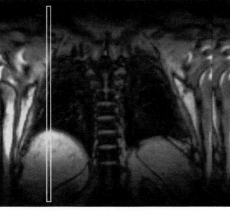

Figure 18.5. Illustration of the placement of a pair of 90- and 180-degree pulses to generate a one-dimensional projection navigator echo to track craniocaudal motion of the diaphragm.

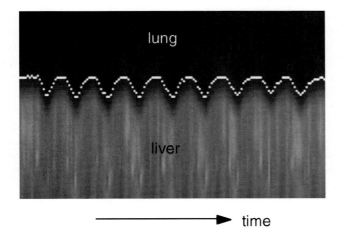

Figure 18.6. Each column of this image is a 1-D Fourier transform of the navigator echo obtained using the spin-echo technique. Multiple columns acquired with a repetition time of 200 msec are displayed. The horizontal axis is time. These columns demonstrate the signal intensity of the 90- to 180-degree pulse intersection column through the liver (high signal, lower part of the image) and lung (low signal, upper part of the image). The boundary is detected using an edge detection algorithm and marked by a bright dot in each column that provides information of diaphragmatic displacement during respiration.

the coronary arteries. Figure 18.7 illustrates a close correlation between the craniocaudal motion of the coronary artery and the diaphragm displacement. This plot was obtained by reconstructing images at different gating levels during the respiratory cycle. Wang et al. (53) studied this relationship by acquiring images with breathholds at different time frames of the respiratory cycle. A close correlation was also found.

Left diaphragmatic motion should correlate more closely to heart motion than right diaphragmatic motion, although the difference appeared to be insignificant in the study by Korin et al. (45). When a spin echo technique is used to acquire navigator echoes, it is dif-

ficult in some subjects in practice to place the 90- and 180-degree pulses on the left side without intersecting the heart because of the proximity of the heart to the chest wall. In these cases, the navigator echo beam has to be placed in the right side of the thoracic space.

The interference of the navigator echo pulses with the heart is not a problem if a 2-D excitation pulse is used to create the navigator echo because of the small flip angle used. This type of navigator echo can be placed on the heart itself. This allows for more direct measure of coronary artery motion. The navigator echo is typically placed on the edge of the free wall of the left ventricle, as shown in Figure 18.8. When the navigator echo beam is in an oblique orientation, the craniocaudal motion of the heart can be determined by correcting for the beam angulation.

Various methods have been used to determine the respiratory motion from navigator echo signals, including edge detection (2), cross-correlation (43,46,54), and least-squares methods (28,44). The edge detection method uses a signal-intensity threshold to determine the edge of the object. A low-pass filter is usually first applied to the navigator echo to remove spikes in the data before edge detection. Both the cross-correlation and least-squares methods compare the current navigator echo to remove spikes in the data before edge detection. Both the cross-correlation and least-squares methods compare the current navigator echo profile with a range of shifts with a reference profile. With the correlation method, the shift that results in the maximal correlation between the current and the reference profiles is taken as the estimated displacement between the current position and reference position. With the least-squares method, the shift with the smallest squared difference between the current and reference profiles is taken as the estimated displacement between the current position and reference position.

In a study involving seven normal volunteers, the uses of the least-squares and edge-detection methods

Figure 18.7. Plot demonstrating the correlation between the SI motion of the diaphragm and the displacement of the cross-section of the proximal LAD ($r = 0.991$). This plot was generated from a 2-D segmented gradient-echo sequence with retrospective respiratory gating. Twenty acquisitions were obtained and images were reconstructed at seven points of the respiratory cycle. Dashed line is the line of regression ($Y = 1.017X - 0.88$).

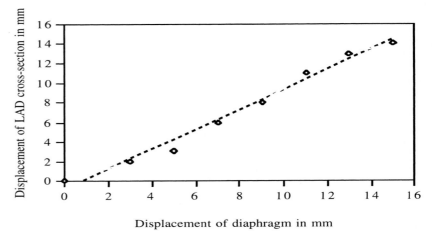

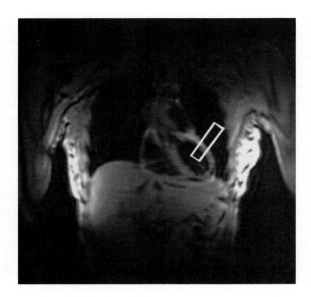

Figure 18.8. The position of a 2-D selective navigator beam that can be placed directly on the heart itself to track the respiratory motion of the edge of the left ventricular free wall.

for the detection of diaphragmatic motion from navigator echoes were found to give equivalent results in delineating coronary arteries in most of the volunteers (31). Although it is not statistically significant because of the limited number of studies, the least-squares method was found to be superior to edge detection in two of the seven volunteers. In a separate study using computer simulation and human volunteers to compare cross-correlation and least-squares methods, it was found that the least-squares algorithm demonstrated better reliability than the correlation method for measuring motion from navigator echo data (55). Further studies are needed to compare the performance of the three methods, investigate the difference between them, and to determine which method is the most robust when applied in a large patient population.

Algorithms Used for Respiratory Gating

An illustration of the data acquisition process for respiratory gating is shown in Figure 18.9. After a trigger de-

lay time, a navigator echo is acquired, followed by the collection of a segment of the raw data of the MR coronary angiogram in middiastole. These data are accepted for eventual reconstruction if the position of the respiration as determined by the navigator echo falls within the gate window. The measurement is repeated n times before the next segment of the raw data is measured. There are a number of approaches to perform the actual respiratory gating. The differences between the approaches include when these decisions are made, and how the number of repetitions n and the gate window are determined.

Prospective Gating
In this approach, the decision to accept or reject data for image reconstruction is made during data acquisition, based on a gate window chosen before the start of the scan (28,46,47). The collection of each segment of data is repeated until it is found to be within the gate window. The number of repetitions (n) is variable for each segment of data and depends on the breathing pattern. This guarantees that all data used for image reconstruction are within the gate window. The disadvantage is that the gate window has to be determined before the start of the scan and remains fixed, without taking into consideration the actual breathing pattern during the data acquisition process. On one hand, this may result in prolonged imaging time if the gate window was too narrow and/or there is a significant change of breathing pattern or bulk motion of the subject during imaging. On the other hand, if the gate window is too wide, the resultant image will be suboptimal in terms of motion artifact removal.

Retrospective Gating

A schematic diagram of retrospective respiratory gating is shown in Figure 18.10. In this approach, the decision to accept the data is made after they are all collected (2,31). The gate window, therefore, can be chosen after the acquisition, giving flexibility of changing this window at the time of image reconstruction, taking the actual breathing pattern during data acquisition into consideration. By reconstructing multiple sets of images at

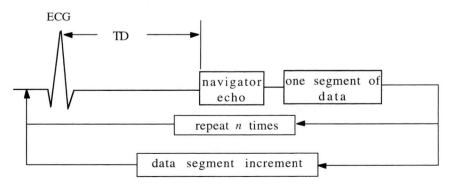

Figure 18.9. Schematic diagram of imaging coronary arteries with respiratory gating. TD: trigger delay time. For prospective gating, n is variable, data acquisition is repeated until a respiratory signal within the gate window is found. For retrospective gating, n is fixed. In the hybrid approach (DVA), n is variable and is in the outer loop.

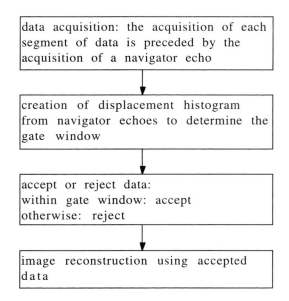

Figure 18.10. Generic diagram of retrospective respiratory gating.

different gate windows, coronary arteries at different phases of the breathing cycle can be delineated. In addition, for multiple overlapping scans, the same gating centers can be used retrospectively to register the slabs. The disadvantage of the method is that the number of repetitions is fixed and has to be determined prior to data acquisition. This will result in an unequal number of repetitions for different segments of data used in image reconstruction, reducing the time efficiency of the method.

With retrospective respiratory gating, the acquisition of each segment of data is repeated n times in n consecutive heartbeats so that the total imaging time of the segment will be greater than the duration of a respiratory cycle. Assuming a respiratory period of 3–4 seconds, five acquisitions of each segment of the data (in five heartbeats) will ensure full coverage of the respiratory cycle. If the subject has a long respiratory cycle or erratic breathing pattern, the number of repetitions for

the collection of each segment of data will need to be increased, resulting in a relatively long imaging time, especially for a 3-D scan.

The gate window is determined from a histogram of the number of distinct data segments as a function of the respiratory position, as shown in Figure 18.11. The peak position of the histogram is selected as the center of the gate window, the width of the window is either set to ±1 mm of the gate center (assuming the spatial resolution of the navigator echo is 1 mm) (31) or such that at least 90% of all the segments has at least one repetition within the gate window (2). If none of the repetitions of certain data segments lays within the gate window, the repetitions of these data segments obtained at respiratory positions closest to the gate window would be used for image reconstruction.

Diminishing Variance Algorithm (DVA)
A third approach of respiratory gating is a hybrid method between prospective and retrospective approaches, referred to as the diminishing variance algorithm (22). In the scheme, the entire k-space is first covered with a sequential mode. At the end of the first pass of k-space, a histogram will be constructed. The data segment that is farthest from the center of the histogram will subsequently be reacquired. The histogram will then be updated. This process is repeated until certain stopping criteria are reached. This hybrid approach seems to be more time efficient and flexible than either the prospective or retrospective gating methods. It is also unfortunately more demanding on the imaging system and more complex to implement. It requires real-time histogram processing and decision making. A comparison of the major features of the prospective, retrospective, and the hybrid respiratory gating methods is shown in Table 18.1.

Respiratory Feedback Triggering
A respiratory feedback monitoring system using navigator echoes has been used to collect data with multiple breathholds (26,54,56,57). The system initiates a signal to instruct subjects to suspend their breath when the

Figure 18.11. An example histogram of the number of distinct phase-encoding lines as a function of relative diaphragm positions detected using the navigator echo signal. If more than one acquisition of a phase-encoding line corresponds to the same diaphragm position, only one acquisition will be counted. In this particular example, 144 phase-encoding lines and six excitations were obtained. A maximum of 136 different lines were found to correspond to one diaphragm position, which is taken as the gate center. This leads to an excellent, high-resolution reconstruction of the coronary arteries.

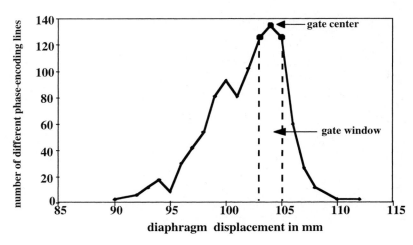

Table 18.1. Comparison of various respiratory gating approaches.

	No. of repetitions	Gate window
Prospective gating	Variable	Fixed
Retrospective gating	Fixed	Variable
Hybrid gating (DVA)	Variable	Variable

diaphragmatic displacement falls within a preset window. This method has proven effective in volunteer studies. It is, however, still limited by the patient's ability to cooperate. This may ultimately become a limiting factor for general clinical use of the approach.

Coronary Imaging Using Respiratory Gating

In the previous section, we discussed the basic principles of respiratory gating and various approaches of respiratory gating. In this section, results of coronary artery imaging using respiratory gating will be presented. Computer simulation results on stenosis detection in the presence of residual motion will also be presented.

2-D Imaging

Respiratory gating has been applied to remove the need for breathhold in 2-D coronary artery imaging. The 2-D imaging technique itself remains the same. By removing the constraint on acquisition time, however, there is a larger freedom to choose the scan parameters. Figure 18.12 shows an example of 2-D images of the RCA obtained with prospective navigator gating, with the navigator located at the edge of the free wall of the left ventricle. By using respiratory gating and adaptive navigator correction, the misregistration between imaging slices due to variability in breathhold positions is removed (49).

Respiratory gating resulted in equal or better image quality compared with that of breathhold with a similar effective scan time (47,58,59). When an increase in scan time is acceptable, the spatial resolution can be increased together with an increase of number of signal averages to preserve the SNR ratio. Oshinksi et al. (47,58) showed improved visualization of branch vessels and questionable vessel segments using such a prolonged acquisition time with a 0.5 mm in-plane resolution.

Prospective respiratory gating in combination with 2-D MR coronary artery imaging was also applied by Sachs et al. with spiral k-space trajectories in combination with DVA (22).

3-D Imaging

A fast 3-D gradient-echo sequence for coronary artery imaging is illustrated in Figure 18.13. Sequence parameters include: TR/TE = 8/3 msec, slice thickness = 2 mm, 16–32 partitions/cardiac cycle with centrally re-

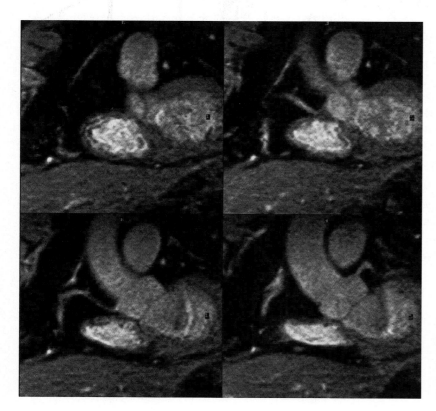

Figure 18.12. Four slices in the same oblique orientation parallel to the proximal right coronary artery of a healthy volunteer. The images were obtained with a 2-D technique using prospective respiratory gating with a 2-D navigator echo beam located on the left ventricle.

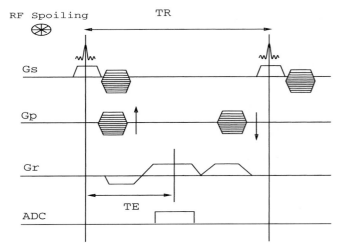

Figure 18.13. Sequence diagram of a fast 3-D gradient-echo sequence for coronary artery imaging. G_s = slice gradient; G_p = phase-encoding gradient; G_r = readout gradient.

ordered partition encoding. A constant flip angle of 15 degrees was initially used for each partition-encoding step (2,11). A variable flip angle series of 20–90 degrees for each partition-encoding loop was used to increase the blood signal and to improve signal uniformity (31).

In an initial study comparing coronary artery delineation with and without respiratory gating, gated images represent a significant improvement over nongated images. Two-dimensional breathhold scans, however, still showed better delineation of coronary arteries than did the gated 3-D images (2). Figure 18.14 illustrates this comparison with a representative example of the left coronary artery. The thick slab in the 3-D technique resulted in saturation of the MR signal from blood, causing a loss of contrast. In a preliminary clinical trial comparing this early version of the technique with X-ray contrast angiography, a low sensitivity of detecting significant coronary artery stenoses (38%) was reported (30). Some of the technical problems with this initial

study included a relatively high signal bandwidth and a long data acquisition window per cardiac cycle (260 msec for 32 partitions), resulting in severe image blur from cardiac motion.

An improved gradient subsystem allowed a lower signal bandwidth, more symmetric readout, and a higher spatial resolution (on the order of $1.2 \times 1.0 \times 2$ mm^3). The data acquisition time per cardiac cycle was reduced to 120 msec with 16 partitions and variable flip angles were used to maximize blood signal. With five repetitions per phase-encoding step, the imaging time for each scan was 8–16 minutes (with R–R intervals ranging from 0.6 to 1.2 seconds). A comparison of 3-D coronary artery images with and without retrospective respiratory gating is presented in Figure 18.15. In a study involving 12 normal volunteers (31), retrospective respiratory gating was found to improve significantly image quality and coronary artery definition over nongated scans (both single acquisition and multiple signal averaged acquisition) in conjunction with a 3-D gradient-echo sequence.

One of the major advantages of 3-D imaging is the acquisition of thin and contiguous slices that are completely registered in slice positions. These images can be postprocessed by MPR or maximum intensity projection (MIP) to view the coronary arteries in different planes and orientations. Figure 18.16 shows four consecutive slices from a 3-D data set acquired with retrospective respiratory gating. One can follow these images and visualize the origin of the left main coronary artery, the bifurcation of the left main artery to the LAD and left circumflex (LCx) branches, and the more distal portions of the LAD and LCx arteries. Images generated by MPR are shown in Figure 18.17, where long portions of coronary arteries are visualized. By performing MPR to a 3-D data set, cross-sectional coronary arteries can be obtained to visualize the lumen area change (Fig. 18.18).

By acquiring multiple, partially overlapped 3-D slabs, the entire heart can be covered. The length of four major coronary arteries contiguously visible in a study with

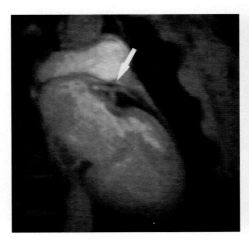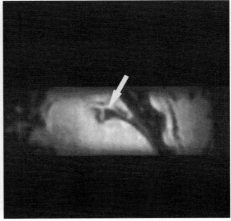

Figure 18.14. Comparison of 2-D breathhold image (left panel) showing the left coronary arteries (arrow) and the equivalent plane in a 3-D respiratory gated data set (right panel) obtained in the same healthy volunteer. (Reprinted, with permission, from Hofman et al. (2).)

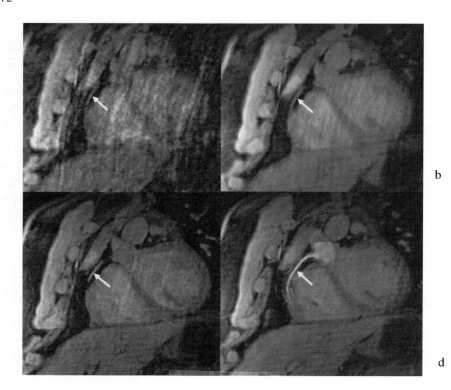

a

b

c

d

Figure 18.15. A comparison of representative coronary artery images obtained without and with retrospective respiratory gating. (a) An image from a data set acquired using a 3-D gradient-echo sequence with one acquisition. Note the poor image quality due to respiratory motion. The RCA is barely visible (arrow). (b) The same slice position as in (a), but obtained by averaging over five acquisitions. The image quality is improved over (a), but blurring of the RCA (arrow) still remains. (c) With retrospective respiratory gating, the definition of the RCA (arrow) is greatly improved over (a) and (b). (d) By segmenting RCA in consecutive slices of the gated data set and superimposing the RCA projection to one partition slice, a long portion of the RCA (arrow) is delineated. (Reprinted with permission from Li et al. (31).)

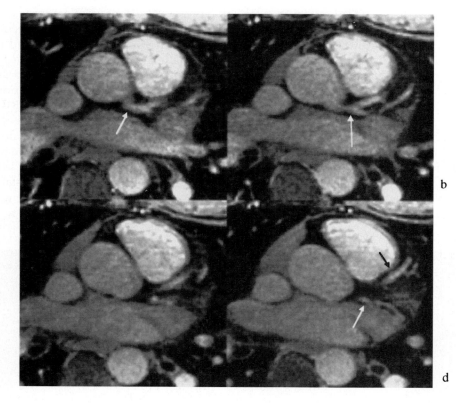

a

b

c

d

Figure 18.16. Four contiguous images acquired using a 3-D sequence with retrospective gating delineating the left coronary arteries. One can follow the left coronary artery from its origin to more distal portions by looking through the slices. Note the excellent visibility of the coronary arteries despite the curvature of the vessel. The left main (LM) coronary artery (arrow) is shown in (a); the bifurcation (arrow) of the LM to the LAD and LCx coronary arteries in (b); and the more distal portions of LAD (black arrow) and LCx (white arrow) in (c,d). (Reprinted with permission from Li et al. (31).)

Figure 18.17. MPR images of a 3-D data set to depict (a), the left coronary arteries, and (b), the right coronary artery. (Reprinted with permission from Li et al. (31).)

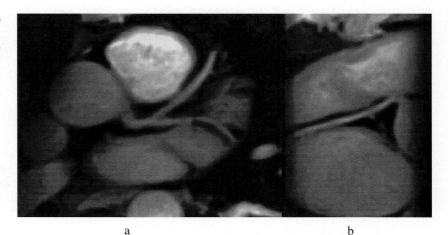

a   b

five normal volunteers using retrospective respiratory gating is listed in Table 18.2. Two projection images from different angles obtained from a volunteer are shown in Figure 18.19. The images were created after background tissues were removed manually. Note that the definition of distal coronary arteries is inferior to that of the proximal portions of coronary arteries. This is because distal coronary arteries generally have smaller diameters and experience an increased motion from respiration (60). They are also more adjacent to myocardium and cardiac chambers than proximal coronary arteries. This is especially the case for the left circumflex coronary artery. Higher resolution (i.e., a voxel size of approximately 1 mm³) is required to define the coronary arteries better.

Clinical trials with modified retrospective respiratory gating demonstrated improved capability of detecting significant coronary artery stenoses (32,34). Details of the clinical trials and practical problems with the technique are discussed in other chapters of the book.

Several methods of improving respiratory gating have been suggested, including *k*-space–weighted gat-

ing (48) and motion-matched phase reordering (61). These and other modifications will make respiratory gating more robust and clinically applicable.

Simulations

Respiration-related motion artifacts are significantly reduced by respiratory gating. Nevertheless, there is still residual motion that could cause image blur at the boundary of coronary arteries. To demonstrate that in principle significant coronary artery stenoses can still be detected in the presence of certain residual motion during data acquisition, computer simulations were performed to investigate the effect of motion on lumen definition. From Figure 18.20, a 30% concentric stenosis can still be clearly visualized in the presence of 1-mm motion during data acquisition with a vessel diameter as small as 3 mm. When the vessel diameter reduces to 2 mm the narrowing is no longer visible because of the motion blur.

Two important factors that affect the motion blur of

Figure 18.18. (a) The cross-sectional cut through the normal lumen of the LAD (arrow), and (b) the cross-sectional cut through the stenosis (arrow). The solid lines on the top of the two images illustrate the orientations from which MPR images were generated. The apparent signal loss pointed by the arrow in (b) indicates the presence of a significant LAD stenosis by comparing with the normal luminal signal in (a). (Reprinted with permission from Li et al. (31).)

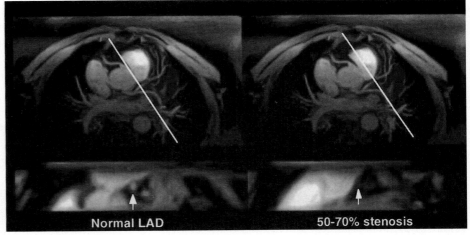

a   b

Table 18.2. Length of contiguously visible coronary arteries (*n* = 5).

	Left main	Left anterior descending	Left circumflex	Right coronary artery
Length (mm)	11.5 ± 0.4	115.9 ± 19.7	97.2 ± 12.5	125.9 ± 18.8

Reprinted, with permission, from Li et al., Ref. 31.
Note: Results are expressed as mean ± standard deviation.

coronary arteries are the direction of motion with respect to vessel axis and the in-plane resolution. As illustrated in Figure 18.21, more image blur occurs when motion direction is perpendicular to vessel axis than parallel to vessel. In addition, with the same voxel size (1 mm³), there is less image blur with better in-plane resolution (0.5 × 0.5 mm³). These issues need to be carefully studied to design optimal strategies of imaging coronary arteries using respiratory gating.

Other Applications of Respiratory Gating

We have presented examples of respiratory-gated imaging of coronary arteries. This approach should be readily applicable to other imaging tasks. One application of respiratory gating is coronary artery flow quantification (62) to remove the constraints imposed by the duration of a breathhold.

In coronary flow quantification, it is required to acquire data throughout the cardiac cycle, whereas for angiographic applications only a middiastolic image is obtained. This results in a larger sensitivity of the technique to the cardiac motion of the arteries because image blurring will occur when there is severe in-plane displacement within the acquisition window. For a breathhold approach, a typical acquisition window for a coronary flow acquisition will be around 120 msec. It has been shown that the coronary arteries move as much as 6–14 mm during this period, depending on the artery segment studied (63). The magnitude of motion is about twice as large for the proximal right as for the proximal left coronary artery. The acquisition window, therefore, should be much smaller to obtain flow data in the coronary arteries with

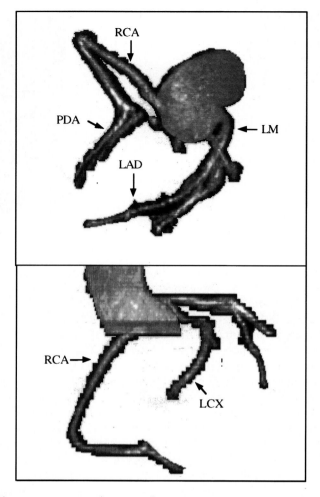

Figure 18.19. Visualization of a 3-D coronary artery tree from two different orientations. The original images were acquired using a 3-D sequence with retrospective respiratory gating. Multiple 3-D slabs with 40% overlap were obtained to cover the entire heart. The background tissue (myocardium and heart chambers) were manually removed before projection. (Reprinted with permission from Li et al. (31).)

a high spatial resolution. Respiratory gating permits a decrease of the duration of the acquisition window at the cost of overall scan time. A second reason for a small acquisition window, and thus a high temporal resolution, is that it permits acquisitions of the full phasic information of the coronary flow throughout the cardiac cycle.

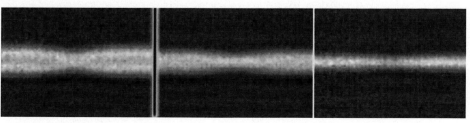

4 mm   3 mm   2 mm

Figure 18.20. Visualization of vessel lumen narrowing in the presence of 1-mm motion perpendicular to vessel axis. The resolution of the image is 1 × 1 × 1 mm³. The vessel model has a 30% concentric diameter stenosis in the midsegment. Vessel diameters are labeled under the image.

Figure 18.21. Delineation of a coronary artery stenosis with different resolution and motion direction by computer simulation. The vessel has a 50% concentric stenosis in the midsegment. The lumen diameter is 4 mm.

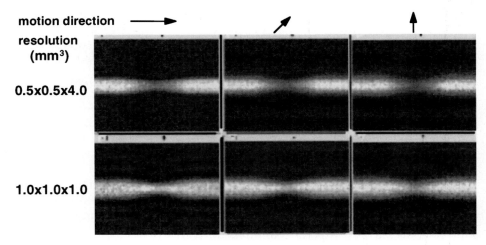

motion direction

resolution (mm³)

0.5x0.5x4.0

1.0x1.0x1.0

Using respiratory gating, coronary flow was measured successfully within the right coronary artery, whereas a breathhold technique failed (64). Figure 18.22 shows cross-sectional images of the RCA during early systole obtained using a breathhold technique and using respiratory gating. This figure illustrates that the blurring resulting from the large acquisition window in the breathhold technique can be removed using respiratory gating. This technique has been validated with intravascular Doppler in humans.

In gradient-echo cardiac cine imaging, breathhold significantly improves image quality. When complete coverage of the heart is required to calculate ejection fractions, however, the potential mismatch of slice positions acquired from separate breathhold periods may cause inaccuracy of the global function index calculation. If a respiratory gating approach is used, images from different scans will be better registered because they are reconstructed at the same phase of the breathing cycle.

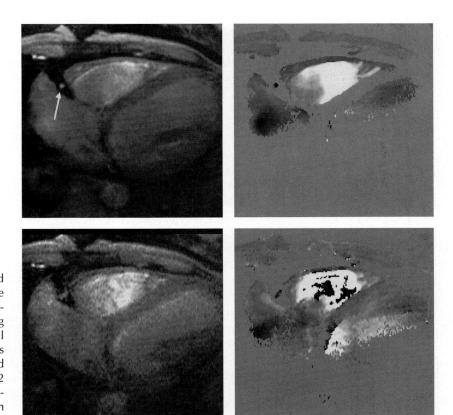

Figure 18.22. Magnitude images (left) and through-plane velocity maps (right) in a plane perpendicular to the right coronary artery (arrow) all obtained in the same subject during early systole, a time point with substantial movement of the coronary arteries. Top panels show data obtained with a respiratory-gated technique with an acquisition window of 32 msec, whereas the bottom panels were obtained using a breathhold technique with an acquisition window of 126 msec.

Further Developments in Nonbreathhold Coronary Artery Imaging

Motion Correction Using Navigator Echoes

In addition to respiratory gating, navigator echo data can also be used for motion correction through image processing (43,44,65,66). This method requires an accurate model of the object motion and has proven effective for lower abdominal organs. Initial attempts for MR coronary angiography failed (2), but later studies by Wang et al. (67) using a calibration factor between diaphragm motion and coronary motion showed some success. This calibration factor is clearly not constant over a large patient population. The major problem with this method is that it assumes translational motion of the whole object, which is a simplification of the actual complicated motion patterns of the heart during respiration. Hence, this method has not found widespread applications in cardiac imaging.

Real-time shift of the excitation slice according to respiratory motion has been proposed to image coronary arteries (49,68). This and other motion correction methods, if proven feasible, will result in significant improvement in time efficiency over simple respiratory gating. It is also possible that a combination of gating and motion correction may provide an optimal approach. Gating is performed here to limit the heart displacement to a narrow range. A correction is applied to reduce the remaining blurring for the data within this window. The gate window will reduce the errors of the simplified translational motion model used with the correction algorithm.

Combination of Both 2-D and 3-D Techniques

Both 2-D and 3-D techniques have advantages and disadvantages for coronary artery imaging. The major advantage of 2-D imaging is high blood signal from the inflow enhancement effect. The disadvantages include the relatively thick imaging slice and the difficulty of acquiring contiguous slices. Three-dimensional imaging, on the other hand, can provide thin and inherently contiguous slices. Problems with 3-D data acquisition include blood spin saturation and a relatively long imaging time, especially with respiratory gating. Variations of subject's breathing pattern during this period may explain the inconsistency in image quality in some patient studies using the technique. A shorter imaging time using faster data acquisition techniques (e.g., segmented echo-planar sequence) may provide a solution (27). Targeted data acquisitions with thin slab and/or small field-of-view (FOV) can also reduce imaging time for a 3-D sequence (35,69).

Contrast-Enhanced Coronary Artery Imaging

Early success has been demonstrated in contrast-enhanced coronary artery imaging using conventional extravascular contrast agents (33,70). The development of new intravascular contrast agents, such as MS-325 (EPIX Medical, Inc., Cambridge, MA) (71), opened the door for further improvement in blood signal-to-noise and spatial resolution (72,73). This and other intravascular contrast agents may prove necessary for the diagnosis of distal coronary artery stenosis, especially with a 3-D imaging technique. With the help of an intravascular contrast agent, the current advantage of higher inflow contrast in 2-D techniques over 3-D techniques will vanish. This topic will be discussed in detail in other chapters of the book.

Summary and Conclusion

Technical development, animal studies, and clinical trials have demonstrated that it is now feasible to image coronary arteries and detect significant stenoses without the need for breathhold. The major advantages of nonbreathhold imaging are the patient-friendliness and the ability to obtain high resolution images (both 2-D and 3-D). Nonbreathhold techniques will also permit high spatial and temporal resolution, high signal-to-noise, complete registration of slice positions acquired from different scans, and the possibility of 3-D data acquisition with high spatial resolution and large volume coverage, which are crucial for coronary artery visualization. Further evaluation and developments are needed to improve various respiratory gating and motion correction techniques to make them a powerful clinical tool for coronary artery imaging.

Acknowledgments. The authors thank Richard D. White, MD, for Figure 18.3 and Pamela K. Woodard, MD, for Figure 18.18. D.L. and E.M.H. acknowledge the support of NIH grant R01-HL-38698 for the work.

References

1. Manning WJ, Li W, Boyle NG, Edelman RR. Fat-suppressed breathhold magnetic resonance coronary angiography. Circulation 1993;87:97–104.
2. Hofman MBM, Paschal CB, Li D, Haacke EM, van Rossum AC, Sprenger M. MRI of coronary arteries: 2D breath-hold versus 3D respiratory gated acquisition. J Comput Assist Tomogr 1995;19:56–62.
3. Alfidi RJ, Masaryk TJ, Haacke EM, et al. MR angiography of peripheral, carotid, and coronary arteries. Am J Roentgenol 1987;149:1097–109.
4. Paulin S, von Schulthess GK, Fossel E, Krayenbuehl HP, Higgins CB. MR imaging of the aortic root and proximal coronary arteries. Am J Roentgenol 1987;148:665–70.
5. Vered Z, Kenzora J, Gutierrez F. Noninvasive evaluation

of the left main coronary artery in man with magnetic resonance imaging. Am J Noninvas Cardiol 1990;4:154–58.

6. Cho ZH, Mun CW, Friedenberg RM. NMR angiography of coronary vessels with 2D planar image scanning. Magn Reson Med 1991;20:134–43.

7. Dumoulin CL, Souza SP, Darrow RD, Adams WJ. A method of coronary MR angiography. J Comput Assist Tomogr 1991;15:705–10.

8. Edelman RR, Manning WJ, Burstein D, Paulin S. Coronary arteries: breathhold MR angiography. Radiology 1991;181:641–43.

9. Burstein D. MR imaging of coronary artery flow in isolated and in vivo hearts. J Magn Reson Imag 1991;1:337–46.

10. Meyer CH, Hu BS, Nishimura DG, Macovski A. Fast spiral coronary artery imaging. Magn Reson Med 1992;28:202–13.

11. Li D, Paschal CB, Haacke EM, Adler LP. Coronary arteries: three-dimensional MR imaging with fat saturation and magnetization transfer contrast. Radiology 1993;187:401–6.

12. Manning WJ, Li W, Edelman RR. A preliminary report comparing magnetic resonance coronary angiography with conventional angiography. N Engl J Med 1993;328:828–32.

13. Duerinckx AJ, Urman MK. Two-dimensional coronary MR angiography: analysis of initial clinical results. Radiology 1994;193:731–38.

14. Pennell DJ, Bogren HG, Keegan J, Firmin DN, Underwood SR. Assessment of coronary artery stenosis by magnetic resonance imaging. Heart 1996;75:127–33.

15. Edelman RR, Manning WJ, Pearl J, Li W. Human coronary arteries: projection angiograms reconstructed from breathhold two-dimensional MR images. Radiology 1993;187:719–22.

16. Doyle M, Scheidegger MB, DeGraaf RG, Vermeulen J, Pohost GM. Coronary artery imaging in multiple 1-sec breath holds. Magn Reson Imag 1993;11:3–6.

17. Wielopolski PA, Scharf JG, Edelman RR. Multislice coronary angiography within a single breath hold (abstr.). J Magn Reson Imag 1994;4 (Suppl.):80.

18. Lenz GW, Haacke EM, White RD. Retrospective cardiac gating: a review of technical aspects and future directions. Magn Reson Imag 1989;7:445–55.

19. Paschal CB, Haacke EM, Adler LP, Finelli DA. Magnetic resonance coronary artery imaging. Cardiovasc Intervent Radiol 1992;15:23–31.

20. Paschal CB, Haacke EM, Adler LP. Three-dimensional MR imaging of the coronary arteries: preliminary clinical experience. J Magn Reson Imag 1993;3:491–500.

21. Li D, White RD, Adler LP, Haacke EM. Three-dimensional cardiovascular MR imaging: initial clinical experience. Proceeding of the Society of Magnetic Resonance in Medicine Twelfth Meeting, 1993:556.

22. Sachs TS, Meyer CH, Irarrazabal P, Hu BS, Nishimura DG, Macovski A. The diminishing variance algorithm for real-time reduction of motion artifacts in MRI. Magn Reson Med 1995;34:412–22.

23. Dougherty L, Schnall MD, Holland GA, Greenman BL, Axel L. Fast 3D imaging of coronary arteries using Gd-DTPA enhancement. Proceedings of the Society of Magnetic Resonance, Third Scientific Meeting and Exhibition. Nice, France, 1995:1397.

24. Li D, Haacke EM, Shelton ME, Kaushikkar S. Magnetic resonance imaging of coronary arteries. Cor Art Dis 1995;6:368–76.

25. Haacke EM, Li D, Kaushikkar S. Cardiac MRI: concepts and techniques. Top Magn Reson 1995;7:200–17.

26. Wang Y, Grimm RC, Rossman PJ, Debbins JP, Riederer SJ, Ehman RL. 3D coronary MR angiography in multiple breathholds using a respiratory feedback monitor. Magn Reson Med 1995;34:11–16.

27. Wielopolski PA, Manning WJ, Edelman RR. Single breathhold volumetric imaging of the heart using magnetization-prepared 3D segmented echo-planar imaging. J Magn Reson Imag 1995;5:403–10.

28. Wang Y, Rossman PJ, Grimm RC, Riederer SJ, Ehman RL. Navigator-echo-based real-time respiratory gating and triggering for reduction of respiratory effects in 3D coronary imaging. Radiology 1996;198:55–60.

29. Stillman AE, Wilke N, Li D, Haacke EM, McLachlan S. Ultrasmall superparamagnetic iron oxide to enhance MRA of the renal and coronary arteries: studies in human patients. J Comput Assist Tomogr 1996;20:51–55.

30. Post JC, van Rossum AC, Hofman MBM, Valk J, Visser CA. Three-dimensional respiratory-gated MR angiography of coronary arteries: comparison with conventional coronary angiography. Am J Roentgenol 1996;166:1399–404.

31. Li D, Kaushikkar S, Haacke EM, et al. Coronary arteries: three-dimensional MR imaging with retrospective respiratory gating. Radiology 1996;201:857–63.

32. Muller MF, Fleisch M, Kroeker R, Chatterjee T, Meier B, Vock P. Proximal coronary artery stenosis—three-dimensional MRI with fat saturation and navigator echo. J Magn Reson Imag 1997;7:644–51.

33. Goldfarb JW, Edelman RR. Coronary arteries: breathhold, gadolinium-enhanced, three-dimensional MR angiography. Radiology 1998;206:830–34.

34. Woodard PK, Li D, Haacke EM, et al. Detection of coronary stenoses on source and projection images using three-dimensional MR angiography with retrospective respiratory gating: preliminary experience. Am J Roentgenol 1998;170:883–88.

35. Yang GZ, Gatehouse PD, Keegan J, Mohiaddin RH, Firmin DN. Three-dimensional coronary MR angiography using zonal echo planar imaging. Magn Reson Med 1998;39:833–42.

36. Bailes DR, Gilderdale DJ, Bydder GM, Collins AG, Firmin DN. Respiratory ordered phase encoding (ROPE): a method for reducing respiratory motion artifacts in MR imaging. J Comput Assist Tomogr 1985;9:835–38.

37. Haacke EM, Patrick JL. Reducing motion artifacts in two-dimensional Fourier transform imaging. Magn Reson Imag 1986;4:359–76.

38. Chien D, Atkinson DJ, Edelman RR. Strategies to improve contrast in turboFLASH imaging: reordered phase encoding and k-space segmentation. J Magn Reson Imag 1991;1:63–70.

39. Atkinson D, Edelman R. Cineangiography of the heart in a single breathhold with a segmented TurboFLASH sequence. Radiology 1991;178:359–62.

40. Haacke EM, Lenz GW, Nelson AD. Pseudo-gating: elimination of periodic motion artifacts in magnetic resonance imaging without gating. Magn Reson Med 1987;4:162–74.

41. Runge VM, Clanton JA, Partain CL, James AEJ. Respiratory gating in magnetic resonance imaging at 0.5 Tesla. Radiology 1984;151:521–23.

42. Ehman RL, McNamara MT, Pallack M, Hricak H, Higgins CB. Magnetic resonance imaging with respiratory gating: techniques and advantages. Am J Roentgenol 1984;143:1175–82.

43. Ehman RL, Felmlee JP. Adaptive technique for high-definition MR imaging of moving structures. Radiology 1989;173:255–63.

44. Felmlee JP, Ehman RL, Riederer SJ, Korin HW. Adaptive motion compensation in MRI: accuracy of motion measurement. Magn Reson Med 1991;18:207–13.

45. Korin HW, Ehman RL, Riederer SJ, Felmlee JP, Grimm RC. Respiratory kinematics of the upper abdominal organs: a quantitative study. Magn Reson Med 1992;23:172–78.

46. Sachs TS, Meyer CH, Hu BS, Kohli J, Nishimura DG, Macovski A. Real-time motion detection in spiral MRI using navigators. Magn Reson Med 1994;32:639–45.

47. Oshinski JN, Hofland L, Mukundan S, Dixon WT, Parks WJ, Pettigrew RI. Two-dimensional coronary MR angiography without breathholding. Radiology 1996;201:737–43.

48. Weiger M, Bornert P, Proksa R, Schaffter T, Haase A. Motion-adapted gating based on k-space weighting for reduction of respiratory motion artifacts. Magn Reson Med 1997;38:322–33.

49. McConnell MV, Khasgiwala VC, Savord BJ, et al. Prospective adaptive navigator correction for breathhold MR coronary angiography. Magn Reson Med 1997;37:148–52.

50. Hinks RS. Monitoring echo gating (MEGA) for the reduction of motion artifacts (abstr.). Magn Reson Imag 1988;6(Suppl.):48.

51. Hardy CJ, Bottomley PA, O'Donnell M, Roemer P. J Magn Reson 1988;77:233.

52. Pauly J, Nishimura D, Macovski A. A k-space analysis of small-tip-angle excitation. J Magn Reson 1989;81:43–56.

53. Wang Y, Riederer SJ, Ehman RL. Respiratory motion of the heart: kinematics and the implications for spatial resolution of coronary MR imaging. Magn Reson Med 1995;33:713–19.

54. Liu Y, Riederer SJ, Rossman PJ, Grimm RC, Debbins JP, Ehman RL. A monitoring, feedback, and triggering system for reproducible breathhold MR imaging. Magn Reson Med 1993;30:507–11.

55. Wang Y, Grimm RC, Riederer SJ, Ehman RL. Algorithms to extract motion information from navigator echoes. Proceedings of the Society of Magnetic Resonance, Third Scientific Meeting and Exhibition. Nice, France, 1995:751.

56. Wang Y, Grimm RC, Rossman PJ, Debbins JP, Riederer SJ, Ehman RL. Coronary MR angiography in multiple breathholds using a respiratory feedback monitor. Magn Reson Med 1995;34:11–16.

57. Wang Y, Christy PS, Korosec FR, et al. Coronary MRI with a respiratory feedback monitor: the 2D imaging case. Magn Reson Med 1995;33:116–21.

58. Oshinski JN, Hofland L, Mukundan S, Dixon WT, Parks WJ, Pettigrew RI. Respiratory gated coronary magnetic resonance angiography compares favorably with breathhold imaging. Proceedings of the Society of Magnetic Resonance, Third Scientific Meeting and Exhibition. Nice, France, 1995:22.

59. McConnel MV, Khasgiwala VC, Savord BJ, et al. Comparison of real-time navigator gating to other respiratory motion suppression techniques for magnetic resonance coronary angiography. International Society of Magnetic Resonance in Medicine, Fourth Scientific Meeting and Exhibition. New York, 1996:450.

60. Wang Y, Grist TM, Korosec FR, et al. Respiratory blur in 3D coronary MR imaging. Magn Reson Med 1995;33:541–48.

61. Jhooti P, Keegan J, Gatehouse PD, et al. 3D coronary imaging with phase reordering for optimal scan efficiency. International Society of Magnetic Resonance in Medicine, Sixth Annual Meeting. Sydney, Australia, 1998:318.

62. Li D, Kaushikkar S, Haacke EM, Dhawale P. Coronary artery flow quantification using segmented phase contrast sequence with retrospective respiratory gating. Proceedings of the Society of Magnetic Resonance, Third Scientific Meeting and Exhibition. Nice, France, 1995:320.

63. Hofman MB, Wickline SA, Lorenz CH. In-plane motion of the left coronary arteries during the cardiac acquisition time window for flow quantification. International Society of Magnetic Resonance in Medicine, Fourth Scientific Meeting and Exhibition. New York, 1996:452.

64. Hofman MB, Visser FC, van Rossum AC, Vink QM, Sprenger M, Westerhof N. In vivo validation of magnetic resonance blood volume flow measurements with limited spatial resolution in small vessels. Magn Reson Med 1995;33:778–84.

65. Korin HW, Felmlee JP, Ehman RL, Riederer SJ. Adaptive technique for three-dimensional MR imaging of moving structures. Radiology 1990;177:217–21.

66. Felmlee JP, Ehman RL, Riederer SJ, Korin HW. Adaptive motion compensation in MR imaging without use of navigator echoes. Radiology 1991;179:139–42.

67. Wang Y, Johnston DL, Riederer SJ, Ehman RL. Adaptive motion correction for real-time navigator gated coronary MR angiography. International Society of Magnetic Resonance in Medicine, Fourth Scientific Meeting and Exhibition. New York, 1996:175.

68. Danias PG, McConnell MV, Khasgiwala VC, Chuang ML, Edelman RR, Manning WJ. Prospective navigator correction of image position for coronary MR angiography. Radiology 1997;203:733–36.

69. Wielopolski PA, van Geuns RJM, de Feyter PJ, Oudkerk M. VCATS, MR coronary angiography using breath-hold volume targeted acquisitions. International Society of Magnetic Resonance in Medicine, Sixth Meeting. Sydney, Australia, 1998:14.

70. Zheng J, Li D, Bae KT, Woodard PK, Haacke EM. Three-dimensional gadolinium-enhanced coronary MR angiography: initial experience. J Cardiovasc Magn Reson 1999;1(1):33–42.

71. Lauffer RB, Parmelee DJ, Dunham SU, et al. MS-325: albumin-targeted contrast agent for MR angiography. Radiology 1998;207:529–38.

72. Li D, Dolan B, Walovitch RC, Lauffer RB. Three-dimensional MR imaging of coronary arteries using an intravascular contrast agent. Magn Reson Med 1998;39:1014–18.

73. Stuber M, Botnar RM, McConnell MV, et al. Coronary artery imaging with the intravascular contrast agent MS-325. International Society of Magnetic Resonance in Medicine, Sixth Meeting. Sydney, Australia, 1998:316.

19
MR Navigators and Their Use in Cardiac and Coronary Imaging

Peter G. Danias and Warren J. Manning

Introduction

Magnetic resonance (MR) imaging of the cardiovascular system has always been challenging. Ventricular contraction results in a complex cardiac motion that includes caudal displacement primarily of the base, with simultaneous translation on the horizontal plane and rotation around the long axis of the heart (1). In addition, bulk cardiac motion occurs due to craniocaudal respiratory diaphragmatic displacement and chest wall expansion during free breathing. Imaging without motion compensation invariably results in image degradation (Fig. 19.1). Early imaging techniques were technically limited and not able to account for bulk cardiac motion related to respiration (2–5). Although ventricular contraction can effectively be "frozen" by gating image acquisition from the surface EKG, the absence of a clear triggering signal during the respiratory cycle and the inconsistent depth of inspiration among sequential breathing cycles render respiratory gating more challenging. In order to compensate for respiratory motion artifacts, oversampling with signal averaging was employed early on. Following advances that allowed k-space segmentation (6–8), it became possible to implement a breathhold imaging to suspend respiratory motion.

Although a 16–20-second breathhold can be usually tolerated well by volunteers and motivated patients, patients with cardiac and/or pulmonary disease often cannot comply with prolonged breathholding. It has been reported that 16% of hospitalized patients are unable to perform even short repeated breathholds, whereas the majority of inpatients or outpatients with cardiac and/or lung disease are unable to sustain prolonged breathholds (9). At the same time, advances in MR technology (magnets, gradients, coils) have allowed for higher resolution imaging, but new sequences frequently require breathholding up to 30–40 seconds (10–13), which is impractical for clinical use. As an alternative to breathholding, coached breathing has been proposed, so that image data would be acquired during periods of suspended breathing, at the same time-point of the respiratory cycle (14,15). The need for considerable patient training and cooperation, and the significant operator involvement, are limitations both for breathhold and coached-breathing techniques. In addition, registration errors frequently occur when serial image acquisitions are performed during different depths of inspiration, corresponding to different diaphragmatic positions (Fig. 19.2) (15,16). Such errors are of particular importance for coronary magnetic resonance angiography (MRA) because discontinuities of the coronary vessels due to image plane misregistration could be erroneously interpreted as focal stenoses. Finally, poor breathholding technique results in motion artifacts and image degradation (Fig. 19.3) (16,17), limiting the use of possible image enhancements such as 3-D imaging, signal averaging, and high-resolution imaging.

To overcome problems associated with suspended breathing and to allow for free (unrestricted) breathing, respiratory belts (bellows) have been used to monitor chest wall expansion and gate data acquisition (18,19). This technique, however, is not consistently reliable because the temporal relationship between chest wall expansion and intrathoracic or intraabdominal organ position is not constant. A more direct technique to monitor respiratory motion is with the use of navigator beams. The word *navigator* has been in use since the fifteenth century and originates from the latin verb *navigare*, from navis (= ship) and agere (= drive) (20). Although navigators were initially introduced to monitor respiratory motion and to gate image acquisition accordingly,

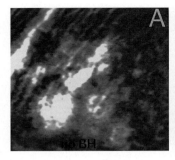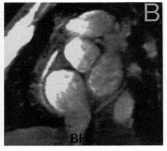

Figure 19.1. Segmented 2-D gradient-echo coronary MRA of the right coronary artery (double oblique coronal projection), acquired (A) without respiratory compensation and (B) during breathholding. Free breathing results in image degradation from motion artifacts. (Reprinted with permission from Wang (16).)

advances have allowed the active guidance of image acquisition, better justifying the word *etymology*.

Physics/Implementation

Several navigator sequences have been described and are currently used. The description of the theoretical properties—advantages and disadvantages of each sequence—is beyond the scope of this chapter and the interested reader is referred elsewhere (21–26). The underlying principle relies on the excitation of a narrow beam of tissue along the axis of primary motion. Similar to M-mode echocardiography, data analysis is then performed along the axis of this beam. If this beam is positioned in such a way as to traverse tissues with different MR-specific properties, a sharp interface within this beam can be detected, corresponding to the tissue border. With sampling at consecutive time points, the exact position of the interface (tissue border) can be measured by comparing each (new) position with a predefined reference. For example, if a vertical navigator is positioned through the dome of the right hemidiaphragm, a sharp interface can be detected between liver and lung. During freebreathing this interface moves caudally during inspiration and cranially during expiration (Fig. 19.4). If the reference position is ac-

quired so as to correspond to the end-expiratory position, all subsequent diaphragmatic positions can be measured by the navigator in relation to this reference (i.e., end-expiration). A variety of intrathoracic and intraabdominal structures can be used for detection of respiratory motion in coronary magnetic resonance imaging (MRI). Our laboratory has compared the effect of different navigator locations on image quality for coronary MRA, using a 2-D segmented *k*-space approach (27). Diaphragmatic and left ventricular navigators performed equally well; however, because positioning of the diaphragmatic navigator is less operator dependent and technically less demanding, and because of image artifacts associated with certain types of navigators (see later), most centers utilize this approach.

A 2-D selective excitation can be used to generate the navigator beam and readout is performed in only one direction. Depending on the nature of the sequence, the operator prescribes either the position of the navigator beam itself (Fig. 19.5) or two planes the intercepting line of which corresponds to the navigator beam (Fig. 19.6). The navigator sequences can be implemented before, after, or both before and after image data acquisition. The timing of the navigator sequence relative to the imaging sequence is dependent on the hardware design of the MR scanner. Rejection/acceptance of image data can be performed either retrospectively or prospectively depending on the timing of the navigator sequence in relation to image data acquisition.

The readout of the excited beam is in one only direction (along the axis of the beam); this eliminates the need for any phase-encoding steps and can be performed in a short time (20–60 msec). Potential limitations of navigator sequences include the following:

1. Although relatively short, the time spent for excitation and analysis of navigator position can be prohibitively long for certain types of studies. For example, when navigators are used to correct image position during breathholding for cine left ventricular function studies (28), delaying the image acquisition for more than 40 msec following the QRS complex may result in erroneous measurement of the end-diastolic volume and ejection fraction (29).

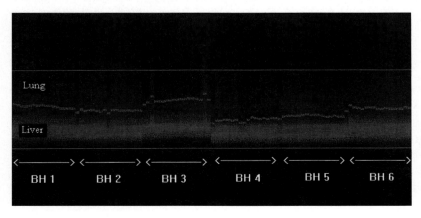

Figure 19.2. Diaphragmatic position of a normal volunteer in six serial breathholds (BH). The lung–liver interface is detected with a navigator beam positioned vertically at the dome of the right hemidiaphragm. Variable depth of breathholding results in variable diaphragmatic position.

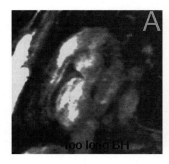
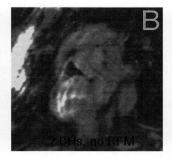
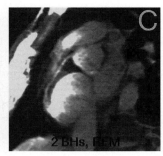

Figure 19.3. Proximal right coronary artery in a double oblique projection. Image degradation occurs with poor breathholding (BH) technique. (A) The subject was unable to sustain an 18 heartbeat breathhold. (B) Two 10-heartbeat breathholds without respiratory feedback monitoring (RFM) were used to repeat the scan. Misregistration resulted in image degradation. (C) The two breathholds were repeated with feedback monitoring. Improved slice registration resulted in better image quality. (Reprinted with permission from Wang (16).)

Figure 19.4. Diaphragmatic position of a normal volunteer assessed with a navigator beam during free breathing. Positive values represent expiratory diaphragmatic positions, and negative values inspiratory ones. Sampling of the diaphragmatic position is performed once in every cardiac cycle. The position of a typical 4-mm gating window is also indicated.

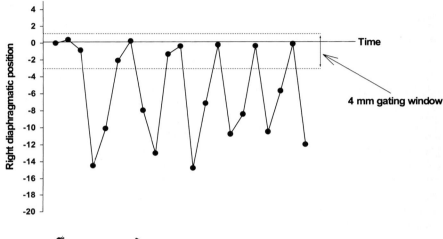

Figure 19.5. Diagram showing the positioning of a cylindrical navigator on the dome of the right hemidiaphragm, using coronal (left panel) and transverse (right panel) scout images. AAo = ascending aorta, DAo = descending aorta, LL = left lung, LV = left ventricle, Nav = navigator, RHD = right hemidiaphragm, RL = right lung, RV = right ventricle.

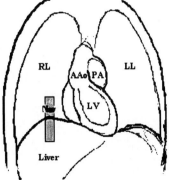

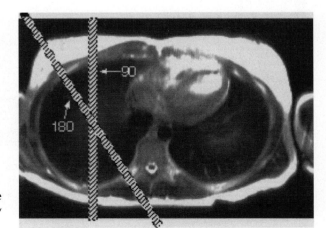

Figure 19.6. Positioning of a navigator (intersecting planes) on the dome of the right hemidiaphragm, using a coronal image. (Courtesy of James W. Goldfarb, Ph.D., Boston.)

2. Use of high-excitation flip angle for the navigator beam (e.g., typically used in crossing-plane navigators and certain applications of cylindrical navigators), result in loss of tissue magnetization at the location of the navigator. This is of particular importance when the navigator crosses the imaging region-of-interest. An exaggerated example of such an effect is shown in Figure 19.7: Increase of the navigator flip angle to 180 degrees creates an image artifact at the position of the navigator.

3. Cylindrical navigators may be susceptible to off-resonance effects on fat signal excited by higher-order harmonics.

Navigators and Respiratory Physiology

Navigators offer a unique tool to noninvasively quantitate respiratory diaphragmatic kinematics. Even though similar information can be obtained by fluoroscopy, this would require significant radiation exposure. Gamma-scintigraphy has also been used (30), but it has significantly lower spatial resolution than does MRI, and is it also associated with radiation exposure. Although ultrasonography overcomes limitations of these methods (31), it is unsuitable for prolonged studies and is largely operator dependent. Use of external monitoring devices (e.g., mouth spirometry, chest-wall plethysmography, or direct subject observation) use indirect indexes to measure diaphragmatic excursion. Taylor et al. (32) studied the respiratory kinematics in 10 volunteers during free breathing in supine position over 35 minutes, using MR navigator sequences through the dome of the right hemidiaphragm. This study confirmed that the *end-expiratory* dwell time of the right hemidiaphragm is almost threefold greater than the corresponding *end-in-*

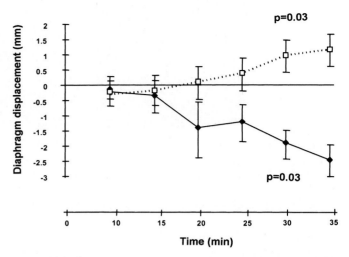

Figure 19.8. Average end-expiratory diaphragm position plotted against time for subjects in whom end-expiratory position drifts up (– □ –, $n = 5$) and in whom it drifts down (-◆-, $n = 4$). Error bars represent standard error of the mean. Zero represents calculated end-expiratory point for first respiratory trace. Analysis of variance (ANOVA) for linear trend p values are shown. (*From*: MR navigator-echo monitoring of temporal changes in diaphragm position implications for MR coronary angiography. Taylor et al., *J Magn Reson Imag* 1997. Reprinted by permission of Wiley-Liss, Inc., a subsidiary of John Wiley & Sons, Inc.)

spiratory dwell time. In addition, the end-expiratory diaphragmatic position was found to have greater stability than the end-inspiratory one (standard deviation 1.9 mm vs. 5.9 mm, respectively). The authors also reported that during prolonged recumbence, the diaphragm tends to drift (usually in a cephalad direction). This drift may have implications for scans in which imaging time exceeds a few minutes (Fig. 19.8).

Our laboratory has also used diaphragmatic navigators to assess breathholding and to evaluate the effect of supplemental oxygen administration and hyperventilation on the breathhold duration (33). It was noted in a study including 10 volunteers that during breathholding, the diaphragm drifted (2–16 mm) toward a cephalad direction in all subjects, and this drift was proportionately greater in the first 10 seconds of breathholding. These observations have direct implications for imaging that requires high degrees of intrathoracic or intraabdominal organ stability.

Navigator Gating Strategies for Coronary MRA

Retrospective Navigator Gating

With this implementation, navigator data are acquired (and analyzed) *after* the acquisition of image data in each cardiac cycle (Fig. 19.9). If for a certain cardiac cycle the tissue interface is within the preset gating window from the reference position (usually end-expiration), then data are accepted. If not, data are rejected. Several cen-

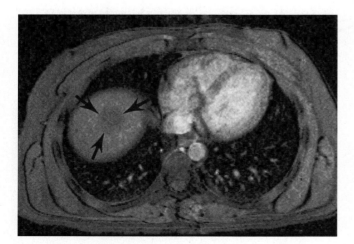

Figure 19.7. Artifact from a navigator beam positioned at the dome of the right hemidiaphragm (arrows). To make this image, the excitation angle of the navigator sequence was increased to 180 degrees.

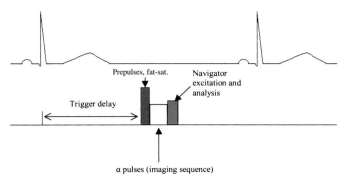

Figure 19.9. Retrospective navigator gating. The navigator sequence follows image data acquisition.

ters have investigated the use of retrospective navigator gating. The application of this technique for coronary MRA was first described in normal volunteers by Hofman et al. (34), who evaluated MR coronary arteriograms of 10 subjects and compared a 2-D breathhold approach with a 3-D navigator gated technique. In that study, both techniques were able to visualize the proximal parts of the coronary arteries with comparable vessel length and vessel diameter values. Images obtained with breathholding, however, were "sharper" than those obtained with respiratory gating. It should be noted, however, that the acquisition window (per cardiac cycle) was threefold *longer* for the 3-D navigator gated approach; this would result in more cardiac motion during the 3-D acquisition window (35,36).

In a subsequent study by Li et al. (37), 3-D coronary MRA was performed in 12 healthy volunteers and 1 patient with coronary disease, using retrospective diaphragmatic navigator gating. These investigators measured the length of the coronary vessels visible with this technique, which was greater by a factor of 2, compared with previous reports. Upon direct comparison of gated with ungated images, the authors concluded that navigator respiratory gating significantly improved image quality.

A number of studies have also examined the application of retrospective navigator gating in patients with coronary disease. Post et al. (38) prospectively compared the 3-D navigator-gated coronary MRA with data from conventional X-ray coronary angiography in 20 patients. Although the length of the coronary vessels seen was significantly smaller than the study by Li et al. (37), these investigators reported high interobserver agreement (0.92, $k = 0.65$) and a high specificity (95%) of detecting coronary stenoses with coronary MRA. Müller et al. (39–41) have also used retrospective diaphragmatic navigator gating to evaluate coronary stenoses in patients with coronary disease. The authors reported high sensitivity (83%) and specificity (93%) in detecting coronary stenoses, although only 83% of the stenoses were detected and interpretable by coronary MRA. The same

group has also reported on the feasibility of this navigator-gated 3-D technique to evaluate recurrent coronary stenoses in patients undergoing balloon angioplasty (41).

All of these investigations have utilized retrospective navigator gating, with the navigator positioned at the dome of the right hemidiaphragm. This location is arbitrary, however, and is not a requirement for this approach.

Finally, retrospective navigator gating has been implemented with a phase-contrast quantification technique to measure blood flow in the right coronary artery (RCA) in six normal volunteers (42), and compared with standard breathhold acquisition. In this study, navigator-gated acquisitions provided consistently better image quality, particularly in systole and early diastole; thus, they appeared to be more robust than breathholding for flow measurements throughout the whole cardiac cycle. Similar results were reported by Post et al. (43) in eight patients who underwent conventional angiograms and Doppler flow measurements of the RCA with angiographically normal vessels. These investigators showed a good correlation ($r = 0.9, p < 0.005$) between coronary MRA and Doppler measurements.

Prospective Navigator Gating

With prospective navigator gating, the navigator excitation and analysis is performed *prior* to image data acquisition (Fig. 19.10). Similar to retrospective gating, if the tissue interface is determined to be within the prespecified gating window relative to the reference position, image data are accepted. If not, data are rejected.

The application of prospective navigator gating for coronary MRA was first described by Oshinski et al. (17). These investigators compared the use of respiratory gating with breathholding for coronary MRI in 20 healthy volunteers and 11 patients with coronary disease. For respiratory gating, two techniques were used: respiratory bellows and navigator gating. The authors suggested that respiratory gating with two signal averages had better image quality and signal-to-noise than breathholding. Navigator-gated images also had significantly better image quality (~20%) compared with the respiratory-belt gated images.

Information from navigator respiratory monitoring acquired prospectively, can be used for feedback to the subject during imaging. Using this approach for breathhold imaging combined with audio or visual feedback signals, Wang et al. have reported improved slice registration for 2-D (16) and 3-D (44) coronary MRA in volunteers. The same group (45) also described the use of a leading and a trailing navigator positioned at the posterior part of the diaphragm for 3-D coronary MRA in six healthy volunteers. A combination of prospective navigator gating (leading navigator) and retrospective

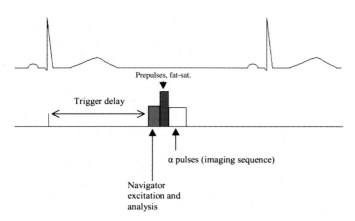

Figure 19.10. Prospective navigator gating. The navigator sequence precedes image data acquisition.

gating (trailing navigator) was compared against triggered acquisition with a coached breathing scheme (breathholding with feedback monitoring), having a two-signal average acquisition during free breathing as the reference for comparison. Both gated and triggered acquisitions were found to be similar to each other and significantly better than continuous (nongated) acquisitions.

Prospective navigator gating has also been applied for coronary flow measurements. Oshinski et al. (46) have studied flow in the RCA using a prospective navigator-gated phase-contrast technique in both a phantom model and eight volunteers. The investigators found a good accuracy for MR phantom flow rate measurements, and were also able to demonstrate the biphasic flow pattern in the RCA in the volunteers.

Navigator Gating with Prospective Slice Correction for Coronary MRA

This technique represents a refinement of the prospective navigator-gated approach. With this method, navigator position measurements are performed prospectively (i.e., *prior* to image data acquisition) and data from the analysis of the navigator position are prospectively incorporated to shift the slice position by adjusting the frequency of the slice-selective excitation, read-out frequency, and phase-encoding offset. The theoretical advantage of this technique is that because image data are corrected for position, a larger gating window can be used, and thus scan time efficiency (i.e., percentage of excitations that are accepted) can potentially improve.

When prospective real-time slice correction is used in combination with breathholding using a 2-D approach, slice registration significantly improves compared with standard 2-D imaging without navigator correction. In a study of 10 volunteers, we have previously shown that prospective navigator correction reduces registration er-

rors by approximately 50% (47). During free breathing, the application of slice correction algorithms in combination with prospective diaphragmatic navigator gating was also shown to improve image quality significantly, compared with navigator-gated images, using the same 2-D approach (48). This approach allows for use of larger gating windows without adverse effects on image quality, thereby increasing scan efficiency. Indeed, in our experience (48), the use of a diaphragmatic navigator with a 5-mm gating window and with prospective slice correction results in image quality similar to breathholding and to gated-only acquisitions with a 3-mm gating window, but with double the scan efficiency (i.e., half the imaging time). This approach can be also implemented with 3-D imaging techniques (Fig. 19.11).

These data have been confirmed by Oshinski et al. (49), who also found that using a diaphragmatic navigator with a 4–5-mm gating window with slice tracking (correction) image quality was similar to diaphragmatic navigator gating along with a 2-mm gating window. Bornstedt et al. (50) have also shown that when a constant gating window is used, the application of correction algorithms can improve image quality over navigator gating alone.

Limitations of Navigator Approaches

In addition to the physical limitations of navigators that have previously been discussed the implementation of navigators for coronary MRA has additional potential limitations. For good image quality, it is important that acquisition of the reference navigator is obtained at the end-expiratory position and while the patient/volunteer is breathing quietly. Although information from a respiratory belt or a preliminary set of navigator data can be used to determine this position, obtaining a good reference navigator may be challenging and requiring operator expertise. Furthermore, during MR scanning, diaphragmatic drift is common (31,32), and this results in a shift of the end-expiratory position. The use of a "fixed" gating window results in a significant decrease of scan efficiency and in acquisition of data during periods of fast diaphragmatic motion, which result in motion artifacts and image degradation. Although shifting the gating window to track the diaphragmatic drift may improve efficiency, it may also introduce data registration errors.

Current correction algorithms (for implementation with slice correction techniques) assume a constant relationship between diaphragmatic and cardiac motion (51); however, such a constant relationship throughout the respiratory cycle, among different respiratory cycles in the same individual, and among individuals, is unlikely. Bornstedt (50) has shown that the use of a con-

Figure 19.11. Coronary MRA in a normal volunteer. Serial transverse slices at the level of the aortic root, using a 3-D TFE sequence with prospective navigator gating with slice correction. The navigator beam was positioned on the right hemidiaphragm and a 5-mm gating window was used. The plane resolution is 0.7 × 1.0 mm. Portions of the left anterior descending (curved arrow), left circumflex (LCx) (arrowhead), and right coronary artery (straight arrow) are noted.

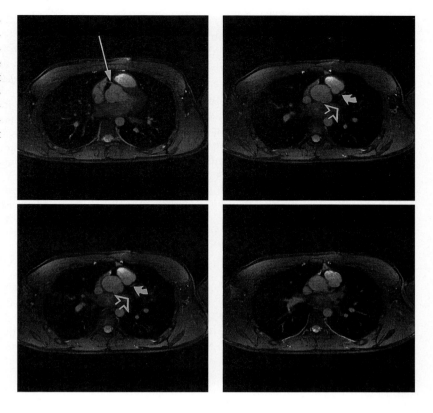

stant algorithm may actually result in worsening of image quality. We have investigated the relationship between cardiac and diaphragmatic position in normal volunteers and found that it is patient-specific, and may also vary within each subject depending on the gating window used (52). These data suggest that the use of individualized correction algorithms might be needed for the image detail required for coronary MRA.

Future Perspectives

The use of navigators for coronary MRA has been developed with new technologic advances. The use of multiple navigators has been described (53), and offers the potential to adjust slice position in both the craniocaudal direction (primary axis of motion) as well as in the anteroposterior and lateral directions. Although the anteroposterior and lateral displacement of the heart are proportionately smaller than the craniocaudal motion, adjustments for these motions may provide an incremental benefit in image quality for coronary MRA. Indeed, this technique has been applied for coronary MRA with promising results (54).

Other advances relate to more efficient uses of the information derived by the navigators. One of these approaches has been termed *diminishing variance algorithm* (DVA) and claims to overcome some of the previous acceptance–rejection algorithm limitations (55). With DVA approaches, a preliminary data set is acquired during free breathing, with navigator position information linked to the image data. Then, the most common navigator position is determined (corresponding to the end-expiratory position). Subsequent image data are acquired for those k-space lines that the original navigator position was the farthest away from end-expiration. Image data acquisition continues until the operator is satisfied with the resulting image quality, which is monitored in real time. This method is likely to have optimal scan efficiency, and negates the operator determining of end-expiration to obtain the reference navigator. However, image quality still remains susceptible to bulk patient motion artifacts and "correction" algorithms are more complex.

A Hybrid Phase-Ordered Phase Encoding has also been reported for coronary MRA (56). This technique allows for use of large (10 mm) gating windows to improve scan time efficiency. Data that fall in a narrow range (i.e., 5 mm) around the end-expiratory position are used to fill the central lines of k-space, whereas data from more distant positions are used to fill in outer lines of k-space. This differential weighting of data maximizes the efficiency of the navigator-gated approaches.

Finally, application of individualized correction algorithms for motion correction may have a role, if diaphragmatic navigator detection is to be employed. The improvement in spatial resolution of navigators, and the shortening of the time spent for navigator data acquisition and analysis, also have potential to enhance efficiency for navigator-gated and/or corrected images. Use of contrast media for coronary MRA with navigator gating and/or correction has already been shown to improve the signal-to-noise ratio and image quality in preliminary studies (57,58), whereas the addition of prepulses does not seem to affect the effectiveness of the navigator information (59). The role of navigators in coronary MRA will likely be important for future applications, particularly with evolving fast imaging approaches (54,60). Further advances in this field will likely establish coronary MRA as a significant diagnostic tool for a broad patient population in the years to come.

The winds and waves are always on the side of the ablest navigators.

(Edward Gibbon, 1737–1794)

Acknowledgments. The authors would like to acknowledge Matthias Stuber, PhD, for his helpful comments and review.

References

1. McDonald IG. The shape and movements of the human left ventricle during systole. Am J Cardiol 1970;26:221–30.
2. Lanzer P, Botnivick EH, Schiller NB, et al. Cardiac imaging using gated magnetic resonance. Radiology 1984;150:121–27.
3. Alfidi RJ, Masaryk TJ, Haacke EM, et al. MR angiography of peripheral, carotid and coronary arteries. Am J Roentgenol 1987;149:1097–109.
4. Paulin S, von Schulthess GK, Fossel E, Krayenbuehl HP. MR imaging of the aortic root and proximal coronary arteries. Am J Roentgenol 1987;148:665–70.
5. Lanzer P, Barta C, Botnivick EH, et al. EKG-synchronized cardiac MR imaging: method and evaluation. Radiology 1985;155:681–86.
6. Edelman RR, Manning WJ, Burstein D, Paulin S. Coronary arteries: breath-hold MR angiography. Radiology 1991;181:641–43.
7. Meyer CH, Hu BS, Nishimura DG, Macovski A. Fast spiral coronary artery imaging. Magn Reson Med 1992;28:202–13.
8. Manning WJ, Li W, Boyle NG, Edelman RR. Fat-suppressed breath-hold magnetic resonance coronary angiography. Circulation 1993;87:94–104.
9. Gay SB, Sistrom CL, Holder CA, Suratt PM. Breath-holding capability of adults. Invest Radiol 1994;29:848–51.
10. Grist TM, Pozlin JA, Bianco JA, et al. Measurement of coronary blood flow and flow reserve using magnetic resonance imaging. Cardiology 1997;88:80–89.
11. Globits S, Sakuma H, Shimakawa A, et al. Measurement of coronary blood flow velocity during handgrip exercise using breath-hold velocity encoded cine magnetic resonance imaging. Am J Cardiol 1997;79:234–37.
12. Nitz WR, Stingl D, Kessler W, et al. Blood flow within the internal thoracic mammary arteries: conventional flow quantification versus segmented flow quantification (abstr.). Proc Int Soc Magn Reson Med 1996;1:667.
13. Goldfarb JW, Li W, Griswold MA, et al. Contrast enhanced breath-hold 3D coronary magnetic resonance angiography (abstr.). Proc Int Soc Magn Reson Med 1997;1:441.
14. Doyle M, Scheidegger MB, de Graaf RG, et al. Coronary artery imaging in multiple 1-sec breath-holds. Magn Reson Imag 1993;11:3–6.
15. Liu YL, Riederer SJ, Rossman PJ, et al. A monitoring, feedback, and triggering system for reproducible breath-hold MR imaging. Magn Reson Med 1993;30:507–11.
16. Wang Y, Christy PS, Korosec FR, et al. Coronary MRI with a respiratory feedback monitor: the 2D imaging case. Magn Reson Med 1995;33:116–21.
17. Wang Y, Grist TM, Korosec FR, et al. Respiratory blur in 3D coronary MR imaging. Magn Reson Med 1995;33:541–48.
18. Ehman RL, McNamara MT, Pallack M, et al. Magnetic resonance imaging with respiratory gating: techniques and advantages. Am J Roentgenol 1984;143:1175–82.
19. Oshinski JN, Hofland L, Mukundan S, et al. Two-dimensional coronary MR angiography without breath holding. Radiology 1996;201:737–43.
20. Webster's Ninth New Collegiate Dictionary. Merriam-Webster Inc. Publishers: Springfield, MA, 1988:789.
21. Ehman RL, Felmlee JP. Adaptive technique for high-definition MR imaging of moving structures. Radiology 1989;173:255–63.
22. Korin HW, Felmlee JP, Ehman RL, Riederer SJ. Adaptive technique for three-dimensional MR imaging of moving structures. Radiology 1990;177:217–21.
23. Felmlee JP, Ehman RL, Riederer SJ, Korin HW. Adaptive motion compensation in MRI: accuracy of motion measurement. Magn Reson Med 1991;18:207–13.
24. Sachs TS, Meyer CH, Hu BS, et al. Real-time motion detection in spiral MRI using navigators. Magn Reson Med 1994;32:639–45.
25. Fu ZW, Wang Y, Grimm RC, et al. Orbital navigator echoes for motion measurements in magnetic resonance imaging. Magn Reson Med 1995;34:746–53.
26. Wang Y, Grimm RC, Felmlee JP, et al. Algorithms for extracting motion information from navigator echoes. Magn Reson Med 1996;36:117–23.
27. McConnell MVM, Khasgiwala VC, Savord BJ, et al. Comparison of respiratory suppression methods and navigator locations for MR coronary angiography. Am J Roentgenol 1997;168:1369–75.
28. Chuang ML, Chen MH, Khasgiwala VC, et al. Adaptive correction of imaging plane position in segmented k-space cine cardiac MRI. J Magn Reson Imag 1997;7:811–14.
29. Arai A, Gangireddy C, Abouasali M, Wolff S. 20–35% errors in LV end diastolic volume estimates using FASTCARD. Proc SCMR 1988:9.
30. Wade OL. Movements of the thoracic vage and diaphragm in respiration. J Physiol 1954;124:193–212.
31. Weiss PH, Baker JM, Potchen EJ. Assessment of hepatic respiratory excursion. J Nucl Med 1972;13:758–59.
32. Taylor AM, Jhooti P, Wiessmann F, et al. MR navigator-echo monitoring of temporal changes in diaphragm position: implications for MR coronary angiography. J Magn Reson Imag 1997;7:629–36.

33. Danias PG, Kissinger KV, Stuber M, et al. Breath-hold duration: navigator echo assessment of supplemental oxygen and hyperventilation. Proc SCMR 1998:28.

34. Hofman MBM, Paschal CB, Li D, et al. MRI of coronary arteries: 2D breath-hold vs. 3D respiratory gated acquisition. J Comput Assist Tomogr 1995;19:56–62.

35. Hofman MBM, van Rossum AC, Sprenger M, Westerhof N. Assessment of flow in the right human coronary artery by magnetic resonance phase contrast velocity measurement: effects of cardiac and respiratory motion. Magn Reson Med 1996;35:521–31.

36. Sodickson DK, Chuang ML, Khasgiwala VC, Manning WJ. In-plane motion of the left and right coronary arteries during the cardiac cycle (abstr.). Proc Intern Soc Magn Reson Med 1997;2:910.

37. Li D, Kaushikkar S, Haacke EM, et al. Coronary arteries: three dimensional MR imaging with retrospective respiratory gating. Radiology 1996;201:857–63.

38. Post JC, van Rossum AC, Hofman MBM, et al. Three-dimensional respiratory-gated MR angiography of coronary arteries: comparison with conventional angiography. Am J Roentgenol 1996;166:1399–404.

39. Müller MF, Fleisch M, Kroecker R. Coronary arteries: three-dimensional MR imaging with fat saturation and navigator echo (abstr.). Proc Intern Soc Magn Reson Med 1996;1:160.

40. Müller MF, Fleisch M, Kroecker R, et al. Proximal coronary artery stenosis: three-dimensional MRI with fat saturation and navigator echo. J Magn Reson Imag 1996;7:644–51.

41. Müller MF, Fleisch M, Kroeker R, Chatterjee T, Meier B, Vock P. Proximal coronary artery stenosis: three-dimensional MRI with fat saturation and navigator echo. J Magn Reson Imaging 1997;7:644–51.

42. Hofman MB, van Rossum AC, Sprenger M, Westerhof N. Assessment of flow in the right human coronary artery by magnetic resonance phase contrast velocity measurement: effects of cardiac and respiratory motion. Magn Reson Med 1996;35:521–31.

43. Post JC, Hofman MBM, Piek JJ, et al. Flow assessment in the right coronary artery: navigator-echo-based respiratory-gated MR measurement vs intravascular Doppler guidewire measurement (abstr.). Proc Int Soc Magn Reson Med 1997;1:446.

44. Wang Y, Grimm RC, Rossman PJ, et al. 3D coronary MR angiography in multiple breath-holds using a respiratory feedback monitor. Magn Reson Med 1995;34:11–16.

45. Wang Y, Rossman PJ, Grimm RC, et al. Navigator-echo-based real-time respiratory gating and triggering for reduction of respiration effects in three-dimensional MR angiography. Radiology 1996;198:55–60.

46. Oshinski JN, Hahn PY, Seibert K, Pettigrew RI. Navigator

echo gated coronary flow measurements (abstr.). Proc Int Soc Magn Reson Med 1997;1:108.

47. McConnell MVM, Khasgiwala VC, Savord BJ, et al. Prospective adaptive navigator correction for breathhold MR coronary angiography. Magn Reson Med 1997;37;148–52.

48. Danias PG, McConnell MV, Khasgiwala VC, et al. Prospective navigator correction of image position for coronary MR angiography. Radiology 1997;203:733–36.

49. Oshinski JN, Dixon WT, Salverda P, et al. Magnetic resonance coronary angiography using prospective navigator echo-based slice following. Proc SCMR 1998;39.

50. Nagel E, Bornstedt A, Schnackenburg B, Hug J, Oswald H, Fleck E. Optimization of realtime adaptive navigator correction for 3D magnetic resonance coronary angiography. Magn Reson Med 1999;42:408–11.

51. Wang Y, Riederer SJ, Ehman RL. Respiratory motion of the heart: kinematics and the implications for the spatial resolution in coronary imaging. Magn Reson Med 1995;33:713–19.

52. Danias PG, Stuber M, Botnar RM, Kissinger KV, Edelman RR, Manning WJ. Relationship between motion of coronary arteries and diaphragm during free breathing: lessons from real-time MR imaging. AJR Am J Roentgenol 1999;172:1061–61

53. Sachs T, Meyer C, Hu B, et al. A new approach to respiratory kinematics using navigator echoes. Proc Int Soc Magn Reson Med 1997;463.

54. Sachs TS, Meyer CH, Pauly JM, Hu BS, Nishimura DG, Macovski A. The real-time interactive 3-D-DVA for robust coronary MRA. IEEE Trans Med Imaging 2000;19:73–79.

55. Sachs TS, Meyer CH, Irarrazabal P, et al. The diminishing variance algorithm for real-time reduction of motion artifacts in MRI. Magn Reson Med 1995;34:412–22.

56. Jhooti P, Keegan J, Gatehouse PD, et al. 3D coronary artery imaging with phase reordering for improved scan efficiency. Magn Reson Med 1999;41:555–62.

57. Stuber M, Botnar RM, Danias PG, et al. Contrast agent-enhanced, free-breathing, three-dimensional coronary magnetic resonace angiography. J Magn Reson Imaging 1999;10:790–99.

58. Johansson LO, Hofman MBM, Fischer SE, et al. Intravascular contrast agent improves 3D magnetic resonance coronary angiography in humans. Proc SCMR 1998:50.

59. Botnar RM, Stuber M, Danias PG, Kissinger KV, Manning WJ. Improved coronary artery definition with T2- weighted, free-breathing, three-dimensional coronary MRA. Circulation 1999;99:3139–48.

60. Stuber M, Botnar RM, Danias PG, Kissinger KV, Manning WJ. Breath-hold 3D coronary MRA using real-time navigator technology. J Cardiovasc Magn Reson 1999;1:233–38.

20
Third-Generation Coronary MRA Techniques and Other New Techniques

André J. Duerinckx

Introduction and Overview

Even before the initial preclinical trials with first- and second-generation techniques were completed the need for more user-friendly and less time-consuming coronary magnetic resonance angiographic (MRA) techniques emerged. Interest in this problem has grown significantly in the last several years as witnessed by the number of abstracts on the topic presented at international scientific meetings organized by societies such as the International Society for Magnetic Resonance in Medicine (ISMRM), the North American Society for Cardiac Imaging (NASCI), and the Society for Cardiovascular Magnetic Resonance (SCMR). The creativity of the many researchers in this field has been amazing. In this chapter we will list several of the more promising approaches and propose techniques to solving this problem.

A subset of the many new techniques that have been described will be referred to as the "third-generation coronary MRA techniques." They can be described most simplistically as the "multiple slices in one breathhold" techniques. There is not a single third-generation technique, but several variants, including those without cardiac gating adequate to image portions of coronary bypass grafts. Several third-generation coronary MRA techniques are now being developed that combine some of the user-friendliness of the second-generation techniques with the speed and reliability of the first-generation techniques. Some of these techniques acquire the entire cardiac anatomy in a single breathhold with isotropic resolution. We will summarize some of the more important features of these techniques in this chapter, and refer the reader to other chapters for additional descriptions of techniques (Chap. 3), history (Chap. 4), early clinical applications (Chaps. 10 and 11), and associated techniques (Chap. 21).

Projectional Techniques

Projectional MR coronary angiography techniques use special inversion pulses to manipulate contrast while acquiring one thick slice through the vessel. One such technique has been tested by Wang et al. (1) from the Stanford University group. They used two breathhold acquisitions of a projection two-dimensional (2-D) data set in late diastole that were subtracted. The first one was preceded with a thick selective 180-degree inversion slab applied through the aorta at end systole. The second one was without the inversion.

A variant of this technique was proposed by Edelman et al. and called the "Signal Targeting with Alternating Radiofrequency" (STAR) technique (2). This was extended to an echoplanar version, the echoplanar-STAR (EPISTAR) (3) technique. These projectional techniques with breathholding did not gain widespread acceptance due to difficulties with their implementation (1,2).

Echoplaner Imaging Approaches

"State-of-the-art" gradient hardware has become widely available in new commercial magnetic resonance imaging (MRI) units, providing stronger imaging gradients (> 20 mT/m) and enhanced rise times (slew rates > 80 mT/m/ms). In addition, phased-array coil technology can deliver better signal-to-noise ratios (SNR) over wide field-of-views (FOVs). Together these have made it practical to reduce repetition times (TR) for turboFLASH readouts, effectively increasing the number of lines collected per unit time to provide faster and higher spatial resolution and reliability for breathhold cardiac examinations. High-performance gradient systems have made it possible to produce three-dimensional (3-D) volumetric imaging of the heart using segmented echo planar imaging (EPI) techniques as first described in 1995 by Piotr Wielopolski (4,5). Three-dimensional breathhold coronary MRA using 3-D segmented EPI (4,6) has been demonstrated on 1.5 and 0.5 Tesla MR scanners. The EPI approach to 2-D coronary MRI is so fast that it does not require breathholding; rather, its spatial resolution and SNR are limited (7), which explains the interest in segmented 2-D EPI with breathholding (8) and its extension into 3-D segmented EPI. The 3-D segmented EPI technique (4) was implemented on a noncommercial 1.5 Tesla MR imager (Siemens Medical Systems, Iselin, NJ) with a maximum gradient strength of 38 mT/m and a maximum slew rate of 152 T/m/sec, which is more than what most commercial 1.5 Tesla scanners can achieve today. The technique used fat-suppression and was tested on 15 healthy volunteers only. Six echoes were collected per ratio frequency (RF) excitation (in a time TR = 8.9 msec), with up to Ns = 32 slices, corresponding to an acquisition window of Ns × TR = 285 msec per heartbeat. This required 22 heartbeats per 3-D image set for a 126 × 256 matrix. Slice thickness was 4–12 mm. A repeated breathhold segmented 3-D EPI technique at 0.5 Tesla has also been described (6,9). The 3-D segmented EPI approach may have a great clinical future as EPI technology becomes more readily available on commercial clinical MR imagers.

Free-breathing 3-D coronary MRA with a fast multishot EPI (TFE-EPI) acquisition technique has also been described (10–12).

Higher-Resolution Imaging: Interleaved Spiral Scanning, SMASH, and SENSE Techniques

Several techniques have been proposed to increase the spatial resolution of coronary MRA. The same techniques can also be used to increase temporal resolution for real-time imaging. We will briefly describe three of these techniques.

Three-dimensional interleaved spiral scanning has also been described (13–15), including a first preclinical study of multislice spiral coronary MRA on 18 men and 5 women (16). This implementation used an interleaved spiral sequence. A single spiral interleave was collected over 17 msec. Slice thickness is 5 mm. In-plane resolution was 1.1–1.3 mm. Multislice imaging efficiently used the imaging sequence interval. The 10–20 interleaves for the entire multislice set were acquired on successive cardiac cycles during a single breathhold. Although data for the entire volume was collected over 500–900 msec per cardiac cycle, adjacent-slice acquisitions were temporally offset by only the sequence repetition time of 45 msec. The seqeunce was implemented on a standard 1.5 Tesla Scanner (GE, Signa). Data acquisition was started after early diastole to reduce cardiac motion. Hu et al. were able to

detect 63% of lesions among 27 significant lesions in 18 patients (see also Chap. 13) (16).

SiMultaneous Acquisition of Spatial Harmonics (SMASH) is a new fast-imaging technique that increases MRI acquisition speed by an integer factor over existing fast-imaging methods, without significant sacrifices in spatial resolution or SNR (17). Image acquisition time is reduced by exploiting spatial information inherent in the geometry of a surface coil array to substitute for some of the phase encoding usually produced by magnetic field gradients. This allows for partially parallel image acquisitions using many of the existing fast-imaging sequences. Unlike the data combination algorithms of prior proposals for parallel imaging, SMASH reconstruction involves a small set of MR signal combinations prior to Fourier transformation, which can be advantageous for artifact handling and practical implementation. Savings in image acquisition time has been demonstrated using commercial phased-array coils on two different MRI systems, and larger time savings factors can be expected for appropriate coil designs (17). The SMASH technique has been successfully applied to cardiac MRI (18,19) and coronary MRA (20). Further improvements (e.g., AUTO-SMASH) have also been described (21). This self-calibrating approach is an effective method to increase the potential and the flexibility of rapid imaging with SMASH. With AUTO-SMASH coil sensitivity information required for SMASH imaging is obtained during the actual scan using correlations between undersampled SMASH signal data and additionally sampled calibration signals with appropriate offsets in k-space. The advantages of this sensitivity reference method are that no extra coil array sensitivity maps have to be acquired and that it provides coil sensitivity information in areas of highly nonuniform spin density. This auto-calibrating approach can easily be implemented with only a small sacrifice of the overall time savings afforded by SMASH imaging.

Other fast techniques have been described [e.g., SENSitivity encoding (for convenience: SENSE)] (22–24). As with SMASH this technique uses a reconstruction method that allows for saving phase-encoding steps when an array of receiver coils is used. Sensitivity encoding allows acceleration of cardiac breathhold imaging. The limits of the technique arise from loss in SNR due to undersampling and coil geometry (23).

Third-Generation Coronary MRA Using a 3-D Breathhold Cardiac-Gated TurboFLASH Approach

If single breathhold volumetric imaging of the heart with isotropic resolution is performed, the inspection of such volume data sets using multiplanar reformations

(MPR) can yield information on the optimal double oblique volume orientation to further investigate the entire coronary anatomy with smaller targeted volumes. Wielopolski et al. (5,25) have explored this possibility and taken advantage of the high-performance gradient hardware now available to obtain the highest in-plane resolution and volume coverage possible within the context of a comfortable breathhold. They denominated this approach as volume coronary angiography using targeted scans (VCATS) with the primary goal to cover the coronary anatomy in a few breathholds and to avoid the slice misregistration problems during review that are present with breathhold 2-D coronary MRA (first-generation technique). Other groups have since developed variants of this technique (26,27). We will briefly review some of the key features of the Wielopolski version of this technique (5).

Coronary screening was performed using two 3-D MR pulse sequences with two clearly defined objectives: localization and targeting (5). A volume localizer is used to scan the entire heart volume to provide the necessary input data for the targeted scans of the coronaries VCATS. The procedure for the localization and evaluation of all coronary segments is summarized in the following steps:

1. Use a single end-expiration breathhold 3-D localizer to cover the entire heart.
2. The heart volume localizer data is loaded into the MPR platform and evaluated by focusing on one coronary segment at a time.
3. The optimal double oblique plane and slab position containing the coronary segment of interest is recorded.
4. Slab position and double oblique plane orientation are used for the end-expiration breathhold VCATS.
5. The process is repeated (steps 2–4) until all coronary segments are evaluated.

Scanning was performed on a 1.5T Magnetom Vision platform (Siemens Medical Systems, Erlangen, Germany) (5). The whole-body coil was used for signal excitation. All subjects were positioned supine with a four-channel quadrature body phased-array coil placed over the thorax for signal reception. Sequences were designed to use the maximum gradient strength available, 25 mT/m, and gradient rise times of 300 μsec (83 T/m/sec) in resonant mode for the heart volume localizer and 600 μsec (42 T/m/sec) in nonresonant mode for VCATS, respectively.

VCATS was performed using a double oblique 3-D segmented turboFLASH sequence with TR/TE = 5.3/2.3 msec, which was selected to target each coronary segment. The readout module acquired 21 lines per segment with partial Fourier encoding with an acquisition window of 110 msec per cardiac period. The volume targeted was set to 24 mm. The sequence was tailored to permit a minimum FOV of 230 mm for a 256

matrix using a readout bandwidth of 390 Hz/pixel. Magnetization Transfer Contrast (MTC) radio frequency pulses were applied prior to a single chemical shift fat suppression pulse with the same irradiation time and characteristics as for the heart volume localizer. Seven slice-select phase-encoding steps encoded the volume, and the number of reconstructed sections was freely selectable to ease the review process (default = 16 1.5-mm-thick reconstructed sections). The slice selection profile was optimized to deliver a sharply defined volume with minimal aliasing and SNR loss at the edge sections. An incremental flip-angle series was used to optimize SNR (linear increment, 14–34 degrees). The measurement time was 21 heartbeats using a $126h \times 256$ acquisition matrix (h = partial Fourier encoding). An FOV of 320 mm was selected with a rectangular FOV ratio of 0.75. The trigger delay matched that of the volumetric heart localizer, and the data was acquired during end-expiration.

An example of a 3-D data set obtained with this technique is shown in Figure 20.1. The small volume acquisitions use fat-suppressed 3-D segmented turboFLASH with EKG-gating and fast acquisitions times to allow breathholding. These are EKG-triggered fast implementations of the by-now-established dynamic contrast-enhanced MRA techniques (see upcoming description). These new pulse sequences are now being implemented by some vendors for use on the next generation software release for commercial MR scanners. Exciting preliminary clinical results have been reported (28), and examples are shown in Figure 20.2.

Wielopolski et al. have suggested that breathhold VCATS is a promising alternative for coronary screening if image resolution can be improved by keeping SNR at adequate levels that provide the necessary diagnostic confidence (5). He believes that this may be possible in the near future with the introduction of contrast agents that produce short T1s in blood (< 50 msec) and provide the SNR enhancement necessary. Contrast agents can also provide the fat signal reduction by using a T1-weighted approach that could eliminate the field homogeneity–dependent chemical shift fat suppression.

Third-Generation Coronary MRA Using a 3-D Breathhold Cardiac-Gated TrueFISP Approach

Newer variants of 3-D coronary MRA techniques rely on the pulse sequences developed for real-time cardiac MRI (29,30). Deshpande et al. (31) have described 3-D MR coronary artery imaging using magnetization-prepared EKG-triggered TrueFISP. TrueFISP is Siemens terminology, also called Balanced Fast Field Echo (BFFE) by Philips or Single Shot Free Processing (SSFP)

B

A

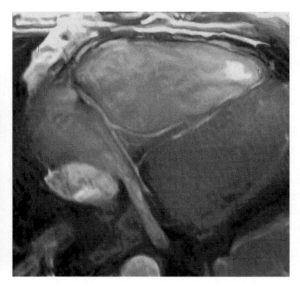

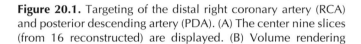

Figure 20.1. Targeting of the distal right coronary artery (RCA) and posterior descending artery (PDA). (A) The center nine slices (from 16 reconstructed) are displayed. (B) Volume rendering integrates the entire course of the distal right coronary artery (RCA). CS = Coronary sinus, MCV = Middle cardiac vein. (Reprinted with permission from Wielopolski (5).)

by General Electric. TrueFISP is a fast imaging approach that gives rise to high signal-to-noise ratio and T1/T2-weighted contrast because it maintains the transverse magnetization within each TR which contributes to the signal intensity. The major problem with TrueFISP has been off-resonance artifacts due to field inhomogeneities. These effects can be minimized by using short TRs with a high-performance gradient system. As a result, TrueFISP has dramatically improved blood signal and contrast over conventional FLASH in cardiac cine imaging. Deshpande et al. (31) investigated the utility of TrueFISP for 3-D coronary artery imaging, but a similar approach could possibly be used for real-time coronary imaging. More information on this 3-D approach will be provided in Chapter 20.

In each cardiac cycle, after the appropriate trigger de-lay, a fat saturation pulse was first applied. This was followed by a prepulse, and 20 dummy pulses to prepare the magnetization to approach a steady state. A segmented TrueFISP sequence was then used to acquire data with a symmetric gradient structure in all three directions. Normal volunteers were studied to compare 3-D TrueFISP and FLASH for coronary artery imaging. The TR was the same for the two sequence (3.8 ms) and each scan was collected within a single breath-hold. Coronary artery SNR was improved by >50% and myocardial signal was significantly suppressed in TrueFISP images, resulting in dramatic improvements in coronary artery visualization, especially in distal portions. Deshpande et al. (31) concluded that TrueFISP is a very promising approach for 3-D breathhold coronary artery imaging.

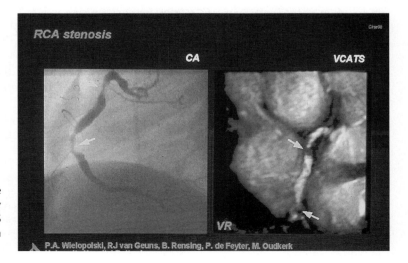

Figure 20.2. Detection of a RCA lesion using the VCATS technique. (A) Conventional X-ray coronary angiogram. (B) 3-D rendering of the RCA using VCATS data. Courtesy of Van Geuns and Wielopolski, with permission.

Dynamic Contrast-Enhanced 3-D Breathhold Noncardiac-Gated TurboFLASH

MR contrast agents will have a dramatic effect on coronary MRA techniques, just as dynamic contrast-enhanced MRA has totally changed the way thoracic and body MRA are performed today. Dynamic contrast-enhanced MRA was first described by Prince in 1993. When first described the acquisition times were very long (more than 1 minute). Much shorter acquisitions allowing breathholding are now utilized (32–41). Breathhold periods of 7–23 seconds for carotid MRA, and pulmonary MRA, are routinely used at some centers. The same non-EKG-triggered technique can be applied for native coronary artery (42) and coronary artery bypass graft (CABG) imaging (43–45).

In order to EKG trigger these MRA pulse sequences for native coronary vessel imaging, one needs to use faster acquisitions rates, k-space data segmentation, data interpolation, and other technical tricks. These 3-D breathhold EKG-triggered MRA techniques are what we described as the "third-generation techniques" (see above).

Contrast Agents for 3-D Breathhold Imaging

Limited work on the use of gadolinium contrast agents with the first-generation techniques has been done (42,46–49). Promising early work with the second-generation techniques has also been performed in animals and humans (50–55). The use of contrast agents with the third-generation coronary MRA techniques seems most promising (56–59).

The initial experience with extravascular MR contrast agents seemed to indicate that very high doses would be needed for first-generation techniques (42,46). With bolus arrival timing to catch the first pass of the gadolinium contrast agent further image-quality improvements have been obtained (improved SNR and contrast-to-noise ratios) for both second- and third-generation techniques (42,60). With the new experimental MR blood pool agents, however, even greater image improvements are being obtained (50–52,61). Sequential breathhold acquisitions, as short as 5–10 seconds, can be obtained with relatively high resolution to image thin 3-D slabs. With several repeated short breathholds this allows patient-friendly high-resolution coverage of large portions of the cardiac and coronary anatomy. It offers the advantage of 3-D acquisitions (with the opportunity for subsequent postprocessing and no misregistration) while taking advantage of the MR contrast agents. The combination of MR contrast agents with coronary MRA techniques may some day allow coronary MRA to out-

perform any other noninvasive coronary imaging technique on all fronts, including spatial resolution and 3-D volume coverage (see also Chaps. 24 and 25).

New Tools for Fast Image Plane Selection: Real-Time Cardiac MRI

Real-time cardiac imaging and fluoroscopy have been discussed and proposed by several investigators (62–65). Real-time cardiac imaging for coronary imaging has been described most recently by Hardy (29,30,64) (see also Chap. 21), and also by others (66–69). Having real-time interactive imaging as an integral component allows quick location of oblique coronary scan planes prior to high-resolution coronary MRA. This offers another very powerful approach to overcoming problems inherent with first-generation techniques.

Hybrid Techniques

Limitations of spatial and temporal resolution of the existing 3-D breathhold techniques can be overcome by using a HYBRID technique, such as volume splitting using prospective real-time navigator technology (70). Using this approach Stuber et al. acquired a 9-cm-thick volume with in-plane resolution of 1.2×2.2 mm can be acquired during five breathholds of 15 sec duration each (70). Other approaches have considered breathhold multislice 2-D segmented gradient-recalled echo (GRE), as well as segmented EPI (71) and spiral (72). Foo et al. (73) have described prospectively gated breathheld spiral coronary artery imaging using vessel tracking, a hybrid real-time technique. Breathholding can also be improved by administering oxygen during the preparation phase (74).

The Future

Third-generation coronary MRA with or without the use of contrast agents and with real-time interactive slice (or slab) positioning will play a prominent role in coronary MRA. Pre-clinical trials of these very promising techniques are now under way (75). These techniques offer immediate feedback to the imager, and are acquired within a breathhold. Hybrid techniques, where navigator echo information is used to reposition sequential 3-D thin-slab acquisitions, could become a very cost- and time-efficient alternative to all other coronary MRA techniques (76,77).

References

1. Wang S, Hu B, Macovski A, Nishimura D. Coronary angiography using fast selective inversion recovery. Magn Reson Med 1991;18:417–23.
2. Edelman RR, Siewert B, Adamis M, Gaa J, Laub G,

Wielopolski P. Signal targeting with alternating radiofrequency (STAR) sequences: application to MR angiography. Magn Reson Med 1994;31:233–38.

3. Edelman RB, Wielopolski P, Schmitt F. Echo-planar MR imaging. Radiology 1994;192:600–12.

4. Wielopolski PA, Manning WJ, Edelman RE. Single breath-hold volumetric imaging of the heart using magnetization-prepared 3-dimensional segmented echo-planar imaging. J Magn Reson Imag 1995;5(4):403–9.

5. Wielopolski P, vanGeuns RJ, deFeyter PJ, Oudkerk M. Breath-hold coronary MR angiography with volume targeted imaging. Radiology 1998;209:209–20.

6. Börnert P, Jensen D. Coronary artery imaging at 0.5 T using segmented 3D echo planar imaging. Magn Reson Med 1995;34:779–85.

7. Pearlman JD, Edelman RE. Ultrafast magnetic resonance imaging: segmented TurboFLASH, echo-planar, and real-time nuclear magnetic resonance. Radiol Clin North Am 1994;32(3):593–612.

8. McKinnon GC. Ultrafast interleaved gradient-echo-planar imaging on a standard scanner. Magn Reson Med 1993;30:609–16.

9. Börnert P. 3D-EPI-imaging of the proximal coronary arteries at 0.5 T (abstr.). In: Book of Abstracts of the Third Meeting of the Society of Magnetic Resonance (SMR) and the Twelfth Annual Scientific Meeting of the European Society for Magnetic Resonance in Medicine and Biology (ESMRMB). Nice, France, August 20–25, 1995.

10. Botnar RM, Stuber M, Kissinger KV, Manning WJ. Isotropic free-breathing 3D coronary MRA (abstr.). In: Society for Cardiovascular Magnetic Resonance, Second Meeting, January 22-24, 1999. Atlanta, 1999:89.

11. Botnar RM, Stuber M, Kissinger KV, Manning WJ. A fast 3D approach for coronary MRA (abstr.). In: Society for Cardiovascular Magnetic Resonance, Second Meeting, January 22–24, 1999. Atlanta, 1999:80.

12. Botnar R, Stuber M, Kissinger KV, Danias PG, Manning WJ. Free-breathing 3D coronary MRA with a fast TFE-EPI acquisition technique (abstr.). In: Book of Abstracts and Proceedings of the Seventh Meeting of the International Society of Magnetic Resonance in Medicine (ISMRM). Philadelphia, May 22–23, 1999.

13. Hu BS, Meyer CH, Macosvki A. Multislice spiral magnetic resonance coronary angiography (#371) (abstr.). In: Printed Program of the Second Meeting of the Society of Magnetic Resonance (SMR). San Francisco, August 6–12, 1994.

14. Brittain JH, Hu BS, Wright GA, Meyer CH, Macovski A, Nishimura DG. Multislice coronary angiography with muscle and venous suppression (#367) (abstr.). In: Printed Program of the Second Meeting of the Society of Magnetic Resonance (SMR). San Francisco, August 7–12, 1994.

15. Irarrazabel P, Sachs T, Meyer C, Brittain J, Nishimura D. Fast volumetric imaging of the heart (abstr.). In: Book of Abstracts of the Third Meeting of the Society of Magnetic Resonance (SMR) and the Twelfth Annual Scientific Meeting of the European Society for Magnetic Resonance in Medicine and Biology (ESMRMB). Nice, France, August 20–25, 1995.

16. Hu BS, Meyer CH, Macovski A, Nishimura DG. Multislice spiral magnetic resonance coronary angiography (ab-

str.). In: Book of Abstracts of the Fourth Meeting of the International Society of Magnetic Resonance in Medicine (ISMRM). New York, April 27–May 3, 1996; Vol. 1: 671.

17. Sodickson DK, Manning WJ. Simultaneous acquisition of spatial harmonics (SMASH): fast imaging with radiofrequency coil arrays. Magn Reson Med 1997;38(4):591–603.

18. Jakob PM, Griswold MA, Edelman RR, Manning WJ, Sodickson DK. Cardiac imaging with SMASH (abstr.). In: Proceedings of the Sixth Scientific Meeting of the International Society for Magnetic Resonance in Medicine (ISMRM), April 18–24, 1998 (paper #16). Sydney, Australia, 1998.

19. Sodickson DK, Stuber M, Botnar RM, Kissinger KV, Manning WJ. SMASH real-time cardiac imaging at echocardiographic frame rates (abstr.). In: Book of Abstracts and Proceedings of the Seventh Meeting of the International Society of Magnetic Resonance in Medicine (ISMRM). Philadelphia, May 22–28, 1999.

20. Sodickson DK, Stuber M, Botnar RM, Kissinger KV, Manning WJ. Accelerated coronary MR angiography in volunteers and patients using double-oblique 3D acquisitions combined with SMASH (abstr.). In: Society for Cardiovascular Magnetic Resonance, Second Meeting, January 22–24, 1999. Atlanta, Georgia, 1999:81.

21. Jakob PM, Griswold MA, Edelman RR, Sodickson DK. AUTO-SMASH: a self-calibrating technique for SMASH imaging. SiMultaneous Acquisition of Spatial Harmonics. Magma 1998;7(1):42–54.

22. Weiger M, Scheidegger MB, Pruessmann KP, Boesiger P. Cardiac real-time acquisition using coil sensitivity encoding (abstr.). In: Proceedings of the Sixth Scientific Meeting of the International Society for Magnetic Resonance in Medicine (ISMRM), April 18–24, 1998 (paper #803). Sydney, Australia, 1998; Vol. 2: 803.

23. Weiger M, Pruessmann KP, Boesiger P, Scheidegger MB. Accelerated cardiac breathhold imaging using coil sensitivity encoding (abstr.). In: Proceedings of the Sixth Scientific Meeting of the International Society for Magnetic Resonance in Medicine (ISMRM), April 18–24, 1998 (paper #799). Sydney, Australia, 1998; Vol. 2.

24. Weiger M, Pruessmann KP, Boesiger P. High performance cardiac real-time imaging using SENSE (abstr.). In: Book of Abstracts and Proceedings of the Seventh Meeting of the International Society of Magnetic Resonance in Medicine (ISMRM). Philadelphia, May 22–23, 1999; Vol. 1.

25. Wielopolski PA, vanGeuns RJM, deFeyter PJ, Oudkerk M. VCATS (volume coronary arteriography using targeted scans), MR coronary angiography using breath-hold volume targeted acquistions (abstr.). In: Proceedings of the Sixth Scientific Meeting of the International Society for Magnetic Resonance in Medicine (ISMRM), April 18–24, 1998 (paper #14). Sydney, Australia, 1998.

26. Kessler W, Achenbach S, Moshage W, Ropers D, Laub G. Coronary arteries: three-dimensional breath-hold MR angiography using a gadolinium-enhanced ultrafast gradient-echo technique (abstr.). In: Proceedings of the Sixth Scientific Meeting of the International Society for Magnetic Resonance in Medicine (ISMRM), April 18–24, 1998 (paper # 315). Sydney, Australia, 1998; Vol. 1: 315.

27. Goldfarb JW, Edelman RR. Coronary arteries: breath-hold, gadolinium-enhanced, three-dimensional MR angiography. Radiology 1998;206(3):830–34.

28. vanGeuns RJM, Wielopolski PA, Rensing B, debruin HG, defeyter PJ, Oudkerk M. Clinical evaluation of breath-hold MR coronary angiography using targeted volumes (abstr.). *In*: Proceedings of the Sixth Scientific Meeting of the International Society for Magnetic Resonance in Medicine (ISMRM), April 18–24, 1998 (paper #324). Sydney, Australia, 1998; Vol. 1: 324.

29. Hardy CJ, Darrow RD, Pauly JM, et al. Interactive coronary MRI. Magn Reson Med 1998;40(1):105–11.

30. Hardy CJ. Real-time cardiovascular MR imaging. *In*: Reiber JHC, vanderWall EE, ed. What's New in Cardiovascular Imaging? Dordrecht: Kluwer Academic Publishers, 1998: 207–19.

31. Deshpande V, Laub G, Simonetti O, et al. 3-D MR coronary artery imaging using magnetization-prepared True-FISP (abstr.). *In*: Book of Abstracts of the First International Workshop on Coronary MR & CT Angiography. Lyon, France, October 1–3, 2000. Organized and published by the North American Society for Cardiac Imaging. Reprinted in Inter J Card Imag 2000;16.

32. Prince MR, Yucel EK, Kaufman JA, Harrison DC, Geller SC. Dynamic gadolinium-enhanced three-dimensional abdominal MR arteriography. J Magn Reson Imag 1993;3: 877–81.

33. Prince MR. Gadolinium-enhanced MR aortography. Radiology 1994;191:155–64.

34. Prince MR, Narasimham DL, Stanley JC, et al. Gadolinium-enhanced magnetic resonance angiography of abdominal aortic aneurysms. J Vasc Surg 1995;21:656–69.

35. Prince MR, Narasimham DL, Jacoby WT, et al. Three-dimensional gadolinium-enhanced MR angiography of the thoracic aorta. Am J Roentgenol 1996;166:1387–97.

36. Prince MR, Arnoldus C, Frisoli JK. Nephrotoxicity of high-dose gadolinium compared with iodinated contrast. J Magn Reson Imag 1996;1:162–66.

37. Cloft HJ, Murphy KJ, Prince MR, Brunberg JA. 3D gadolinium-enhanced MR angiography of the carotid arteries. Magn Reson Imag 1996;14(6):593–600.

38. Johnson DB, Lerner CA, Prince MR, et al. Gadolinium-enhanced magnetic resonance angiography of renal transplants. Magn Reson Imag 1997;15(1):13–20.

39. Meaney JF, Prince MR, Nostrant TT, Stanley JC. Gadolinium-enhanced MR angiography of visceral arteries in patients with suspected chronic mesenteric ischemia. J Magn Reson Imag 1997;7(1):171–76.

40. Foo TK, Saranathan M, Prince MR, Chenevert TL. Automated detection of bolus arrival and initiation of data acquisition in fast, three-dimensional, gadolinium-enhanced MR angiography. Radiology 1997;203(1):275–80.

41. Prince MR, Narisimham DL, Stanley JC, et al. Breath-hold gadolinium-enhanced MR angiography of the abdominal aorta and its major branches. Radiology 1995;197:785–92.

42. Ho VB, Foo TKF, Arai AE, Wolff SD. Gadolinium-enhanced two-dimensional coronary MR angiography using an automated contrast bolus detection algorithm (MR smartprep) (abstr.). *In*: Proceedings of the Sixth Scientific Meeting of the International Society for Magnetic Resonance in Medicine (ISMRM), April 18–24, 1998 (paper #19). Sydney, Australia, 1998 (in press).

43. van Rossum AC, Galjee MA, Post JC, Visser CA. A practical approach to MRI of coronary artery bypass graft patency and flow. Int J Card Imag 1997;13(3):199–204.

44. Vrachliotis TG, Aliabadi D, Bis KG, Shetty AN, London J, Farah J. Breath-hold electrocardiogram-triggered, contrast-enhanced, 3D MR angiography to evaluate patency of coronary artery bypass graft (abstr.). Radiology 1996;201(P):273.

45. Vrachliotis TG, Bis KG, Aliabadi D, Shetty AN, Safian R, Simonetti O. Contrast-enhanced breath-hold MR angiography for evaluating patency of coronary artery bypass grafts. Am J Roentgenol 1997;168(4):1073–80.

46. Duerinckx AJ, Urman M, Sinha U, Atkinson D, Simonetti O. Evaluation of gadolinium-enhanced MR coronary angiography (abstr.). *In*: Seventy-ninth Scientific Assembly and Annual Meeting of the Radiological Society of North America (RSNA). Chicago, November 28–December 3, 1993; Radiology 1993;189(P):278.

47. Stillman AE, Wilke N, Li D, Haacke EM, McLachlan SJ. MRA of renal and coronary arteries using an intravascular contrast agent (abstr.). *In*: Printed Program of the Second Meeting of the Society of Magnetic Resonance (SMR). San Francisco, California, August 6–12: 1994.

48. Saeed M, Wendland MF, Engelbrecht M, Sakuma H, Higgins CB. Contrast-enhanced magnetic resonance angiography in the coronary and peripheral arteries. Acad Radiol 1998;5 Suppl 1:S108–12.

49. Taylor AM, Panting JR, Keegan J, et al. Safety and preliminary findings with the intravascular contrast agent NC100150 injection for MR coronary angiography. J Magn Reson Imag 1999;9(2):220–27.

50. Li D, Dolan RP, Walovitch RC, Lauffer RB. Three-dimensional MRI of coronary arteries using an intravascular contrast agent. Magn Reson Med 1998;39(6):1014–18.

51. Li D, Zheng J, Weinmann H-J, et al. Comparison of intravascular and extravascular contrast agents in coronary artery imaging. (abstr.). *In*: Proceedings of the Sixth Scientific Meeting of the International Society for Magnetic Resonance in Medicine (ISMRM), April 18–24, 1998. Sydney, Australia:1998;Vol 1:17.

52. Stuber M, Botnar RM, McConnell MV, et al. Coronary artery imaging with the intravascular contrast agent MS-325. (abstr.). *In*: Proceedings of the Sixth Scientific Meeting of the International Society for Magnetic Resonance in Medicine (ISMRM), April 18–24, 1998. Sydney, Australia:1998;Vol 1:316.

53. Sakuma H, Goto M, Nomura Y, Kato N, Takeda K, Higgins CB. Three-dimensional coronary magnetic resonance angiography with injection of extracellular contrast medium. Invest Radiol 1999;34(8):503–8.

54. Stuber M, Botnar RM, Danias PG, et al. Contrast agent-enhanced, free-breathing, three-dimensional coronary magnetic resonance angiography. J Magn Reson Imag 1999;10(5):790–99.

55. Zheng J, Bae KT, Woodard PK, Haacke EM, Li D. Efficacy of slow infusion of gadolinium contrast agent in three-dimensional MR coronary artery imaging. J Magn Reson Imag 1999;10(5):800–5.

56. Goldfarb JW, Edelman RR. Coronary arteries: breath-hold, gadolinium-enhanced, three-dimensional MR angiography. Radiology 1998;206(3):830–34.

57. deBruin HG, vanGeuns RJM, Wielopolski PA, deFeyter PJ, Oudkerk M. Improvement of magnetic resonance imag-

ing of the coronary arteries with a clinically available intravascular contrast agent (abstr.). *In*: Book of Abstracts of the First International Workshop on Coronary MR & CT Angiography. Lyon, France, October 1–3, 2000. Organized and published by the North American Society for Cardiac Imaging. Reprinted in Int J Card Imag 2000;16.

58. Kessler W, Laub G, Achenbach S, Ropers D, Moshage W, Daniel WG. Coronary arteries: MR angiography with fast contrast-enhanced three-dimensional breath-hold imaging—initial experience. Radiology 1999;210(2):566–72.

59. Kruger DG, Busse RF, Johnston DL, Ritman EL, Ehman RL, Riederer SJ. Contrast-enhanced 3D MR breathhold imaging of porcine coronary arteries using fluoroscopic localization and bolus triggering. Magn Reson Med 1999; 42(6):1159–65.

60. Kessler W, Laub G, Ropers D, Achenbach S, Moshage W, Bachmann K. Contrast-enhanced 3D breath-hold MRA for the visualization of the coronary arteries in oblique projection angiograms (abstr.). *In*: Proceedings of the Sixth Scientific Meeting of the International Society for Magnetic Resonance in Medicine (ISMRM), April 18–24, 1998. Sydney, Australia, 1998; Vol. 1: 317.

61. Taylor AM, Panting JR, Gatehouse PD, et al. Safety and preliminary findings with an intravascular contrast agent, NC100150 for MR coronary angiography (abstr.). *In*: Proceedings of the Sixth Scientific Meeting of the International Society for Magnetic Resonance in Medicine (ISMRM), April 18–24, 1998. Sydney, Australia, 1998; Vol. 1:18.

62. Kerr AB, Pauly JM, Hu BS, et al. Real-time interactive MRI on a conventional scanner. Magn Reson Med 1997;38(3): 355–67.

63. Spielman DM, Pauly JM, Meyer CH. Magnetic resonance fluoroscopy using spirals with variable sampling densities. Magn Reson Med 1995;34(3):388–94.

64. Hardy CJ, Curwen RW, Darrow RD. Robust coronary MRI by spiral fluoroscopy with adaptive averaging (abstr.). *In*: Proceedings of the Sixth Scientific Meeting of the International Society for Magnetic Resonance in Medicine (ISMRM), April 18–24, 1998 (paper #22). Sydney, Australia, 1998.

65. Hangiandreou NJ, Debbins JP, Rossman PJ, Riederer SJ. Interactive selection of optimal section orientations using real-time MRI. J Magn Reson Imag 1995;34:114–19.

66. Chien D, Heid O, Simonetti O, Laub G. New developments in ultrafast and interactive cardiac MR by Siemens Medical Systems (abstr.). *In*: Twenty-sixth Annual Meeting of the North American Society for Cardiac Imaging. Dallas, 1998.

67. Weiger M, Pruessmann KP, Boesiger P. High performance cardiac real-time imaging using SENSE (abstr.). *In*: Book of Abstracts and Proceedings of the Seventh Meeting of the International Society of Magnetic Resonance in Medicine (ISMRM). Philadelphia, May 22–23, 1999.

68. Sodickson DK, Stuber M, Botnar RM, Kissinger KV, Manning WJ. SMASH real-time cardiac imaging at echocardiographic frame rates. (abstr.). *In*: Book of Abstracts and Proceedings of the Seventh Meeting of the International Society of Magnetic Resonance in Medicine (ISMRM). Philadelphia, May 22–28, 1999.

69. Bundy JM, Laub G, Kim R, Finn JP, Simonetti OP. Real-time data acquisition for LV function (abstr.). *In*: Book of Abstracts and Proceedings of the Seventh Meeting of the International Society of Magnetic Resonance in Medicine (ISMRM). Philadelphia, May 22–23, 1999.

70. Stuber M, Botnar RM, Danias PG, Kissinger KV, Manning WJ. Breathold three-dimensional coronary magnetic resonance angiography using real-time navigator technology. J Cardiovasc Magn Reson 1999;1(3):233–38.

71. Slavin GS, Riederer SJ, Ehman RL. Two-dimensional multishot echo-planar coronary MR angiography. Magn Reson Med 1998;40(6):883–89.

72. Meyer CH, Hu BS, Yang PC, et al. Spiral cardiac imaging with high-performance gradients (abstr.). *In*: Book of Abstracts and Proceedings of the Seventh Meeting of the International Society of Magnetic Resonance in Medicine (ISMRM). Philadelphia, PA, May 22–23, 1999.

73. Foo TK, Ho VB, Hood MN. Vessel tracking: prospective adjustment of section-selective MR angiographic locations for improved coronary artery visualization over the cardiac cycle. Radiology 2000;214(1):283–89.

74. Danias PG, Stuber M, Botnar RM, Kissinger KV, Chuang ML, Manning WJ. Navigator assessment of breath-hold duration: impact of supplemental oxygen and hyperventilation. Am J Roentgenol 1998;171(2):395–97.

75. van Geuns RJ, Wielopolski PA, de Bruin HG, et al. MR coronary angiography with breath-hold targeted volumes: preliminary clinical results. Radiology 2000.

76. Book of Abstracts of the Second Workshop on Coronary MR & CT Angiography, Sept 29–Oct 2, 2001, Chicago, IL. Organized and published by the North American Society for Cardiac Imaging. Reprinted in Int J Card Imag 2001;17:5.

77. Deshpande VS, Shea SM, McCarthy R, Laub G, Simonetti O, Finn JP, Li D. Update on MR 3D True-FISP coronary artery imaging (abstr.). Presented at the Second Workshop on Coronary MR & CT Angiography, Sept 29–Oct 2, 2001, Chicago, IL. Published by the North American Society for Cardiac Imaging in the Inter J Card Imag 2001;17:5.

21
Real-Time Coronary MRI

Christopher J. Hardy

Introduction

Magnetic resonance imaging (MRI) has been utilized to assess a variety of parameters useful for the diagnosis and management of heart disease (1), including left-ventricular function (2), cardiac wall motion (3), myocardial perfusion (4) and strain (5), coronary anatomy (6–13) and flow (14), and even myocardial metabolism (15). This raises the possibility of the development of a comprehensive exam for coronary artery disease, which combines many or all of these assessments within a single exam. In the past the relatively slow speeds of most MRI scanners have necessitated the use of EKG gating and respiratory compensation or breathholding to acquire cardiac images, often requiring tens of minutes per data set, making this possibility unlikely. Advances in gradient and reconstruction hardware and in pulse sequence design, however, have pushed maximum MRI rates into the range of 10 frames per second or better (16,17), making real-time interactive MRI now practical. High-speed MRI should play an important role in the context of an integrated cardiac MR exam, allowing for rapid, interactive progression from one stage of the exam to the next, and should allow the rapid assessment of left ventricular function and wall motion. It should prove especially important for rapid location of oblique coronary scan planes, and for visualization of the proximal coronaries in real time.

Rapid MRI

High-speed MRI has evolved over a number of years, with a variety of pulse sequences employed for applications ranging from angiography to interventional MR (18–20). A method for performing rapid MRI was first proposed by Mansfield and Pykett (21), whose echo-planar imaging (EPI) sequence involved the traversal of all of k-space after a single nuclear magnetic resonance (NMR) excitation. This soon evolved to a form that used blipped gradients on one axis (22,23). The advent of resonant (24) and switched (25–27) gradient power tech-

nology and low-inductance, self-shielded coils (28,29) brought increased imaging speeds with reduced artifacts, producing real-time (28,30) EPI movie loops and relatively high-quality phase-contrast interleaved EPI images (31) of the heart. On the other hand, faster gradient speeds were used to improve bandwidth and thus signal-to-noise ratio (SNR), while keeping imaging speed constant (32). Rapid gradient-echo imaging techniques employing low-tip-angle radio frequency (RF) excitation pulses (33,34) also proved beneficial for cardiac imaging, minimizing some artifacts associated with EPI, such as sensitivity to variations in magnetic field susceptibility, and chemical-shift artifacts.

Hybrid sequences [e.g., RARE (35) and GRASE (36)] used multiple gradient and RF refocusing pulses after an NMR excitation to produce T2-weighted snapshots with reduced sensitivity to chemical shift and field inhomogeneity compared with standard EPI sequences. The use of multiple RF refocusing pulses, however, increased RF heating and MR-signal saturation effects, making these sequences less useful for continuous real-time imaging. Interleaved EPI pulse sequences (31,37) employed multiple excitation pulses with interleaved k-space trajectories (similar to that shown in Fig. 21.1A, with corresponding pulse sequence diagram in Fig. 21.1B) to reduce the echo-train length, and minimize some of the artifacts associated with EPI pulse sequences. Circular EPI trajectories (38) dropped the corners of k-space in order to improve speed, without yielding large sacrifices in spatial resolution. BURST imaging techniques (39) relied on a rapid sequence of RF pulses to generate multiple echoes during a constant readout gradient, removing the need for gradient switching, and producing ultrafast imaging rates, albeit with reduced resolution and SNR and with relatively high sensitivity to motion (40).

Another class of imaging sequence replaced rectilinear k-space trajectories with curved paths that pushed the gradient slew rate more evenly over the entire sequence. The most successful of these has been the spiral trajectory (41,42) and its variant, the interleaved

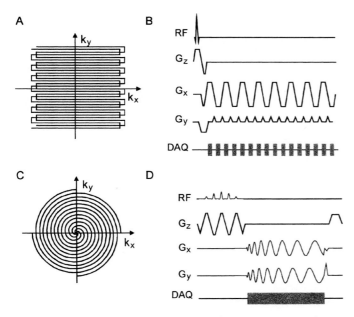

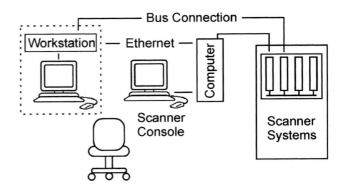

Figure 21.1. Rapid MRI sequences. (A) *k*-space trajectory for interleaved echo-planar sequence. Two interleaves of six-interleaf sequence are shown, with offset on k_x axis for better visibility. (B) Corresponding RF, gradient, and data-acquisition waveforms for one of the interleaves. (C) *k*-space trajectory for interleaved spiral sequence. (D) Corresponding waveforms for one of the interleaves.

spiral, or pinwheel (7,38,42,43). The spiral trajectory can be traversed at a nonuniform rate to produce constant gradient amplitudes or slew rates, thus maximizing bandwidth (44). A pinwheel trajectory and pulse sequence corresponding to one arm of the pinwheel are shown in Figures 21.1C and 21.1D, respectively. The NMR excitation pulse in this sequence is both spatially and spectrally selective (45), allowing the suppression of fat signals, which would otherwise cause blurring in a spiral acquisition. The advantages of reduced readout times gained by interleaving in EPI (31,37) also hold for interleaved spirals. Spirals have the further benefits of good flow characteristics (46) and relative insensitivity to motion (38), making them especially useful for cardiac imaging. Off-resonance and susceptibility effects can affect image quality, however, and measures such as automated field-map calculation and correction in the image reconstruction are generally required to prevent regional image blurring (47).

Real-Time Interactive Cardiac MRI

For high-speed pulse sequences to be utilized to full advantage an imaging system is needed that is capable of rapid reconstruction and real-time image display. Such a system was first developed and demonstrated by Wright et al. (48), who used a workstation and array processor connected to a conventional MR scanner.

Other experimental real-time whole-body MRI systems have since been developed (38,49–52), including those targeting cardiac (38,49) and interventional (51–52) applications. One such system is shown in Figure 21.2. To improve imaging frame rates, a sliding reconstruction technique was introduced (53) that continually incorporates the most recently acquired lines of *k*-space to update the raw data set partially before reconstruction, with new reconstructions performed at a rate faster than the image acquisition rate. This allows the visualization of motion even when the basic repetition rate of the pulse sequence is not real time. The sliding reconstruction method has since also been applied to interleaved-spiral imaging (38). Spirals benefit from the fact that each interleaf samples the same range of spatial frequencies, including the center of *k*-space, providing a uniform response to motion. This is especially true when the interleaves are acquired in "bit-reversed" order rather than sequentially because this causes any motion artifacts to be spread more diffusely (38).

To make best use of these real-time MRI capabilities, it is important to have interactive control of the imaging plane and contrast parameters during real-time imaging. The first step toward such control was made by Holsinger et al., who interactively redirected a gradient-echo pulse sequence by entering new parameter values from the keyboard as the sequence was executing (54). Graphical tools (38,49,55–58) and interfaces to hardware devices (58,59) have also been developed to provide highly intuitive methods for real-time scan-plane prescription, most in the context of cardiac MRI applications. A number of schemes have been employed, all of which can be implemented during continuous imaging, permitting visualization of the beating heart during movement of the scan plane. A scan-plane library (shown in Fig. 21.3A) has been used for rapid storage and retrieval of scan locations, with a different thumbnail image created to represent each location. Scan planes are retrieved by selecting the appropriate thumbnails with the mouse. A colored three-dimensional (3-D)

Figure 21.2. Workstation-based research platform for interactive cardiac MRI.

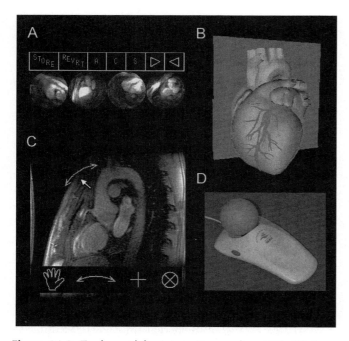

Figure 21.3. Tools used for interactive cardiac MRI. (A) Scan-plane library allows rapid storage and retrieval of scan locations. (B) Semitransparent plane embedded in colored 3-D heart model reflects real-time location of current scan plane. (C) Colored icons can be dragged across imaging window to rotate or offset scan plane in real time, as shown for in-plane rotation. (D) Six-dimensional controller can be twisted or pushed to rotate or offset scan plane in any direction.

heart model (58,60) with a semitransparent embedded plane (Fig. 21.3B) has also been utilized to track the location of the imaging plane in real time, to enable the user to stay better oriented during interactive imaging. In another scheme, scan-plane prescription from within the real-time-imaging window has been effected by "pushing" on various regions of the current image with the mouse to tilt the scan plane about its center (55). On the other hand, various colored icons can be dragged across the real-time imaging window (Fig. 21.3C) to reorient or offset the scan plane relative to its current location (58). Six-dimensional controllers (Fig. 21.3D) have also been used to rotate or offset the scan plane in real time, by twisting or pushing in any direction as if the heart itself were being manipulated, with icons moving across the window to indicate the type, direction, and extent of motion. The advantage of these kinds of methods is that they are very intuitive: They allow users to keep their eyes fixed on the imaging window during scan prescription, and they furnish essentially instantaneous visual feedback (via screen graphics) beyond that provided by the new images themselves.

Real-time interactive MRI should prove extremely useful for rapid localization of coronary scan planes prior to EKG-gated coronary MRA. The acquisition of complete 3-D segmented gradient-echo data sets (8) to

visualize the coronary arteries can be both time consuming and sensitive to motion, even with use of multiple breathholding or respiratory gating. Single-slice, transverse, or oblique imaging (6) requires repetitive positioning of the scan plane at multiple locations along the coronary tree, with gated breathheld imaging at each location. In an alternate hybrid approach, real-time interactive imaging is first used to locate an optimal oblique coronary scan plane [e.g., a left anterior oblique (LAO) caudal view of the right coronary artery, or Gruentzig view of the left-anterior-descending artery]. A limited number of contiguous oblique slices can then be acquired around that plane within a breathhold with use of multislice spiral (61) or two-dimensional (2-D) segmented gradient-echo (58,62) imaging, or with an oblique 3-D segmented gradient-echo technique (13). Finally, if needed, a limited reformat of the data can be performed to produce images from relatively long sections of the coronaries. This approach yields relatively rapid visualization of portions of the coronary tree. Figure 21.4 shows a series of MRIs captured from a real-time video segment, displaying the proximal right coronary artery. Visualization of the coronaries is good enough with this real-time spiral pulse sequence to al-

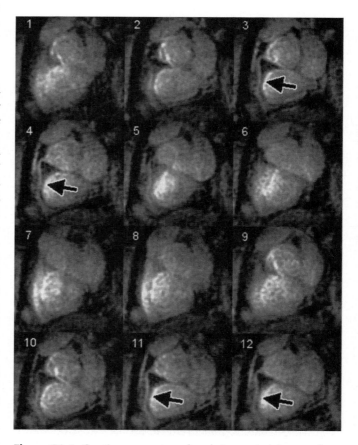

Figure 21.4. Continuous series of real-time spiral images from a normal volunteer, showing proximal right coronary artery (arrows) in selected frames.

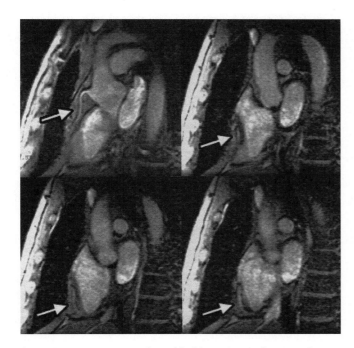

Figure 21.5. Contiguous breathheld, EKG-gated MRIs of proximal right coronary artery (arrows) from a normal volunteer, acquired after localization of scan plane.

low interactive prescription of optimal oblique planes in as little as 10 seconds (58). Breathheld, EKG-gated images of four contiguous oblique slices from a normal volunteer are shown in Figure 21.5.

Conclusions

With improvements in gradient and reconstruction hardware, pulse sequence design, and user interface, real-time interactive cardiac MRI has now become practical. This tool should play a key role in the development of a flexible staged cardiac MRI exam that can be run in a variety of settings. Real-time capabilities should benefit coronary MRI in particular, enabling relatively rapid and robust visualization of the vessels. A number of advances currently on the horizon promise to increase the effectiveness of MRI further in the diagnosis and management of coronary artery disease. More gains in reconstruction and display speed appear likely as low-cost computer processing power continues to increase. Gradient speeds will probably show continued improvement as well, although they may soon be approaching limits set by human physiology. Further refinement of MR pulse sequences is likely, with real-time capabilities being exploited to change the way clinically relevant parameters are measured.

A variety of intravascular MR contrast agents are under development. These offer the promise of relatively high-contrast, high-resolution coronary MRA, providing greatly improved coronary visualization. Because these agents remain in the blood pool for relatively long periods, precise synchronization of the MR pulse sequence to the contrast injection is not necessary, and data can be collected over a longer interval of time. Early results have shown the potential benefits of MR stress testing for detecting and assessing the physiologic significance of coronary disease, with MRI pulse sequences employed to measure rapidly (e.g., coronary flow before and during stress). MRI may prove useful as well for characterizing the morphology and composition of coronary plaques, for the purpose of assessing vulnerability to thrombosis. Regardless of which of these applications of coronary MRI demonstrates the most utility, real-time imaging seems likely to play an increasing role in the cardiovsacular MRI exam of the future.

References

1. Van der Wall EE, Vliegen HW, De Roos A, Bruschke AVG. Magnetic resonance imaging in coronary artery disease. Circulation 1995;92:2723–39.
2. Van Rossum AC, Visser FC, Sprenger M, Van Eenige MJ, Valk J, Roos JP. Evaluation of magnetic resonance imaging for determination of left ventricular ejection fraction and comparison with angiography. Am J Cardiol 1988;62: 628–33.
3. White RD, Cassidy MM, Cheitlin MD, et al. Segmental evaluation of left ventricular wall motion after myocardial infarction: magnetic resonance imaging versus echocardiography. Am Heart J 1988;115:166–75.
4. Atkinson DJ, Burstein D, Edelman RR. First-pass cardiac perfusion: evaluation with ultrafast MR imaging. Radiology 1990;174:757–62.
5. Zerhouni EA, Parish DM, Rogers WJ, Yang A, Shapiro EP. Human heart: tagging with MR imaging: a method for noninvasive assessment of myocardial motion. Radiology 1988;169:59–63.
6. Edelman RR, Manning WJ, Burstein D, Paulin S. Coronary arteries: breath-hold MR angiography. Radiology 1991; 181:641–43.
7. Meyer CH, Hu BS, Nishimura DG, Macovski A. Fast spiral coronary artery imaging. Magn Reson Med 1992;28: 202–13.
8. Li D, Paschel CB, Haacke EM, Adler LP. Coronary arteries: three dimensional MR imaging with fat saturation and magnetization transfer contrast. Radiology 1993;187:401–6.
9. Manning WJ, Li W, Boyle NG, Edelman RR. Fat-suppressed breath-hold magnetic resonance coronary angiography. Circulation 1993;87:94–104.
10. Pennell DJ, Bogren HG, Keegan J, Firmin DN, Underwood SR. Assessment of coronary artery stenosis by magnetic resonance imaging. Heart 1996;75:127–33.
11. Duerinckx AJ, Urman MK. Two-dimensional coronary MR angiography: analysis of initial clinical results. Radiology 1994;193:731–38.
12. Sakuma H, Caputo GR, Steffens JC, et al. Breath-hold MR cine angiography of coronary arteries in healthy volunteers: value of multiangle oblique imaging planes. Am J Roentgenol 1994;163:533–37.
13. Wielopolski PA, van Geuns RM, de Feyter PJ, Oudkerk M.

Breath-hold coronary MR angiography with volume targeted imaging. Radiology 1998;209:209–19.

14. Poncelet BP, Weisskoff RM, Wedeen VJ, Brady TJ, Kantor HW. Time of flight quantification of coronary flow with echo-planar MRI. Magn Reson Med 1993;30:447–57.

15. Weiss RG, Bottomley PA, Hardy CJ, Gerstenblith G. Regional myocardial metabolism of high-energy phosphates during isometric exercise in patients with coronary artery disease. N Engl J Med 1990;323:1593–600.

16. Feinberg D. Fast MRI sequence design. In: Syllabus of the ISMRM Fast MRI Workshop, Monterey, October 27–29, 1997. Berkeley: International Society for Magnetic Resonance in Medicine, 1997:1–5 (abstr.).

17. Schmitt F. Gradient hardware considerations for fast MRI. In: Syllabus of the ISMRM Fast MRI Workshop, Monterey, October 27–29, 1997. Berkeley: International Society for Magnetic Resonance in Medicine, 1997:6–13 (abstr.).

18. Cohen MS, Weisskoff RM. Ultra-fast imaging. Magn Reson Imag 1991;9:1–37.

19. Riederer SJ. Real-time imaging. In: Potchen EJ, Siebert JE, Haacke EM, Gottschalk A, eds. Magnetic Resonance Angiography: Concepts and Applications. St. Louis: Mosby, 1993:288–96.

20. Zientara GP. Fast imaging techniques. In: Jolesz FA, Young IR, eds. Interventional MR: Techniques and Clinical Experience. London: Martin Dunitz Ltd, 1998:25–52.

21. Mansfield P, Pykett IL. Biological and medical imaging by NMR. J Magn Reson 1978;29:355–73.

22. Young IR. Nuclear magnetic resonance systems. US patent no. 4,355,282, priority date August 1979.

23. Edelstein WA, Hutchison JMS, Johnson G, Redpath TWT, Mallard JR. Methods of producing image information from objects. US patent no. 4,451,788, priority date March 1980.

24. Rzedzian RR, Pykett IL. Instant images of the human heart using a new, whole-body MR imaging system. Am J Roentgenol 1987;149:245–50.

25. Hutchison JMS, Edelstein WA, Johnson G. A whole-body NMR imaging machine. J Phys E: Sci Instrum 1980;13:947–55.

26. Mueller OM, Roemer PB, Park JN, Souza SP, Watkins RD. A 4-switch GTO speed-up inverter for fast-scan MRI. In: Proceedings of the SMRM Eleventh Annual Meeting. Berlin, August 8–14, 1992. Berkeley: Society of Magnetic Resonance in Medicine, 1992:589 (abstr.).

27. Ideler KH, Nowak S, Borth G, Hagen U, Hausmann R, Schmitt F. A resonant multipurpose gradient power switch for high performance imaging. In: Proceedings of the SMRM Eleventh Annual Meeting. Berlin, August 8–14, 1992. Berkeley: Society of Magnetic Resonance in Medicine, 1992:4044 (abstr.).

28. Chapman B, Turner R, Ordidge RJ, et al. Real-time movie imaging from a single cardiac cycle by NMR. Magn Reson Med 1987;5:246–54.

29. Roemer PB, Edelstein WA, Hickey JS. Self-shielded gradient coils. In: Proceedings of the SMRM Fifth Annual Meeting, Montreal, August 19–22, 1986. Berkeley: Society of Magnetic Resonance in Medicine, 1986:1067–68 (abstr.).

30. Rzedzian RR. Real time MRI at 2.0 Tesla. In: Proceedings of the SMRM Seventh Annual Meeting. San Francisco, August 20–26, 1988. Berkeley: Society of Magnetic Resonance in Medicine, 1988:247 (abstr.).

31. McKinnon GC, Debatin JF, Wetter DR, Von Schulthess GK. Interleaved echo planar flow quantitation. Magn Reson Med 1994;32:263–67.

32. Reeder SB, McVeigh ER. The effect of high performance gradients on fast gradient echo imaging. Magn Reson Med 1994;32:612–21.

33. Henrich D, Haase A, Matthaei D. 3D-snapshot FLASH NMR imaging of the human heart. Magn Reson Imag 1990;8:377–79.

34. Frahm J, Merboldt KD, Bruhn H, Gyngell ML, Hanicke W, Chien D. 0.3-Second FLASH MRI of the human heart. Magn Reson Med 1990;13:150–57.

35. Hennig J, Naureth A, Friedburg H. RARE imaging: a fast imaging method for clinical MR. Magn Reson Med 1986;3:823–33.

36. Oshio K, Feinberg DA. GRASE (gradient- and spin-echo) imaging: A novel fast MRI technique. Magn Reson Med 1991;20:344–49.

37. McKinnon GC. Ultrafast interleaved gradient-echo-planar imaging on a standard scanner. Magn Reson Med 1993;30:609–16.

38. Kerr AB, Pauly JM, Hu BS, et al. Real-time interactive MRI on a conventional scanner. Magn Reson Med 1997;38:355–67.

39. Hennig J, Meuri M. Fast imaging using BURST excitation pulses. In: Proceedings of the SMRM Seventh Annual Meeting. San Francisco, August 20–26, 1988. Berkeley: Society of Magnetic Resonance in Medicine, 1988:238 (abstr.).

40. Jakob PM, Griswold M, Sodickson DK, Edelman RR. BURST imaging: new acquisition strategies. In: Syllabus of the ISMRM Fast MRI Workshop. Monterey, October 27–29, 1997. Berkeley: International Society for Magnetic Resonance in Medicine, 1997:162 (abstr.).

41. Likes RS. Moving gradient zeugmatography, US patent no. 4,307,3434, filed August 1979.

42. Meyer CH, Spielman D, Macovski A. Spiral fluoroscopy. In: Proceedings of the SMRM Twelfth Annual Meeting. New York, August 14–20, 1993. Berkeley: Society of Magnetic Resonance in Medicine, 1993:475 (abstr.).

43. Hardy CJ, Bottomley PA. 31P spectroscopic localization using pinwheel NMR excitation pulses. Magn Reson Med 1991;17:315–27.

44. Hardy CJ, Cline HE. Broadband nuclear magnetic resonance pulses with two-dimensional spatial selectivity. J Appl Phys 1989;66:1513–16.

45. Meyer CH, Pauly JM, Macovski A, Nishimura D. Simultaneous spatial and spectral selective excitation. Magn Reson Med 1990;15:287–304.

46. Nishimura DG, Irarrazabal P, Meyer CH. A velocity k-space analysis of flow effects in echo-planar and spiral imaging. Magn Reson Med 1995;33:549–56.

47. Irarrazabal P, Meyer CH, Nishimura DG, Macovski A. Inhomogeneity correction using an estimated linear field map. Magn Reson Med 1996;35:278–82.

48. Wright RC, Riederer SJ, Farzaneh F, Rossman PJ, Liu Y. Real-time MR fluoroscopic data acquisition and image reconstruction. Magn Reson Med 1989;12:407–15.

49. Hardy CJ, Darrow RD, Nieters EJ, et al. Real-time acquisition, display, and interactive graphic control of NMR cardiac profiles and images. Magn Reson Med 1993;29:667–73.

50. Crelier GR, Fischer SE, Arm E, Kunz P, Boesiger P. Real-time image reconstruction system for interactive magnetic resonance acquisition. *In*: Proceedings of the SMRM Twelfth Annual Meeting. New York, August 14–20, 1993. Berkeley: Society of Magnetic Resonance in Medicine, 1993:506 (abstr.).

51. Schenck JF, Jolesz FA, Roemer PB, et al. Superconducting open-configuration MR imaging system for image-guided therapy. Radiology 1995;195:805–14.

52. Hardy CJ. High-speed interactive imaging for MRT. *In*: Proceedings of the SMR Third Meeting. Nice, August 19–25, 1995. Berkeley: Society of Magnetic Resonance, 1995:489 (abstr.).

53. Riederer SJ, Tasciyan T, Farzaneh F, Lee JN, Wright RC, Herfkens RJ. MR fluoroscopy: technical feasibility. Magn Reson Med 1988;8:1–15.

54. Holsinger AE, Wright RC, Riederer SJ, Farzaneh F, Grimm RC, Maier JK. Real-time interactive magnetic resonance imaging. Magn Reson Med 1990;14:547–53.

55. Hardy CJ, Darrow RD. Interactive slice prescription schemes for rapid MR imaging of coronary arteries. *In*: Proceedings of the SMR Second Meeting. San Francisco, August 6–12, 1994. Berkeley: Society of Magnetic Resonance, 1994:500 (abstr.).

56. Hardy CJ, Darrow RD. Heartscape: an interactive cardiac scan-plane positioner. *In*: Proceedings of the ISMRM Fourth Annual Meeting. New York, April 27–May 3, 1996. Berkeley: International Society for Magnetic Resonance in Medicine, 1996:1496 (abstr.).

57. Debbins JP, Riederer SJ, Rossman PJ, et al. Cardiac magnetic resonance fluoroscopy. Magn Reson Med 1996;36:588–95.

58. Hardy CJ, Darrow RD, Pauly JM, et al. Interactive coronary MRI. Magn Reson Med 1998;40:105–11.

59. Silverman SG, Collick BD, Figueira MR, et al. Interactive MR-guided biopsy in an open-configuration MR imaging system. Radiology 1995;197:175–81.

60. Schroeder W, Martin K, Lorensen W. The Visualization Toolkit, an Object Oriented Approach to Computer Graphics. Englewood Cliffs, NJ: Prentice-Hall, 1996.

61. Meyer CH, Hu BS, Kerr AB, et al. High-resolution multi-slice spiral coronary angiography with real-time interactive localization. *In*: Proceedings of the ISMRM Fifth Annual Meeting. Vancouver, April 12–18, 1997. Berkeley: International Society for Magnetic Resonance in Medicine, 1997:439 (abstr.).

62. Hardy CJ, Dumoulin CL, Darrow RD. MR coronary angiography using a hybrid multi-slice technique with fat/muscle suppression and fluoroscopic localization. *In*: Proceedings of the ISMRM Fifth Annual Meeting. Vancouver, April 12–18; 1997. Berkeley: International Society for Magnetic Resonance in Medicine, 1997:440 (abstr.).

22
Postprocessing and 3-D Visualization Techniques

André J. Duerinckx

Representation of 3-D vascular structures is a complex task, often requiring significant postprocessing not routinely available at clinical sites. The best-known techniques are maximum-intensity projection (MIP) as used with traditional magnetic resonance angiographic (MRA) acquisitions, surface rendering after segmentation, which has become very popular with helical computed tomography (CT) angiography, and multiplanar reconstruction from 3-D data sets. We will not discuss these options in detail given their limited availability at the present time.

Image Display for 2-D Data Sets (First-Generation Techniques)

There are several ways to review the data from a coronary MRA study: individual still images on film or an electronic display (1,2); a "spatial" cine-loop video display of images obtained in sequential planes (3); a "static temporal" cine-loop display of images in one (static) plane obtained throughout the cardiac cycle; or a "dynamic temporal" cine-loop, where an image plane tracks the motion of the heart (dynamic) while following changes throughout the cardiac cycle.

Manning et al. (3) has advocated reviewing data in a "spatial" cine-loop format to evaluate the continuity of vessels better and to improve detection of lesions. Other cardiologists may also find cine-loop review an easier approach to data analysis. Most radiologists, however, feel quite comfortable with still images. Cardiologists or others using cine-loops should be aware of the following problem. Experience has shown that a significant number of patients and volunteers cannot perform consistent breathholding, and that the diaphragm position can vary significantly between consecutive breathholds (4). Many techniques have been developed to address

this (5–7), and a 3-D data acquisition with respiratory gating may be a solution. CINE loop review of data is probably ideal for those patients with perfectly consistent breathholds (see discussion on limitations and artifacts later); however, review of individual still images is also sufficient if an adequate number of images have been acquired.

"Spatial" cine-loop video display (i.e., displaying a sequence of images on a video screen acquired in sequential parallel planes) as advocated by Manning et al. should not be confused with "temporal" cine-loops. We will define two types of "temporal" video loops. The first one is a "dynamic temporal" cine-loop acquired during multiple breathholds. This requires tracking of vessels as they move during the cardiac cycle (by repeating all the localizer image acquisitions for each cardiac phase), and actually following vessels as they move. This technique is ideal when performing flow quantification in vessels (see later) or when studying the appearance of coronary arteries during peak-systole (8). This is different from "static temporal" cine-loops where images are acquired in one plane throughout the cardiac cycle, with vessels moving in and out of the plane. The use of static temporal cine-loop coronary MRA has been advocated to facilitate the distinction between arteries and veins. A study by Hundley et al. (9) in humans with infarcted arteries showed how MR-derived "static temporal" cine-loop studies of the coronary arteries can help confirm the presence of antegrade flow and distinguish between venous and arterial flow. Their imaging parameters were: field-of-view (FOV) from 22 to 26 cm, with corresponding pixel sizes of 1.0 to 1.2 mm in the phase-encoding direction and 0.8 to 1.0 mm in the readout direction. Slice thickness was 8 mm. By viewing the images in a cine loop, they were able to facilitate the differentiation of arteries and veins by visualizing flow in arteries during early diastole.

Image Postprocessing for 3-D Data Sets (Second- and Third-Generation Techniques)

Representation of 3-D vascular structures is a complex task, often requiring significant postprocessing not routinely available at clinical sites. The best-known techniques are: MIP as used with traditional MRA acquisitions; surface rendering after segmentation, which has become very popular with helical CT angiography; and multiplanar reconstruction from 3-D data sets. We will not discuss these options in detail given their limited availability at the present time.

Three-dimensional rendering of coronary arteries is one type of postprocessing that requires segmentation of the data (10,11). To execute this 3-D rendering routine, "seeds" are placed in both the left and right coronary vessels, and thresholds are set to discriminate individual coronary vessels from adjacent structures (10). Segmentation of the left coronary system with its many branches is much more involved than the right coronary artery (RCA) segmentation. Edelman et al. (12) have also described a technique to render projection MRAs depicting a substantial length of human coronary arteries from sequential two-dimensional (2-D) breathhold images. They applied the technique to five normal volunteers and 10 patients.

Other aspects of post-processing are discussed in the April 1998 issue of the *Journal of Roentgenology* (13–17) and by de Koning et al. (18). More discussion on this topic can also be found in the next chapter (Chap. 23) and in the article by Achenbach et al. on "Visualization of the coronary arteries in three-dimensional reconstructions using respiratory gated magnetic resonance imaging" (19).

Virtual Endoscopy

With the advent of more powerful computers and more interactive fast computer graphics, the virtual fly-through of the coronary arteries has become possible using either CTA or MRA data sets (20).

References

1. Duerinckx AJ, Urman M. Two-dimensional coronary MR angiography: analysis of initial clinical results. Radiology 1994;193:731–38.
2. Pennell DJ, Keegan J, Firmin DN, Gatehouse PD, Underwood SR, Longmore DB. Magnetic resonance imaging of coronary arteries: technique and preliminary results. Br Heart J 1993;70(4):315–26.
3. Manning WJ, Li W, Edelman RR. A preliminary report comparing magnetic resonance coronary angiography with conventional angiography. N Engl J Med 1993;328: 828–32.
4. Duerinckx AJ, Urman MK, Atkinson DJ, Simonetti OP, Sinha U, Lewis B. Limitations of MR coronary angiography (abstr.). *In*: Printed Program of the First Meeting of the Society of Magnetic Resonance (SMR). Dallas, March 5–9, 1994; J Magn Reson Imag 1994;4:81.
5. Sachs TS, Meyer CH, Hu BS, Kohli J, Nishimura DG, Macovski A. Real-time motion detection in spiral MRI using navigators. Magn Reson Med 1994;32(5):639–45.
6. Liu YL, Rossman PJ, Grimm RC, Debbins JP, Ehman RL, Riederer SJ. Comparison of two breath-hold feedback techniques for reproducible breath holds in MRI (abstr.). *In*: Printed Program of the First Meeting of the Society of Magnetic Resonance (SMR). Dallas, March 5–9, 1994; J Magn Reson Imag 1994;4(P):61.
7. Liu YL, Riederer SJ, Rossman PJ, Grimm RG, Debbins JF, Ehman RL. A monitoring, feedback, and triggering system for reproducible breath-hold MR imaging. Magn Reson Med 1993;30:507–11.
8. Duerinckx AJ, Atkinson D. Coronary MR angiography during peak-systole (abstr.). *In*: Book of Abstracts of the Third Meeting of the Society of Magnetic Resonance (SMR) and the Twelfth Annual Scientific Meeting of the European Society for Magnetic Resonance in Medicine and Biology (ESMRMB). Nice, France, August 20–25, 1995; Vol. 3, p. 1396.
9. Hundley WG, Clarke GD, Landau C, et al. Noninvasive determination of infarct artery patency by cine magnetic resonance angiography. Circulation 1995;91:1347–53.
10. Doyle M, Scheidegger MB, DeGraaf RG, Vermeulen J, Pohost GM. Coronary artery imaging in multiple 1-sec breath holds. Magn Reson Imag 1993;11:3–6.
11. Börnert P, Jensen D. Coronary artery imaging at 0.5 T using segmented 3D echo planar imaging. Magn Reson Med 1995;34:779–85.
12. Edelman RR, Manning WJ, Pearlman J, Wei L. Human coronary arteries: projection angiograms reconstructed from breath-hold two-dimensional MR images. Radiology 1993;187(3):719–22.
13. Rogers LF. The heart of the matter: noninvasive coronary artery imaging (editorial). Am J Roentgenol 1998;170: 841.
14. Duerinckx AJ, Lipton MJ. Noninvasive coronary artery imaging using CT and MR imaging (comment) [see comments]. Am J Roentgenol 1998;170(4):900–2.
15. Achenbach S, Moshage W, Ropers D, Bachmann K. Curved multiplanar reconstructions for the evaluation of contrast-enhanced electron beam CT of the coronary arteries. Am J Roentgenol 1998;170:895–99.
16. Woodard PK, Li D, Haacke EM, et al. Detection of coronary stenosis on source and projection images using three-dimensional MR angiography with retrospective respiratory gating: preliminary experience. Am J Roentgenol 1998;170:883–88.
17. Shimamota R, Suzuki J-i, Nishikawa J-i, et al. Measuring the diameter of coronary arteries on MR angiograms using spatial profile curves. Am J Roentgenol 1998;170:889–93.
18. de Koning PJH, van der Geest RJ, Reiber JHC. Enhanced visualization and quantification of 3D contrast enhanced MRA (abstr.). *In*: Book of Abstracts of the First International Workshop on Coronary MR & CT Angiography.

Lyon, France, October 1–3, 2000. Organized and published by the North American Society for Cardiac Imaging. Reprinted in: Intnal J Card Imag 2000;16(3):190.

19. Achenbach S, Kessler W, Moshage WE, et al. Visualization of the coronary arteries in three-dimensional reconstructions using respiratory gated magnetic resonance imaging. Cor Art Dis 1997;8(7):441–48.

20. Geiger B, Krishnan A, Bani-Hashemi A, Becker C. Virtual angioscopy of the coronary arteries (abstr.). *In*: Book of Abstracts of the First International Workshop on Coronary MR & CT Angiography. Lyon, France, October 1–3, 2000. Organized and published by the North American Society for Cardiac Imaging. Reprinted in: Int J Card Imag 2000; 16(3):190.

23

MR of Coronary Artery Lesions Using an Interleaved Multiple Slice Image Acquisition Technique

M.B. Scheidegger

Introduction

Chapter Survey

Aspects of an alternative method for coronary artery imaging using an interleaved multiple slice image acquisition technique will be discussed and results will be presented in this chapter. The method bases on magnetic resonance (MR) data acquisition over an approximately 10-minute period using a dedicated breathing pattern. The entire cardiac cycle is used for data acquisition.

We will give a short and noncomplete survey of varying MR data acquisition techniques for coronary artery magnetic resonance angiography (MRA) based on how the approaches deal with breathing motion. The proposed multiple slice technique is then explained in detail, together with two display techniques for the resulting data sets. The proposed technique will be compared with other approaches described in this book.

A series of images and results will also be presented, together with a complete list of imaging parameters of the described acquisition method.

Motivation

Direct imaging of the coronary arteries by X-ray contrast angiography represents the gold standard for the assessment of coronary artery disease (CAD), and images of the coronary arteries of adequate quality for interventional requirements are generally produced only with this modality. The findings of this imaging procedure are used for therapy planning, percutaneuous transluminal coronary angioplasty (PTCA), bypass surgery, and medication therapy.

This technique, however, is invasive requiring catheterization, is expensive, carries a small risk, and is not well suited for repeated examinations.

PTCA plays a central role in treatment of coronary artery disease. The diagnostic angiography and the treatment by PTCA are increasingly done in one single session; thus, high-quality diagnostic images are available at no extra cost or intervention.

Approximately 20% of all contrast angiographies, however, result in normal findings (1). Furthermore, only about one quarter of all contrast angiographies lead to PTCA, the large majority of which remain diagnostic [information based on (2), data from Germany]. With improved medication therapies this could change toward even a smaller percentage resulting in an angioplastic intervention. A large and possibly growing number of patients, therefore, could benefit from a noninvasive examination, if a suitable technique were present.

Noninvasive visualization of the coronary arteries would be a major step forward for two reasons:

- First, for the noninvasive diagnosis of coronary artery disease in patients at high risk.
- Second, for repeated follow-up examinations after coronary interventions (e.g., PTCA or bypass surgery).

Technical Requirements for Imaging of Coronary Artery Lesions

Requirements for the two major clinical applications mentioned earlier are slightly different: A follow-up study after, for example, a PTCA, requires good intra-subject reproducibility. Consecutive measurements in a time series have to be compared with each other. Diagnosis of coronary artery disease with MR as the only imaging method requires much more: A potential lesion must be discriminated against method deficiencies [i.e., magnetic resonance imaging (MRI) artifacts].

- *Resolution.* Any method must be compared against the gold standard. The image resolution achievable with contrast angiography is on the order of 0.14–0.2 mm, with 0.2–0.3 mm obtained in practice. Angioplastic interventions are possible in the major epicardial vessels. Smaller peripheral vessels, though usually well displayed in conventional contrast angiography, are rarely treated due to their small size with respect to the catheter dimensions, as well as the accessibility of the stenosis, and they are generally also less life-threatening. The question arises, therefore, whether the highest resolution achieved with contrast angiography is really needed in all cases for MR examinations. For a clear depiction of a 50% (area) stenosis in a 2-mm diameter vessel, an image resolution in the order of 0.25–0.3 mm is necessary, with complete absence of imaging artifacts. For a detection of a 75% stenosis, a resolution of 0.5 mm suffices. This results in voxel volumes (assuming isotropic imaging) of 0.01 mm^3, or 0.125 mm^3, respectively. This seems far away from the 2–3 mm^3 usually obtained in conventional MRI of the heart, or even still far away from the 1 mm^3 image resolution obtained in high-resolution MR coronary artery imaging.

- *Image Artifacts.* It is usually the artifact level rather than the nominal image resolution that sets a limit for the resolution that can actually be obtained in the heart. These artifacts are mainly caused by motion: blood velocity in the chambers, heart motion, and respiratory motion. Unless data for an examination of the coronary arteries can be obtained in less than 50 msec, which does not seem to be feasible in the near future, MRI acquisitions rely on the motion to be perfectly periodic so that measurements can be triggered or gated. Very high reproducibility of heart motion and heart position, therefore, is needed. It is this reproducibility of the cardiac motion and the respiratory heart motion that mainly determines the image quality that can be achieved.
- *Contrast.* The larger epicardial vessels are largely embedded in fat. A good fat suppression is therefore needed. For the medial to distal left anterior descending coronary artery, running adjacent to the myocardial muscle of the left ventricle good image contrast between artery and myocardial tissue is also necessary.
- *Display.* The algorithm generally used for display of vessels measured by MR, the maximum intensity projection (MIP) algorithm (18) cannot be used for the coronary arteries because they would be covered within large bright areas of chamber blood. A quick visual impression of the coronary arteries is best obtained by looking at the cine movie across all slices. Alternative versions of displaying vessel data to the user are needed. This chapter will describe two attempts to work out the essential information about a single coronary artery into one image.

MR Coronary Angiography Techniques

Classification of MRI Techniques for Coronary Angiography

Respiratory motion is usually neglected in conventional MRI of the heart with relatively low image resolution in the order of 2–3 mm. Heart displacement by respiration, however, is in the range of 1–2 cm, and is, therefore, considerably larger than the diameter of the coronary arteries. Thus, a precise control of respiratory heart motion is crucial for MR coronary angiography. A number of approaches have been proposed in the past: Data for a single image entity [normally corresponding to a single MR slice image, or to a small volume in three-dimensional (3-D) acquisition] can be acquired:

1. in a single heartbeat
2. in a single breathhold
3. over multiple breathhold periods or breathing cycles

In the following different techniques for MR coronary angiography are sorted according to the type of breathing motion control because this is the most difficult problem to overcome. Early approaches (3,4) did not deal with respiratory motion appropriately, and the progress made over the last few years can be attributed to a good deal of attention paid to the control of the respiratory motion of the heart.

Techniques with Image Acquisition in a Single Heartbeat

Provided the data for a single image entity could be acquired in less than 50 msec, motion artifacts by both cardiac and respiratory motion would not occur.

It is currently possible, however, to acquire one single MR slice image in as little as 50 msec only with single-shot echo-planar image (EPI) acquisition techniques and the use of a special gradient system. Poncelet et al. (5) used EPI to measure coronary blood flow velocities. The spatial resolution of single-shot echo-planar imaging in the heart, however, is usually on the order of approximately 2–4 mm, which is similar to the diameter of the examined vessels and is thus insufficient to distinguish normal from stenotic segments accurately. In our own work with real-time cardiac MRI images can be acquired in approximately 60 msec with an image resolution of approximately 2.7 × 3.5 mm. Although there are absolutely no breathing artifacts, coronary arteries can be sometimes but not always visualized. Extensive improvements in image resolution are needed to use single-shot EPI techniques for MR coronary artery imaging.

Techniques with the Image Acquisition of a Single (or a Few) Slices in One Single Breathhold Period

Edelman et al. (6–8) and Macovski et al. (9–10) developed approaches with breathholding that allowed an image acquisition within a single apnea phase of approximately 12–25 seconds. During this interval one single-slice image of approximately 4-mm thickness and an in-plane resolution of about 1.5 mm^2 is acquired. A corresponding k-space–segmented gradient echo sequence was described by Edelman et al. in 1991 (6). Eight to 10 phase-encoding profiles are measured in a time interval of approximately 100–120 msec during a single diastole, and 10–20 heartbeat intervals are needed for a single (or a few) slice images. Repetitive apnea phases are thus necessary to complete an image data set for display of the proximal coronary arteries. Artifact-free high-quality images are obtained, and the number of slices or breathhold periods, respectively, can be kept to a minimum with suitable slice orientation. This approach has so far been quite successful because the contrast generated in the images by inflow is high, and there are no considerable breathing motion artifacts. A number of authors have used, evaluated, and further developed this approach, and they have published patient studies [see (11–13) for a noncomplete list].

There have also been several other imaging techniques published quite early that also base on breathholding (14).

These are nevertheless long apnea phases for cardiac patients. One problem is that it is difficult to reproduce precisely the inspiration level and thus the slice position with respect to the heart. Thus, it is a robust method to make single (or a few) images during one breathhold period. The difficulty of this approach is the proper definition of the image orientation. It is not always easy to locate the desired parts of the coronary arteries, specifically if the position of the heart varies from one breathhold to the next. This problem is overcome in acquisition strategies that image a volume.

Image Acquisition Over Multiple Respiratory Cycles or Multiple Short Breathhold Periods (Repeated Short Breathholds, Triggering or Gating Techniques, Navigator Techniques)

All imaging techniques that acquire data for a single image entity over more than one inspiration phase fall in this category. The requirements in imaging speed are largely removed when compared with the first two categories. Imaging can last several minutes, and long breathholds are not necessary.

The imaging techniques that fall into these categories are:

1. multiple breathholds for one or more image slices
2. respiratory triggering
3. respiratory gating

Triggering and gating approaches base on information about the inspiration level. This information can be provided by non-MR devices; most commonly, a pneumatic chest belt is used for that purpose. On the other hand, more accurate breathing information can be obtained by additional MR measurements (so-called navigator echoes) to track the motion caused by respiration.

The main problem to be solved for this category of measurement techniques is the reproducibility of the heart position with respiration. Displacements by respiration during the acquisition of a k-space data set directly lead to large artifacts in the single images.

The techniques in categories c2 and c3 can be used with two-dimensional (2-D) or with 3-D image acquisition techniques (15–20). Some of the 3-D image acquisitions have been performed without respiratory motion control, but a large number of signal averages (at least eight) were acquired. Approaches with triggering and gating are discussed in detail elsewhere in this book.

We will now focus on the problems and possibilities created by imaging techniques based on the acquisition of data over multiple breathholds (i.e., the imaging techniques under category c1, where data for every image slice are acquired over multiple short breathholds or inspiration/exhalation cycles).

Coronary Artery MRA with an Interleaved Multiple Slice Acquisition Technique

Breathing Scheme

Instead of long apnea phases a breathing scheme (Fig. 23.1) is used that has been adapted to the natural breathing rhythm (21). The MR signals are acquired approximately every fourth heartbeat during a short apnea phase of approximately 2 seconds. The patient is allowed to breathe in and out normally, but tries to keep the inspiration level after relaxed exhalation for approximately 2 seconds (arrow "stop" in Fig. 23.1). As soon as the MR signal acquisition with its gradient noise (arrow "MR" in Fig. 23.1) is over, the next breathing interval begins.

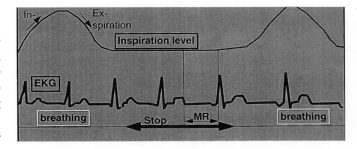

Figure 23.1. Breathing scheme with repeated short apnea phases. The solid line depicts the inspiration level as measured with a pneumatic chest belt. Also shown is the electrocardiogram trace, which is used for triggering of the MR experiment. The breathhold scheme is adapted to the normal breathing rhythm, with a short inspiration–exhalation phase, followed by a breathing pause of approximately 2 seconds duration (arrow "STOP"). During this pause the MR signal acquisition takes place (arrow "MR"). The presented time sequence is repeated every four heartbeats.

The target breathing frequency is 15 cycles/minute. The number of heartbeats, therefore, waited after the MR measurement is adjusted depending on the heart rate of the patient. Correct breathing is monitored with a pneumatic chest belt measuring the extent of the chest circumference (solid line in Fig. 23.1) and displayed to the MR operator.

MRI Sequence

Conventional MR equipment and sequences rather than ultrafast imaging can be used with such breathing schemes. The scheme is well suited for multiple slice acquisition techniques (21–23): MR signals of one phase-encoding step are obtained for all slices within one diastole. The slice arrangement and the acquisition timing for all of the image slices are presented in Figure 23.2. Data for the first slice are acquired at the apex of the heart during early diastole, or even during systole. The slice then moves in a linear sequence from the apex toward the base of the heart during diastole. At end diastole shortly before the next R-wave the last slice is acquired at the level of the ascending aorta, distally to the orifices of the coronary arteries.

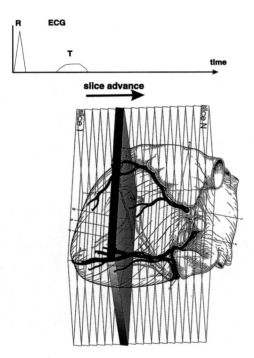

Figure 23.2. Slice arrangement and acquisition timing for all image slices. Data for the first slice are acquired at the apex of the heart during early diastole. The slice then moves in a linear sequence from the apex toward the base of the heart during diastole. At end diastole shortly before the next R-wave in the EKG the last slice is acquired at the level of the ascending aorta, distally to the orifices of the coronary arteries. Slices overlap each other for an improved contrast between inflowing blood in the coronary arteries and surrounding myocardial tissue.

To enhance the contrast between coronary arteries and surrounding tissue, slices overlap each other, causing partial saturation of the overlapping portions (24). With a slice acquisition interval of 15 msec, 30–70 slices are acquired with a slice thickness of 3.5 mm and an overlap of 1.5 mm.

The MR signal of myocardium thus stems from a 2-mm thick slice, whereas signals from blood in the coronary arteries flowing mainly in the opposite direction of the slice movement originate from a 3.5-mm thick portion due to inflow (22).

With the overlapping slices an image contrast is generated between inflowing blood in the coronary arteries and myocardium. Signals from blood moving parallel to the slice movement direction are suppressed to a certain extent. To reduce motion artifacts first-order flow compensation is applied, resulting in an echo time of 7.5 msec, an imaged area of 180×250 mm, and an in-plane resolution of 1 mm^2. All of our examinations have been performed on a commercial 1.5 Tesla whole body Philips Gyroscan ACS-II MR Scanner. A special heart quadrature surface coil was used, and the patients were placed in the prone position. The image volume of 60–140-mm thickness is positioned to cover as much of the proximal coronary arteries as possible; in most cases, the whole heart was covered.

Approximately 180 such "inspire-exspire-wait" cycles are needed for one full data set corresponding to the acquisition of 180 phase-encoding steps, resulting in an acquisition time of 9–13 minutes. The total examination time is approximately 30 minutes. Data for each slice are acquired at a different time in diastole, but data for every single slice image are always acquired at the same time point within diastole so that periodic heart motion does not blur the individual images.

The acquisition window is thus shortened to the readout period for one gradient echo (i.e. to a few milliseconds). As long as there is no jitter uncertainty in the R-wave detection, and the cardiac motion is perfectly reproducible, there will be no blur in the images due to the width of the acquisition window, which is now too short for cardiac motion to cause image artifacts.

In this work we assume that the variation in diameter of the coronary arteries is small over the cardiac cycle. This assumption allows imaging throughout the cardiac cycle (i.e., even in time points with high cardiac motion, such as during contraction or rapid filling). As long as there is sufficient blood flow for the generation of inflow contrast, there is no disadvantage of making use of the whole cardiac cycle for imaging instead of only a short period during diastase in diastole; thus, the efficiency of imaging is increased.

Fat Suppression

The proximal parts of the coronary arteries are largely embedded in fat; therefore, fat signal suppression is essential for good image contrast to enhance local image contrast, and to avoid chemical shift artifacts. The fat signal suppression is accomplished by narrow-band selective saturation pulses on the fat resonance. These pulses, however, last 15 msec each on systems with a field strength of 1.5 Tesla. Fat suppression is therefore more costly in the proposed multislice sequence, which uses all available time in the cardiac cycle for imaging, and a constant fat signal suppression is required throughout the cardiac cycle. As a solution to this time problem it is proposed to sacrifice the constant fat suppression and to apply only one fat suppression pulse every 100 msec. This results in a varying degree of fat suppression in consecutive images (22). In phantoms and in patient examinations an average reduction of the amplitude of the fat signal by a factor of 7.5 could be achieved. This fat suppression factor is roughly sufficient, largely increasing the image contrast in areas with coronary arteries. As shown later in Figure 23.8 the varying degree of fat suppression over consecutive images can be seen at the chest wall.

Image Display

The slice overlap generates a rather low contrast between coronary arteries and myocardial tissue. The algorithm generally used for display of vessels measured by MR, the maximum intensity projection algorithm (25)

cannot be used for the coronary arteries, since they would be covered within large bright areas of chamber blood. A quick visual impression of the coronary arteries is best obtained by looking at the cine movie across all slices. Also final decisions about the status of the coronary arteries were only based on the inspection of the original source images.

The need for a "one-image"-visualization of the coronary arteries does remain. Edelman et al. (26) used local maximum intensity projection procedures, where larger bright areas as for instance blood pools in heart chambers are marked by the operator and "cut" out of the image.

In the next two sections we will describe two different attempts for a "one-image"-visualization, which should resemble a projection view commonly obtained in conventional X-ray contrast angiography. By using dedicated software both approaches allow to perform several types of measurements on the coronary tree (e.g. length or diameter measurements), as well as the determination of the cross-sectional area of the coronary artery.

Curved Planar Reformat ("Vessel Tracking Reformat")

In curved planar reformatting, the centerline of the vessel of interest has to be defined, and marked manually by the operator. The user is offered a slice perpendicular to the current position in the path and two images along the vessel (i.e. perpendicular to the first image). This situation is demonstrated in Figures 23.3.

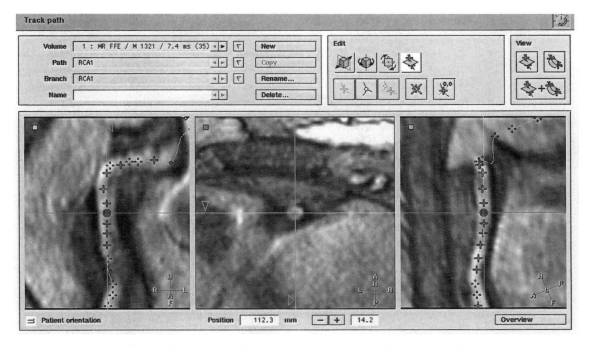

Figure 23.3. *Curved planar reformat ("vessel tracking reformat").*

Figure 23.3 (middle) shows the slice perpendicular to a right coronary artery, and the user marks the middle of the vessel. The perpendicular views, the images on the left and on the right, serve to confirm that the choice of the vessel center is correct; fine adjustments can be made on these perpendicular images. A vessel can usually be tracked in a few minutes, and the calculation of the vessel tracking projections lasts a few seconds.

Figure 23.4 demonstrates the construction of the path follow reformat plane: A suitable projection plane is automatically chosen by the computer, shaded in gray in Figure 23.4A. The algorithm constructs a plane that is oriented orthogonal to the projection plane and passes through the selected path [see middle part, (B) in Fig. 23.4]. This constructed plane is now folded out into the display plane to yield the curved planar reformat view, or a "vessel tracking reformat," shown in the right (C) part of Figure 23.4.

Although any plane may be used for the projection of the path, a plane is initially selected that will optimally show the curvature of the path. The user can rotate this plane horizontally and vertically later, as demonstrated in Figure 23.5a. The middle of the vessel has sometimes not been found exactly. The curved reformatted plane, therefore, can now be offset slightly from the centerline, as shown in Figure 23.5b. Small offsets will now slightly alter the appearance of the vessel in the vessel tracking reformat view. It will generally be improved in certain vessel segments, and worsened in others. Moving through a number of different offsets quickly gives a good impression of the vessel diameter along the whole coronary artery. Figure 23.6 explains the effect of these small offsets. If the middle point of a

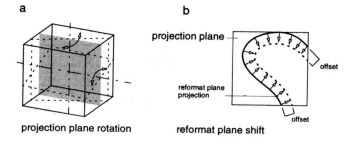

Figure 23.5. Although any plane may be used for the projection of the path, a plane is initially selected that will optimally show the curvature of the path. The user can rotate this plane horizontally and vertically later, as demonstrated in (a). This rotation will alter the appearance of the vessel in the reformatted plane, generally changing its curvature as well as the orientation to neighboring objects. The middle of the vessel has sometimes not been found exactly. The curved reformatted plane, therefore, can now be offset slightly from the centerline, as shown in (b). Small offsets will now slightly alter the appearance of the vessel in the vessel tracking reformat view. It will generally be improved in certain vessel segments, and worsened in others. Moving through a number of different offsets quickly gives a good impression of the vessel diameter along the whole coronary artery.

vessel is not found exactly, the reconstructed plane does not pass through the center of the vessel. If one assumes a circular cross-section, the diameter of the vessel will be rendered too small in the vessel-tracking projection. Adding or subtracting small offsets can locally correct for this effect. The algorithm used is available on a commercial Easy Vision CT/MR workstation (Philips Medical Systems, Best, The Netherlands), based on a SUN computer (SUN 5, Palo Alto, CA).

The procedure for coronary arteries is defined as follows: The starting point for the vessel path is set in the ascending aorta, well above the aortic valve, and above the orifices of the coronary arteries. The path initially follows the middle of the ascending aorta for a few centimeters. Path points are then defined toward a coronary orifice, and the particular vessel of interest is followed, as long as it is well defined. The procedure has to be performed separately for each artery of interest. We usually examined the right coronary artery from orifice to bifurcation into right posterior descending branch and the right interventricular coronary artery, and, if possible, followed one of these branches. On the left coronary artery tree, we concentrated on setting a path from the aorta, through the left main coronary artery, and then along the left anterior descending coronary artery. The left circumflex artery was often not defined well enough in the original images to be traced reliably.

Examples of vessel tracking projections of coronary arteries will be shown later in Figures 23.12 and 23.14.

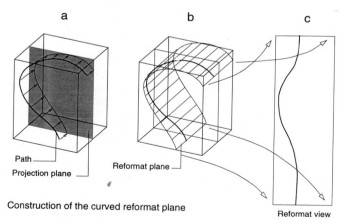

Construction of the curved reformat plane

Figure 23.4. Construction of the path follow reformat plane. A suitable projection plane is automatically chosen by the computer, shaded in gray in (a). The algorithm constructs a plane that is oriented orthogonal to the projection plane and passes through the selected path (see middle part, b). This constructed plane is now folded out into the display plane to yield the curved planar reformat view, or a "vessel-tracking reformat," shown in the right part of (c).

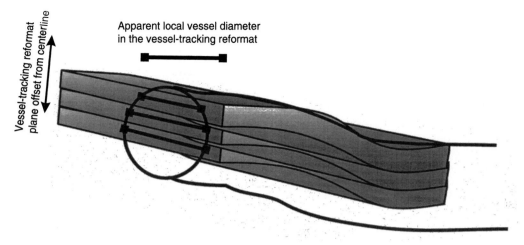

Figure 23.6. The effect of small offsets of the found vessel center (relate to Fig. 23.5B). If the middle point of a vessel is not found exactly, the reconstructed plane does not pass through the center of the vessel. If a circular cross-section is assumed, the diameter of the vessel will be rendered too small in the vessel-tracking projection. Adding or subtracting small offsets (i.e., reconstructing planes shaped identically to the original one, but with a plane offset in the plane projection direction) can locally correct for this effect.

3-D Reconstruction

As an alternative to the vessel-tracking projection we explored displays of coronary arteries by segmentation and 3-D object rendering. A semiautomatic segmentation of the coronary arteries was performed on a computer workstation (VAXstation 4000/90, Digital Equipment, Maynard, USA). In a first step, the vessel contours are determined semi-automatically slice by slice (27). This contouring procedure results in a contour set for a short piece of the ascending aorta, the right coronary artery (RCA), the left main coronary artery with its two main branches (left circumflex, left anterior descending coronary artery), and, if possible, short segments of further side branches.

The contour finding algorithm (27,28) is an iterative procedure, starting with an initial contour guess provided by the user, for which the most probable contour is approached step by step. The probability criterion contains the following aspects:

- the signal intensity outside of the contour (within the surrounding fat, adjacent myocardial tissue) should be low
- the signal intensity inside the contour should be as high as the expected flow-enhanced vascular signal
- the contour points should not deviate too much from the contour points of the previous iteration
- contour points in the neighborhood of other contour points are favored

All of these aspects are weighted such that rapid convergence is achieved. In relatively straight segments of the RCA with predominantly through-plane flow, automatic contouring produces good contour sets. The left main, the proximal left anterior descending, and the circumflex arteries require manual corrections because they contain longer segments laying within the image plane, and thus exhibit much lower image contrast. At vessel branches and at sites of severe stenoses operator input is required to aid the contouring algorithm.

The segmented arteries plus a short piece of the ascending aorta are then displayed on the same workstation with a 3-D visualization package specially designed for surface reconstruction of contour-based 3-D objects (29). The reconstructed vessels can be rotated freely into any desired view.

Normal RCAs usually exhibited enough contrast to be segmented automatically. The left main (LM), the left anterior descending (LAD), and the left circumflex artery (LCx) required user interaction. The segmented arteries together with a short piece of the ascending aorta are then reconstructed and displayed with a 3-D presentation package on the same workstation. The reconstructed vessels can be rotated into any desired view (see Figure 23.15).

How Does the Presented Method Differ from More Widespread Acquisition Techniques?

In the Timing of the Acquisition During the Heart Cycle

The entire cardiac cycle is used for imaging in the multiple-slice acquisition strategy. Data for a single slice, however, are acquired within a few milliseconds, always at the same time point within the cardiac cycle. As long as the patient has a regular heartbeat, the periodic heart motion does not blur the images. Because the acquisition lasts only a few milliseconds, data acquisition even during periods of fast heart motion is not affected by motion, and data can be gathered during systole and diastole. Assuming that the diameter of the coronary arteries does not change largely over the cardiac cycle, scanning in both systole and diastole increases efficiency.

In the "single-slice, single breathhold" approach data are acquired over a time window with relatively little cardiac motion. This time window is placed in diastole, and usually lasts on the order of 100 msec (11). It is too long to image (e.g., during systole), which would lead to large image artifacts. This fact has also been noted by Hofmann et al. for quantitative flow measurements in the coronary arteries over the entire cardiac cycle (30), as well as for flow measurements (31).

The heart is a three-dimensional moving structure; consequently, a four-dimensional type of acquisition (three object dimensions and time) is needed if imaging is performed over the cardiac cycle. The proposed multislice imaging sequence acquires data in three spatial dimensions (multiple 2-D slices), but uses the entire cardiac cycle for this purpose. As a result, the time axis (motion during the cardiac cycle) is mapped onto the third spatial dimension in the data set (i.e., the through-plane direction). Apical slices are acquired in systole and early diastole, equatorial and basal slices during mid- and late diastole. This results in a geometrical distortion of the coronary artery tree. This effect, however, does not lead to image blurring or artifacts because data for a single slice are always acquired at the same time point in the cardiac cycle. The consequence is merely a distortion, most pronounced in the distal segments of the coronary artery tree.

In Inflow Contrast
Imaging a single slice with a high pulse angle and a short repetition time, as done in the "single-slice, single breathhold" approach, results in a large inflow contrast even for low velocities. Static tissue is largely suppressed and contributes little signal. The multiple-overlapping-slice technique generates a much lower contrast between inflowing blood in the coronary arteries and myocardial tissue. This is a major disadvantage of the proposed technique. The inflow contrast is also restricted to one inflow-direction, whereas signals from inflowing spins from the opposite direction are largely suppressed.

Because all the time within one heartbeat interval is used for acquiring the approximately 50 slices, there is no time left to include prepulses to enhance image contrast between myocardial tissue and blood in the coronary arteries. Such contrast-enhancing prepulses [e.g., T_2-saturating sequence proposed by Brittain (32), or the use of MTC prepulses are much easier incorporated in the "single-slice, single breathhold" technique.

In Slice Orientation with Respect to the Coronary Arteries
Although single slices are measured in the multislice approach, essentially a volume is acquired. Because the in-

flow contrast is low, coronaries are best imaged if they cut perpendicularly through the slices. The slice stack is positioned (see Fig. 23.2) to incorporate as much of the coronary artery tree in the imaged area, and at the same time so that the most important segments are more or less perpendicular to the slices.

In contrast to this setup, the number of slices to be acquired is minimized for the "single-slice, single breathhold" technique, and for this purpose, longer segments of the coronary arteries are imaged "in-plane."

In Ease of Use
Therefore typically 45–50 slices are acquired with a volume of 250 mm $\times$ 180 mm $\times$ (90 . . . 100) mm. With such a large imaging volume the proximal parts of the coronary arteries are always imaged. It is therefore very easy to position the imaging volume; no extensive experience in imaging coronary arteries nor very good knowledge of the coronary anatomy of the operator is required.

This is in contrast to the very popular and also successful "single-slice, single breathhold" approach where one slice is imaged per single breathhold, and breathholds are repeated. Because the number of breathholds that a patient can perform is limited, the correct slice positioning has to be found within a few tries. This job is often further complicated if the level of inspiration is not always the same over consecutive breathholds.

Initial Clinical Applications

If we regard (1) noninvasive diagnosis of coronary artery disease in patients at high risk, and (2) repeated examinations after coronary interventions (e.g., PTCA or bypass-surgery as the two major possible applications), then the latter is less demanding. Our attempts were therefore initially concentrated on the repeatability of the MR examination for follow-up studies after PTCA.

A number of volunteers without any symptoms for coronary artery disease were examined. Patients with known coronary artery disease have been imaged, usually 1 day before treatment of the coronary artery lesion with PTCA, to evaluate whether the stenotic lesion could be identified with the MR procedure. Another MR examination was performed 1–8 days after the intervention. One to four follow-up examinations were performed in these patients, normally 3, 6, and 12 months after PTCA, for the detection of restenosis.

Details of the Image Acquisition Technique

Table 23.1 lists all the imaging parameters in detail. For better readability the parameters were grouped into "geometry," "hardware and patient," "contrast and timing," and "motion and others." It should be possible to fully copy the approach from this list.

Figure 23.7 shows image sections of 27 consecutive images from an examination with 70 acquired slices. The 27 images cover almost the full length of the right coronary artery. The display order is (from upper left = image 1 to lower right = image 27) from base to apex. In the first and the second image the orifice of the RCA is depicted. Imaging of the RCA is usually successful from orifice to the distal bifurcation. A segment of the right posterior descending coronary artery is also visible in the presented case. In this early case the acquisition was performed without fat suppression. The use of an "opposite-phase" echo time (i.e., fat and water are out of phase, at an echo time of 6.9 ms on a 1.5 Tesla system), however, helps to distinguish the RCA from adjacent tissue in the ventricular groove in this case. Data are taken from a patient with a severe lesion in the proximal LAD, and an unobstructed RCA.

Figure 23.8 shows a similar data set of an RCA now with the proposed fat suppression pulse once every 100 msec. Fat suppression largely increased the vessel contrast for the RCA. Small side branches (best seen in the middle row) start to be visible for a short distance. The varying degree of fat suppression is evident at the fat layer of the chest wall; however, fat suppression appears to be sufficient for the intended purpose.

Figures 23.9A–C show three single-slice images of the proximal part of the LAD coronary artery of a 53-year-old patient with a high-grade stenosis in that vessel segment. The stenosis is visible as a short segment of signal loss, or uncertainty of the vessel status in Figure 23.9A. The image in Figure 23.9A was acquired 1 day before treatment of the stenosis with PTCA. Figures 23.9B,C represent images from the MR examination 1 day after the PTCA, and 6 months later, respectively. An open vessel is found in both images, with just a slight impression of narrowing in the acquisition 6 months after treatment.

Table 23.1. Imaging parameters.

Parameter group	Parameter	Value (range)
Geometry	Field-of-view	250 × 180 (mm)
	Slice thickness acquisition	3.5 (mm)
	Effective slice thickness static tissue	2 (mm)
	Slice overlap	1.5 (mm)
	Slice acquisition order	Linear order from apex toward base
	Image resolution	0.97 × 1.02 (mm)
	Image matrix	256
	Acquisition strategy	Multiple slices
	Number of slices	50 at heart rate of 60 bpm
	Scan percentage	95%
Hardware and Patient	Coil	Circular surface coil (diam. 20 cm) or quadrature surface coil
	Patient position	Prone
	Breathing monitoring	Pneumatic chest belt
	Magnet	1.5 Tesla
	HW used	Philips Gyroscan ACS-II or Philips Gyroscan ACS/NT
Contrast and Timing	Pulse angle	85 degrees
	Technique	Gradient echo
	Partial echo	yes
	Partial echo factor	0.63
	Echo time	Approx. 7.5 msec, dep. on angulation
	Half scan	no
	Fat suppression	yes
	Fat suppression pulses	Frequency-selective (SPIR)
	Fat suppression sequence	One fat-suppression pulse every 100 msec
	Number of phase-encoding profiles	171
	Scan duration	11.4 min at heart rate 60 bpm 9.1 min at heart rate 75 bpm
	Time interval between the acquisition of 2 slices	17 msec
Motion and others	Cardiac synchronization	EKG triggering
	Trigger delay	From 8 to 250 msec (systolic and diastolic acquisition or diastolic acquisition only)
	Heartbeats/data acquisition (= repetition time)	Usually one heart cycle acquisition every four heartbeats, depending on heart rate
	Special calibration step	Automatic localized shimming; for fat-suppression pulses

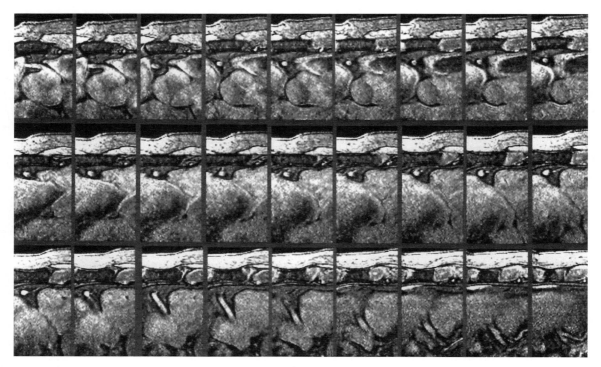

Figure 23.7. Image sections of 27 consecutive images from an examination with a total of 70 acquired slices. The 27 images cover a long part of the RCA. The display order is (from upper left = image 1; to lower right = image 27) from base to apex. In the first and the second image the orifice of the RCA is depicted. Imaging of the RCA is usually successful from orifice to the distal bifurcation. A segment of the right posterior descending coronary artery is also visible in the presented case. Note that no longer vessel segments are visible, the acquisition slice orientation is oriented as perpendicular to the vessel as possible, in order to maximize inflow contrast. However, this acquisition strategy asks for reformatting or postprocessing steps of the original image data.

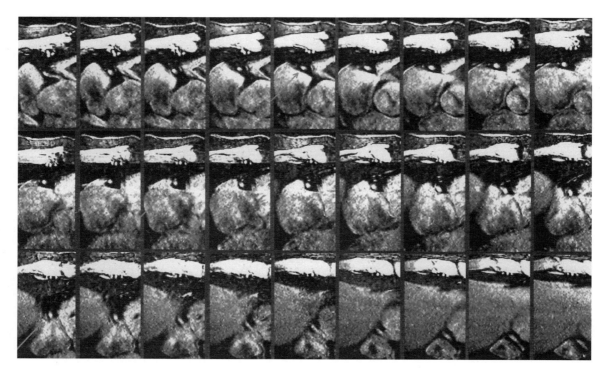

Figure 23.8. Image sections of 27 consecutive images from an examination with a total of 60 acquired slices. The 27 images cover the full length of the right coronary artery from orifice to the distal bifurcation. This coverage of the RCA is very typical. The display order is (from upper left = image 1, to lower right = image 27) from base to apex. In the first and the second image the orifice of the RCA is depicted. Compared with Figure 23.7, where no fat suppression was used (but 70 images could be acquired), this data set was acquired with the frequency-selective fat saturation pulse (but only 48 images could be acquired). Note the varying degree of fat suppression over the consecutive images, which is sufficient in all images to largely enhance vessel contrast. Small side branches of the RCA start to be visible (e.g., images 12–18 in the middle row), although they are usually too small to be tracked and reliably displayed.

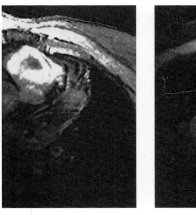
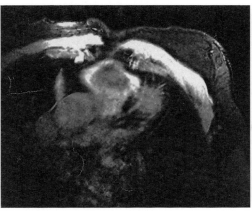
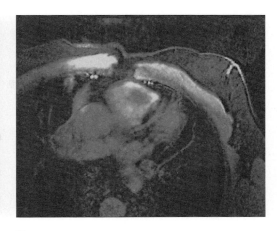

A   B   C

Figure 23.9. Unprocessed source images from three examinations of the same patient. The image in (A) was acquired 1 day before treatment of the high-grade stenosis of the left anterior descending coronary artery. Note that the vessel is shown only over a short segment in each image slice acquired. In order to show a slightly longer segment, three consecutive image slices have been added and displayed as a sum image, done for all images in A–C. This summation causes some additional image blurring, not present in the originally acquired images. (B) presents the sum image from the acquisition 1 day after the treatment of the stenosis with PTCA. There seems to be a slight shadow at the originally stenosed location, but the success of the treatment is clearly visible. The result from the examination late after PTCA, after 6 months, is shown in (C). The vessel remained open over the 6 months, and no restenosis could be detected.

Figures 23.10 and 23.11 represent the corresponding contrast angiography projections, before and immediately after PTCA, with superimposed diameter evaluation plots.

In Figure 23.12 a vessel-tracking reformat image is presented, in comparison with a corresponding contrast angiography projection, shown in Figure 23.13. The presentation of the normal nonstenosed vessel in this example is limited to the first 5 cm of the proximal RCA in the contrast angiography, whereas the MR vessel-tracking reformat shows a much longer segment of the RCA; approximately 13 cm are visible. On the left part the reconstructed image along the path is shown. Please note that the unfolding of a tortuous 3-D path onto a plane results in displaying larger structures in the heart in a very distorted fashion. A distorted part of the ascending aorta is visible in the upper right of the image, with the orifice of the RCA. The path then follows the RCA until the distal bifurcation and then a further 2 cm along the right interventricular branch, until the vessel

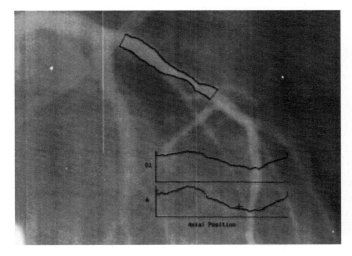

Figure 23.10. Conventional contrast angiography image of the stenosis case shown in Figure 23.9A. The image is presented after automatic edge detection, and the detected vessel diameter and the calculated vessel cross-sectional area are plotted along the vessel in the lower right part of the figure. This high-grade stenosis was subsequently treated with PTCA.

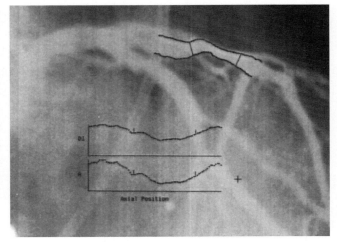

Figure 23.11. Conventional contrast angiography image of the case in Figure 23.9, acquired immediately after the treatment of the stenosis. This image corresponds to the MRI in Figure 23.9B, which was acquired 1 day later.

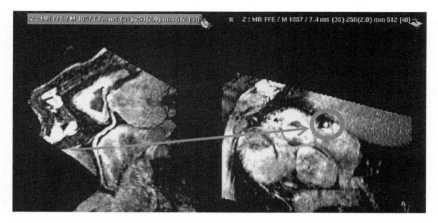

Figure 23.12. Demonstration of a typical result of the vessel-tracking reformat procedure. On the left part the reconstructed image along the path is shown. Please note that the unfolding of a tortuous 3-D path onto a plane results in displaying larger structures in the heart in a very distorted fashion. In the upper right of the image a distorted part of the ascending aorta is visible, with the orifice of the RCA. The path then follows the RCA until the distal bifurcation and then a further 2 cm along the right interventricular branch, until the vessel leaves the stack of acquired images. The right-hand image displays a reformatted image *perpendicular* to the vessel at the marked location. The RCA is marked in the circle. Using this feature, the true vessel cross-section can be displayed, and vessel diameter and vessel cross-sectional area can be derived. This feature is unique for MR because only MR acquires a truly 3-D data set, and the vessel cross-section can be assessed in its true shape without any assumptions. The orientation of this image is not self-explanatory, but the computer program allows one to measure the distance along the path. In the case shown, the cross-section displayed is located 6.8 cm distal to the orifice of the RCA.

leaves the stack of acquired images. The right-hand image displays a reformatted image *perpendicular* to the vessel at the marked location. The RCA is marked in the circle. Using this feature, the true vessel cross-section can be displayed, and vessel diameter and vessel cross-sectional area can be derived. This feature is unique for MR because only MR acquires a truly 3-D data set, and the vessel cross-section can be assessed in its true shape without any assumptions. The computer program allows to measure the distance along the path. In the case shown, the cross-section displayed is located 6.8 cm distal to the orifice of the RCA.

In Figures 23.14A–D and 23.15A–D vessel tracking reformat views of the LAD coronary artery of the case in Figures 23.9A,C are shown. The reformat view from the pretreatment scan (Fig. 23.14 A–D) is of doubtable quality. The left parts in the Figures 23.14A–D show the image plane along the vessel, and the high-grade stenosis is visible. The right parts of Figure 23.14A–D present the cross-sectional view through the vessel at the location marked with the bar in the left parts of the figures. The following locations are shown: immediately proximal of the stenosis (A), right through the center of the stenosis (B), approximately 4 mm distal to the stenosis (C), and finally approximately 2 cm distal to the stenosis.

The vessel cross-section is marked with a circle in all images. Flow signal is clearly visible proximal to the stenosis. The vessel is barely visible in the stenosis. The cross-sectional area, and, with this, the degree of vessel narrowing cannot be determined due to signal loss at the location of the stenosis.

Reconstitution of the vessel signal is observed 4 mm distal to the stenosis (C), as well as 2 cm distal to the stenosis (Fig. 23.14D).

Figures 23.15A–D present the vessel-tracking reformat from the examination 6 months after PTCA. The left parts in Figures 23.15A–D show the image plane along the vessel, and the good definition of the vessel without considerable narrowing at the site of the former stenosis can be noted.

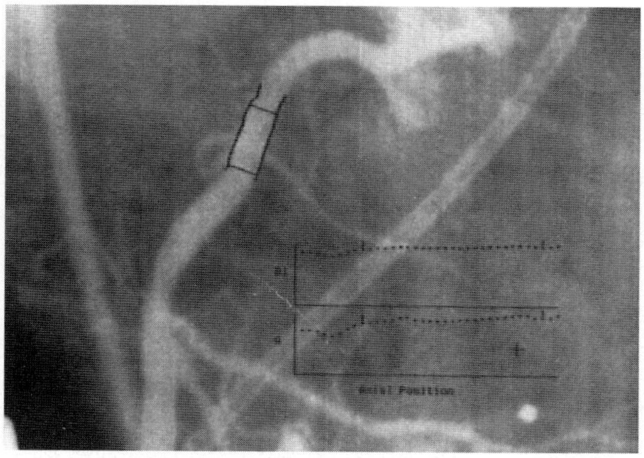

Figure 23.13. Conventional contrast angiography image of the RCA shown in Figure 23.12. The unwinding procedure of the coronary artery in MR vessel-tracking reformat makes the comparison in a well-defined orientation difficult. The position in centimeters along the vessel has to serve as a measure for direct comparison of vessel segments.

Figure 23.14. Vessel tracking reformat display of the left anterior descending coronary artery of the case in Figure 23.9. The left parts in (A–D) show the image plane along the vessel. The high-grade stenosis is visible, although this image stack is of rather low quality. The right parts of (A–D) show the cross-sectional view through the vessel at the location marked with the bar in the left parts of the figures. (A) right: Cross-section immediately proximal of the stenosis. The vessel cross-section is visible, marked with the circle. (B) right: Cross-section through the center of the stenosis. The vessel is barely visible. The cross-sectional area, and, with this, the degree of vessel narrowing cannot be determined due to signal loss at the location of the stenosis. (C) right: Cross-section of the vessel approximately 4 mm distal to the stenosis. Reconstitution of the vessel signal is observed. (D) right: Cross-section approximately 2 cm distal to the stenosis. Full reconstitution of the vessel signal (as in all images, marked with a circle).

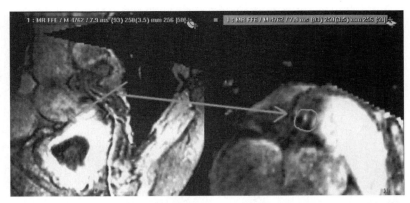

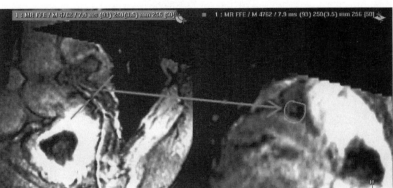

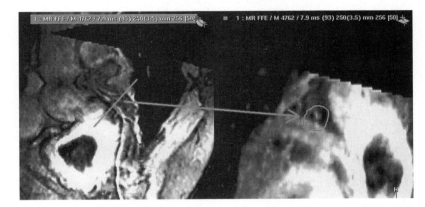

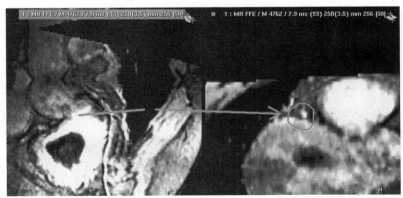

A

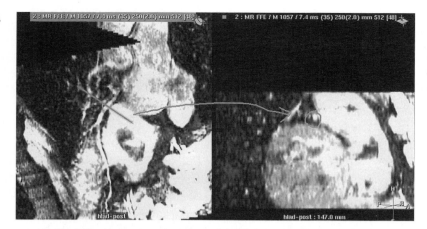

B

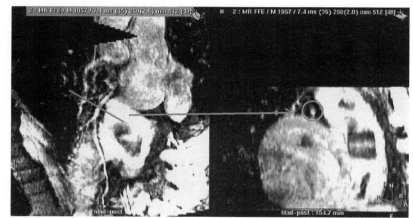

C

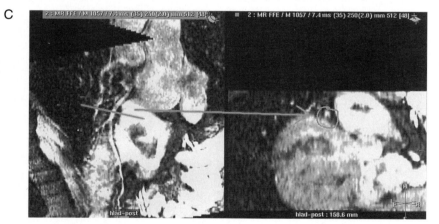

D

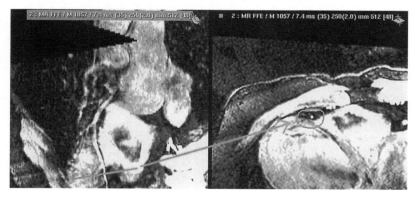

Figure 23.15. Vessel-tracking reformat display of the left anterior descending coronary artery of the case in Figure 23.9. Data are taken from the examination 6 months after treatment of the stenosis with PTCA. The left parts in (A–D) show the image plane along the vessel, and the good definition of the vessel without considerable narrowing at the site of the former stenosis can be noted. A slight shadow is still visible at this vessel location. The right parts of (A–D) show the cross-sectional view through the vessel at the location marked with the bar in the left parts of the figures. The vessel is marked with a circle in each of the images. (A) Cross-sectional image 8 mm proximal of the site of the former stenosis. Cross-section right through the location of the former stenosis. The vessel cross-sectional area is not remarkably different from the area as seen in (A) right, and (C) right. Cross-section (C) right is located 8 mm downstream of the old stenosis. (D) right shows the vessel cross-section approximately 7 cm distal to the site of the former stenosis, to show that the cross-section in a further distal location is still very well defined in these MR data sets.

There seems to be a slight "shadow" visible at the site of the former stenosis, more pronounced than in the examination 3 months ago (not shown), but the diameter of the vessel at that location was not changed when compared with the examination 1 day after the treatment.

The right parts of Figures 23.15A–D show the cross-sectional view through the vessel at the location marked with the bar in the left parts of the figures. The vessel is marked with a circle in each of the images.

The following locations are shown: 8 mm proximal to the site of the former stenosis (A), right through the center of the stenosis (B), approximately 8 mm distal to the stenosis (C), and finally approximately 7 cm distal to the stenosis (D), to show that the cross-section in a further distal location is still very well defined in these MR data sets.

The vessel cross-sectional area at the site of the former stenosis (Figure 23.15B, right) is not remarkably different to the area as seen in Figure 23.15A, right, and 23.15C, right.

A 3-D reconstruction of the coronary artery tree of a 48-year-old patient with one-vessel disease is presented in Figure 23.16. The MR examination was performed 4 months after successful PTCA of the proximal LAD. An

open vessel was found initially; however, restenosis occurred 4 months later that had to be treated again with a second PTCA. The stenosis (arrow) is displayed as a short segment of an occluded vessel. This is explained by signal loss at the stenosis, which is caused by high blood flow velocities and a high spatial velocity gradient, respectively. The second PTCA was again successful and the result could be documented by MRA.

Diameter Evaluation

Conventional contrast angiograms were acquired in all cases during the intervention. Proximal (approximately 10 mm after the orifice) and distal (20–30 mm and 40–50 mm distal to the orifice) vessel diameters (D) were determined with both magnetic resonance and quantitative coronary angiography (QCA). Figure 23.17 shows the diameter evaluation procedure for MRI. Single MRI were selected. First, a sinc-interpolation algorithm (Fourier interpolation) of a selected region onto a grid of 0.1×0.1 mm was performed. The vessel boundaries were then drawn manually on a computer workstation using a program designed for that purpose. The diameter was then measured 10 times over a length of approximately 5–8 mm, and the single measurements were averaged. In Figure 23.17 the diameter of a normal proximal segment of an RCA is evaluated approximately 10 mm distal to the orifice. Only normal nonstenosed vessel segments were included for this comparison because the diameter could not be estimated in stenotic segments due to signal loss across the lesion in the MR images.

Quantitative evaluation of coronary angiograms was performed with a semi-automatic computer system (33–35). The system is based on a 35-mm film projector (Tagarno 35 CX), a slow-scan CCD-camera for image digitization, and a computer work station (Apollo DN 3000) for image storage and processing. Contour detection was carried out with use of a geometric–densitometric edge detection algorithm (36). The diameter of the three major coronary vessels (LAD, LCx, and RCA) was measured from one to three end-diastolic cine frames over a length of approximately 5 mm. The computer traced this segment automatically and calculated the mean diameter over this segment. For each vessel segment measurements in different projections were obtained and averaged. Calibration was performed automatically by using the proximal part of the 8F Judkins catheter as a scaling device.

Forty-four vessel segments were measured. The correlation coefficient amounted to $r = 0.76$, the regression line $D_{MR} = 0.71 D_{QCA} + 0.8$ (mm). The mean difference was 0.2 mm and the standard deviation of the mean difference 0.4 mm. In general, small coronary diameters were overestimated by MRA. This can be explained by partial volume effects and with an image blur by remaining respiratory movements.

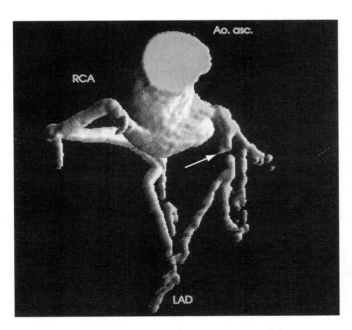

Figure 23.16. Three-dimensional reconstruction of the coronary artery tree of a 48-year-old patient with coronary one-vessel disease. The MR examination was performed 4 months after successful PTCA of the proximal LAD. An open vessel was found initially; however, 4 months later restenosis occurred which had to be treated again with a second PTCA. The stenosis (arrow) is displayed as a short segment of an occluded vessel. This is explained by signal loss at the stenosis, which is caused by high blood flow velocities and a high spatial velocity gradient, respectively. Only a few millimeters downstream of the stenosis, there is full-signal reconstitution.

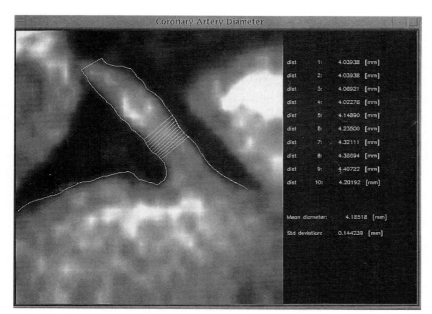

Figure 23.17. Demonstration of the procedure for the determination of the vessel diameters from single MR images. First, a sinc-interpolation algorithm (Fourier interpolation) of a selected region onto a grid of 0.1 × 0.1 mm was performed. The vessel boundaries were then drawn manually on a computer workstation using a program designed for that purpose (i.e., see the white line in the image). The diameter was then measured 10 times over a length of approximately 5–8 mm (the 10 white lines), and the single measurements were averaged. In this example the diameter of a normal proximal segment of an RCA is evaluated approximately 7 mm distal to the orifice. Only normal non-stenosed vessel segments were included for this comparison because the diameter could not be estimated in stenotic segments due to signal loss across the lesion in the MRIs.

Figures 23.18 and 23.19 show examples of the diameter comparison. Orifices and bifurcations served as landmarks in the coronary vessel tree for matching the location of the diameter measurements. Figures 23.18A,B demonstrate a measurement pair in the distal right coronary artery just proximal to the bifurcation into the right posterior descending branch and the right interventricular coronary artery. Diameter measurements account for 3.5 mm (MR) versus 3.3 mm (angiography). Because the MRI represents a single slice image, only a short piece of the artery is visible, and its location can be determined only from the context of adjacent images, which are not shown. In Figures 23.19A,B a similar comparison is shown in the proximal LAD coronary artery (diameter values obtained are 2.5 mm for the MRI and 2.3 mm for the contrast angiography technique).

Perspectives

What Has Been Achieved So Far?

Coronary Vessels

Several studies (6,7,8,11,13,15–23) have shown that a reasonably good MRA is obtained in a majority of patients or examinations, although the reported degree of success shows a wide variation. According to the experience with the procedure outlined in this chapter (i.e., multiple-interleaved slices, the proximal two thirds of the coronary arteries can be usually visualized reliably in the majority of patients (with the exception of the LCx artery). The best results are generally obtained in the RCA due to its proximity to the chest wall, and to the surface coil, respectively. Patients are put into prone position; therefore, the anterior parts of the heart are very close to the coil. Results are somewhat less good for the

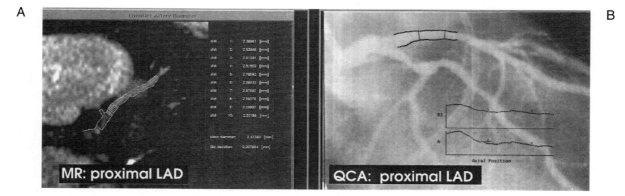

Figure 23.18. Vessel diameter comparison MR versus QCA. An example in the LAD coronary artery, approximately 2–3 cm distal to the bifurcation of the left main coronary artery into LAD and LCx coronary artery. (A) Measurement in the MR image, diameter = 2.5 mm. (B) Measurement with QCA, diameter = 2.3 mm.

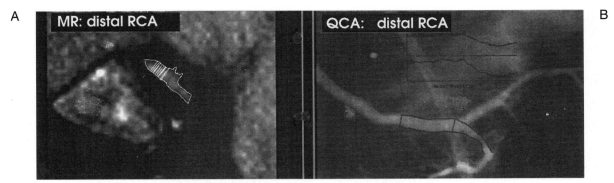

Figure 23.19. Vessel diameter comparison MR versus QCA. An example in the distal RCA, immediately proximal to the bifurcation into right posterior descending coronary artery (which has a stenosis in this case, demonstrated with contrast angiography), and the right interventricular branch. (A) Measurement in the MR image, diameter = 3.5 mm. (B) Measurement with QCA, diameter = 3.3 mm.

LAD coronary artery, and are rather unreliable for the LCx. This is due to the large distance of the LCx to the surface coil on the chest wall. It may also be affected by the relatively large motion of the lateral and inferior segments of the heart at the basal level.

Reproducibility
One of the main problems of earlier attempts to image coronary arteries was the reproducibility of the image quality over different examinations. The image quality now appears to be sufficiently reproducible over repeated examinations of the same patient in follow-up examinations; however, a constant, high-quality image is still not achieved in all patient examinations, and a considerable patient-to-patient variation of the MRI quality remains. This seems to be caused mainly by the varying success of reproducing the breathing motion pattern, and appears to be the main challenge in a further development of MRA of the coronary arteries.

Limitations in Spatial Resolution/Contrast
The spatial resolution for the visualization of high-grade coronary stenoses averages between insufficient and borderline, sometimes already about sufficient. The resolution for an accurate delineation of a moderate stenosis is clearly insufficient.

Using surface coils, at present, an in-plane resolution of 1×1 mm with approximately 2-mm-thick slices can be obtained. This spatial resolution is sufficient to image the proximal segments of the main coronary arteries. It is also sufficient to distinguish between a completely normal vessel and a severe proximal lesion. High-grade stenoses often exhibit considerable signal loss within and a few millimeters downstream of the constriction. Signal loss is therefore a major contributor to stenosis visibility. This fact is pronounced in the presented data with an echo time used of approximately 7 msec. Signal loss helped to locate stenoses in the current studies. A reliable stenosis detection, however,

should base on imaging the "true" vessel lumen, not on imaging signal loss in a stenosis.

The MRI resolution, however, is not sufficient for imaging the more distal segments or smaller side branches, and is also not sufficient for accurate rating of mild to moderate stenoses of less than 50% reduction in cross-sectional vessel area, and it is still very low when compared with contrast angiography. An improvement may be achieved with intravascular contrast agents, selectively lowering the T_1-relaxation time of blood. It is expected that such agents will largely improve image contrast, and that they can be used in clinical routine in a few years.

Breathing Motion Artifacts
Previous evaluations confirmed that even highly motivated volunteers have difficulties with the long apneic phases to reproduce the same diaphragm position over the consecutive long breathholds. If data for one slice are obtained in one apneic phase, varying degrees of inspiration of different breathholds lead to a series of images that are partly misaligned. With the presented multislice technique, however, a congruent 3-D volume is acquired with excellent vessel continuity (21–23).

The price to pay for the perfect vessel continuity is an increased artifact level in the individual images, caused by slight variations in the inspiration level across consecutive short breathholds.

With only one exception all volunteers and all patients understood the breathing scheme easily and breathing errors were relatively rare. Nobody complained about shortness of breath because the breathhold scheme resembles normal breathing. Because they are required for the methods in References (6–13) longer repetitive breathhold periods can often be too strenuous for cardiac patients. Moreover, heart rate can vary as a consequence of the apnea, leading to image artifacts.

When compared with the long breathhold techniques the MR technique presented in this chapter for visualization of the coronary arteries is associated with a slightly improved signal-to-noise ratio, or a slightly better image resolution can be obtained, respectively.

The detection of too long or too short heartbeat intervals and the repetition of the corresponding measurements can be easily achieved with the currently used multiple slice technique, or with any other technique which combines data from different breathing cycles into one image (triggering, gating, navigators), whereas for long breathhold schemes a further prolongation of the already long apnea phases would result.

Image quality is highly reproducible with the current technique during repeated examinations in the same patient. Nevertheless, respiration is still the main source of artifacts. It reduces the resolution and causes the image quality to vary considerably across the patient population. A "feedback" of the inspiration level to the patient (18–20) could possibly improve the reproducibility of the inspiration level over the repetitive apnea phases in cooperative patients, leading to an image quality improvement. Nevertheless, faster imaging techniques are still needed for the reduction of the total scan time, which in turn is always helpful in improving image quality with lesser breathing motion artifacts.

Image Display

The *segmentation* of the coronary arteries is currently only possible on a semiautomatic basis; therefore, it is associated with a considerable observer dependence. Nevertheless, the 3-D reconstructions helped to locate potential lesions quickly. The final assessment of the critical vessel segments was done always on the basis of the *original MRIs*. A fully automated vessel segmentation would solve this problem, but the local image contrast would have to be improved considerably.

Vessel-tracking reformatted appears to be a good compromise between the two extreme forms of data display: raw image viewing and semiautomatic segmentation. It does not touch the original data in any way. The only operation performed is a form of reformatting volume data for display along a path defined by the operator. The definition of the vessel path itself is operator dependent. Acquiring multiple curved reformat view along the path with small offsets and then adding these images may reduce such a remaining operator dependence to a minimum.

Short- and Long-Term Goals in Coronary MRA

The short-term usefulness of noninvasive MR coronary angiography can be seen in follow-up examinations after treatment of coronary artery lesions with PTCA or bypass surgery. It seems to be a valuable tool for this task, restricted for the time being to the large epicardial vessels close to the orifice, specifically in (the majority of) patients in which good images can be obtained be-cause the image quality over different examinations of the same patient varies very little.

In patients with good image quality the results from MR coronary angiography may allow to circumvent coronary angiography especially after successful PTCA (restenosis). In a few cases in our studies, if an open vessel was found by MR in the follow-up examinations after PTCA, and the image quality was good, we omitted further diagnostic evaluation with X-ray contrast angiography.

The long-term goal, however, is the improvement of the MR technique to allow a noninvasive diagnosis of coronary artery disease in patients at high risk. For this task, the MR technique needs many further refinements. The spatial resolution for this purpose is currently still insufficient, and further developments in both hardware and acquisition techniques are necessary. We estimate that an approximate doubling of the effective spatial resolution in the heart should be sufficient for this goal.

References

1. Johnson LW, Lozner EC, Johnson D, et al. Coronary arteriography 1984–1987: a report of the registry of the Society for Cardiac Angiography and Interventions. I: results and complications. Cath Cardiovasc Diag 1989;17:5–10.
2. Stehling MK, von Smekal A, Reiser M. MRI of the coronary arteries: possibilities and limits: a comparative presentation with reference to coronary angiography, echocardiography and electron beam tomography (in German). Radiologe 1994;34:462–68.
3. Paulin S, von Schulthess GK, Fossel E, Krayenbuehl HP. MR imaging of the aortic root and proximal coronary arteries. Am J Roentgenol 1987;148:665–70.
4. Underwood SR. Imaging of acquired heart disease. *In*: Underwood SR, Firmin DN, eds. Magnetic resonance of the cardiovascular system. London: Blackwell, 1991:41–67.
5. Poncelet BP, Weisskoff RM, Wedeen VJ, Brady TJ, Kantor H. Time of flight quantification of coronary flow with echo-planar MRI. Magn Reson Med 1993;30:447–57.
6. Edelman RR, Manning WJ, Burstein D, et al. Coronary arteries: breath hold MR angiography. Radiology 1991;181:641–43.
7. Manning WJ, Li W, Edelman RR. A preliminary report comparing magnetic resonance coronary angiography with conventional angiography. N Engl J Med 1993;328:828–32.
8. Manning WJ, Li W, Boyle NG, Edelman RR. Fat-suppressed breath-hold magnetic resonance coronary angiography. Circulation 1993;87:94–104.
9. Meyer CH, Hu BS, Nishimura DG, Macovski A. Fast spiral coronary artery imaging. Magn Reson Med 1992;28:202–13.
10. Sang SJ, Hu BS, Macovski A, Nishimura DG. Coronary angiography using fast selective inversion recovery. Magn Reson Med 1991;18:417–23.
11. Pennell DJ, Keegan J, Firmin, DN, Gatehouse PD, Underwood SR, Longmore DB. Magnetic resonance imaging of coronary arteries: technique and preliminary results. Br Heart J 1993;70:315–26.

12. Duerinckx AJ, Urman MK. Two-dimensional coronary MR angiography: analysis of initial clinical results. Radiology 1994;193:731–38.

13. Duerinckx AJ. MR angiography of the coronary arteries. Top Magn Reson Imag 1995;7:267–85.

14. Cho ZH, Mun CW, Friedenberg RM. NMR angiography of coronary vessels with 2-D planar image scanning. Magn Reson Med 1992;20:134–43.

15. Li D, Paschal CB, Haacke EM, Adler LP. Coronary arteries: three-dimensional MR imaging with fat saturation and magnetization transfer contrast. Radiology 1993;187:401–6.

16. Paschal CB, Haacke EM, Adler LP. Three-dimensional MR imaging of the coronary arteries: preliminary clinical experience. J Magn Reson Imag 1993;3:491–500.

17. Post JC, van Rossum AC, Hofman MB, Valk J, Visser CA. Three-dimensional respiratory-gated MR angiography of coronary arteries: comparison with conventional coronary angiography. Am J Roentgenol 1996;166:1399–404.

18. Liu YL, Riederer SJ, Rossman PJ, Grimm RC, Debbins JP, Ehman RL. A monitoring, feedback, and triggering system for reproducible breath-hold MR imaging. Magn Reson Med 1993;30:507–11.

19. Wang Y, Christy PS, Korosec FR, Alley MT, Grist TM, Polzin JA, et al. Coronary MRI with a respiratory feedback monitor: the 2D imaging case. Magn Reson Med 1995; 33:11–16.

20. Wang Y, Rossman PJ, Grimm RC, Riederer SJ, Ehman RL. Navigator-echo-based real-time respiratory gating and triggering for reduction of respiration effects in three-dimensional coronary MR angiography. Radiology 1996; 198:55–60.

21. Doyle M, Scheidegger MB, Pohost GM. Coronary artery imaging in multiple 1-sec breath holds. Magn Reson Imag 1993;11:3–6.

22. Scheidegger MB, Muller R, Reiser M. Magnetic resonance angiography: methods and its applications to the coronary arteries. Technol Health Care 1994;2:255–65.

23. Scheidegger MB, Stuber M, Boesiger P, Hess OM. Coronary artery imaging by magnetic resonance. Herz 1996; 21(2):90–96.

24. Matsuda T, Doyle M, Pohost GM. Slice thickness reduction by partial overlapping presaturation. Magn Reson Med 1992;24:358–63.

25. Rossnick S, Kennedy D, Laub G. Three dimensional display of blood vessels in MRI. In: Proceedings of the IEEE

Computers in Cardiology Conference. Piscataway, NJ: IEEE, 1986:193–96.

26. Edelman RR, Manning WJ, Pearlman J, Li W. Human coronary arteries: projection angiograms reconstructed from breath-hold two-dimensional MR images. Radiology 1993;187:719–22.

27. Ruegsegger P, Muench B, Felder M. Early detection of osteoarthritis by 3D computed tomography. Technol Health Care 1993;1:53–56.

28. Münch B. 3D-Analyse von Knietomogrammen. Ph.D. Thesis Nr. 9459, ETH Zurich, Switzerland, 1991.

29. Müller R, Hildebrand T, Rüegsegger P. Non-invasive bone biopsy: a new method to analyse and display the three-dimensional structure of trabecular bone. Phys Med Biol 1994;39:145–64.

30. Hofman MB, Visser FC, van-Rossum AC, Vink QM, Sprenger M, Westerhof N. In vivo validation of magnetic resonance blood volume flow measurements with limited spatial resolution in small vessels. Magn Reson Med 1995; 33:766–77.

31. Scheidegger MB, Hess OM, Boesiger P. Assessment of coronary flow over the cardiac cycle and diastolic-to-systolic flow ration with correction for vessel motion. Proceedings of the Second Annual Meeting of the Society of Magnetic Resonance, Berkeley, 1994.

32. Brittain JH, Hu BS, Wright GA, Meyer CH, Macovski A, Nishimura DG. Coronary angiography with magnetization-prepared T2 contrast. Magn Reson Med 1995;33: 689–96.

33. Villari B, Hess OM, Meier Ch, et al. Regression of coronary artery dimensions after successful aortic valve replacement. Circulation 1992;85:972–78.

34. Buechi M, Hess OM, Kirkeeide RL, et al. Validation of a new automatic system for biplane quantitative coronary arteriography. Int J Card Imag 1990;5:93–103.

35. Suter TM, Buechi M, Hess OM, Haemmerli-Saner C, Gaglione A, Krayenbuehl HP. Normalization of coronary vasomotion after percutaneous transluminal coronary angioplasty. Circulation 1992;85:86–92.

36. Kirkeeide RL, Gould KL, Parsel L. Assessment of coronary stenoses by myocardial perfusion imaging during pharmacologic vasodilation. VII: validation of coronary flow reserve as a single integrated functional measure of stenosis severity reflecting all its geometric dimensions. J Am Coll Cardiol 1988;7:103–13.

24
Contrast Agents for Coronary MRA

André J. Duerinckx

The use of extracellular magnetic resonance (MR) contrast agents is increasing dramatically in all types of body magnetic resonance angiography (MRA) applications (1). A similar trend is developing for coronary MRA. This chapter provides a brief introduction to the topic. The ultimate role of contrast agents for coronary MRA is yet unknown. Thus we opted to keep this chapter rather brief and refer mostly to the peer- reviewed literature on this subject (2).

Most coronary artery MRA images have proton-density-weighted contrast as a direct consequence of the wait interval introduced by the cardiac synchronization. Therefore the signal from stagnant blood, blood clot, or plaque can recover completely and appear as an integral part of the coronary artery (appearing isointense), especially when signal-to-noise ratio (SNR) and resolution are not adequate (3). Contrast agents or preparation pulses (MTC or T2prep) would be very helpful to avoid this problem, and are both being investigated. It is known that coronary artery lumens appear thinner on contrast-enhanced MR images when compared to pre-contrast-enhanced images. This seems to suggest that without contrast the vessel wall and the blood cannot always be distinguished. It may also explain why certain types of coronary lesions are missed with coronary MRA (4,5). Black-blood imaging offers a totally different but complementary approach to this problem (6).

Contrast agents for MRA will cause a dramatic T1 shortening in blood and can yield high-quality breathhold MRA. Using a blood pool agent which remains in the blood for a longer period of time than an extracellular agent facilitates the acquisition of images. Wielopolsi et al. (3), Lorenz et al. (2), and especially Johansson et al. (7) provide excellent further discussions of these topics. We refer the reader to these articles. Lorenz et al. (2) reviewed various methods that have been proposed to improve signal-to-noise and contrast-to-noise ratios in MR coronary imaging with an emphasis on the role of T1-shortening contrast agents, both extracellular and intravascular.

The Use of Contrast Agents for Coronary MRA

Limited work on the use of extracellular and intravascular contrast agents with the first-generation techniques has been done (8–12). Promising early work with the second-generation techniques has also been performed in animals and humans (13–18). The use of contrast agents with the third-generation coronary MRA techniques appears promising and is discussed in more detail (19–22).

The Use of Contrast Agents with Third-Generation Techniques

MR contrast agents will probably have the most effect on third-generation coronary MRA techniques because they are very similar to the dynamic contrast-enhanced MRA techniques used for thoracic and body MRA today. These techniques can be used to image native coronary artery (11) and coronary artery bypass grafts (CABG) (23–25). In order to EKG-trigger these MRA pulse sequences for native coronary vessel imaging, one needs to use faster acquisitions rates, k-space data segmentation, data interpolation, and other technical tricks.

The initial experience with extracellular MR contrast agents seemed to indicate that very high doses would be needed for first-generation techniques (8,11). With bolus arrival timing to catch the first pass of the gadolinium contrast agent further image quality improvement have been obtained (improved signal-to-noise and contrast-to-noise ratios) for both second- and third-generation techniques (11,26). With the new experimental MR blood pool agents, however, even greater image improvements are being obtained (13–15,19,27). Sequential breathhold acquisitions, as short as 5–10 seconds, can be obtained, with relatively high-resolution, to image thin 3-D slabs. With several repeated short breathholds this allows patient-friendly high-resolution coverage of large portions of the cardiac and coronary anatomy. It offers the advantage of 3-D acquisitions (with the opportunity for subsequent postprocessing and no misregistration) while taking advantage of the MR contrast agents.

The Future

The combination of MR contrast agents with coronary MRA techniques will most likely allow coronary MRA to out perform any other noninvasive coronary imaging technique on all fronts, including spatial resolution and 3-D volume coverage, as indicated by early results in animals (28) and humans.

As stated by Lorenz et al. (2), although much progress has been made in recent years in techniques for imaging the coronary arteries, ultimate clinical success remains unproved. Success will depend on synergistic developments in MR acquisition techniques, respiratory compensation methods, post-processing techniques, and contrast agents to develop a workable solution for reliable coronary imaging across a wide range of patients. Research is actively being performed to further evaluate this potential use of MR contrast agents (29,30).

References

1. Prince MR, Grist TM, Debatin JF. 3D Contrast MR Angiography, second ed. Berlin: Springer-Verlag, 1999.
2. Lorenz CH, Johansson LO. Contrast-enhanced coronary MRA. J Magn Reson Imag 1999;10(5):703–8.
3. Wielopolski PA, van Geuns RJ, de Feyter PJ, Oudkerk M. Coronary arteries. Eur Radiol 2000;10(1):12–35.
4. Duerinckx AJ. Coronary MR angiography. In: Cardiac MR Imaging, LM Boxt, guest ed. MRI Clin North Am 1996; 4(2):361–418.
5. Duerinckx AJ. MRI of coronary arteries. Inter J Card Imag 1997;13(3):191–97.
6. Stuber M, Manning WJ. Black-blood coronary MRA (abstr.). In: Book of Abstracts of the First International Workshop on Coronary MR & CT Angiography. Lyon, France, October 1–3, 2000. Organized and published by the North American Society for Cardiac Imaging. Reprinted in Inter J Card Imag 2000;16.
7. Johansson LO, Fischer SE, Lorenz CH. Benefit of T1 reduction for magnetic resonance coronary angiography: a numerical simulation and phantom study. J Magn Reson Imag 1999;9(4):552–56.
8. Duerinckx AJ, Urman M, Sinha U, Atkinson D, Simonetti O. Evaluation of gadolinium-enhanced MR coronary angiography (abstr.). In: Seventy-ninth Scientific Assembly and Annual Meeting of the Radiological Society of North America (RSNA). Chicago, November 28–December 3, 1993; Radiology 1993;189(P):278.
9. Stillman AE, Wilke N, Li D, Haacke EM, McLachlan SJ. MRA of renal and coronary arteries using an intravascular contrast agent (#944) (abstr.). In: Printed Program of the Second Meeting of the Society of Magnetic Resonance (SMR). San Francisco, August 6–12, 1994.
10. Saeed M, Wendland MF, Engelbrecht M, Sakuma H, Higgins CB. Contrast-enhanced magnetic resonance angiography in the coronary and peripheral arteries. Academic Radiol 1998;5:108–12.
11. Ho VB, Foo TKF, Arai AE, Wolff SD. Gadolinium-enhanced two-dimensional coronary MR angiography using an automated contrast bolus detection algorithm (MR smartprep) (abstr.). In: Proceedings of the Sixth Scientific Meeting of the International Society for Magnetic Resonance in Medicine (ISMRM), April 18–24, 1998 (paper #19). Sydney, Australia, 1998 (in press).
12. Taylor AM, Panting JR, Keegan J, et al. Safety and preliminary findings with the intravascular contrast agent NC100150 injection for MR coronary angiography. J Magn Reson Imag 1999;9(2):220–27.
13. Li D, Dolan RP, Walovitch RC, Lauffer RB. Three-dimensional MRI of coronary arteries using an intravascular contrast agent. Magn Reson Med 1998;39(6):1014–18.
14. Li D, Zheng J, Weinmann H-J, et al. Comparison of intravascular and extravascular contrast agents in coronary artery imaging. (abstr.). In: Proceedings of the Sixth Scientific Meeting of the International Society for Magnetic Resonance in Medicine (ISMRM), April 18–24, 1998 (paper #17). Sydney, Australia, 1998; Vol. 1: 17.
15. Stuber M, Botnar RM, McConnell MV, et al. Coronary artery imaging with the intravascular contrast agent MS-325. (abstr.). In: Proceedings of the Sixth Scientific Meeting of the International Society for Magnetic Resonance in Medicine (ISMRM), April 18–24, 1998 (paper #316). Sydney, Australia, 1998; Vol. 1: 316.
16. Sakuma H, Goto M, Nomura Y, Kato N, Takeda K, Higgins CB. Three-dimensional coronary magnetic resonance angiography with injection of extracellular contrast medium. Invest Radiol 1999;34(8):503–8.
17. Stuber M, Botnar RM, Danias PG, et al. Contrast agent-enhanced, free-breathing, three-dimensional coronary magnetic resonance angiography. J Magn Reson Imag 1999;10(5):790–99.
18. Zheng J, Bae KT, Woodard PK, Haacke EM, Li D. Efficacy of slow infusion of gadolinium contrast agent in three-dimensional MR coronary artery imaging. J Magn Reson Imag 1999;10(5):800–5.
19. Goldfarb JW, Edelman RR. Coronary arteries: breath-hold, gadolinium-enhanced, three-dimensional MR angiography. Radiology 1998;206(3):830–34.
20. de Bruin HG, van Geuns RJM, Wielopolski PA, de Feyter PJ, Oudkerk M. Improvement of magnetic resonance imaging of the coronary arteries with a clinically available intravascular contrast agent (abstr.). In: Book of Abstracts of the First International Workshop on Coronary MR & CT Angiography. Lyon, France, October 1–3, 2000. Organized and published by the North American Society for Cardiac Imaging. Reprinted in Inter J Card Imag 2000;16.
21. Kessler W, Laub G, Achenbach S, Ropers D, Moshage W, Daniel WG. Coronary arteries: MR angiography with fast contrast-enhanced three-dimensional breath-hold imaging—initial experience. Radiology 1999;210(2):566–72.

22. Kruger DG, Busse RF, Johnston DL, Ritman EL, Ehman RL, Riederer SJ. Contrast-enhanced 3D MR breathhold imaging of porcine coronary arteries using fluoroscopic localization and bolus triggering. Magn Reson Med 1999; 42(6):1159–65.

23. van Rossum AC, Galjee MA, Post JC, Visser CA. A practical approach to MRI of coronary artery bypass graft patency and flow. Intl J Card Imag 1997;13(3):199–204.

24. Vrachliotis TG, Aliabadi D, Bis KG, Shetty AN, London J, Farah J. Breath-hold electrocardiogram-triggered, contrast-enhanced, 3D MR angiography to evaluate patency of coronary artery bypass graft (abstr.). Radiology 1996; 201(P):273.

25. Vrachliotis TG, Bis KG, Aliabadi D, Shetty AN, Safian R, Simonetti O. Contrast-enhanced breath-hold MR angiography for evaluating patency of coronary artery bypass grafts. Am J Roentgenol 1997;168(4):1073–80.

26. Kessler W, Laub G, Ropers D, Achenbach S, Moshage W, Bachmann K. Contrast-enhanced 3D breath-hold MRA for the visualization of the coronary arteries in oblique projection angiograms (abstr.). *In*: Proceedings of the Sixth Scientific Meeting of the International Society for Magnetic Resonance in Medicine (ISMRM), April 18–24, 1998 (paper # 317). Sydney, Australia, 1998; Vol. 1: 317.

27. Taylor AM, Panting JR, Gatehouse PD, et al. Safety and preliminary findings with an intravascular contrast agent, NC100150 for MR coronary angiography. (abstr.). *In*: Proceedings of the Sixth Scientific Meeting of the International Society for Magnetic Resonance in Medicine (ISMRM), April 18–24, 1998 (paper #18). Sydney, Australia, 1998; Vol. 1: 18.

28. Johansson LO, Nolan NM, Taniuchi M, Fischer SE, Wickline SA, Lorenz CH. High resolution magnetic resonance coronary angiography of the entire heart using a new blood-pool agent NC100150 injection: comparison with invasive x-ray angiography in pigs. J Cardiovasc Magn Reson 1999;2(1):139–44.

29. Li D, Green J, McCarthy R, Yinchou, Finn JP. MR coronary artery imaging with IV injection of contrast agent and 2D projection imaging (abstr.). Presented at the Second Workshop on Coronary MR & CT Angiography, Sept 29–Oct 2, 2001, Chicago, IL. Published by the North American Society for Cardiac Imaging in the Inter J Card Imag 2001; Vol. 17:5.

30. Book of Abstracts of the Second Workshop on Coronary MR & CT Angiography. Chicago, IL, Sept 29–Oct 2, 2001. Organized and published by the North American Society for Cardiac Imaging. Reprinted in: Inter J Card Imag 2001: Vol. 17:5.

25
Intravascular Contrast Agents for Cardiac MRI

Arthur E. Stillman, Norbert Wilke, and Michael Jerosch-Herold

At the present time, all FDA-approved intravenous contrast agents may be classified as being "extracellular." The prototypical example is Gd-DTPA. These contrast agents have found widespread applications throughout the body. They have been used in the heart to assess myocardial perfusion (1,2), delineate infarcts (3,4), improve the detection of the endocardial border for MR cine (5), and improve visualization of coronary artery grafts (6,7). Intravascular contrast agents have been developed and are currently undergoing clinical evaluation. A list of the intravascular contrast agents currently under clinical investigation is provided in Table 25.1. Unlike the extracellular agents, these contrast media are largely confined to the intravascular compartment. Given the success of the extracellular agents, it is reasonable to ask, what benefit might be anticipated given the more limited biodistribution of this new class of contrast media? To answer this question, one first must consider the differences in biodistribution.

The extracellular agents distribute first into the intravascular compartment and subsequently into the interstitial space (8). Thus, there is both vascular and tissue enhancement. The relative contribution of each depends on the size of these compartments as well as the time after injection that enhancement is measured. Leakage from the intravascular compartment enters the interstitial space. Elimination is largely via the kidneys and hence has a vascular route. Thus, contrast must exit the interstitial space to the vascular compartment in order to be eliminated.

Myocardial Perfusion

With the so-called first pass of an extracellular contrast agent after a bolus injection, there is first enhancement of the blood pool with rapid leakage into the interstitial space. In order to separate these two processes, the initial (upslope) portion of the tissue signal-intensity curves are used to provide a measure of myocardial perfusion (9). If leakage into the interstitial compartment is negligible, the area of the signal intensity time curve provides a measure of the myocardial blood volume. With extracellular agents, there is significant leakage even during the first pass for normal or higher blood flow. Thus, it is not possible to determine both the myocardial blood volume and interstitial leakage readily. By contrast, intravascular agents have the advantage that the leakage may be neglected in nonischemic myocardium. In this way both myocardial perfusion and blood volume can be separately assessed. Because these are regulated differently, intravascular contrast agents have a distinct advantage in understanding pathophysiology. It is unknown at this time, however, how this additional information might impact clinically.

Myocardial Infarction

It has long been recognized that infarcts exhibit late enhancement following injection with extracellular agents (10). This enhancement is due to both increased leakage from the vascular compartment as well as an increased distribution volume from loss of cell membrane integrity. Injured but viable myocardium might still demonstrate late enhancement, but this is due to the leakage and increased interstitial volume (edema) (11). We are unaware of any studies of infarction using intravascular contrast agents. We anticipate, however, that because there is less baseline enhancement of normal myocardium with intravascular agents, injured or infarcted myocardium should be more conspicuous. Viability determination can be expected to remain problematic on the basis of late enhancement alone. Moreover, because of the leakage effect, determination of myocardial blood volume in severely ischemic regions using intravascular contrast media can be expected to be problematic as well.

Table 25.1. MR contrast agents for coronary angiography.

Contrast agent	Manufacturer	Characteristics
Gadomer-17	Schering AG, Berlin, Germany	Dendritic contrast agent with molecular weight of 30 kD that contains 24 Gd complexes at the surface of dendrimer
AngioMark (MS-325)	EPIX Inc., Boston & Mallinckrodt	Highly protein bound after injection (80–96%) bound in human plasma
Clariscan™ (NC100150)	Nycomed SA, Oslo, Norway	Ultrasmall particle, superparamagnetic iron oxide contrast agent with high T_1 and T_2^* relaxivities
Combidex (Ferrumoxan, AMI-227, AMI Code 7227)	Advanced Magnetics Inc., Boston	Superparamagnetic iron oxide contrast agent with high T_1 and T_2^* relaxivities

MR Cine

Both extracellular (5) and intravascular (12) contrast agents have been used to improve the endocardial border definition in magnetic resonance (MR) cine. These images may suffer loss of blood pool contrast from saturation effects when there is insufficient inflow of fresh spins into the imaging plane. This is particularly a problem in patients with low cardiac outputs or if long axis images are obtained where spin refreshment is less than short axis slices (cf. Fig. 25.1). Contrast media diminish the saturation of the blood and thereby maintain good myocardial–blood pool contrast. The intravascular contrast agents have a distinct advantage in this regard because they enhance myocardium to a much lesser degree and have a longer blood pool half-life. As shown in Figure 25.2, the improved myocardial–blood pool contrast facilitates edge detection that is required for automated segmentation of the endocardial border to determine chamber volumes and ejection fraction and minimizes the need for manual editing. For this reason we expect that intravascular blood pool agents will find widespread application once approved for clinical use.

Coronary Angiography

The principle value of intravascular contrast agents for angiography is the relative lack of tissue enhancement. Thus, there is great vessel-to-background image contrast; however, these agents fail to discriminate arteries from veins and a superposition of arteries and veins results. This is problematic for diagnostic purposes in most body areas, but it is less of an issue for the coronary vessels because of the more simple anatomy.

Both two-dimensional (2-D) and three-dimensional (3-D) methods have been used for MR coronary angiography. The 3-D methods have the advantage of less operator dependence, but they suffer from relatively long scan times and saturation of the blood signal. Long scan times result in respiratory motion artifact. This can be minimized by use of a navigator pulse to monitor diaphragm motion (13). The saturation problem is readily solved with intravascular contrast media (cf. Fig. 25.3) (14–16).

Although it is clear that intravascular contrast agents improve coronary MRA, there still is insufficient spatial resolution with current techniques to identify stenoses even under ideal conditions. As shown in Figure 25.4,

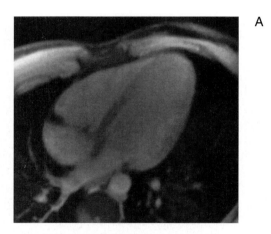

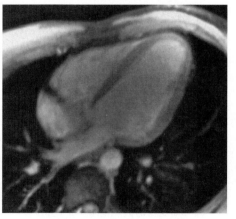

Figure 25.1. Long axis image of the heart (A) precontrast and (B) postcontrast (AMI-227). Note the relative saturation of the blood pool in the precontrast image. The same window settings were used in these figures. The endocardial borders are more clearly defined with a blood pool contrast agent. (*From*: Use of an intravascular T1 contrast agent to improve MR cine myocardial-blood pool definition in man. Stillman et al., *J Magn Reson Imag* 1997. Reprinted with permission of Wiley-Liss, Inc., a subsidiary of John Wiley & Sons, Inc.)

A

B

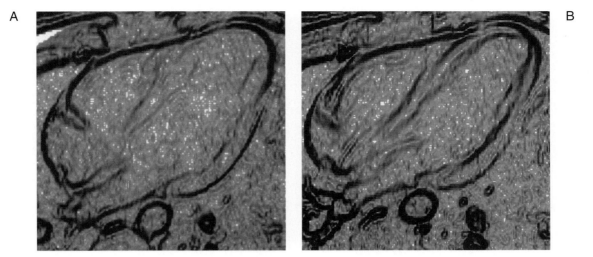

Figure 25.2. The same images shown in Figure 25.1 have been postprocessed with an edge-enhancing Sobel filter. This filter makes use of gradients in the image similar to those used in au-tomated computer programs that segment the blood pool. The edge strength is clearly stronger in the postcontrast image (B).

A

B

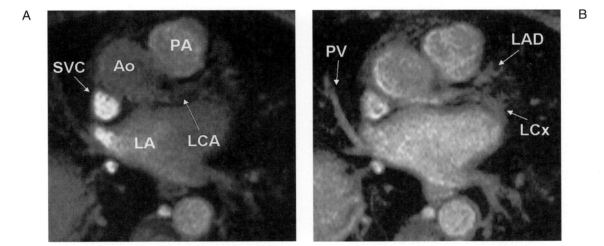

Figure 25.3. Axial image from a 3-D MRA data set (A) precontrast and (B) postcontrast (AMI-227). The blood pool is not saturated and the LAD coronary artery is more clearly seen following contrast. (Reprinted with permission from Stillman et al. (14).)

A

B

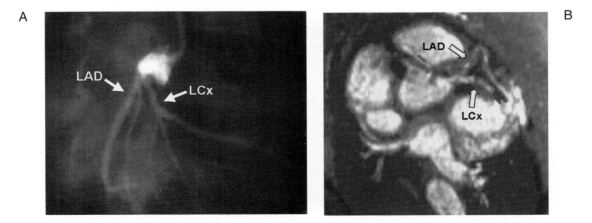

Figure 25.4. (A) X-ray angiogram showing a 25% stenosis of the LAD and 37% stenosis of the LCx in a pig model. The arrows indicate the ligated areas. (B) Three-dimensional MRA in the same animal after injection of Nyocmed (NC100150) does not clearly depict these stenoses. (Courtesy of Debiao Li.)

A

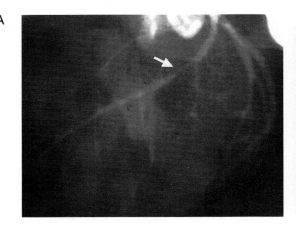

B

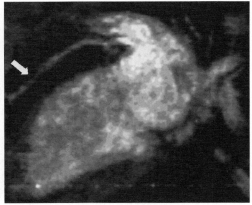

Figure 25.5. (A) X-ray angiogram showing a 65% stenosis of the LAD in another pig. (B) Three-dimensional MRA in the same animal after injection of Nyocmed (NC100150) shows the corresponding narrow area. It appears that the threshold for detection is between 40 and 65%. (Courtesy of Debiao Li.)

3-D magnetic resonance angiography (MRA) with intravascular contrast media (Clariscan™, Nycomed NC100150) failed to visualize clearly a 25% stenosis of the left anterior descending (LAD) and 37% stenosis of the left circumflex (LCx) in a pig model. A 65% stenosis of the LAD was identified in another animal (Fig. 25.5). Thus, it appears that the threshold for detection of stenosis is somewhere between 40 and 65%. Although mild narrowing of the coronary vessels may not be clinically significant in terms of ischemia, soft plaque rupture is known to precipitate acute myocardial infarct. These soft plaques need not cause significant narrowing prior to rupture. Thus, there is considerable emphasis being placed now on plaque characterization and morphology. Further technological advancement will be required before coronary MRA can be relied upon for this purpose.

References

1. Wilke N, Jerosch-Herold M, Wang Y, et al. Myocardial perfusion reserve: assessment with multisection, quantitative, first-pass MR imaging. Radiology 1997;204(2):373–84.
2. Jerosch-Herold M, Wilke N. MR first pass imaging: quantitative assessment of transmural perfusion and collateral flow. Int J Card Imag 1997;13(3):205–18.
3. Steffans JC, Sakuma H, Bourne MW, Higgins CB. Magnetic resonance imaging in ischemic heart disease. Am Heart J 1996;132(1 Pt. 1):156–73.
4. Dendale P, Franken PR, Block P, Pratikakis Y, De Roos A. Contrast enhanced and functional magnetic resonance imaging for the detection of viable myocardium after infarction. Am Heart J 1998;135(5 Pt. 1):875–80.
5. Pennell DJ, Underwood SR, Longmore DB. Improved cine MR imaging of left ventricular wall motion with gadopentetate dimeglumine. J Magn Reson Imag 1993;3(1):13–19.
6. Vrachliotis TG, Bis KG, Aliabadi D, Shetty AN, Safian R, Simonetti O. Contrast-enhanced breath-hold MR angiography for evaluating patency of coronary artery bypass grafts. Am J Roentgenol 1997;168(4):1073–80.
7. Wintersperger B, Engelmann M, von Smekal A, et al. Patency of coronary bypass grafts: assessment with breath-hold contrast-enhanced MR angiography-value of a non-electrocardiographically triggered technique. Radiology 1998;208:345–51.
8. Weinmann HL, Laniado M, Mutzel W. Pharmacokinetics of Gd-DTPA/dimeglumine after intravenous injection into healthy volunteers. Physiol Chem Phys Med NMR 1984;16:167–72.
9. Wilke N, Jerosch-Herold M, Stillman AE, et al. Concepts of myocardial perfusion imaging in magnetic resonance imaging. Magn Reson Q 1994;10(4):249–86.
10. Wolfe CL, Moseley ME, Wikstrom MG, et al. Assessment of myocardial salvage after ischemia and reperfusion using magnetic resonance imaging and spectroscopy. Circulation 1989;80:969–82.
11. Rogers WJ, Kramer CM, Geskin G, et al. Contrast enhanced MRI early after reperfused MI predicts late functional recovery (abstr. 3164). In: Programs and Abstracts from the Sixty-ninth Scientific Sessions of the American Heart Association, New Orleans, 1996.
12. Stillman AE, Wilke N, Jerosch-Herold M. Use of an intravascular T1 contrast agent to improve MR cine myocardial–blood pool definition in man. J Magn Reson Imag 1997;7(4):765–67.
13. Li D, Kaushikkar S, Haacke EM, et al. Coronary arteries: three-dimensional MR imaging with retrospective respiratory gating. Radiology 1996;201(3):857–63.
14. Stillman AE, Wilke N, Li D, Haacke M, McLachlan S. Ultrasmall superparamagnetic iron oxide to enhance MRA of the renal and coronary arteries: studies in human patients. J Comput Assist Tomogr 1996;20(1):51–55.

15. Li D, Zheng J, Weinmann H-J, et al. Comparison of intravascular and extravascular contrast agents in coronary artery imaging. Proceedings of the Third Meeting of the International Society for Magnetic Resonance in Medicine. Sidney, Australia, 1998.

16. Stuber M, Botnar RM, McConnell MV, et al. Coronary artery imaging with the intravascular contrast agent MS-325. Proceedings of the Third Meeting of the International Society for Magnetic Resonance in Medicine. Sidney, Australia, 1998.

26
Alternatives to Coronary MRA

André J. Duerinckx

Many imaging tools exist to directly evaluate the coronary artery anatomy: computed tomography (see Chap. 28), coronary magnetic resonance angiography (MRA), echocardiography (both transthoracic and transesophageal), intravascular ultrasound (see Chap. 29), and invasive X-ray coronary angiography, which is today's gold standard. Coronary CT angiography (CTA) can now be performed using both electron-beam computed tomography (EB-CT) (1–5) and cardiac-gated multislice CT (6–9). CTA and MRA appear very close competitors for the same application. However, unlike EB-CT or multislice CT, coronary MRA does not require iodinated contrast agents or X-ray radiation and has the potential to become a more widespread and easy-to-use cardiac screening tool.

In the next chapter (Chap. 28), Achenbach et al. review the performance of EB-CT for coronary artery visualization (2,3,5,10–16). Achenbach et al. also published their results on the value of EB-CT for the noninvasive detection of high-grade coronary artery stenoses and occlusions in the *New England Journal of Medicine* (3). EB-CT was performed in 125 patients. Technical problems impaired image quality in 124 (25%) of the 500 coronary arteries studied in 125 patients. In 19 patients (15%) no vessel could be evaluated, and in another 28 patients (22%) one, two, or three vessels could not be evaluated. In the remaining coronary arteries with adequate image quality the sensitivity for detection of a high-grade stenosis ($\geq$ 75% diameter narrowing) or occlusion was 92% (69 of 75 lesions or occlusions), and the specificity was 94%. Obviously, with technical problems in 25% of patients, the 92% sensitivity figure is artificially elevated. A more realistic figure would be anywhere between 34% and 92%. The 34% sensitivity corresponds to the worst-case scenario in which each of the 125 vessel segments that could not be evaluated has a lesion. It is important for potential users of this technology to consider the implications of a 25% nonvisualization rate.

Multislice CT offers a less expensive alternative to EB-CT both for coronary calcium screening and for 3-D coronary artery imaging (6,8,9,15). During the first International Workshop on Coronary MR and CTA, held in Lyon, France, October 1–3, 2000, and organized by the North American Society for Cardiac Imaging (with abstracts required in the *International Journal of Cardiac Imaging*, Vol. 16) the latest developments in multislice CTA and EB-CT for coronary angiography were discussed and debated. Below we provide detailed information from only two of the many presentations at this symposium, and refer to the workshop proceedings for more information.

Ohnesorge et al. (8) developed a new method for cardiac investigations with a four-slice CT system using retrospectively EKG-gated spiral scanning. Scan and reconstruction techniques are optimized for motion-free cardiac volume imaging for high-resolution coronary CTA. Data acquisition and spiral reconstruction techniques are optimized with regard to both temporal resolution and volume coverage. The entire heart may be scanned with 1-mm slices within a single breathhold and reconstructed with a temporal resolution up to 125 msec. For coronary CTA examinations continuous volume images are reconstructed in the diastolic phase of the cardiac cycle. Additional systolic reconstructions can be used for cardiac function evaluation. Ohnesorge et al. (8) demonstrated that EKG-gated four-slice spiral scanning with 1-mm slices and submillimeter image increment can provide isotropic volume data within a single breathhold for high resolution 3-D evaluations of the coronary arteries. First patient studies indicate that coronary stenosis correlated to calcified and noncalcified arthero-sclerotic plaques may be reliably detected for low to moderate heart rates. Cardiac function analysis is possible based on end-diastolic and end-systolic reconstructions from the same data set. They conclude that the first clinical results indicate the potential of multislice CT for high resolution coronary CTA and cardiac function evaluation.

Van Geuns et al. (9) postulated that although in clinical cardiology computed tomography (CT) is presently only used for evaluation of congenital and acquired disease of the aorta, because of the increased rotation speed and the development of new detector systems the use of CT in cardiology may change in the near future. They investigated the possibilities of retrospective EKG-gated quarter-second multislice spiral CT and performed several phantom and patient studies. For the phantom studies they used seven models of coronary artery stenoses. Within a phantom of a 3-mm-thick vessel a stenosis with a residual lumen of 0.25, 0.5, 0.75, 1.0, 1.5, 2.0, or 2.5 mm was created. These phantoms were filled with diluted ionated contrast and studied on a Spiral CT Scanner (Somatom Plus 4 VolumeZoom, Siemens, Erlangen, Germany). This CT scanner is able to obtain four slices of 1.25 mm thickness with an acquisition time of 250 msec using a pitch of 1.5. The EKG of a healthy volunteer was used for retrospective cardiac gating, with a time delay set to middiastole. Image reconstruction was performed with a field-of-view (FOV) of 150×150 mm using a matrix of 512×512, resulting in a pixel size of 0.29×0.29 mm. For patient studies five patients with angiographically proven nondiseased coronary arteries and one patient with significant stenosis were studied with the same imaging protocol. The phantom studies of Van Geuns et al. (9) showed the ability to obtain nearly artifact-free images using the retrospective reconstruction algorithm with an acquisition time of 250 ms. However, the selected pixel size was insufficient to be able to distinguish the 90% stenosis from a total occlusion. In the patient studies the proximal coronary arteries were visualized in all patients including the patient with the proximal coronary artery stenosis. From these initial experiences with retrospective EKG-gated multislice spiral CT Van Geuns et al. (9) conclude that there are enormous potentials from this technique in the diagnosis of atherosclerotic coronary artery disease.

In Chapter 28, Nicosia and Fitzgerald review the use of intravascular ultrasound for coronary lesion evaluation. Such approach is much more invasive than MR or EB-CT, and as such is not a direct competitor, but could be used as a gold standard for imaging and flow measurements. In the year 2000, cardiac-gated multislice CT has emerged as a very serious competitor for both EB-CT and MRI/MRA. The jury is still out as to which imaging modality will ultimately prevail. This topic continues to be hotly debated at many cardiac imaging meetings (17).

References

1. Achenbach S, Kessler W, Moshage WE, et al. Visualization of the coronary arteries in three-dimensional reconstructions using respiratory gated magnetic resonance imaging. Coron Artery Dis 1997;8(7):441–48.
2. Achenbach S, Moshage W, Ropers D, Bachmann K. Comparison of vessel diameters in electron beam tomography and quantitative coronary angiography. Int J Card Imag 1998;14(1):1–7; discussion 9.
3. Achenbach S, Moshage W, Ropers D, Nossen J, Daniel WG. Value of electron-beam computed tomography for the noninvasive detection of high-grade coronary artery stenoses and occlusions. N Engl J Med 1998;339(27): 1964–71.
4. Brenner P, Wintersperger B, von Smekal A, et al. Detection of coronary artery bypass graft patency by contrast enhanced magnetic resonance angiography. Eur J Cardiothorac Surg 1999;15(4):389–93.
5. Chernoff DM, Ritchie CJ, Higgins CB. Evaluation of electron beam CT coronary angiography in healthy subjects. Am J Roentgenol 1997;169(1):93–99.
6. Becker CR, Knez A, Leber A, et al. Initial experiences with multi-slice detector spiral CT in diagnosis of arteriosclerosis of coronary vessels [see comments]. Radiologe 2000;40(2):118–22.
7. Hu H. Multi-slice helical CT: scan and reconstruction. Med Phys 1999;26(1):5–18.
8. Ohnesorge B, Flohr T, Becker CR, Knez A, Reiser MF. ECG-gated multi-slice cardiac volume CT for coronary CT angiography—initial experience. (abstr.). In: Book of Abstracts of the First International Workshop on Coronary MR & CT Angiography. Lyon, France, October 1–3, 2000. Organized and published by the North American Society for Cardiac Imaging. Reprinted in: Inter J Card Imag 2000;16.
9. van Geuns RJ, van Ooijen PMA, Nieman K, Rensing BJ, Oudkerk M, de Feyter PJ. Initial results with retrospective ECG gated quarter second multi-slice spiral CT (abstr.). In: Book of Abstracts of the First International Workshop on Coronary MR & CT Angiography. Lyon, France, October 1–3, 2000. Organized and published by the North American Society for Cardiac Imaging. Reprinted in Inter J Card Imag 2000;16.
10. Schmermund A, Baumgart D, Adamzik M, et al. Comparison of electron-beam computed tomography and intracoronary ultrasound in detecting calcified and noncalcified plaques in patients with acute coronary syndromes and no or minimal to moderate angiographic coronary artery disease. Am J Cardiol 1998;81(2):141–46.
11. Schmermund A, Rensing BJ, Sheedy PF, Bell MR, Rumberger JA. Intravenous electron-beam computed tomographic coronary angiography for segmental analysis of coronary artery stenoses. J Am Coll Cardiol 1998;31(7):1547–54.
12. Baumgart D, Schmermund A, Goerge G, et al. Comparison of electron beam computed tomography with intracoronary ultrasound and coronary angiography for detection of coronary atherosclerosis. J Am Coll Cardiol 1997;30(1):57–64.
13. Achenbach S, Moshage W, Bachmann K. Detection of high-grade stenosis after PTCA using contrast-enhanced electron beam CT. Circulation 1998.
14. Achenbach S, Moshage W, Bachmann K. Noninvasive coronary angiography by contrast-enhanced electron beam computed tomography. Clin Cardiol 1998;21(5):323–30.
15. Achenbach S, Moshage W, Ropers D, Bachmann K. Curved multiplanar reconstructions for the evaluation of contrast-enhanced electron beam CT of the coronary arteries. Am J Roentgenol 1998;170:895–99.
16. Reddy GP, Chernoff DM, Adams JR, Higgins CB. Coronary artery stenoses: assessment with contrast-enhanced electron-beam CT and axial reconstructions. Radiology 1998;208(1):167–72.
17. Book of Abstracts of the Second Workshop on Coronary MR & CT Angiography. Chicago, IL, Sept 29–Oct 2. Organized and published by the North American Society for Cardiac Imaging. Reprinted in: Inter J Card Imag, 2001; Vol. 17:5.

27

Coronary Angiography by EB-CT

Stephan Achenbach, Werner Moshage, and Daniel M. Chernoff

Introduction

Electron-beam computed tomography (EB-CT, also called cine computed tomography (CT) or ultrafast CT) is a cross-sectional imaging technique similar to conventional computed tomography (1,2). With EB-CT, image acquisition is achieved without rotation of an X-ray tube, the mechanical movement of which limits the imaging speed of conventional CT scanners. Instead, X-rays are generated by an electron beam that is electronically focused and deflected to sweep over target rings that are arranged in a semicircular manner around the patient; an array of detectors on the opposite side of the patient serves to record X-ray attenuation (see Fig. 27.1). This arrangement permits image acquisition in as little as 50 msec, at least 10-fold faster than conventional CT (1,2).

Due to its unique combination of high spatial and temporal resolution and the fact that image acquisition can be synchronized with the electrocardiogram, EB-CT is ideally suited for imaging of the coronary arteries. To date, coronary imaging by EB-CT has mainly been applied to visualize and quantify calcification of the coronary arteries. This so-called calcium screening has been shown to permit early and reliable diagnosis of coronary artery disease (3–6). Quantitative analysis of coronary calcifications in EB-CT also has high prognostic value (7,8).

Since 1995, several groups have used EB-CT in combination with intravenous injection of contrast agents to visualize the inner lumen of the coronary arteries and in this way permit direct imaging of coronary artery stenoses and occlusions (9–13). This chapter will summarize the imaging protocols, methods of data evaluation, and clinical results, as well as the problems and future perspectives of EB-CT coronary angiography.

Imaging Protocol

In order to visualize the coronary arteries by EB-CT, a volume data set of the heart is acquired within one breathhold. To achieve maximal vasodilation, nitrates may be given prior to the investigation (e.g., 0.8 mg of nitroglycerine s.1.). Image acquisition is done in the scanner's high-resolution single-slice mode with an acquisition time of 100 msec per image and an image matrix of 512 × 512. A field of view of 15–18 cm permits cardiac imaging with highest possible spatial resolution, but exact positioning of the volume data set as well as careful timing of contrast injection are crucial to achieve optimal image quality. The following three-step imaging protocol has proven useful.

Determination of Heart Position

The patients are investigated head first in supine position. To locate the heart position, the scanner's multislice mode is used to acquire eight axial cross-sections of the chest (7-mm slice thickness, 4-mm gap after every other section) without contrast enhancement. The position of the ascending aorta is determined on these cross-sections (9,10).

Measurement of Contrast Agent Transit Time

Exact timing of contrast injection is important to achieve optimal image quality. Several methods can be used to estimate the circulation time, including the injection of magnesium sulfate or indocyanine green. The most reliable measurements, however, can be achieved by test injection of contrast agent (9,11). A bolus of 10 ml of contrast agent is injected intravenously (4 ml/sec). After a delay of 10 seconds, 10 axial cross-sections of the

A

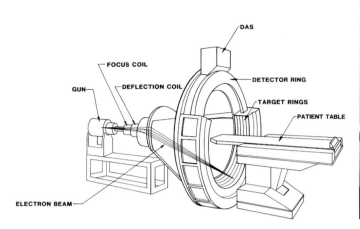

B

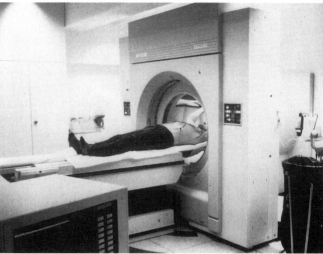

Figure 27.1. (A) Setup of the electron beam CT scanner. An electron beam, created by an electron gun, is focused and deflected by a series of electromagnets to sweep across the target rings

arranged in a semicircular manner around the patient, where the X-rays are created. (B) Investigation of a patient by EB-CT.

chest at the level of the ascending aorta are acquired in single-slice mode (acquisition time 100 msec), triggered to the EKG at 80% of the R–R interval with one imaging acquisition following every other heartbeat. In this way, a time–density curve within the ascending aorta can be obtained covering 20 heartbeats, and the exact contrast agent transit time from injection to maximum

enhancement in the aortic root can be measured (see Fig. 27.2). In addition, this serves to double-check the positioning of the following volume data set.

Volume Data Set

Due to the tortuous course of the coronary arteries, it is not possible to visualize the coronary vessels within one image. A volume data set of the heart, therefore, has to be acquired with evaluation of the coronary arteries by off-line postprocessing. Forty axial cross-sections of the heart are typically acquired within one breathhold, with one image following every heartbeat at 80% of the R–R interval. A 3-mm slice thickness with a table feed of 2 mm between slice acquisitions generates overlapping cross-sections. If larger volumes have to be covered (as, for example, in patients with bypass grafts), contiguous cross-sections without overlap are acquired. From 120 to 160 ml of contrast agent (30–35% iodine) are injected at a rate of 4 ml/second. From the initiation of contrast injection to the acquisition of the first image, a delay is maintained according to the individually determined contrast agent transit time (usually 15–25 seconds). Some authors have reported using 1.5-mm slice thickness without overlap (13). This reduces the covered volume to a 6-cm slab. Other authors, based on phantom studies, have suggested the use of the scanner's multi-slice mode to acquire eight quasi-parallel 8-mm thick cross-sections within 50 msec, and by using a table feed of 2 mm, to generate a set of heavily overlapped images with reconstruction of virtual cross-sections with smaller slice thickness by complex postprocessing techniques (14).

Figure 27.2. Time-density curve obtained in the aortic root after bolus injection of contrast agent. The first acquisition is started 10 seconds after the injection, subsequent acquisitions are obtained after every other heartbeat. Peak density in the aorta (110 HU) is observed 15 seconds after the injection.

Data Evaluation

In the cross-sectional images of the heart obtained during and after contrast injection, the mean CT density within the coronary arteries is about 165–200 Hounsfield Units (HU), whereas the mean density of the myocardium (85–100 HU) and connective tissue (−100 HU) are significantly lower (9–11). This permits selective visualization of the coronary artery lumen filled with contrast agent. In the contrast-enhanced EB-CT scans, the coronary arteries can be clearly identified in the cross-sectional axial images (see Fig. 27.3). Due to the tortuous course of the coronary vessels, however, detection and grading of coronary arteries using the axial images can be very difficult. For this reason, various forms of image reconstruction are applied, usually after transferring the volume data to a computer workstation.

Multiplanar Reconstruction

The continuous volume data set permits generation of secondary images in arbitrary planes by postprocessing, so-called multiplanar reconstructions (MPR). These reconstructions require no thresholding and all information concerning different CT attenuations is preserved. Due to the anisotropic nature of the volume data set, the spatial resolution of the generated multiplanar reconstructions depends on orientation: the closer the orientation to the axial plane, the higher the spatial resolution of the reconstructed images. In order to visualize long segments of the curved coronary arteries within one image, multiplanar reconstructions are generated in oblique and double-oblique planes (13). Several views in different planes have to be rendered to cover the complete course of each coronary vessel (see Fig. 27.4).

In order to depict the complete course of the coronary arteries in one single image, "curved" multiplanar reconstructions can be used. For these reconstructions, the coronary artery is depicted in a curved plane that follows the course of the coronary vessel through the volume data set (see Fig. 27.4). Although oblique, double-oblique, and curved multiplanar reconstructions can be rendered very quickly with dedicated software, the technique is limited by the fact that separate reconstructions are necessary for every coronary artery and that side branches are not visualized.

Shaded Surface Display

The "shaded surface display" (SSD) is a three-dimensional (3-D) rendering technique. All pixels below a certain threshold are discarded and the remaining pixels are shaded according to a lighting model and depth from the observer to preserve depth information (see Fig. 27.5). In EB-CT of the coronary arteries, the reconstruction threshold is usually chosen at 80–100 HU for optimal discrimination between the contrast-enhanced vessel lumen and

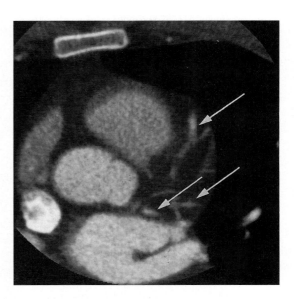

Figure 27.3. Axial EB-CT image. Cross-sections of the coronary artery lumen can clearly be seen after the injection of contrast agent (arrows).

the surrounding connective tissue, even though systematic investigation of the optimal reconstruction threshold (which may vary from patient to patient) have not been conducted. Because portions of the coronary vessels can be obscured by the pulmonary trunk and atrial appendages, manual segmentation (image editing) must be performed before the coronary arteries can be visualized in an SSD reconstruction (see Figs. 27.5 and 27.6). The reconstructions are rendered from different angles to show all parts of the coronary artery system. By further segmentation, everything but the coronary arteries can be removed to obtain reconstructions of the isolated coronary artery tree (see Fig. 27.5).

Drawbacks of the shaded surface display technique include: (1) all information concerning the density of structures above the reconstruction threshold is lost in the reconstruction process; (2) manual editing is a potential cause of errors and can be very time consuming, particularly if a display of the isolated coronary arteries is attempted. New imaging software that permits "real-time" 3-D reconstructions may eliminate the need for manual segmentation and may greatly speed up the image evaluation process.

Maximum Intensity Projection

Maximum intensity projection (MIP) renderings are two-dimensional (2-D) projection images in which each pixel is assigned a gray-scale value corresponding to the maximum pixel CT attenuation observed along a ray projected through the volume data (see Figs. 27.5 and 27.6). In these reconstructions, spatial information is lost due to overlap and projection, but information concerning density of contrast and calcifications within

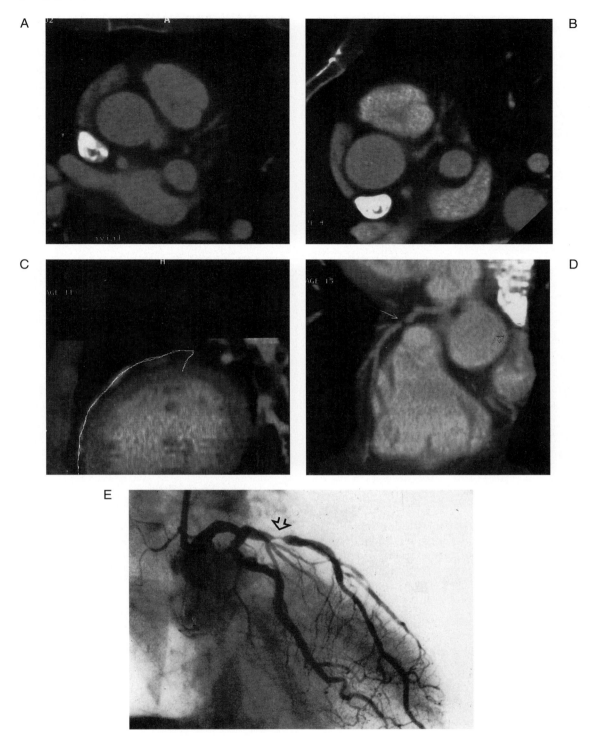

Figure 27.4. (A) Axial contrast-enhanced EB-CT image. A short segment of the left anterior descending coronary artery is visualized. (B) Oblique multiplanar reformation. A longer section of the LAD is visualized, but several reconstructions would be necessary to cover the complete course of the LAD. (C,D) By reconstructing a secondary image along a curved plane that follows the course of the LAD through the volume data set (C), a "curved multiplanar reconstruction" is created (D). This permits visualization of the complete course of the LAD within one image. A stenosis in the proximal LAD is recognized and confirmed by conventional angiography (E).

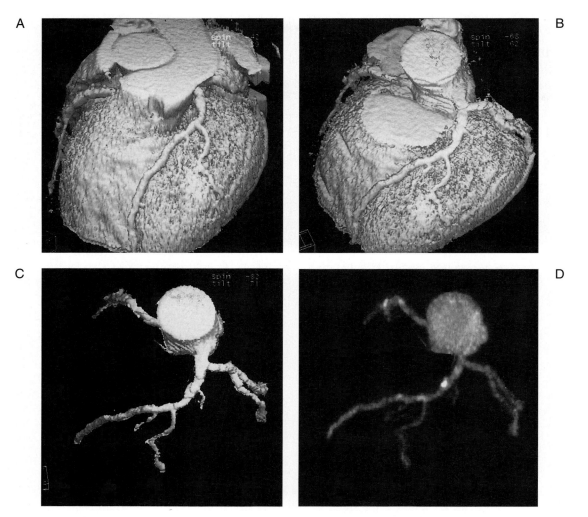

Figure 27.5. (A) Three-dimensional SSD reconstruction of the complete heart. The chest wall has been removed by segmentation. The pulmonary trunk and atrial appendages cover parts of the coronary arteries. A reconstruction threshold of 80 HU has been used. (B) After manual segmentation to remove the pulmonary trunk and atrial appendages, all parts of the coronary vessels can be seen. (C) Further segmentation yields an isolated reconstruction of the coronary artery tree. (D) Maximum intensity projection. The same raw data as for the SSD reconstruction in (C) was used. In this 2-D projection technique, coronary calcifications can be visualized in the course of the coronary arteries. (Reproduced with permission from Achenbach (10).)

the coronary arteries is retained. Some manual editing is usually required and can be time consuming. Maximum intensity projection (MIP) reconstructions have to be rendered from various angles to compensate for overlap and in their appearance, they resemble fluoroscopic angiograms.

Results of Patient Studies

The studies of EB-CT coronary angiography that have been published to date comprise approximately 160 patients and healthy subjects (11–13,15,16). In unselected patient groups, the studies are technically adequate for evaluation in about 80–90% of cases (12,15).

In 11 healthy volunteers, Chernoff et al. determined the length of the continuously visualized coronary artery lumen (11). They found mean values of 65 mm for the left anterior descending (LAD) coronary artery, 45 mm for the left circumflex (LCx), and 58 mm for the right coronary artery (RCA). These values compare favorably to similar investigations by magnetic resonance imaging (MRI) (17–20). The determination of the mean coronary artery diameters measured by EB-CT in these 11 subjects yielded no significant difference to normal value reported in the literature (11).

Measurement of coronary artery diameters in EB-CT shaded surface display reconstructions of 10 patients with coronary artery disease yielded a correlation of $r = 0.83$ to the diameter measured at identical sites by quan-

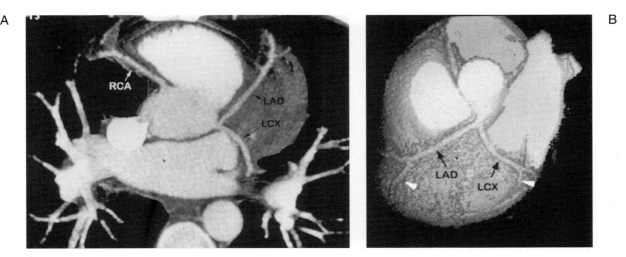

Figure 27.6. (A) Maximum intensity projection of the coronary arteries in a healthy volunteer. Some parts of the heart which would have obscured the coronary arteries were removed by manual segmentation. (B) Surface rendering (shaded surface display) of the same subject. (Reproduced with permission from Chernoff et al. (11).)

titative coronary angiography (21). Due to better image quality, a closer correlation was found for the left main and LAD coronary artery ($r = 0.87$). Partial volume effects lead to underrepresentation of very small coronary arteries and stenotic segments in the EB-CT reconstructions, whereas a tendency toward overestimation of the diameter of large coronary vessels and bypass grafts was observed (21).

Concerning the detection of coronary artery stenoses and occlusions, overall sensitivities ranging from 74 to 90% and specificities from 91 to 95% were found in comparisons of EB-CT to conventional X-ray coronary angiography (9,12,13,16). Fig. 27.7 shows an example of a high-grade stenosis in the LAD coronary artery in comparison with conventional angiography, as well as the result following coronary angioplasty. Although the results for the left main and LAD coronary artery are uniformly good, with sensitivities usually well above 90% (9,12,13,16), the results are worse for the RCA, and especially the LCx coronary artery, with both concerning technically adequate visualization of the vessels and detection of significant coronary artery stenoses.

Electron-beam computed tomography (EB-CT) also seems well suited for the demonstration of short- and long-term success of coronary revascularization: In 40 patients, it could be shown that restenoses following coronary angioplasty can be detected with a sensitivity of 100% by EB-CT (22), and both occlusions and high-grade stenoses of coronary artery bypass grafts were detected with 100% sensitivity in a group of 25 patients

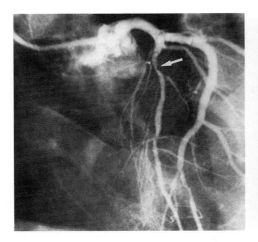

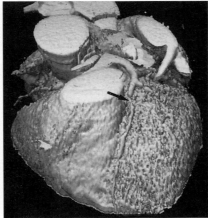

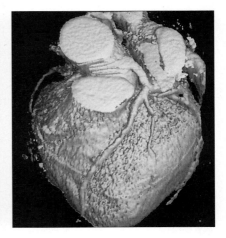

A B C

Figure 27.7. Patient with a high-grade stenosis of the left anterior descending coronary artery in angiography (A) and EB-CT (B). After angioplasty, normalization of the lumen diameter is documented by EB-CT (C). (Reproduced with permission from Moshage et al. (9).)

A
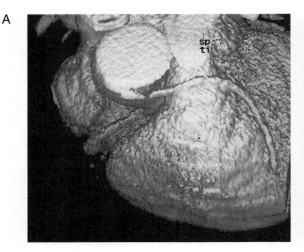

B
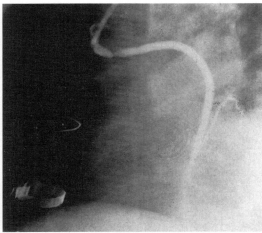

Figure 27.8. High-grade stenosis in a bypass graft to the left anterior descending coronary artery in EB-CT (A) and coronary angiography (B). (Reprinted from Am J Cardiol, volume number 79,

Achenbach et al., "Noninvasive, three-dimensional visualization of coronary artery bypass grafts by electron beam tomography," pages 856–61, copyright 1997, with permission from Excerpta Media, Inc.)

(see Fig. 27.8) (23). Although the value of EB-CT coronary angiography as a screening method for coronary artery stenoses is still limited due to reduced image quality especially of the LCx coronary artery, its application in the evaluation of patients after coronary revascularization seems clinically feasible.

Limitations of EB-CT Coronary Angiography

The major potential limitations of EB-CT coronary angiography in its present form are motion artifacts, difficulties in segmentation of the coronary arteries, problems with EKG synchronization, and poor discrimination between the contrast-filled coronary lumen and wall calcifications. In the published studies, the image quality obtained in about 10–15% of vessels was too poor for evaluation, ranging from 6% for the proximal LAD coronary artery to 26% for the proximal LCx coronary artery. Several factors contribute to degraded image quality. Motion artifacts affect mainly the right and left circumflex coronary artery in their midsegments (see Fig. 27.9). Faster scan rates are necessary to eliminate these artifacts because the current scan time of 100 msec in the high-resolution mode is insufficient to prevent motion artifacts completely from cardiac pulsations (24). In addition, the LCx and to a lesser extent the RCA have close anatomical relationships to venous structures, such as the coronary sinus and atrial appendages, that can be a potential source of error in manual segmentation of the data sets. All vessel segments can be affected by EKG synchronization or respiration artifacts. These artifacts can be detected in surface display reconstructions because they

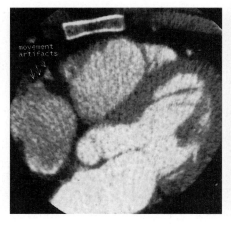

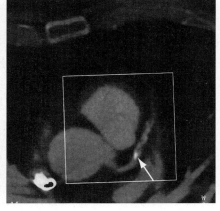

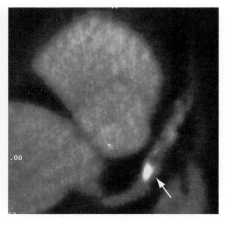

A   B   C

Figure 27.9. Artifacts and problems in EB-CT coronary angiography. Movement artifact of the right coronary artery (A). Patient with heavy calcifications of the LAD (arrow) which make evaluation of the contrast-enhanced scans impossible (B,C).

produce step artifacts of the surface of the heart, but they may be difficult to detect and cause false-positive detection of stenoses in other forms of image reconstruction. Finally, calcifications of the coronary vessels have a similar or higher CT density than the contrast-enhanced vessel lumen and can therefore cause false-negative results in shaded surface display reconstructions (see Fig. 27.9). They have also been cited as a cause for false-positive results in multiplanar reconstructions (13).

Comparison of EB-CT and MR Coronary Angiography

As compared with MR coronary angiography, EB-CT has several advantages. The spatial resolution is superior to that of most MRI sequences, and the overall acquisition time is considerably shorter. Conventional MR coronary angiography sequences require repeated breathholds (17,25,26) with severe misregistration of sections due to the patient's inability to hold his or her breath at a consistent level of inspiration (18). New navigator-echo–based respiratory-gated sequences can eliminate the need for repeated breathholds (20,27,28), but they are not yet widely available, and in order to fill k-space completely, image data cannot be exclusively limited to expiration so that some motion artifacts persist. Patients with metallic implants are excluded from MRI and claustrophobia can be a problem. Magnetic resonance angiography (MRA), however, has a major advantage in that it can be performed without injection of contrast agent and does not involve exposure to ionizing radiation. In addition, the availability of MR scanners is vastly superior to that of EB-CT systems.

Future Prospects for EB-CT Coronary Angiography

In order to improve the results of EB-CT coronary angiography, modifications of the scanner would be desirable. Shorter scan times would reduce motion artifacts. Improved in-plane spatial resolution would help reduce partial volume effects and might permit discrimination of coronary calcifications and lumen by introducing an additional upper threshold for reconstruction. As long as only one scan can be acquired in every cardiac cycle, the number of scans that make up the volume data set cannot be significantly increased because the breathhold cannot be extended over more than 30–40 seconds. This also further prevents reduction of the slice thickness; therefore, simultaneous acquisition of several cross-sections would be desirable.

Acquisition of a static volume data set might not even be the best and only way to investigate stenoses of the coronary arteries. Very promising results have been reported for time–density measurements in the coronary arteries after bolus injection of contrast agent using the scanner's multislice mode to investigate the patency of coronary artery stents (29,30). These results warrant further investigation.

Summary

Due to its high temporal resolution, EB-CT is well suited for cardiac imaging. Although the major cardiac application of EB-CT to date has been detection and quantification of coronary calcifications, studies have demonstrated that cardiac EB-CT in combination with intravenous injection of contrast agent permits imaging of the coronary vessel lumen and detection of coronary artery stenoses and occlusions. Results obtained for the left main and LAD coronary artery, as well as for venous bypass grafts, correlate well with conventional angiography, whereas motion artifacts and anatomic difficulties currently reduce the diagnostic value for the right and especially left circumflex coronary arteries. Even though improvements in scanner design and in the investigation protocol are warranted, clinical applications of the method (e.g., in the followup after coronary revascularization) seem possible.

In the year 2000, cardiac-gated multislice CT has emerged as a very serious competitor for both EB-CT and MRI/MRA. The jury is still out as to which imaging modality will ultimately prevail. This topic continues to be hotly debated at many cardiac imaging meetings.

References

1. Boyd D, Gould RG, Quinn J, Sparks R, Stanley R, Hermannsfeldt W. A proposed cardiac 3-D densitometer for easy detection and evaluation of heart disease. IEEE Trans Nucl Sci 1979;26:2724–27.
2. Gould RG. Principles of ultrafast computed tomography: historical aspects, mechanisms, and scanner characteristics. *In*: Stanford W, Rumberger JA, eds. Ultrafast Computed Tomography in Cardiac Imaging: Principles and Practice. Mt Kisco, NY: Futura, 1993:1–16.
3. Agatston AS, Janowitz WR, Hildner FJ, Zusmer NR, Viamonte M, Detrano R. Quantification of coronary artery calcium using ultrafast computed tomography. J Am Coll Cardiol 1990;15:827–32.
4. Breen JF, Sheedy PF, Schwartz RS, et al. Coronary artery calcification detected with ultrafast CT as an indication of coronary artery disease. Radiology 1992;185:435–39.
5. Budoff MJ, Georgiou D, Brody A, Agatston AS, Kennedy J, Wolfkiel C, et al. Ultrafast computed tomography as a diagnostic modality in the detection of coronary artery disease. Circulation 1996;93:898–904.
6. Rumberger JA, Sheedy PF, Breen JF, Fitzpatrick LA, Schwartz RS. Electron beam computed tomography and coronary artery disease: scanning for coronary artery calcification. Mayo Clin Proc 1996;71:369–77.
7. Arad Y, Spadaro LA, Goodman K, Lledo-Perez A, Sherman S, Lerner G, et al. Predictive value of electron beam

computed tomography of the coronary arteries. Circulation 1996;93:1951–53.

8. Detrano R, Hsiai T, Wang S, Puentes G, Fallavolita J, Shields P, et al. Prognostic value of coronary calcification and angiographic stenoses in patients undergoing coronary angiography. J Am Coll Cardiol 1996;27:285–90.

9. Moshage W, Achenbach S, Seese B, Bachmann K, Kirchgeorg M. Coronary artery stenoses: three-dimensional imaging with electrocardiographically triggered, contrast agent-enhanced, electron-beam CT. Radiology 1995;196:707–14.

10. Achenbach S, Moshage W, Bachmann K. Coronary angiography by electron beam tomography. Herz 1996;21: 106–17.

11. Chernoff DM, Ritchie CJ, Higgins CB. Evaluation of electron beam CT coronary angiography in healthy subjects. Am J Roentgenol 1997;169:93–99.

12. Budoff MJ, Oudiz RJ, Zalace CP, Baksheshi H, Goldberg SL, Rami TG, et al. Intravenous three dimensional coronary angiography using contrast enhanced electron beam computed tomography. J Am Coll Cardiol 1997;29:393A.

13. Nakanishi T, Ito K, Imazu M, Yamakido M. Evaluation of coronary artery stenoses using electron-beam CT and multiplanar reformation. JCAT 1997;21(1):121–27.

14. Thomas PJ, McCollough CH, Ritman E. An electron-beam approach for transvenous coronary angiography. JCAT 1995;19(3):383–89.

15. Achenbach S, Moshage W, Ropers D, Nossen J, Bachmann K. Non-invasive coronary angiography by electron beam tomography: methods and clinical evaluation in the follow-up after PTCA. Z Kardiol 1997;86:121–30.

16. Achenbach S, Moshage W, Nossen J, Ropers D, Seese B, Janáen G, et al. Nichtinvasive Koronararteriendarstellung mittels Elektronenstrahltomographie-Vergleich zur Koronarangiographie bei 100 Patienten. Z Kardiol 1997; 86(Suppl. 2):205.

17. Manning WJ, Li W, Boyle NG, Edelman RR. Fat-suppressed breath-hold magnetic resonance coronary angiography. Circulation 1993;87:94–104.

18. Duerinckx AJ, Atkinson DP, Mintorovitch J, Simonetti OP, Vrman MK. Two-dimensional coronary MRA: limitations and artifacts. Eur Radiol 1996;6:312–25.

19. Pennell DJ, Keegan J, Firmin DN, Gatehouse PD, Underwood SR, Longmoore DB. Magnetic resonance imaging of coronary arteries: technique and preliminary results. Br Heart J 1993;70:325–26.

20. Hofman MBM, Paschal CB, Li D, Haacke EM, van Rossum AC, Sprenger M. MRI of coronary arteries, 2D breath-hold versus 3D respiratory gated acquisition. JCAT 1995;19: 56–62.

21. Achenbach S, Moshage W, Ropers D, Bachmann K. Comparison of vessel diameters in electron beam tomography and quantitative coronary angiography. Int J Card Imag 1998;Vol 14(1):1–7.

22. Achenbach S, Moshage W, Bachmann K. Electron beam tomography for the non-invasive detection of restenosis after coronary angioplasty. Am J Card Imag 1996;10(Suppl. 1):6.

23. Achenbach S, Moshage W, Ropers D, Nossen J, Bachmann K. Noninvasive, three-dimensional visualization of coronary artery bypass grafts by electron beam tomography. Am J Cardiol 1997;79(7):856–61.

24. Ritchie CJ, Godwin JD, Crawford CR, Stanford W, Anno H, Kim Y. Minimum scan speed for the suppression of motion artifacts in CT. Radiology 1992;185:37–42.

25. Manning WJ, Li W, Edelman RR. A preliminary report comparing magnetic resonance coronary angiography with conventional angiography. N Engl J Med 1993;328: 828–32.

26. Pennell DJ, Bogren HG, Keegan J, Firmin DN, Underwood SR. Assessment of coronary artery stenosis by magnetic resonance imaging. Heart 1996;75:127–33.

27. Post JC, van Rossum AC, Hofman MBM, Valk J, Visser CA. Three-dimensional respiratory-gated MR angiography of coronary arteries: comparison with conventional coronary angiography. Am J Roentgenol 1996;166:1399–404.

28. Wang Y, Rossman PJ, Grimm RC, Riederer SJ, Ehman RL. Navigator-echo-based real-time respiratory gating and triggering for reduction of respiration effects in three-dimensional coronary MR angiography. Radiology 1996; 198:55–60.

29. Schmermund A, Haude M, Baumgart D, Gorge G, Gronemeyer D, Seibel R, et al. Non-invasive assessment of coronary Palmaz-Schatz stents by contrast enhanced electron beam computed tomography. Eur Heart J 1996;17:1546–53.

30. Schimpf SC, Sehnert CA, Schmermund A, Eberl R, Seibel RM, Gronemeyer DH. Noninvasive perfusion measurements in stents in coronary arteries, with electron-beam tomography. J Am Coll Cardiol 1997;29(2)(Suppl. A):517.

28

Intravascular Ultrasound. A "Look Inside" Coronary Arteries: Clinical Applications and Future Directions

Antonino Nicosia, Ali Hassan, and Peter J. Fitzgerald

Introduction

Intravascular ultrasound (IVUS) has been a major development in the imaging of the coronary arteries and has greatly expanded our knowledge about coronary artery disease and coronary interventions. The direct visualization of the vessel wall and the atherosclerotic plaque has offered valuable qualitative information into both the morphology and tissue characteristics of the diseased arterial wall, occult to angiography. Furthermore, the use of the miniaturized catheters (2.9–3.2 F) has permitted accurate on-line quantitative information regarding lumen size, vessel size, and plaque burden for assessment of progression–regression of atherosclerosis and the guidance of coronary interventions. It is likely that continued technical developments will enhance and define the clinical role of intravascular ultrasound in coronary interventional practice because this tool becomes a permanent part of the catheter lab inventory.

Limitations with Angiography

For the past three decades angiography has been the gold standard for evaluating patients with coronary artery disease. Angiography describes a planar two-dimensional (2-D) silhouette of a contrast-filled lumen and provides an overall map of the distribution of the coronary arteries and the location of atherosclerotic narrowings; however, advances in catheter-based therapies have highlighted some basic limitations of angiography. It has been clear for years from pathologic studies that the extent of coronary atherosclerosis is underestimated by the angiogram (1). The presence of a plaque on angiography relies on seeing a segment that is narrowed compared with an adjacent reference segment, believed by angiography to be free of disease. By intracoronary ultrasound, it is now known that, due to diffuse nature of atherosclerosis, the "normal" reference segment has on average 35–40% of its cross-sectional area occupied by plaque (2,3). Thus, accurately quantitating a stenosis using a reference segment poses problems for the angiographer (Fig. 28.1).

Furthermore, even in locations where the angiogram shows a definitive narrowing, the amount of plaque actually present is much greater than would be predicted on the basis of the measured lumen diameters alone. Indeed, intravascular ultrasound has confirmed the observations first made by Glagov et al. that there is a remodeling process with increasing plaque accumulation whereby the vessel expands to accommodate the plaque load (4). The remodeling effect cannot be visualized by angiography because it is not possible to visualize the plaque and the outer vessel boundary directly. It has been suggested that discrete coronary artery lesions only become apparent angiographically when they occupy more than 40% of the vessel area; the accumulation of plaque above a threshold of 40% of vessel area overcomes the ability of the vessel to compensate further (5–7). Intravascular ultrasound studies, however, have shown that the extent of vessel dynamics in a given artery is an even more complicated process that may be quite variable with segments revealing positive remodeling (expansion), no change, and/or negative remodeling (shrinkage) (8) (Fig. 28.2).

The introduction of quantitative coronary angiography (QCA) has had a tremendous impact in interventional cardiology and in studies of progression–regression of atherosclerosis because it offered the opportunity to standardize absolute measurements of the lumen, rather than relative values of percent stenosis. Ostial stenoses or lesions at bifurcations, however, may be insufficiently visualized because of catheter wedging, vessel overlapping,

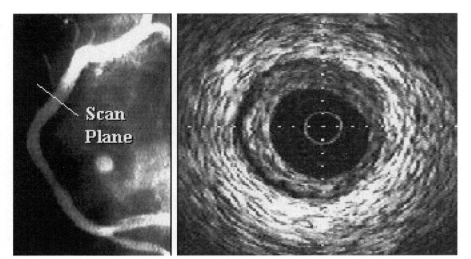

Figure 28.1. Example of quantitating a stenosis.

or foreshortening. This is particularly common when assessing the left main stem either at its origin, which may be behind the catheter tip, or its bifurcation, where the left anterior descending, circumflex, and intermediate vessels arise. Furthermore, the problems with accurate angiographic quantitation are frequently accentuated after coronary intervention due to plaque fracture and the subsequent appearance of a hazy lumen (9).

Despite these limitations, angiography remains the standard road-map for the assessment of coronary stenoses and the angiographic appearance is routinely used to determine the success of an interventional procedure. In several trials, however, angiography has failed to elucidate the mechanism for lumen improvement after an interventional procedure clearly. For example, the Coronary Angioplasty versus Excisional Atherectomy Trial (CAVEAT) and Canadian Coronary

Atherectomy Trial (CCAT) (10,11) are two trials primarily focused on coronary atherectomy. Both these studies demonstrated an improvement in lumen size by angiography with debulking by directional atherectomy compared with balloon dilatation. Despite a marginal improvement after 6-month followup in these patients, however, death and non–Q-wave myocardial infarction were also significantly higher. Other trials have suggested a disparity between angiographic result and clinical outcome [e.g., the Benestent (Belgium and the Netherlands Stent)-I trial (12), pharmacological restenosis trials (13), and the multicenter lipid-lowering trials (14), in which significant reductions in cardiovascular events have not correlated with change in angiographic dimensions at follow up]. These studies suggest that in order to make important prognostic assessment of therapeutic success in complicated lumen morphologies (e.g., after DCA) or in order to visualize subtle changes

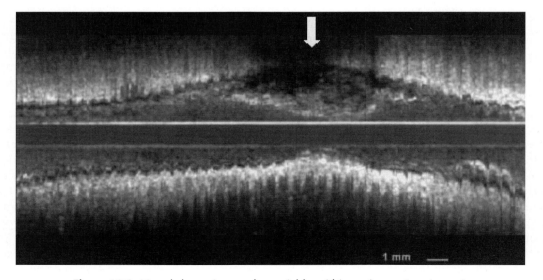

Figure 28.2. Vessel dynamics can be variable within a given artery (arrow).

in lumen geometries following a regression strategy, more accurate information on lumen, vessel, and plaque composition and distribution will be required. A "look inside" by IVUS may provide some answers.

Normal Coronary Arteries

An appreciation of the coronary anatomy and its relationship to structures "outside" the artery is important to the accurate interpretation and orientation of intravascular ultrasound images. Advances in image quality and improved tissue penetration has allowed the use of perivascular structures in addition to side-branches as reference points for tomographic and axial positioning (Fig. 28.3).

By intravascular ultrasound imaging, the most common appearance of the epicardial coronary vessels is a "three-layers" appearance due to the muscular composition of the medial layer. The inner layer is a relatively bright layer of plaque/intima (usually 150–200 μm thick in the adult); it consists of endothelial cells and a subendothelial layer of smooth muscle cells and fibro-blasts in a connective tissue matrix. The intermediate layer is a thin darker layer of media (the medial thickness ranges from 125 to 350 μm, but in the presence of plaque it may be considerably thinner or involuted and replaced by plaque) (15). The outer layer is brighter adventitia (which can extend from 300 to 500 μm); for the most part it is not possible to discriminate the adventitia from periadvential structures because they have similar echoreflectivity. The three-layered appearance by in-

travascular ultrasound occurs due to the acoustic impedance between each of the adjacent layers. It is thus dependent on the intima being of sufficient size to be identified with the current generation of ultrasound transducers and on the presence of a sufficient acoustic interface between media and adventitis (16). The threshold of intimal thickening required to resolve a definite intimal layer is 160 μm. Because the average intimal thickness in 40-year-old males is 200 μm, it is evident that a high proportion of even angiographically normal segments in adults have a three-layered appearance (17). Furthermore, over a given coronary artery segment, the three-layered appearance may alternate with a two-layered appearance due to the relative content of elastin and collagen. Thus, a three-layered appearance may be lost in the left main stem and at the proximal part of the right coronary artery (RCA) due to the increase in elastin content in transition from the highly elastic aortic root in these segments (Fig. 28.4).

Abnormal Vessels

Early Plaque Accumulation

The earliest accumulation of atherosclerotic plaque consists of a typical homogenous, intermediate echo-intensity intimal thickening. A common site for initial plaque accumulation occurs at branch points and bifurcations (most typically at the outer side). The greater cross-section area, the bending effect, and the reduced wall thickness are factors related to the accumulation of a plaque at the "hips" (18,19). IVUS has also confirmed the pathological reports, showing that a common site of early accumulation of atherosclerotic plaque is the segment proximal to a myocardial bridging. In a study in which information from IVUS and pressure measurements were combined, it was concluded that disturbance of blood flow and high wall stress proximal to myocardial bridging was a main contributor to the development of atherosclerosis in the segment proximal to the bridge (20).

Mild-to-Moderate Disease

With mild-to-moderate accumulations of plaque the process of remodeling becomes evident on intravascular ultrasound imaging (4–7). Positive remodeling and vessel expansion occur most often in the midportion of epicardial vessels away from branches that tend to stabilize the vessel geometry. The mid-LAD is a common site for observing vessel compensation. The greater accumulation of the plaque, the greater the complexity of plaque types that may be appreciated by ultrasound. *Calcification* is commonly seen by intravascular ultrasound as a bright echo with shadowing behind often associated with a reverberation artifact in the area of the

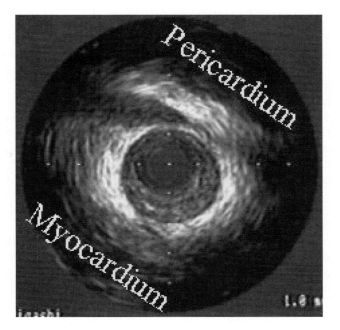

Figure 28.3. Use of pericardium and myocardium as reference points for tomographic and axial positioning.

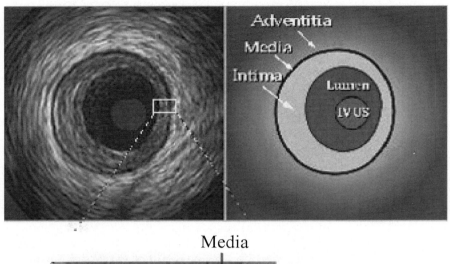

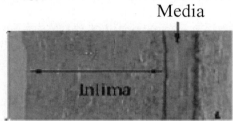

Media

Intima

Adventitia

Figure 28.4. Angiographically normal segments can have a three-layered appearance.

shadow. This is due to oscillation of the ultrasound beam back and forward between calcium and transducer. Calcification is seen much more commonly in intracoronary ultrasound than by fluoroscopy. In the guidance by ultrasound imaging for decision endpoints (GUIDE) trial (Phase I), 70% of target lesions had areas of calcium by ultrasound, compared with 40% of angiograms (21). Calcification may be graded from absent (0) to severe (3+) by the extent of the arc of calcium (22). In general a calcium score of 180 is required before there is a sufficient mass of calcium to be detected on fluoroscopy. The calcium may be distributed in the plaque in several ways: deep deposit in an arc at the intima–media border, or as superficial deposits, located directly at the luminal surface (Fig. 28.5).

Fibrous plaque has an intermediate echodensity between less echodense media or lipid and more echoreflective calcium. Such fibrous plaques with similar brightness to adventitia may then be described as hard or soft (with respect to the gray scale), depending on the presence or absence of shadowing behind the plaque, which relies on the relative amount of collagen and elastin contained in the plaque substances (Fig. 28.5).

Fatty plaques are usually more echolucent because they usually have a high content of lipid tissue that is poorly echoreflective; when large they may be appreciated as lipid pools. Because shadowing in relation to a fibrous plaque may be misinterpreted as a lipid collection, however, there is a tendency to classify plaques containing lipids broadly as *fibrofatty* (Fig. 28.5).

Identification of *thrombus* is one of the most difficult aspects of intravascular ultrasound imaging because it is frequently mistaken for soft plaque (23). It often appears as a scintillating or sparkling lobulated mass, undulating in a separate manner from the movement of the artery. Where the blood flow is significantly impaired, the backscatter of blood may be sufficiently intense to mimic for thrombus or soft plaque. Advanced signal analysis of the radiofrequency pattern may help to provide a rational and objective criteria to differentiate thrombus from fibrofatty plaque (24). In general, IVUS is very poor discriminating thrombus within a target segment. Angioscopy is far superior; however, IVUS examination within a stented segment makes thrombus recognition more favorable. The large signal reflectance from the metal struts provides a stand-off reference which allows thrombus to be easily distinguished from tissue prolapse and plaque protrusion.

Several groups have compared IVUS-determined tissue characteristics with actual histology. Based on the experience of Hodgson et al. on the histologic analysis of directional atherectomy samples, soft plaque, characterized by echolucent homogenous echoes, correlated with lipid deposits and highly cellular tissues (25). Hard plaques, characterized by echo density similar to the ad-

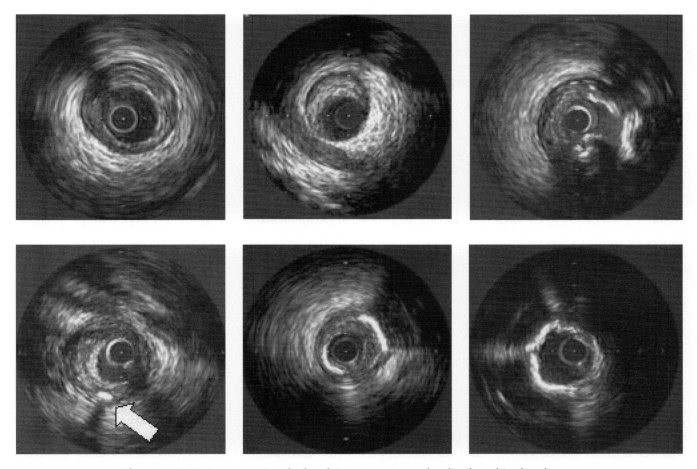

Figure 28.5. Various ways in which calcium (arrow) may be distributed in the plaque.

ventitia, correlated with relatively acellular fibrous tissue. Rasheed et al. reported that patients with unstable angina have a high proportion of soft plaque, whereas patients with stable chronic angina have a preponderance of calcified and hard plaque (26). Using postmortem specimens, De Feyter et al. showed that echolucent (lipid-rich coronary) plaques are prone to rupture, and that rupture and superimposed thrombosis are the primary mechanisms causing acute coronary syndromes (27).

Applications in Interventions

With the development of catheters as small as 2.9 F, intravascular ultrasound may be used to assess lesions prior to interventions and to formulate a strategy of lesion-targeted therapy based on plaque distribution and characteristics. In general, the two most important factors influencing the device selection are the plaque load or burden, and the extent and severity of calcification. With an extensive plaque load, a debulking strategy by directional coronary atherectomy has become

common in interventional practice. At the same time, an arc of superficial calcium of more than 180 degrees and located at the luminal surface has been associated with an inability to cut with a directional atherectomy device and causes difficulty in expanding a stent to full caliber (28). In these cases, high-speed rotational atherectomy has become increasingly used to ablate superficial calcium in lesions with a large plaque load, either as a stand-alone procedure or in preparation for further treatment strategies (29).

Furthermore, as highlighted earlier, ostial lesions or lesions at branches may be difficult to assess by angiography. The ability of intravascular ultrasound to characterize lesions and modify strategies accordingly has been assessed in the study of Mintz et al., in which 313 target lesions underwent intravascular ultrasound resulting in a change of therapy in 40% of cases (28). In this study a strategy for device selection was suggested: Lesions with significant superficial calcium were treated with rotablation, excimer laser, or surgery; eccentric noncalcified lesions underwent directional atherectomy; dissections were stented; thrombotic vein grafts were treated with thrombolysis and/or extraction atherectomy;

and fibrotic vein grafts were often stented after balloon dilatation.

Guidance During Interventions

The most widespread use of preprocedure intravascular ultrasound is in choice, guiding and monitoring the use of different interventional devices, as an invaluable complement to the angiographic assessment. In the future, IVUS may help triage lesions between a surgical approach and intervention, and it may provide valuable insights into targeting anastomotic sites in the era of minimally invasive surgical approaches.

Balloon Angioplasty

For balloon angioplasty, IVUS provides a direct visualization of the stretching and tearing processes that are key to lumen expansion (30,31). An initial in vitro study (32) assessed that the dissection of the plaque and the presence of arterial flaps that protruded into the lumen were a common finding after balloon angioplasty. The studies of Honye et al. (33) and Gerber et al. (34) have confirmed that tearing or fracturing, rather than compression, of the plaque occurs in 60–80% of coronary angioplasty cases (33,35). In these studies, a classification of the dissection patterns have been proposed, based on the extent and the depth of such tears. The presence of calcium in a coronary lesion determines the response of the artery to balloon dilatation. In one study of patients after balloon angioplasty of peripheral and coronary vessels, it was concluded that intralesional localized calcium played a direct role in promoting dissection by increasing shear stress within the plaque at the junction between tissue types with different elastic properties (35).

IVUS can be also used during interventional procedures in order to measure lumen and vessel area accurately at both the lesion site and at the reference segment, allowing the operator to size angioplasty balloons more exactly. In a key study of 223 coronary vessels treated by a Palmatz-Schatz stent, directional atherectomy or laser balloon angioplasty, the major procedural determinant of restenosis was the acute luminal gain, leading to the "bigger is better" hypothesis (36). Accurate balloon sizing is central to achieving the largest acute lumen gain after balloon angioplasty. A recent study (37) of the Clinical Outcomes of Ultrasound Trial (CLOUT) suggests that balloons may be sized more aggressively than conventional practice without increasing the acute complication rates. Balloons with a diameter halfway between the lumen and media-to-media dimension of the reference segment (as determined by ultrasound) were used safely and resulted in significantly larger postprocedure lumens than the conventional, angiographically guided approach. Using less balloons and achieving a "stentlike" result may be valuable in today's cost-conscious cath-lab.

Directional Coronary Atherectomy (DCA)

This plaque-debulking technique involves the use of a balloon-supported directional cutting device or atherectomy catheter. Ultrasound studies have shown that despite the excellent angiographic appearance following treatment with directional atherectomy, the actual plaque burden remaining behind is quite large. The value of adjunct IVUS imaging is that it can direct the cutting device to the area of largest plaque load and can identify the presence of superficial calcification that is a relative contraindication to the use of the cutting device. As in the case of PTCA, the GUIDE trial demonstrated that lower residual plaque burdens with DCA (percentage of plaque area) correlated with better long-term outcomes (38).

Both the orientation of the cutting device as well as the morphologic characteristics of the plaque determine the success of the procedure that is best achieved using ultrasound imaging. In a study of 170 patients with successful ultrasound-guided atherectomy (39), the arc of calcium was the most consistent predictor of success by any of the ultrasound criteria (e.g., postatherectomy lumen area, cross-sectional narrowing, or percentage of plaque removal). Several IVUS studies have suggested that plaque extraction may only account for 60–66% of lumen enlargement, with the remainder being due to expansion or Dottering (30,40).

Given that the amount of plaque removal leads to an increase in acute lumen and that the IVUS may be used to guide appropriate cutting, the optimal atherectomy restenosis study (OARS) was designed to introduce an aggressive DCA strategy (<15% residual diameter stenosis). The study was designed to see if a lower residual plaque area by ultrasound translates into a reduced restenosis rate at follow up (41). A residual percent plaque area of 55.6% was achieved by this aggressive IVUS-guided approach and the restenosis rate was 30.3%, a value that is well behind the 50% restenosis rate of the CAVEAT trial. The adjunctive balloon angioplasty following coronary atherectomy study (ABACAS) was a prospective randomized multicenter trial in Japan to evaluate whether more aggressive debulking by IVUS-guided DCA followed by adjunctive balloon angioplasty can reduce the restenosis rate without any increase in complication rates. The final results of the trial showed that with IVUS guidance, aggressive cutting can safely achieve optimal angiographic results with low residual plaque mass, and this was associated with a low restenosis rate.

Aggressive cutting, on the other hand, is associated with a greater frequency of deep wall cutting (Fig. 28.6). De Cesare et al. (43) showed that all the patients with

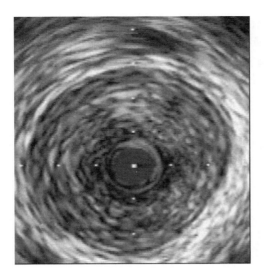 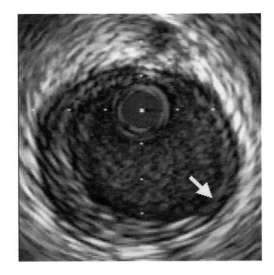

Figure 28.6. An example of deep wall cutting (arrow).

angiographic ectasia had media, adventitia, or both present in the atherectomy specimens and that the restenosis tends to occur more often in patients with marked ectasia after coronary atherectomy. A new combined imaging/atherectomy device may allow one to obtain a more aggressive debulking, reducing the amount of deep cuts and subsequent intimal injury (44).

High-Speed Rotational Atherectomy

Rotational atherectomy uses a rotating diamond-coated burr to abrade atherosclerotic plaque at a speed as high as 200,000 rpm. Intravascular ultrasound studies of high-speed rotational atherectomy have confirmed that selective cutting of noncompliant (especially calcified) plaque is an operative mechanism of this device. In a study of 28 patients Mintz et al. (45) showed that a distinct, circular intimalumen interface was achieved following rotablation with the lumen size 20% larger than the largest burr used, without damage to the media and dissections. Kovach et al. (46) confirmed that rotablation causes lumen enlargement by selective ablation of hard plaque with rare arterial expansion. Both studies showed that a significant residual plaque load was present after initial rotablation, indicating the need for adjunctive balloon angioplasty or stenting to achieve an adequate final lumen area. Intravascular ultrasound can be highly useful during this procedure in helping to determine the sequence of burr upsizing and in predicting the risk of perforation. In everyday practice, superficial calcium not apparent to angiography is amenable to successful rotablation if the calcium arc is more than 180 degrees and extends more than half of the lesion length. This lesion-specific initial debulking strategy may then be supplemented by a final intervention (e.g., stenting) to obtain the largest acute lumen gain.

Coronary Stenting

In the past few years a marked increase in the use of intracoronary stenting has been seen, guided by the assumption that achieving a large acute lumen gain (47,48) could have modified the restenosis process. A 29% rate of subacute thrombosis with a high rate of bleeding complications dampened the first era of the stent deployment. Indeed, IVUS studies help tremendously in this "early" era, suggesting that stents that appeared to be well deployed by angiography were not always completely expanded, and the metal struts were not always apposed to the vessel wall. In a landmark study of 359 patients (49), IVUS has been used to guide stent deployment and showed that adjunct high-pressure balloon dilatation (mean pressure of 15 atmospheres) and larger balloon selection achieved superior expansion and drastically reduced the subacute thrombosis rate. This pivotal IVUS-guided study led to the "high-pressure" stent deployment era and eventually provided the basis for reduced anticoagulation protocols.

Over the past few years many different criteria for optimal stent expansion by ultrasound imaging have been proposed, with all of them trying to reach the goal of achieving a stent expansion that was not less than 70–80% of the reference segments (49,50). In addition for adequate stent expansion, it is imperative that apposition to the vessel wall is achieved at the time of stent expansion. The widespread use of IVUS in the past few years has been justified by the attempt to achieve an optimal stent expansion and apposition, which cannot be easily determined by angiography, especially in the setting of radiolucent stent strut material. The use of high-pressure balloon dilatations and the confirmation by IVUS of adequate stent expansion and apposition have reduced stent thrombosis, made a favorable impact on stent restenosis, and provided the rationale to reduce the anticoagulation protocol (49).

Following stent deployment it has been noted that the metal struts can cause injuries at the margins of the stent (marginal dissections or edge tears) due to the impact of the stent struts on the unrecognized reference plaque adjacent to the stented area. IVUS is the only method to document these tears accurately. The STRUT registry (51) documented an incidence of edge tears of 12%. It is still unclear if the operator should try to cover all the tears, or just proceed to a further stent deployment only in case of deep mobile flaps extending into the media that protrude into the lumen (Fig. 28.7). To evaluate objectively whether ultrasound-guided stent deployment results in an additional clinical benefit over angiography alone, several multicenter randomized trials have been designed to access the clinical and/or angiographical benefit associated with the routine use of IVUS during stent deployment. The CRUISE trial (51) and the AVID trial (52), recently completed, have been consistent in showing a significant reduction (up to 45%) of the restenosis rate of lesions treated by intravascular ultrasound guided stent implantation (51), especially in large vessels (>3.5 mm diameter) and in saphenous vein grafts (52). Furthermore, in the MUSIC study (50) the systematic use of Intravascular Ultrasound during Palmaz-Schatz stent implantation led to a restenosis rate of 9.7%.

Intravascular ultrasound can also help guiding therapy of in-stent restenosis that remains a clinical problem. Several strategies have evolved to deal with in-stent restenosis, such as repeat balloon angioplasty using a noncompliant balloon, or, alternatively, high-speed rotational atherectomy sized within the measured minimum stent area by ultrasound or excimer laser angioplasty.

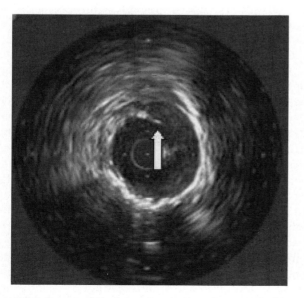

Figure 28.7. Deep mobile flaps (arrow) protruding into the lumen.

Restenosis and Vascular Remodeling after Interventions

Following an interventional procedure, 20–50% of the lesions show an angiographic restenosis at 6 months. It has become apparent that the two are the main mechanism of the restenosis process: (1) an aggressive tissue response to injury—intimal hyperplasia—that for many years was believed by many investigators to be the main mechanism; (2) shrinkage or negative remodeling of the treated segment. In one published study of 209 patients evaluated by serial ultrasound and angiography pre- and postintervention and at 6 months follow up after intervention, it was showed that a total of 73% of the reduction in lumen area at follow up was due to a decrease in vessel size, with the remainder due to an increase in plaque area. During follow up, only 22% of patients showed an increase in total vessel area accommodating the raised plaque area (positive remodeling) (53).

An IVUS trial (serial ultrasound restenosis, SURE) has been reported and has assessed the relative contribution of neo-intimal hyperplasia and vessel remodeling to late lumen loss after balloon angioplasty and directional atherectomy. They showed that the late loss correlated closely with the reduction in vessel area, suggesting that the geometric remodeling was the main mechanism determining restenosis (54).

Cardiac Allograft Vasculopathy

Cardiac allograft vasculopathy (CAV) is a unique form of coronary artery disease that develops early after transplantation (55,56). It is characterized by being more diffuse, involving smaller vessels, in addition to the epicardial vessels, and correlates with poor graft outcome and impaired survival rates (57). Coronary angiography has been the gold standard to detect the allograft vasculopathy; however, a few studies clearly demonstrated the low sensitivity of conventional angiography due to the diffuse pattern and rapid progression of this vasculopathy, especially within the first year after transplantation.

By IVUS, both the lumen parameters as well as quantitative and qualitative information about the plaque can be obtained. Intravascular ultrasound studies elucidated why the angiographic disease pattern in these patients is different compared with native coronary artery disease. Considerable concentric intimal thickening with a relatively homogeneous plaque type is typically seen in transplanted hearts, in contrast with a mixed and eccentrically distributed plaque burden, exemplifying the coronary artery disease (48,58). Rickenbacher et al. investigated the incidence of CAV over time (up to 15 years) using ultrasound in 174 transplant recipients. The mean intimal thickening was significantly higher 1 year after transplantation with progression of disease within the first several years. Calcification in plaques of these patients, an entity rarely seen in the first years after transplantation, increased especially after the sixth year (59). When predictors of the development of IVUS-detected vasculopathy were analyzed, donor undersize (<20% of recipient by weight), donor smoking history, and duration after transplantation were independently correlated with the overall amount of thickness (60).

The critical issue of whether the extent of IVUS-detected vasculopathy correlates with clinical outcome was also studied by the Stanford group. In this study, intimal thickening was considered pathological when it exceeded 0.3 mm. Intimal thickening of more than 0.3 mm correlated with an inferior survival and also with impaired freedom from cardiac death and retransplantation, regardless of angiographic evidence of cardiac allograft vasculopathy (61). These results indicate the feasibility and importance of ultrasound monitoring and suggest that this method might be used for the annual investigation of transplant patients because changes in therapeutic strategies could potentially be drawn from ultrasound results.

Future Developments

To avoid exchanging catheters and to provide an on-line guidance during the interventional procedures new combined imaging/therapeutic devices are being developed. A combined imaging and balloon catheter (Oracle Micro, Endosonic Corp.) has a complete over-the-wire design and consists of a low-compliance polyethylene balloon and a 64-element transducer located at the proximal site of the balloon. It operates at a frequency of 20 MHz (62). This design would also allow a stent to be crimped onto the balloon, thus facilitating "on-board" ultrasound guidance.

A combined imaging/atherectomy device has been developed and has undergone initial clinical testing. Initial testing has suggested that ultrasound-guided directional atherectomy appears to be feasible technically and may allow one to obtain a more aggressive debulking, reducing the amount of deep cuts and subsequent intimal injury (44). Human trials have demonstrated effective debulking with extremely low subintimal injury.

Intravascular ultrasound provides just a cross-sectional display of the arterial dimensions and pathology. Three-dimensional reconstruction of IVUS images offers an even more comprehensive insight into the spatial distribution of vascular structures and the longitudinal extent of arterial disease (63). Different techniques of three-dimensional reconstruction have been developed, differing mainly in the image acquisition (continuous motorized pull-back or stepwise EKG-gated pull-back) (64) and segmentation. The segmentation step identifies structures of interest according to a certain gray-scale scene. Three methods currently used are: (1) the threshold method which identifies different structures based on the definition of thresholds in the gray scale of ul-

trasound images (65); (2) the acoustic quantification method (66), which discriminates between the blood pool and the vessel wall, using an algorithm for statistical pattern recognition (Echoquant, Indec, Sunnyvale, CA); (3) the contour-detection method (67), which is based on the application of a minimum cost algorithm (initially developed for the quantitative coronary angiography) and permits the identification of the intimal leading edge and the external contour of the total vessel. Several factors, however, including general problems of ICUS as well as specific limitations of 3-D reconstruction can limit the quality of the final reconstruction (68). Current 3-D reconstructions are partially artificial because the true spatial position of the imaging catheter tip is not recorded, and the reconstruction is based on the false assumption that the path of the transducer through the artery is a straight line. Vessel curvatures with a radius of less than 5 cm cause a significant distortion of the reconstructed image, leading to over- or underestimation of certain portions of the plaque. It is likely that technical solutions to these problems will be found in the near future, and that this technique will ultimately provide a new standard for volumetric lumen and vessel measurements.

One of the biggest current limitations of IVUS is the inability to discriminate in a reliable way between certain plaque subtypes and to recognize thrombus. One approach to this problem has been the use of the raw radiofrequency signal, which is reflected back from the plaque to the transducer and diverted to a computer, before being translated into images. The amplitude and frequency data in the radiofrequency signal is compared with a known statistical profile for a given tissue subtype. Advances in imaging processing may allow the direct and tempestive visualization of particular subtypes of vulnerable plaque (e.g., a thin fibrous cap covering a lipid core), opening a new era of research into the causes and prevention of myocardial infarction.

References

1. Tobis JM, Mallery J, Mahon D, Lehman K, Zalesky P, Griffith J, et al. Intravascular ultrasound imaging of human coronary arteries in vivo: analysis of tissue characterization with comparison to in-vitro histological specimens. Circulation 1991;83:319–26.
2. Mintz GS, Painter JA, Pichard AD, Kent KM, Satler LF, Popma JJ, et al. Atherosclerosis in angiographically "normal" coronary artery segments: an intravascular ultrasound study with clinical correlations. J Am Coll Cardiol 1995;25(7):1479–85.
3. Yock PG, Fitzgerald PJ, Popp RL. Intravascular ultrasound. Sci Am 1995;2:68–77.
4. Glagov S, Weisenberg E, Zarins CK, Stankunavicius R, Kolettis GJ. Compensatory enlargement of human atherosclerotic arteries. N Engl J Med 1987;316:1371–75.
5. Kakuta T, Currier JW, Haudehschild CC, Ryan TJ, Faxon

DP. Differences in compensatory vessel enlargement, not intimal formation, account for restenosis after angioplasty in the hypercholesterolemic rabbit model. Circulation 1994;89;2809–15.

6. Post MJ, Borst C, Kuntz RE. The relative importance of arterial remodeling compared with intimal hyperplasia in lumen renarrowing after ballon angioplasty. Circulation 1994;89:2816–21.

7. Currier JW, Faxon DP. Restenosis after percutaneous transluminal coronary angioplasty: have we been aiming at the wrong target? J Am Coll Cardiol 1995;25:516–20.

8. Pasterkamp G, Borst C, Post MJ. Atherosclerosis arterial remodeling in the superficial femoral artery: individual variation in local compensatory enlargement response. Circulation 1996;93:1818–25.

9. Topol EJ, Nissen SE. Our preoccupation with coronary luminology: the dissociation between clinical and angiographic findings in ischemic heart disease. Circulation 1995;92:2333–42.

10. Topol EJ, Leya F, Pinkerton CA, Whitlow PL, Hofling B, Simonton CA, et al. A comparison of coronary angioplasty with directional atherectomy in patients with coronary artery disease. The CAVEAT study group. N Engl J Med 1993;329;221–27.

11. Adelman AG, Cohen EA, Kimball BP, Bonan R, Ricci DR, Webb JG. A comparison of directional atherectomy with balloon angioplasty for lesions of the left anterior descending coronary artery. N Engl J Med 1993;329;228–33.

12. Serruys PW, de Jaegere P, Kiemeneij F, Macaya C, Rutsch W, Heyndrickx G, et al., for the Benestent Study Group. A comparison of balloon expandable stent implantation with balloon angioplasty in patients with coronary artery disease. N Engl J Med 1994;331:489–95.

13. Emanuelsson H, Beatt KJ, Bagger JP, Balcon R, Heikkila J, Piessens J, et al., for the European Angiopeptin Study Group. Long-term effects of angiopeptin treatment in coronary angioplasty. Circulation 1995;91:1689–96.

14. Brown BG, Zhao XQ, Sacco DE, Albers JJ. Lipid lowering and plaque regression: new insights into prevention of plaque disruption and clinical events in coronary disease. Circulation 1993;87;1781–90.

15. Waller BF. The eccentric coronary atherosclerotic plaque: morphologic observations and clinical relevance. Clin Cardiol 1989;12:14.

16. Picano E, Landini L, Lattanzi F, et al. Time domain echo pattern evaluations from normal and atherosclerotic arterial walls: a study in vitro. Circulation 1988;3:654.

17. Fitzgerald PJ, St. Goar FG, Connolly RJ, Pinto FJ, Billingham ME, Popp RL, Yock PG. Intravascular ultrasound imaging of coronary arteries: is three layers the norm? Circulation 1992;86:154–58.

18. Bassiouny HS, Zarins CK, Kadowaki MH, Glagov S. Hemodynamic stress and experimental aortoiliac atherosclerosis. J Vasc Surg 1994;19:426–34.

19. Giddens DP, Zarins CK, Galgov S. The role of fluid mechanics in the localization and detection of atherosclerosis. J Biomech Eng 1993;115(4B0):588–94.

20. Ge J, Erbel R, Gorge G, Haude M, Meyer J. High wall shear stress proximal to myocardial bridging and atherosclerosis: intracoronary ultrasound and pressure measurements. Br Heart J 1995;73(5):462–65.

21. GUIDE trial investigators. IVUS-determined predictors of restenosis in PTCA and DCA: final report from the GUIDE trial, Phase II (abstr.). J Am Coll Cardiol 1996;27:156A.

22. Farb A, Virmani R, Atkinson JB, Kolodgie FD. Plaque morphology and pathologic changes in arteries from patients dying after coronary balloon angioplasty. J Am Coll Cardiol 1990;16:1421–29.

23. Siegel RJ, Ariani M, Fishbein MC, Chae JS, Park JC, Maurer G, et al. Histopathologic validation of angioscopy and intravascular ultrasound. Circulation 1991;84:109–17.

24. Metz JA, Preuss P, Komiyama N, Ramo P, Haywood G, Gullestad L. Discrimination of soft plaque and thrombus based on radiofrequency analysis of intravascular ultrasound (abstr.). J Am Coll Cardiol 1996;27(Suppl. A);200A.

25. Rasheed Q, Dhawale P, Anderson J, Hodgson J. Intracoronary ultrasound-defined plaque composition: computer-aided plaque characterization and correlation with histologic samples obtained during directional atherectomy. Am Heart J 1995;129:631–37.

26. Rasheed Q, Nair RN, Sheehan HM, Hodgson JM. Coronary artery plaque morphology in stable angina and subsets of unstable angina: an in vivo intracoronary ultrasound study. Int J Card Imag 1995;11(2):89–95.

27. de Feyter PJ, Ozaki Y, Baptista J, Escaned J, Di Mario C, de Jagere PP. Ischemia-related lesion characteristics in patients with stable or unstable angina: a study with intracoronary angiography and ultrasound. Circulation 1995;92(6):1408–13.

28. Mintz GS, Pichard AD, Kovach JA, Kent KM, Satler LF, Javier SP. Impact of preintervention intravascular ultrasound imaging on transcatheter treatment strategies in coronary artery disease. Am J Cardiol 1994;73:423–30.

29. Ellis SG, Popma JJ, Buchbinder M, Franco I, Leon MB, Kent KM. Relation of clinical presentation, stenosis morphology, and operator technique to the procedural results of rotational atherectomy-facilitated angioplasty. Circulation 1994;89:882–92.

30. Di Mario C, Gil R, Camenzind E, Ozaki Y, von Birgelen C, Umans V. Quantitative assessment with intracoronary ultrasound of the mechanisms of restenosis after percutaneous transluminal coronary angioplasty and directional coronary atherectomy. Am J Cardiol 1995;75:772–77.

31. Baptista J, Di Mario C, Ozaki Y, Escaned J, Gil R, de Feyter PJ, et al. Impact of plaque morphology and composition on the mechanism of lumen enlargement using intracoronary ultrasound and quantitative angiography after balloon angioplasty. Am J Cardiol 1996;77(2):115–21.

32. Tobis JM, Mallery JA, Gessert J, Griffith J, Mahon D, Bessen M, et al. Intravascular ultrasound cross-sectional arterial imaging before and after balloon angioplasty in vitro. Circulation 1989;80:873–82.

33. Honye J, Mahon DJ, Jain A, White CJ, Ramee SR, Wallis JB, et al. Morphological effects of coronary balloon angioplasty in-vivo assessed by intravascular ultrasound imaging. Circulation 1992;85:1012–25.

34. Gerber TC, Erbel R, Görge G, Ge J, Rupprecht H-J, Meyer J. Classification of morphological effects of percutaneous transluminal coronary angioplasty assessed by intravascular ultrasound. Am J Cardiol 1992;70;1546–54.

35. Fitzgerald PJ, Ports TA, Yock PG. Contribution of localized calcium deposits to dissection after angioplasty: an

observational study using intravascular ultrasound. Circulation 1992;86:64–70.

36. Kuntz RE, Safian RD, Levine MJ, Reis GJ, Diver DJ, Baim DS. Novel approach to the analysis of restenosis after the use of three new coronary devices. J Am Coll Cardiol 1992;19:1493–99.

37. Stone GW, Hodgson JM, St Goar FG, Frey A, Mudra H, Sheehan H, et al., for the Clinical Outcomes with Ultrasound Trial (CLOUT) Investigators. Improved procedural results of coronary angioplasty with intravascular ultrasound-guided balloon sizing: the CLOUT pilot trial. Circulation 1997;95(8):2044–52.

38. The GUIDE trial investigators. Lumen enlargement following angioplasty is related to plaque characteristics: a report from the GUIDE trial (abstr.). Circulation 1992; Suppl. I:I–531.

39. Matar FA, Mintz GS, Pinnow E, Javier SP, Popma JJ, Kent KM. Multivariate predictors of intravascular ultrasound end points after directional coronary atherectomy. J Am Coll Cardiol 1995;25:318–24.

40. Nakamura S, Mahon D, Leung C, Maheswaran B, Gutfinger D, Yang J. Intracoronary ultrasound imaging before and after directional coronary atherectomy: in vitro and clinical observations. Am Heart J 1995;129:841–51.

41. Lansky AJ, Mintz GS, Popma JJ, Pichard AD, Kent KM, Satler LF, et al. Remodeling after directional coronary atherectomy (with and without adjunct percutaneous transluminal coronary angioplasty): a serial angiographic and intravascular ultrasound analysis from the Optimal Atherectomy Restenosis Study. J Am Coll Cardiol 1998; 32(2):329–37.

42. Suzuki T, Hosokawa H, Katoh O, Fujita T, Ueno K, Takase S, et al. Effects of adjunctive balloon angioplasty after intravascular ultrasound-guided optimal directional coronary atherectomy: the results of adjunctive balloon angioplasty after coronary atherectomy study (ABACAS). J Am Coll Cardiol 1999;34(4):1028–35.

43. De Cesare NB, Popma JJ, Holmes DR, Dick RJ, Whitlow PL, King SB, et al. Clinical angiographic and histologic correlates of ectasia after directional coronary atherectomy. Am J Cardiol 1992;69:314–19.

44. Fitzgerald PJ, Belef M, Connolly AJ, Sudhir K, Yock PG. Design and initial testing of an ultrasound-guided directional atherectomy device. Am Heart J 1995;129(3):593–98.

45. Mintz GS, Potkin BN, Keren G, Satler LF, Pichard AD, Kent KM, et al. Intravascular ultrasound evaluation of the effect of rotational atherectomy in obstructive atherosclerotic coronary artery disease. Circulation 1992;86:1383–1393.

46. Kovach JA, Mintz GS, Pichard AD, Knet KM, Popma JJ, Satler LF, et al. Sequential intravascular ultrasound characterization of the mechanisms of rotational atherectomy and adjunct balloon angioplasty. J Am Coll Cardiol 1993; 22:1024–32.

47. Fischman DL, Leon MB, Baim D, Schatz RA, Savage MP, Penn I, et al., for the Stent Restenosis Study Investigators. A randomized comparison of coronary stent placement and balloon angioplasty in the treatment of coronary artery disease. N Engl J Med 1994;331:496–501.

48. Serruys PW, de Jaegere P, Kiemeneij F, Macaya C, Rutsch W, Heyndrickx G, et al., for the Benestent Study Group. A comparison of balloon expandable stent implantation with balloon angioplasty in patients with coronary artery disease. N Engl J Med 1994;331:489–95.

49. Colombo A, Hall P, Nakamura S, Almagor Y, Maiello L, Martini G, et al. Intracoronary stenting without anticoagulation accomplished with intravascular ultrasound guidance. Circulation 1995;91:1891–97.

50. de Jagere P, Mudra H, Figulla H, Almagor Y, Doucet S, Penn I, et al. Intravascular ultrasound-guided optimized stent deployment: immediate and 6-month clinical and angiographic results from the Multicenter Ultrasound Stenting In Coronaries Study (MUSIC Study). Eur Heart J 1998;19(8):1214–23.

51. Oshima A, Hayase M, Metz J, Bailey SR, Baim DS, Cleman MW, et al. Final results of the Can Routine Ultrasound Influence Stent Expansion Study (CRUISE). Circulation 2000, in press.

52. Russo R, Attubato M, Davidson C, DeFranco A, Fitzgerald P, Iaffaldano R, et al. Angiography versus intravascular ultrasound-directed stent placement: final results from AVID (abstr.). Circulation 1999;100:I-234.

53. Mintz GS, Popma JJ, Pichard AD, Kent KM, Satler LF, Wong SC, et al. Arterial remodeling after coronary angioplasty: a serial intravascular ultrasound study. Circulation 1996;94:35–43.

54. Kimura T, Kaburagi S, Tamura T, Yokoi H, Nakagawa Y, Yokoi H. Remodeling of human coronary arteries undergoing coronary angioplasty or atherectomy. Circulation 1997;96(2):475–83.

55. Griepp RB, Stinson EB, Bieber CP, Reitz BA, Copeland JG, Oyer PE, et al. Control of graft atherosclerosis in human heart transplant recipients. Surgery 1977;81:262–69.

56. Uretsky BF, Murali S, Reddy PS, Rabin B, Lee A, Griffith BP, et al. Development of coronary artery disease in cardiac transplant receiving immunosuppressive therapy with cyclosporine and prednisone. Circulation 1987;76: 827–34.

57. Velican D, Velican C. Comparative study on age-related changes and atherosclerotic involvement of the coronary arteries of male and female subjects up to 40 years of age. Atherosclerosis 1981;38:39–50.

58. Chenzbraun A, Pinto FJ, Alderman EL, Botas J, Oesterle SN, Schroeder JS, et al. Distribution and morphologic features of coronary disease in cardiac allografts: an intracoronary ultrasound study. J Am Soc Echocardiogr 1995; 8(1):1–8.

59. Rickenbacher PR, Pinto FJ, Chenzbraun A, Botas J, Lewis NP, Alderman EL. Incidence and severity of transplant coronary artery disease early and up to 15 years after transplantation as detected by intravascular ultrasound. J Am Coll Cardiol 1995;25:171–77.

60. Rickenbacker PR, Pinto FJ, Lewis NP, Hunt SA, Gamberg P, Alderman EL. Correlation of donor characteristics with transplant coronary artery disease as assessed by intracoronary ultrasound and coronary angiography. Am J Cardiol 1995;76(5):340–45.

61. Koegh AM, Valantine HA, Hunt SA, Scroeder JS, McIntosh N, Oyer PE, et al. Impact of proximal and midvessel discrete coronary artery stenoses on survival after heart transplantation. J Heart Lung Transplant 1992;11:892–901.

62. Mudra H, Klauss V, Blasini R, Schuhlen H, Klauss V, Richardt G, et al. Ultrasound guidance of Palmaz-Schatz

intracoronary stenting with a combined intravascular balloon catheter. Circulation 1994;90:1252–61.

63. Matar FA, Mintz GS, Douek P, Farb A, Virmani R, Javier SP. Coronary artery lumen volume measurement using three-dimensional intravascular ultrasound; validation of a new technique. Cath Cardiovasc Diag 1994;33:214–20.

64. von Birgelen C, de Very EA, Mintz GS, Nicosia A, Bruining N, Li W, et al. ECG-gated three-dimensional intravascular ultrasound: feasibility and reproducibility of the automated analysis of coronary lumen and atherosclerotic plaque dimensions in humans. Circulation 1997;96(9):2944–52.

65. Rosenfield K, Losordo DW, Ramaswamy K, Pastore JO, Langevin RE, Razvi S, et al. Three-dimensional reconstruction of human coronary and peripheral arteries from images recorded during two-dimensional intravascular ultrasound examination. Circulation 1991;84:1938–56.

66. Prati F, Dimario C, Gil R, von Birgelen C, Camenzind E, Montauban van Swijndregt WJ, et al. Usefulness of on-line three-dimensional reconstruction of intracoronary ultrasound for guidance of stent deployment. Am J Cardiol 1996;77(7):455–61.

67. Li W, von Birgelen C, Di Mario C, Boersma E, Gussenhoven EJ, van der Putten N, et al. Semiautomatic contour-detection for volumetric quantification of intracoronary ultrasound. Proc Comp Cardiol, IEEE Computer Society Press, 1994:277–80.

68. Roelandt JRTC, Di Mario C, Pandian NG, Li W, Keane D, Slager CJ. Three-dimensional reconstruction of intracoronary ultrasound images: rationale, approaches, problems and directions. Circulation 1994;90:1044–55.

29
The Future of Cardiac MRI

André J. Duerinckx

Cardiac magnetic resonance imaging (MRI) is the newest noninvasive imaging technique to be used for the evaluation of patients with ischemic heart disease (1–3). MRI can be used to study myocardial viability, myocardial ischemia, cardiac function and metabolism, and coronary artery anatomy and flow (4). The recent scientific and clinical advances have been such that several small medical societies have started to focus almost exclusively on cardiovascular MRI (5). Each year the North American Society for Cardiac Imaging (www.nasci.org), the Society for Cardiovascular Magnetic Resonance (www.scmr.org), the Council on Cardiovascular Radiology of the American Heart Association and the International Society of Magnetic Resonance in Medicine organize multiple educational events to instruct imagers and practitioners (mostly radiologists and cardiologists) about the potential value of cardiac MRI for patients with ischemic heart disease. In 1999 the Committee for Cardiovascular Imaging, a joint effort of the American College of Radiology, the Radiological Society of North America, the American Roentgen Ray Society, and the American Board of Radiology, was created to address this renewed interest from the radiology community in cardiovascular imaging. One of the first actions of the committee was to create new courses on cardiovascular imaging which are being offered four times a year throughout the United States, with the first one held in June 23–25, 2000, in Chicago (www.acr.org). Recent dramatic improvements in the technology (i.e., newer and better cardiac MRI pulse sequences) and the efforts to teach the performance of coronary magnetic resonance angiography (MRA) to more end-users (radiologists and cardiologists) are both important.

For a variety of reasons most practitioners and imagers are often reluctant to utilize cardiac MRI in the routine workup of patients with ischemic heart disease. In general, these physicians lack exposure to and training in cardiac MRI. Furthermore, these examinations are technically difficult and there is the need for cardiac gating which lengthens the duration of the MR study setup time. Large clinical studies which may prove the utility of MRI for ischemic heart disease are only now being performed or planned. But most important perhaps, as pointed out by Higgins (4), a key component of the MR evaluation of ischemic heart disease, namely coronary MRA, has not yet reached a sufficient level of technical maturity. Unfortunately, cardiac MRI technology is evolving so fast that most clinical trials cannot be completed before a technique becomes obsolete, thus creating the perception that the technology is not mature. Coronary MRA is one of the best examples of such recent technological evolutions in cardiac MRI. The early coronary MRA techniques appeared very promising (6), but because they acquired only one image per breathhold, were limited to 2-D acquisitions and required operator skills. These techniques never gained widespread use (7–9). Improved coronary MRA techniques employing navigator echoes, also referred to as "second-generation coronary MRA techniques," followed, and allowed free-breathing and increased spatial resolution followed (10–13). Later, third-generation techniques allowed the acquisition of a 3-D volume within one breathhold (14). Hybrid techniques offer the greatest hope for fast and efficient coronary MRA with adequate spatial and temporal resolution (15–17). Although these newer coronary MRA techniques are nearly as easy to employ as a conventional computed tomography (CT) scanner, the average practitioner is not comfortable with this constant change and evolution in MR techniques. The use of cardiac MRI for the direct evaluation of myocardial viability and myocardial ischemia has seen a similar dramatic evolution.

Cardiac MRI has become such a vast field that it is impossible to make general statements about its future, except to say that its importance will keep increasing. Cardiac anatomy, function and myocardial viability evaluation are all very important applications, and will one day be part of the "one-stop" noninvasive comprehensive cardiac MRI examination (2,18). In this chapter we will limit our comments about the future of cardiac MRI to those that relate to coronary vessels.

The Need to Provide Noninvasive Coronary MRA

As mentioned in Chapter 1, atherosclerosis—specifically, coronary artery disease—is the most common cause of adult mortality in the Western hemisphere. Cardiac

imaging represents an enormous percentage of all diagnostic imaging procedures. In 1993 an estimated $1.67 billion (or 32% of all costs for imaging) was spent in the United States by Medicare (Part B) for reimbursement of the 10 most common imaging procedures, which are all primarily cardiovascular in nature (19). Atherosclerosis remains an elusive, progressive, and devastating disease, despite the enormous investment of research dollars by government and industry. Invasive selective coronary angiography has long been and is still the gold standard for defining the site and severity of stenotic lesions in the coronary arteries. The functional significance of lesions can be determined with myocardial perfusion tests with and without stress using nuclear cardiology, echocardiography, or MRI. In the more recent literature, the importance of the mechanisms involved in plaque formation and rupture as well as thrombus formation has been emphasized. Plaque histology and plaque stability are and should be critical factors in predicting the importance of a small plaque or a coronary lesion for future events. Nevertheless, in the day-to-day practice of cardiology, the traditional criteria of lesion stenosis and physiological significance of lesion severity (coronary flow reserve) are still routinely used.

Thus, for the day-to-day clinical practice of cardiology, the need to image the coronary vessel's lumen and to exclude the presence of significant coronary lesions remain. Conventional X-ray coronary angiography is used today almost exclusively for the direct visualization of the coronary lumen. Intravascular ultrasound has provided an alternative, but it is still very invasive. Noninvasive alternatives, such as echocardiography (for infants and some pediatric patients), electron-beam computed tomography (EB-CT) angiography, multislice CT angiography and MRA are being evaluated. Electron-beam computed tomography angiography offers a good solution, although it requires the use of X-ray radiation and the injection of a potentially harmful iodinated contrast agent (see Chap. 28). Coronary MRA is less invasive and can be used in a wider patient population (e.g., those with renal failure), but it is excluded in others (e.g., patients with pacemakers). Efforts are being made to teach the performance of coronary MRA to the point where it can be used in many clinical settings with existing commercial MR scanners and pulse sequences (see also Chaps. 4 and 5).

The Future of Cardiac MRI as Seen in 1996 by a Working Group Sponsored by the National Heart, Lung, and Blood Institute

The future role of cardiac MRI has been discussed many times by many groups and authors. One such discussion was held during a meeting on October 28–29, 1996, of a working group sponsored by the National Heart, Lung and Blood Institute (NHLBI) in Bethesda, MD (20). This working group also recommended future work on coronary artery visualization and flow quantification as the number-one high-risk–high-benefit activity for academic researchers and as a special area of emphasis for the NIH. We refer to the full report for more details on other recommendations.

Coronary Plaque and Coronary Vessel Wall Imaging

One should also not forget that in the workup of patients with coronary artery disease the total atherosclerotic burden in the aorta, carotid, and femoral arteries are good predictors of coronary artery disease. A good correlation has been shown between the severity of atherosclerotic disease in one arterial bed and involvement of other vessels. This also opens the potential for more involvement by imagers in noninvasive screening for ischemic heart disease, beyond the already established involvement in coronary calcium screening. Direct characterization with MRI of plaque in larger vessels is already possible (21–24). Measuring the intimal–medial wall thickness in the carotid arteries and the femoral arteries can be easily performed by most radiology practices using ultrasound. This could also become an important parameter in addition to the more traditional screening factors, for the early prediction of coronary artery disease.

Besides these indirect indicators of plaque burden, direct imaging of the coronary wall and plaque is now possible and has been performed by several investigators (25–29). Together these new techniques will provide new tools for risk assessment in patients with ischemic heart disease.

A more general review of the use of cardiac MRI in patients with ischemic heart disease is provided in the next two chapters.

References

1. Stillman AE, Wilke N, Jerosch-Herold M. Myocardial viability. Radiol Clin North Am 1999;37(2):361–78.
2. Kramer CM. Integrated approach to ischemic heart disease: the one-stop shop. Cardiol Clin 1998;16(2):267–76.
3. Shaaban AM, Duerinckx AJ. Magnetic resonance of coronary artery disease in the elderly. Am J Geriatr Cardiol 1999;8(5).
4. Higgins CB. Prediction of myocardial viability by MRI [editorial]. Circulation 1999;99:727–29.
5. Box LM, Lipton MJ. Future direction of cardiovascular research. The North American Society of Cardiac Imaging. Radiology 1998;208(2):283–84.
6. Manning WJ, Li W, Edelman RR. A preliminary report comparing magnetic resonance coronary angiography with conventional angiography. N Engl J Med 1993;328:828–32.

7. Duerinckx AJ, Atkinson DP, Mintorovitch J, Simonetti OP, Urman MK. Two-dimensional coronary MR angiography: limitations and artifacts. Eur Radiol 1996;6(3):312–25.

8. Duerinckx AJ. Coronary MR angiography (invited article). *In:* Cardiac Radiology, LM Boxt, ed.: Radiol Clin North Am 1999;37(2):273–318.

9. Duerinckx AJ, Lipton MJ. Noninvasive coronary artery imaging using CT and MR imaging [comment] [see comments]. Am J Roentgenol 1998;170(4):900–2.

10. Huber A, Nikolaou K, Gonschior P, Knez A, Stehling M, Reiser M. Navigator echo-based respiratory gating for three-dimensional MR coronary angiography: results from healthy volunteers and patients with proximal coronary artery stenoses. Am J Roentgenol 1999;173(1):95–101.

11. Müller MF, Fleisch M, Kroeker R, Chatterjee T, Meier B, Vock P. Proximal coronary artery stenosis: three-dimensional MRI with fat saturation and navigator echo. J Magn Reson Imag 1997;7(4):644–51.

12. Sandstede JJ, Pabst T, Beer M, et al. Three-dimensional MR coronary angiography using the navigator technique compared with conventional coronary angiography. Am J Roentgenol 1999;172(1):135–39.

13. Danias PG, McConnell MV, Khasgiwala VC, Chuang ML, Edelman RR, Manning WJ. Prospective navigator correction of image position for coronary MR angiography. Radiology 1997;203(3):733–36.

14. Wielopolski P, van Geuns RJ, de Feyter PJ, Oudkerk M. Breathhold coronary MR angiography with volume targeted imaging. Radiology 1998;209:209–20.

15. Hundley WG, Hamilton CA, Thomas MS, et al. Utility of fast cine magnetic resonance imaging and display for the detection of myocardial ischemia in patients not well suited for second harmonic stress echocardiography. Circulation 1999;100(16):1697–702.

16. Kessler W, Laub G, Achenbach S, Ropers D, Moshage W, Daniel WG. Coronary arteries: MR angiography with fast contrast-enhanced three-dimensional breathhold imaging—initial experience. Radiology 1999;210(2):566–72.

17. Stuber M, Botnar RM, Danias PG, Kissinger KV, Manning WJ. Breathhold three-dimensional coronary magnetic resonance angiography using real-time navigator technology. J Cardiovasc Magn Reson 1999;1(3):233–38.

18. Bogaert J, Duerinckx AJ, Rademakers FE. Magnetic resonance of the heart and great vessels. Clin Appl (Berlin) 1999.

19. Levin DC, Spettell CM, Rao VM, Sunshine J, Bansal S, Busheé GR. Impact of MR imaging on nationwide health care costs and comparison with other imaging procedures. Am J Roentgenol 1998;170:557–60.

20. Budinger TF, Berson A, McVeigh ER, et al. Cardiac MR imaging: report of a working group sponsored by the National Heart, Lung, and Blood Institute. Radiology 1998;208(3):573–76.

21. Yuan C, Tsuruda JS, Beach KN, et al. Techniques for high-resolution MR imaging of atherosclerotic plaque. J Magn Reson Imag 1994;4(1):43–49.

22. Yuan C, Petty C, O'Brien KD, Hatsukami TS, Eary JF, Brown BG. In vitro and in situ magnetic resonance imaging signal features of atherosclerotic plaque-associated lipids. Arterioscler Thromb 1997;17(8):1496–503.

23. Toussaint JF, LaMuraglia GM, Southern JF, Fuster V, Kantor HL. Magnetic resonance images lipid, fibrous, calcified, hemorrhagic, and thrombotic components of human atherosclerosis in vivo. Circulation 1996;94(5):932–8.

24. Toussaint JF, Southern JF, Kantor HL, Jang IK, Fuster V. Behavior of atherosclerotic plaque components after in vitro angioplasty and atherectomy studied by high field MR imaging. Magn Reson Imag 1998;16(2):175–83.

25. Luk-Pat GT, Gold GE, Olcott EW, Hu BS, Nishimura DG. High-resolution three-dimensional in vivo imaging of atherosclerotic plaque. Magn Reson Med 1999;42(4):762–71.

26. Fayad ZA, Fuster V, Fallon JT, et al. Noninvasive in vivo human coronary artery lumen and wall imaging using black blood MR. (abstr.). *In*: Book of Abstracts and Proceedings of the Eighth Meeting of the International Society of Magnetic Resonance in Medicine (ISMRM 2000 Proceedings Available on CD-ROM). Denver, CO, April 1–7, 2000.

27. Zheng J, Li D, Finn JP, Simonetti O, Cavagna FM. Coronary vessel wall MR imaging: initial experience. (abstr.). *In*: Book of Abstracts and Proceedings of the Eighth Meeting of the International Society of Magnetic Resonance in Medicine (ISMRM 2000 Proceedings Available on CD-ROM). Denver, CO, April 1–7: 2000.

28. Botnar RM, Matthias Stuber, Kissinger KV, Manning WJ. Real-time navigator gated and corrected coronary vessel wall imaging (abstr.). *In*: Cardiovascular Imaging 1999. The 27th Annual Meeting of the North American Society for Cardiac Imaging (NASCI), November 6, 1999, Atlanta, GA: 1999.

29. Botnar RM, Stuber M, Kissinger KV, Manning WJ. In vivo imaging of coronary artery wall in humans using navigator and free-breathing (abstr.). *In*: Book of Abstracts and Proceedings of the Eighth Meeting of the International Society of Magnetic Resonance in Medicine (ISMRM 2000 Proceedings Available on CD-ROM). Denver, CO, April 1–7: 2000.

30

Ischemic Heart Disease: Assessment of Ventricular Function with MRI

Steven Dymarkowski and Jan Bogaert

Introduction

Since Purcell and Bloch published their independent findings in 1946, the nuclear magnetic resonance (NMR) phenomenon has increasingly been used in various branches of modern science as a powerful physico-chemical analytic tool (1,2). It took another 30 years and many more innovations (e.g., the introduction of spatial encoding by Lauterbur) to introduce NMR into the field of clinical imaging (3). Magnetic resonance imaging (MRI) developed rapidly into a clinically useful diagnostic technique and is still constantly evolving, opening perspectives to the examination of different organ systems. In the last decade, cardiac MRI has been added to this expanding array of investigative fields (4,5).

As the motor of the circulatory system, the heart performs a continuous task over more than seven decades, adjusting its output over a more than fivefold range to supply the entire body with oxygen and nutrients. The anatomy and dynamics of the heart have been extensively studied over several centuries, but many of the subtle intricacies still remain unclear. This is related to its highly sophisticated structure involving muscle fiber architecture, collagen matrix, vascularization, innervation, biventricular and pericardial interaction, and global shape (6).

A complete evaluation of a patient with ischemic heart disease has to provide information on the size and shape of the ventricles, in addition to their functional properties. Myocardial damage has to be evaluated and patterns of blood flow and regional metabolism have to be determined. Due to advances in ultrafast imaging, cine-MRI, and cardiac tagging techniques, MRI has provided the field of functional cardiac imaging with an important new tool (7–12). It is fundamentally a three-dimensional (3-D) imaging technique, in which images can be obtained in virtually any orientation with exact knowledge of the location of the imaging plane. This feature permits a hands-on approach to the analysis of the motion and shape of the heart. Although not at its maximum, the best spatial resolution by means of MRI is currently beneath 1 mm for the heart (13,14). By manipulation of sequence parameters, tissue characteristics and properties of the stationary or flowing spins can be determined, thus offering a tailor-made imaging source that can be customized to the patient or the clinical question to be answered. Cardiac MRI is steadily taking its place in clinical practice, providing many answers to aforementioned clinical questions and offering anatomy and an accurate on-line quantitation of functional data sets.

This chapter will provide a clear insight into the aspects of MRI regarding the function of normal and diseased myocardium, especially in patients with coronary artery disease. Along with basic technical issues that are inherent to the technique used, we will review the possibilities of MRI for quantitation of myocardial function in cardiac pathology.

Conventional Imaging of Cardiac Function

Contrast X-Ray Ventriculography

By injecting iodinated contrast medium via an intravascular catheter in the cardiac lumen, projectional images of the left ventricle and other chambers of the heart are obtained. This allows a real-time assessment of the size and shape of the heart chambers throughout the various phases of the cardiac cycle. Determination of the ventricular size at end-diastole and end-systole allows volumetric quantification as well as extraction of functional parameters (e.g., stroke volume, ejection fraction, and cardiac output). Regional wall motion can be qualitatively and quantitatively assessed (15). Up-to-date, contrast ventriculography is often still considered as the gold standard to which other imaging techniques are compared in determining ventricular function. Nevertheless, cardiac catheterization remains an invasive technique in which certain safety standards must be upheld regarding the use of contrast agents and other possible causes of complications. Moreover, ventricular quantification is based on geometric assumptions and not on true volumetric quantifications. This approach may be correct in normal ventricles, but it is questionable in diseased ventricles. Regional wall motion analysis may be incorrect because there is no correction for rigid motion nor for translation or rotation, even with the use of a floating reference system (16,17).

Echocardiography

Transthoracic Echocardiography (TTE)

At this moment, the most frequently used technique to evaluate cardiac function is transthoracic echocardiography (TTE), which has evolved from a mere imaging technique to a nearly complete noninvasive hemodynamic investigation. Its main advantages include wide accessibility, portability, safety, and relatively low cost-price. Echocardiography provides insight into the patient's cardiac anatomy in terms of chamber size, wall thickness, chamber and valvular function, and flow analysis (18,19). All of this information is provided on a real-time basis to the physician. Stress echocardiography (e.g., by means of dobutamine infusion) can be easily performed to detect areas of hypoperfusion and to differentiate between infarcted and dysfunctional but viable myocardium. Despite its great potential and utility, TTE has some limitations. About 30% of patients do not have an adequate echogeneity to permit an adequate diagnosis. In addition, quantification of function with its temporal and regional inhomogeneity remains one of the major issues in cardiac ultrasound. The absence of reference points within the myocardium, poor visualization of the outer myocardial borders, and through-plane motion are other pitfalls, but they are certainly not exclusive to ultrasound because other imaging techniques [e.g., computed tomography (CT) and MRI] suffer from similar difficulties (20,21).

Transesophageal Echocardiography (TEE)

Transesophageal echocardiography (TEE) continues to evolve as an important complementary technique for the diagnosis and management of various cardiovascular disorders (22). Improved transducer technology has expanded the indications to include assessment of ventricular function, especially in the intraoperative setting. Automatic border detection may further simplify the quantitative approach of TEE-guided assessment of ventricular function. Another area in which the technique continues to develop is valvular disease, especially for planimetry of the aortic valve area in aortic stenosis (23). The technique continues to be used in the evaluation of endocarditis, especially prosthetic valve

involvement, and for the evaluation of the patient with a potential cardiac source of emboli.

For monitoring of left ventricle (LV) function and wall motion of patients in intensive care units the transesophageal approach is most often used (24). The left ventricle can be scanned by the transesophageal approach in the long-axis and in cross-sections by the transgastric approach. They correspond to the apical four-chamber and left parasternal cross-sectional imaging of the heart. All segments representing the three coronary arteries can be imaged by using the transgastric approach in the papillary short-axis view. Recording in this position has been found to be highly reproducible. Only localized ischemia of the apex of the ventricle may be missed. The rotation and translocation of the heart remain a problem methodologically using the cross-section images of the heart, but the LV papillary muscles and the septal-right ventricular (RV) borders can be used as landmarks. In addition to the semiquantitative analysis a quantitative calculation using computers is also possible.

Absolute contraindications to the performance of TEE include a history of or current pathologic conditions of the esophagus along with recent esophageal operations. In patients with relative contraindications (e.g., unstable angina, esophageal varices, or active upper gastrointestinal bleeding) an individual assessment must be made before TEE is performed. Complications associated with TEE can be related to the probe, to the procedure, or to drugs used during the examination.

Radionuclide Imaging

Various noninvasive nuclear imaging techniques provide valuable information regarding infarct site and size, regional and global ventricular function, myocardial perfusion, metabolic function and viability, and myocardial salvage after reperfusion in patients with acute coronary syndromes (25–30). This information is valuable to clinicians in streamlining diagnostic and therapeutic decision making for critically ill cardiac patients.

With the availability of new technetium-99m pertechnetate (^{99m}Tc) perfusion tracers, nuclear cardiology imaging techniques can provide information on myocardial blood flow and LV function from a single imaging session (31,32). Ejection fraction, regional wall motion, and changes in wall thickness can be measured and specificity can be improved by gating the images, without increasing the acquisition time. The ability to use conventional gamma cameras to image important positron emission tomography (PET) radiotracers (e.g., fluorodeoxyglucose) similarly allow cost-effective and widespread applications of PET technology (33). Thus, new radiotracers and imaging techniques in nuclear cardiology provide incremental and cost-effective diagnostic information in the assessment of coronary artery disease.

A drawback of ^{99m}Tc radionuclide angiography is the limitation on the number of sequential studies or views that can be obtained because of restrictions on patient radiation exposure. Another problem is the difficulty in determining the myocardial boundaries on the images because the edges are not clearly defined (34). This is even more so in regions that have been strongly affected by ischemic changes because these segments appear blurred and faint. In case of arrhythmia, interpretation is even more compromised due to the temporal blurring that occurs during image acquisition (35). As compared with other imaging techniques, resolution is typically 64×64 pixels or 128×128 pixels, which is a relative coarse sampling that renders accurate estimation of ventricular volumes difficult.

Electron-Beam Computed Tomography (EB-CT)

Electron-beam computed tomography (EB-CT) or ultrafast computed tomography is a noninvasive imaging method with a very high spatial and temporal resolution in a design that uses a rapidly moving focused electron beam to perform image acquisition. The principles of EB-CT can be compared with conventional computed tomography. Fast acquisitions and short exposure times (about 50 msec) are the major qualities of EB-CT, allowing multilevel imaging of the heart, quantification of functional parameters, and disorders of the myocardial contraction. Investigations have demonstrated that EB-CT can be used to define the transit of iodinated contrast material through the cardiac chambers and myocardium. Using classical indicator dilution principles and a rapid intravenous injection of iodinated contrast medium, EB-CT can quantify cardiac output, ejection fraction, ventricular volumes, and ventricular mass as well as perform an evaluation of segmental cardiac function and—to a limited extent—myocardial perfusion (36–42). Ventricular function and wall motion has been assessed in rest and during stress conditions with low-dose dobutamine infusion (43,44). In summary, ultrafast CT technology offers a means to define cardiac anatomy, function, and flow rapidly and accurately in a noninvasive way.

On the downside, the technique does require a careful calibration on a subject-to-subject basis prior to quantification of cardiac output. Although global function can be evaluated by EB-CT, beam hardening artifacts may limit the application in all regions of the LV myocardium. EB-CT is also clearly inferior to MRI in assessing cardiac valvular function and the number of clinically available EB-CT scanners is limited (45).

MRI

Compared with other organ systems (e.g., the central nervous system) cardiac MRI is unavoidably compromised by several challenges, which are inherent to the function of the heart itself. Three major issues are: (1) the signal-to-noise ratio, (2) perpetual motion, and (3) flow phenomena. In other words, special hard- and software adaptations have to be engaged to obtain images with an adequate diagnostic quality. Furthermore, if quantitative information is to be obtained, additional issues regarding spatial resolution and choice of imaging sequences must be considered.

The central location of the heart within the chest, surrounded by the very low proton dense lung parenchyma and the large size of the chest, imply that the MR system picks up a great amount of image noise when using the standard body coil. Although no cardiac dedicated coil is currently available, the development and use of separate local radio frequency (RF) receiver coils (body phased-array coil), as a manner to bring the detecting element as near to the organ of interest as possible and to reduce the detection of noise from outside of this organ, has already yielded to a definite improvement over the standard body coils.

The motion of the heart is executed on a timescale that is very fast as compared with the duration necessary for an MRI to be acquired. To avoid motion artifacts, special strategies have to be deployed to image the moving muscle tissue and the moving blood. The basis principle that allows the heart to be imaged using MRI is cardiac gating, also referred to as cardiac triggering (46,47). During the acquisition, an EKG from the patient is collected, which is used to synchronize the effective measurement. The idea is to acquire the different phase-encoded lines that make up the MRI at the exact same timepoint in the cardiac cycle. The success of cardiac gating can be easily understood, if compared with the quality of nongated images; however, gating alone cannot successfully eliminate all motion artifacts, taking into account the problems caused by physiological beat-to-beat variations and arrhythmia. Respiration is another source of motion artifacts. With conventional MRI sequences, the use of multiple measurements will increase the signal-to-noise ratio and the image sharpness. With the advent of faster MRI techniques, which can be performed in breathhold, respiration motion is no longer a major problem, at least in cooperative patients (8).

The third challenge—the flow phenomenon—can be considered as an advantage rather than as a limitation. Flowing blood provides a natural contrast with the myocardium and vessel walls, so that no intravenous contrast material is required for cardiac chamber and vessel opacification (48,49). On spin-echo MRI, flowing blood appears black due to signal void (50). On gradient-echo MRI, flowing blood has a bright appearance due to an inflow enhancement (51). Differentiation between cavity and myocardial wall, however, may be strenuous due to the presence of stagnant blood in hypocontractile ventricles (e.g., idiopathic or ischemic dilated cardiomyopathies). The administration of paramagnetic contrast agents or special MRI techniques (e.g., myocardial tagging, see later) may facilitate the visualization of the myocardial boundaries (52).

Morphologic Assessment

Left Ventricular Volume and Mass

Serial measurements of LV volume and mass are important in the followup of therapeutic interventions in ischemic heart disease and other conditions (53–55). In various animal and phantom studies, as well as in volunteers and patients, MRI has been used to assess and describe the size of the heart chambers and to quantify the myocardial mass. Because of its good spatial resolution and the ability to obtain images in planes well known to cardiologists (cardiac short-axis, four-chamber and two-chamber long-axis views) it has been accepted as a valuable clinical tool. In general a good correlation can be found in comparing MRI with other quantitating techniques such as contrast ventriculography, two-dimensional (2-D) echocardiography, and nuclear imaging (56).

Several approaches and different MRI techniques to quantify LV volume and mass have been described in literature. Estimation of LV volumes and masses can rely on true volumetric quantitation or geometric assumptions. True volumetric quantification based on the Simpson's rule acquires a series of contiguous slices at the same time of the cardiac cycle (e.g., at end-diastole and end-systole) through the left ventricle (e.g., in the cardiac short-axis) (Fig. 30.1) (57,58). In contrast to other techniques such as echocardiography, the inner and outer myocardial borders are clearly identifiable on MRI. The area of each slice (representing the blood pool or

representing the myocardium) is measured and multiplied by the slice thickness. The sum of all these volumes yields, respectively, the volume of the ventricular cavity or the myocardial mass. The major advantage of this approach is the independency of any geometric model. Several studies have been performed to validate this method in clinical practice, both in healthy volunteers and in diseased myocardium, showing excellent correlation with cineangiography and 2-D echocardiography (57,59–61). Geometric assumptions, on the other hand, compare the left ventricle with a simple or more complex geometric model (e.g., an ellipsoid volume, a half ellipsoid, or a prolate ellipse). The main advantages of this method are its simplicity and the parallel that can be drawn to similar measurements in cardiac ultrasound and contrast ventriculography (62–64). It is, however, necessary to realize that these calculations are made based on certain geometric assumptions. These assumptions do not account for geometric distortions in case of pathology (e.g., ischemia or normal anatomical variations due to trabecular endocardial structure and papillary muscles). Debatin and colleagues compared the previously mentioned approaches and found that the multislice summation (i.e., Simpson's rule) was significantly more accurate than the area–length algorithm (65).

Spin-echo MRI provides a detailed tomographic evaluation of the heart and can be considered as a highly accurate and reproducible technique for quantification of LV mass and volume (66). This technique, however, is time-consuming and the multislice single-phase approach is less practical because each image slice is obtained at a different time phase of the cardiac cycle. With the advent of fast MRI techniques (e.g., turbo spin-echo, HASTE, and echo-planar imaging), one or several (up to 12) cardiac slices can be obtained during a single breathhold period of 15 seconds (Figs. 30.2 and 30.3) (10,67). This approach both reduces the imaging time considerably and the images are obtained during the same period of the cardiac cycle, usually during diastole. Gradient-echo techniques (i.e., cine MRI) are another means to determine the ventricular mass and volume, and are particularly interesting to assess global and regional ventricular function. This technique combines the high temporal resolution of normal tomographic MRI with a high temporal resolution. Variants of this technique (i.e., snapshot gradient-echo method) have been proposed as a rapid and accurate technique for assessing ventricular masses (68).

Some studies report an underestimation of end-systolic and end-diastolic volumes in MRI (69). Determining factors in these calculations are without doubt attributable to slower flow in the end-diastolic phase, in which the distinct interface between the blood pool and the endocardium becomes less apparent and there is difficulty in defining the correct short-axis and base of the apex during the filling phase of the heart. Nevertheless,

Volumetric Quantification

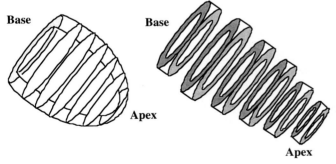

Figure 30.1. True volumetric quantification of the LV based on the Simpson's rule. The true volume of the LV can be acquired by means of contiguous short-axis views encompassing the entire LV. The area of each slice (representing the blood pool or representing the myocardium) is measured and multiplied by the slice thickness. The sum of these volumes yields, respectively, the volume of the ventricular cavity or the myocardial mass.

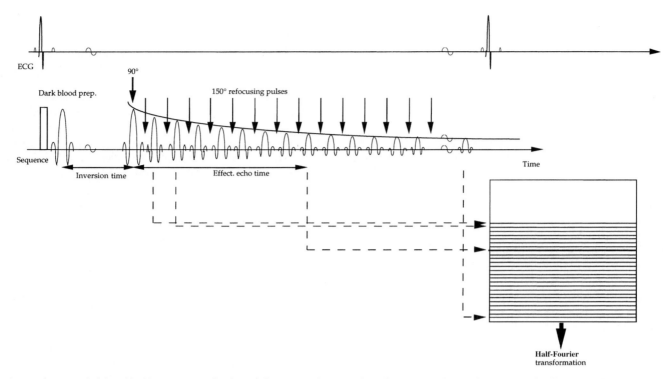

Figure 30.2. Dark-blood half-Fourier single-shot turbo spin-echo (HASTE) MRI. After two dark blood preparation pulses and one 90-degree excitation pulse, half of the *k*-space is filled by mul- tiple refocusing pulses. This approach allows to obtain one MRI image of every second heartbeat. In this way, the entire heart can be studied in less than 1 minute.

interstudy variability has repeatedly been reported as being low by different observers, with values as low as 5% for stroke volume, end-diastolic volume, and end-systolic volume (70,71). In one study, conducted by Pat-tynama and co-workers, the importance of interexami-nation variance was tested using variance component analysis in two subjects who underwent 20 serial ex-aminations (69). Comparison of two techniques used— multislice spin-echo imaging and cine MRI—yielded to

high rates of reproducibility. The interexamination vari-ance was found to be the single most important con-tributor to overall variance, whereas interobserver and intraobserver variability remained low.

In summary, MRI is very likely the gold standard for estimation of LV volume and mass (72). The volumetric approach especially yields highly accurate and repro-ducible results, whereas methods based on geometric as-sumptions are less time-consuming but also less accurate.

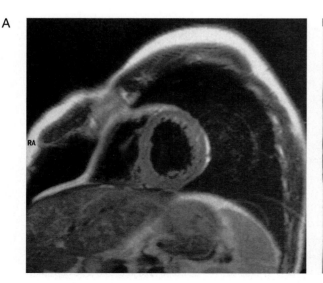

A

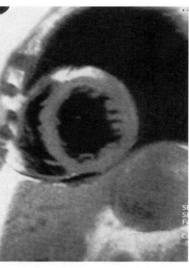

B

Figure 30.3. Cardiac short-axis view in a normal vol-unteer. Comparison be-tween the turbo spin-echo MRI sequence (A) and the dark blood HASTE se-quence (B).

Right Ventricular (RV) Volume and Mass

Relatively few studies have concentrated on measuring RV volume and mass, and evidence for validation of in vivo measurements are virtually nonexistent (73,74). In comparison to the left ventricle, quantitation of RV size is less obvious. Due to its unique anatomical configuration, it does not correspond to any geometric model. Comparison of MRI data with other methods is also difficult because of blood pool superposition in contrast ventriculography and poor echogeneity of a major part of the patient population in cardiac ultrasound. Right ventricular volume measurements have been validated in animals and in humans with radionuclide ventriculography and indicator dilution techniques (68,74). Furthermore, studies comparing RV and LV stroke volumes and ejection fractions have been shown to demonstrate near equal values (60,74). Investigations to perfect the geometric quantitation of the RV are currently ongoing. Application of the modified Simpson's rule approach shows considerably good correlation between in vivo measurements and RV casts (74). Furthermore, low interobserver and interstudy variability definitely points to the direction of this approach being valid (75). Studies by Culham et al. and Kondo et al. using multislice MRI and MR velocity mapping have found statistical significant agreement between pulmonary flow and RV ejection fraction (76,77). To summarize, these data certainly show that MRI provides accurate measurements of RV volume measurements.

Functional Assessment

Global Ventricular Function

Flow-compensated gradient-echo MRI sequences, with short repetition times and small flip angles, enable one to study the heart two-dimensionally at several time phases during the cardiac cycle (i.e., single-slice multiphase approach) (78–80). For instance, with a repetition time (TR) of 40 msec and a heart rate of 60 bpm, 25 images can be acquired. The entire set of images can be loaded into an endless cine loop providing information on dynamic cardiac processes (e.g., the myocardial contraction or the valve function). Cine MRI possesses a good contrast between the blood pool and the myocardial wall, displaying the former with higher signal intensity, thus actually resembling contrast ventriculography. Because of these distinct contrast interfaces, a good distinction of the endo- and epicardial wall is possible. This approach allows the study of the regional wall motion and myocardial wall thickening and, similarly, as described in the morphologic assessment of LV and RV, ventricular volumes can be determined at end-diastole and end-systole, which allows the quantification of the global cardiac ventricular function and cardiac indexes.

The conventional cine MRI technique obtains one k-space line per heart cycle, but has more recently found that it is possible to obtain several k-space lines during each beat by means of the segmented gradient-echo technique (8). Because more k-space lines are picked up within one cycle, the duration of the measurement shortens with a factor equal to the amount of k-lines acquired. This implies that the measurements can be executed in breathhold. In this approach, however, a compromise has to be found between the total acquisition window (temporal resolution) and the duration of breathholding. Bogaert and colleagues found that in obtaining eight k-lines per heartbeat and using a matrix of 256×128, the k-space was filled after 16 heartbeats (Fig. 30.4) (61,81). Depending on the heart rate this results in a breathhold period of about 12–15 seconds. The entire ventricle can thus be encompassed in 12–14 minutes (Figs. 30.5 and 30.6). This technique offers a good compromise between length of breathholding and image

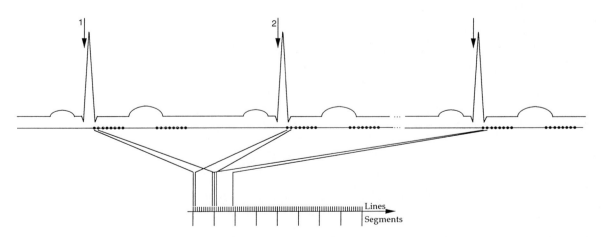

Figure 30.4. Segmented k-space cine MRI technique. Rather than acquiring one k-line each heartbeat, eight k-lines are acquired each heartbeat. With a 256×128 matrix, the k-space is filled in 16 heartbeats, which can be obtained in a breathhold.

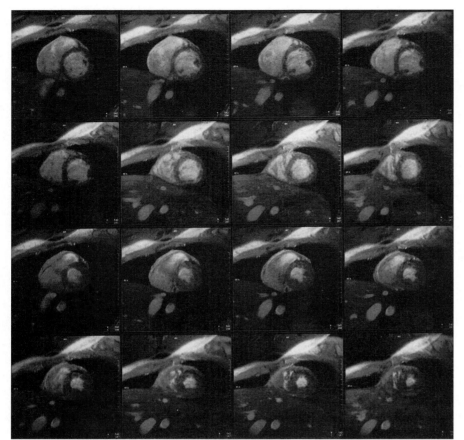

Figure 30.5. Quantification of global LV function in a 25-year-old female healthy volunteer. Contiguous short-axis images are obtained from LV base to LV apex at end-diastole and end-systole, using the segmented *k*-space cine MRI sequence. Each slice is studied in one breathhold. The end-diastolic short-axis levels from LV base to LV apex are shown in the two upper rows. The corresponding end-systolic short-axis views are shown in the third and fourth row. This approach allows a fast and accurate quantification of LV end-diastolic and end-systolic volume, stroke volume, ejection fraction, cardiac output, and cardiac indexes. Global LV parameters: EDV: 99.7 mL; ESV: 32.4 mL; SV: 67.3 mL; EF: 67.5%.

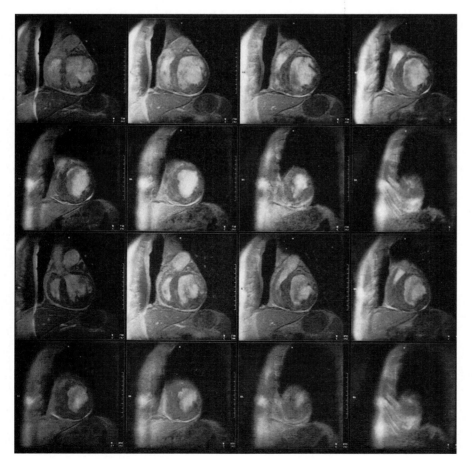

Figure 30.6. Quantification of LV function parameters in a 46-year-old male patient with idiopathic dilated cardiomyopathy, using a similar approach as in Figure 30.5. The LV is slightly dilated and shows a global hypokinetic wall motion. Note areas of marked wall thinning even though other regions show a normal or slightly increased myocardial wall thickness. Global LV parameters: EDV: 119 mL; ESV: 87 mL; SV: 32 mL; EF: 27%.

quality. A longer acquisition window means a lower number of obtainable time phases and a higher risk for cardiac blurring. Further technical improvements (e.g., echosharing) have allowed the doubling of the number of cardiac phases.

Like all sectional imaging modalities, cine MRI is equally affected by partial volume averaging. To determine the extent of this artifact, many investigations have been executed, documenting the reliability of the technique in assessing ventricular size and shape. Buser and colleagues investigated the importance of imaging planes in the evaluation of LV volumes in order to assess whether certain incidences were more vulnerable to partial volume effects than others (82). It had previously been argued that in acquiring axial sections through the heart, partial volume effects caused by the oblique transsection of the ventricle yielded to a greater heterogeneity in volume estimation as compared with sections in the cardiac short-axis. They concluded that both strategies were equally affected by partial volume effects.

In summary, with the advent of fast breathhold cine MRI sequences accurate quantification of global ventricular function and cardiac indexes can be rapidly assessed in a noninvasive manner.

Regional Ventricular Function

Regional Wall Motion and Myocardial Wall Thickening
The ejection of blood by the ventricles is the result of a coordinated contraction of myocytes that are organized in a thick-walled myocardium. Even though excitation of isolated myocytes will lead to a shortening in longitudinal direction and/or to a development of a tensile force, excitation of the myocardium (as a whole) enables the increase of the intraventricular pressure, to reduce the ventricular cavity and to eject blood. The complex intramyocardial fiber arrangement, the complex ventricular geometry and the differences in timing of the excitation-contraction coupling result in complex 3-D wall deformation during systole consisting in a myocardial shortening in the circumferential and longitudinal direction of the ventricle, myocardial wall thickening and shearing motions of the ventricle (e.g., twisting) (83–85).

Several approaches are used to describe and to quantify the wall deformation and motion. Projectional imaging techniques (e.g., contrast ventriculography) rely on the endocardial wall motion, rather than the true myocardial deformation. Segments with abnormal wall motion are described as being hypo-, a-, dys-, or even hyperkinetic. Tomographic or transsectional techniques (e.g., echocardiography and cine MRI), in contrast, allow a meticulous measurement of wall thickness, systolic wall thickening and wall motion during rest and under stress conditions (86–88). A common limitation of all of the previously mentioned techniques, however,

is that they fail to catch the through-plane motion of the LV because they are 2-D techniques. Techniques to quantify the myocardial deformation three-dimensionally will be described shortly.

In patients with coronary artery disease, myocardial wall segments deprived of oxygen (e.g., myocardial ischemia and myocardial infarction) become hypo- or acontractile. Assessment of regional wall thickening may be more objective than assessment of myocardial wall motion because the latter may be confounded by the arbitrary choice of a centerpoint in the ventricle as a reference (16,89,90). Abnormalities in wall thickening occur very early in ischemia, even before such clinical signs as angina or EKG-abnormalities can be detected, thus providing an important diagnostic marker (90). Wall thickening is known to be an active process, closely associated with the dynamics of myocardial fiber shortening (91). Moreover, the absence or impairment of myocardial wall thickening is closely related to a reduction in subendocardial blood flow, as documented by Gallagher and co-workers (92,93). Lieberman and co-workers found in infarcted canine hearts an abrupt deterioration in systolic thickening in segment containing more than 20% transmural extension of the infarct (90).

To obtain reliable quantitative information about ventricular wall thickening during systole, the short-axis image data sets require further postprocessing. At present, semi-automated delineation programs are available to delineate the endo- and epicardial borders on the end-systolic and end-diastolic images. By constructing equidistant chords perpendicular to a centerline drawn midway between the endo- and epicardial border, the myocardium is divided into subregions (94). The length of each individual chord then defines the wall thickness at both timeframes. To avoid bias, the papillary muscles are excluded from delineation. Wall thickening is then defined as the formula: percent systolic wall thickening = [(end-systolic wall thickness − end-diastolic wall thickness)/end diastolic wall thickness] × 100%. An abnormal degree of wall thickening is defined at separate chords as being smaller than the mean value of a control population minus two times the corresponding standard deviation. The mean end-diastolic thickness of the LV as measured in volunteers is about 10 ± 1 mm. In normal situations a variability can be found in normal thickness of the different segments, but the difference in mean values among segments is commonly not significant. In normal basal circumstances global wall thickening reaches about 55–60% and peaks at midsystole. Regional wall thickening analysis has shown that the percentage thickening even reaches 80% at the low papillary muscle level. After inotropic stimulation (see later) these values become higher in nonischemic tissue.

In patients with myocardial infarction, mean maximal percent thickening in abnormal segments has been

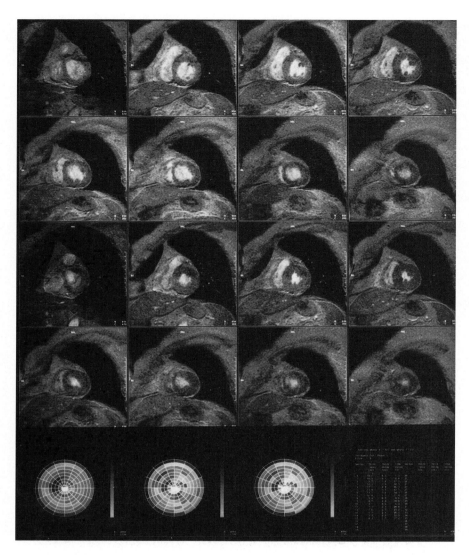

Figure 30.7. Quantification of regional systolic wall thickening in a 59-year-old female patient with a previous myocardial infarction. In the two upper rows are shown the end-diastolic short-axis levels from LV base to LV apex. The corresponding end-systolic short-axis views are shown in the third and fourth row. Note an important wall thinning in the apical part of the interventricular septum, showing both an a- to dyskinetic wall motion pattern as well as a systolic wall thinning. Three bull's eye diagrams are shown in the lower row, representing (from left to right): absolute wall thickness at end-systole, absolute systolic wall thickening, and percentual systolic thickening. Abnormal low values (visible as dark gray regions) for both wall thickness and wall thickening are found in the apical portion of the interventricular septum (ARGUS, Siemens Erlangen, Germany).

reported varying from $5 \pm 3\%$ to $-8 \pm 6\%$, actually indicating systolic wall thinning (Fig. 30.7). Measurements of wall thickening by MRI tagging (see later) have been shown to correlate well with sonomicrometer measurements in the dog (95). In all studies, MRI consistently overestimated the sonomicrometer values. It is possible that the overestimation of trabeculation of the endocardial wall and partial volume effects and flow deceleration during end diastole are responsible for this phenomenon. Sonomicrometers, however, may impair the normal wall thickening, they do not cover the entire thickness of the myocardial wall, and, because they are monodimensional techniques, there is no correction for shear motion of the ventricle (e.g., twisting).

The measurement of systolic wall thickening has considerable clinical implications. A precise discrimination of ischemic and nonischemic myocardium is possible, even more clearly if this technique is supplemented by stress-induced imaging with dobutamine infusion (see later). In addition, regional improvement of wall thickening with

inotropic stimulation ("contractile reserve") has been shown to identify viable myocardium and to predict recovery of function in both acute and chronic ischemic heart disease, as stated by Cigarroa and colleagues (96). The present technique of image acquisition and the use of time-consuming postprocessing algorithms are still subject to improvement. The development of automated border recognition and delineation programs can contribute significantly in the assessment of regional and global myocardial function with regard to wall thickening in patients with suspected ischemic disease.

In summary, regional wall motion and systolic wall thickening can be accurately assessed and quantified by means of (short-axis) cine MRI. Systolic wall thickening is a reliable indicator to discriminate ischemic from nonischemic myocardial segments.

Myocardial Tagging

Principles of Myocardial Tagging. As already mentioned the LV undergoes complex deformations during the cardiac cycle, rendering the analysis of regional function virtually impossible using projectional techniques. Translation and rotation, twisting and torsion along the short axis and shortening of the ventricle as a whole in the long axis plane all occur at subsecond speed. Furthermore, the absence of reference points within the myocardium adds a very important shortcoming to almost all acknowledged dynamic imaging techniques of the heart. To overcome this difficulty, studies using implanted markers have been carried out in a dog model, but also on humans post–heart transplantation (97,98). Problems using this method, among others, were postoperative complications such as inflammation, hemorrhage, fibrosis, and displacement of the markers. Covering of the entire epi- and endocardial wall also proved to be impossible, due to operative inaccessibility. It is clear that although these studies provide clear insight into ventricular contraction, its relevance toward generalized applications is limited (99,100).

A major breakthrough was achieved by Zerhouni and co-workers in 1988 when they introduced the concept of myocardial tagging (7,101). Based on a fairly simple and well-known principle in MRI, this feature has proven to be a very important tool in quantitation of regional wall motion analysis of both LV and RV. Saturation of spins in a certain plane prior to the actual image acquisition is used in many subdisciplines of MRI, mainly to reduce flow-related artifacts. This same technique can also be used to annihilate the MR signal of tissue at specific locations only. The creation of tag lines consists of applying RF pulse in planes perpendicular to the imaging plane prior to the generation of the RF-pulses required for imaging. In this way, the tissue in the tag planes are presaturated and therefore unable to contribute to the information that make up the image(s). During the subsequent acquisition no signal is obtained from the protons in these planes and thus appear as hypointense or black lines. As the heart runs through its cycle, the displacement and deformation of the tagged tissue becomes clearly visible and allows actual myocardial motion to be analyzed and quantitated (Fig. 30.8).

Tag lines do not persist in equal intensity throughout the measurement. After tagging, the saturated spins will steadily return to their basal energy level. The rate of loss of tag visibility is directly related to the T1-relaxation parameters of the heart muscle. Because the T1 value of normal myocardial tissue at 1.5 Tesla is about 800 msec, the tag pulses remain clearly distinct up to 700 msec following the R-pulse of the QRS-complex (7,102). This allows a complete analysis of the total heart cycle in most patients. Tags are usually set down just before end-diastole or mitral valve closure. The sequence is generally triggered by the upslope of the R-wave of the QRS complex, which has an offset to the closing of the atrioventricular valves. This is im-

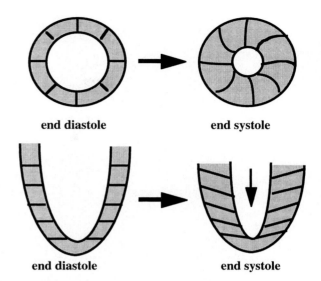

end diastole   **end systole**

end diastole   **end systole**

Figure 30.8. Tags are noninvasively imprinted on the myocardium at end-diastole (left) on the short-axis images (top) and the long-axis images (bottom). During the subsequent systole the tags will deform, displacement depending on the underlying myocardial deformation.

portant because the isovolumetric contraction that follows the mitral valve closure, during which the ventricle builds up pressure to open the aortic valve, is in fact far from isovolumetric and produces a substantial amount of deformation of the ventricular wall. It is therefore important to enscribe the tags during this very short period of time preceding the end-diastolic image, which serves as reference for all others. The precision of tag detection has been estimated to be 0.1 mm, which approximates the position of metallic beads by biplane contrast ventriculography (103,104).

In general, two types of tagging methods have been used. A first type uses specific presaturation planes to define the tags and can use different geometric patterns. In practice, radial or star-shaped tags are applied in the short-axis view and parallel tagging pulse in the long-axis views (Figs. 30.9 and 30.10) (21). The second type of tagging is constructed by two orthogonal sets of parallel stripes that compose a grid-shaped pattern on the image that can again be monitored throughout the cardiac cycle. This technique is described as spatial modulation of magnetization (SPAMM) and was developed by Axel and associates in 1989 (105,106). The grid is generally defined and constructed in a short time, but controlling its exact location on the heart proves to be more difficult.

The tagging principle is compatible with different kinds of imaging sequences (e.g., spin-echo imaging, and conventional and segment k-space gradient-echo sequence measurements) (7,102,107). In current clinical practice, sequences that provide an acceptable compromise between spatial and temporal resolution, signal-

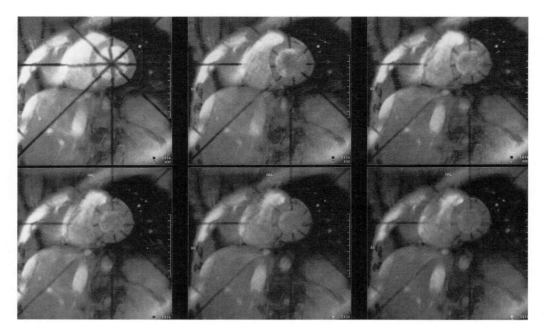

Figure 30.9. Radial myocardial tagging. The tag lines in the short-axis view are radially oriented, crossing each other in the middle of the LV. Above left is shown the LV at end-diastole. During the subsequent cardiac systole, deformation and displacement of the tag lines is directly dependent on the (regional) myocardial deformation.

to-noise ratio and total acquisition time (15–30 minutes) must definitely be preferred.

Strain Analysis. Tagged MR images are in fact 2-D images. This signifies that similar to other nontagged cardiac imaging techniques (e.g., conventional MRI, echocardiography, and contrast ventriculography) they are unable to quantify the through-plane motion of the heart during the cardiac cycle. MR tagging, however, offers the means to quantify the myocardial deformation three-dimensionally. This can be accomplished by acquiring both short- and long-axis tagged MRIs. By

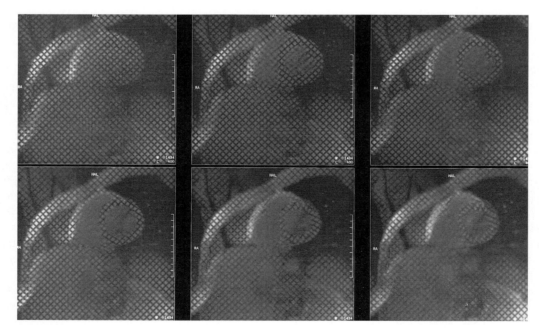

Figure 30.10. Spatial modulation of magnetization (SPAMM) tagging technique. The grid that is placed on the short-axis image at end-diastole (image above left) is deformed during the subsequent systole. One of the main difficulties of the SPAMM technique is the delineation of the endocardial borders at end-diastole.

Figure 30.11. Fusion of 2-D tagged MR images into a 3-D data set. The cardiac short- and long-axis planes are used as imaging as well as tag planes; this double utilization allows the transformation of 2-D information into a real 3-D system. (A) cardiac short-axis planes, (B) cardiac long-axis planes, (C) Cardiac long-axis view with the tags parallel oriented along the cardiac short-axis, (D) cardiac short-axis view with radially oriented tags.

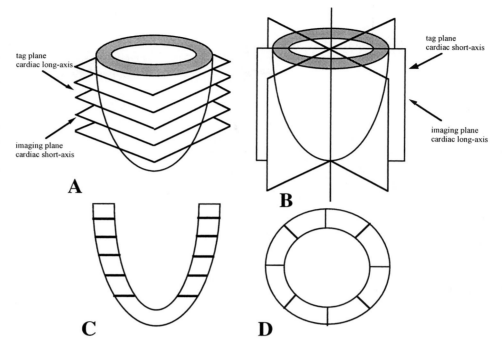

comparing short- and long-axis images in the early end-diastolic phase (before deformation) and aligning the intersection between the tag lines of the different planes, the third dimension can be reconstructed (Fig. 30.11) (108,109).

These 3-D images are thus sliced up by the tag lines of different orientation into small cuboid particles, units of which the individual motion and deformation can be analyzed. The coordinates of the corners of these cuboids (node points) are defined in space by the external XYZ coordinate system at every time point throughout the cardiac cycle at which images were acquired. The XYZ coordinate system is defined by the external magnet and is therefore not optimal to describe and compare the deformation of the myocardial tissue because it is still relative to the external body and not directly to the cardiac ventricle as a unit. In a second step all XYZ coordinates are transferred into a local cardiac coordinate system (RCL) (Fig. 30.12). Two of its axes are oriented tangential to the ventricular wall, and the third is perpendicular to the LV wall. R, C, and L are perpendicular to each other. By definition, the direction of the longitudinal axis is oriented toward the LV base and the radial axis is oriented outward. This RCL coordinate system is specific for each epi- and endocardial node point. Due to the taper of the apex, the radial axis points slightly down and the longitudinal axis slightly outward in this region. To better understand myocardial function, one can use the fiber angles in the subepicardial and subendocardial regions to transform the local coordinate system into a local fiber coordinate system (RFX). Either fiber angles obtained

from pathology examinations in experimental animal studies or from autopsy series in humans can be used. Although the latter method is less accurate, the very stable fiber configuration from one subject to another in different regions of the left ventricle allows the use of a standard set of fiber orientations without a significant loss of accuracy. The direction indicated by F is along the fiber direction parallel to the ventricular surface. The direction of X is the cross-fiber direction, defined as the direction perpendicular to the fiber direction in a plane

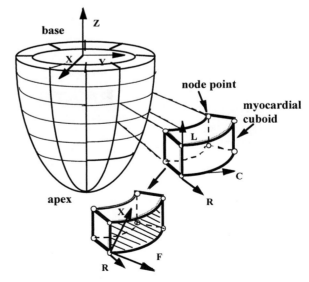

Figure 30.12. Transformation of the XYZ system into a local cardiac (RCL) and a local fiber (RFX) system.

tangential to the ventricular surface. R—the radial coordinate—remains the same as the RCL coordinate system and is perpendicular to the fiber and cross-fiber axis.

Once these reference points are created, analysis of regional functional parameters of the myocardium is performed. The basic principle of which this analysis depends is derived from industrial mechanics and is known as "finite elements method of structural analysis." The ventricle is thus considered to be built up by a finite number of subunits—corresponding to the cuboids created by the tagging planes—also referred to as wall volume elements. Each volume element exerts a certain interaction on its neighboring elements only at the node points within the myocardium. Displacements and forces are exchanged only at these points. In the local fiber coordinate system, the individual displacements and deformations that occur in the cardiac cycle can be exactly defined. They can be best described as strains, further divided in normal and shear strains (Fig. 30.13). Normal strains are displacements that occur along a certain axis in the coordinate system. This results to three strains in the local cardiac coordinate system (RR, CC, LL) and three in the local fiber coordinate system (RR, FF, XX). Shear strains are defined in the plain between two axes of the coordinate system and

describe the deformation of a square to a parallelogram. One of these, the circumferential–longitudinal shear strain (CL)—describes the twisting motion of the ventricle and is closely related to torsion (110,111). A set of algebraic equations derived from mechanics is applied to describe the interindividual relations of forces and displacements within the myocardium.

Tagging allows the regional ejection fraction of each cuboid within the myocardial volume to be estimated, which is similar to calculation of global ejection fraction of the LV by dividing the stroke volume by the end-diastolic volume. The tag lines in the short-axis plane have a common intersection in the center of the ventricle, thus dividing the ventricular cavity in several pie-slice parts. The in- and outward motion during systole and diastole allow calculation of the variation in volume for each part. By subtracting the end-systolic from the end-diastolic volume of these pie slices and dividing the result by the end-diastolic volume, the regional ejection fraction is obtained.

The same measurements can be repeated using the epicardial surface as the base of the triangular sections. By subtracting the former results from the latter, information of wall thickening and thinning is gained. Because of the introduction of semi-automated methods for delineating and calculating ventricular volumes and wall dimensions, much of the pain-staking and time-devouring labor in quantifying these data sets can currently be circumpassed and make this technique clinically more attractive.

The accuracy of MR tagging has been evaluated previously. This technique was already successful in unraveling some major questions about the myocardial function (21,112). The rotational deformation of the LV during systole and the influence of chronotropic, inotropic stimuli and regional ischemia on this rotation was studied by Buchalter and colleagues (110,111). Longitudinal shortening and systolic wall thickening of the LV was accurately quantified (21,95). Rademakers and colleagues stressed the importance of myocardial untwisting during isovolumic relaxation for a normal diastolic function (109). These authors also showed that the transmural interactions during systole lead to a structural rearrangement of the myocardial fibers and to an important subendocardial cross-fiber shortening as a powerful mechanism for extensive systolic wall thickening (i.e., myocardial tethering) (91). The regional myocardial function in patients with hypertrophic cardiomyopathy was studied by several groups (113–116). Dong and colleagues studied the regional LV systolic function in patients with chronic RV pressure overload (117). Finally, McVeigh and colleagues developed noninvasive techniques to study the transmural gradients in myocardial strain (118,119).

Myocardial MRI tagging has been performed in ani-

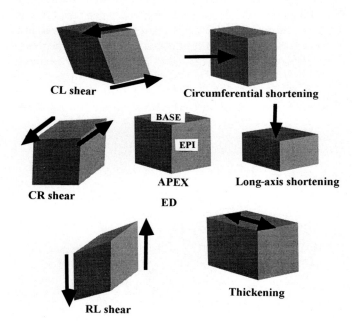

Figure 30.13. Deformation of the myocardial cuboid during systole. The undeformed myocardial cuboid at end-diastole is shown in the middle (ED). During systole the cuboid undergoes a 3-D deformation. Strain analysis allows the decomposition of this deformation into three normal strains shown at the right (i.e., circumferential and longitudinal shortening and wall thickening) and three shear strains shown at the left (i.e., CL shear strain, RL shear strain, and CR shear strain).

mal studies and in patients with myocardial infarction (120–123). Bogaert and co-workers found a significant impairment in myocardial strain in the remote noninfarcted myocardium in patients with a first anterior myocardial infarction (122). Though the mechanism of functional impairment in the remote myocardium remains unclear, it is very likely related to morphologic changes in the infarcted myocardium that increases the work load in the noninfarcted myocardium. The same group evaluated the degree of functional recovery after early revascularization in patients with a transmural myocardial infarction and found a significant recovery of the subepicardial function in the myocardial wall segments showing a match pattern on positron emission tomography (i.e., significant impairment of the myo-cardial blood flow and metabolism) (123). The improvement of the subepicardial myocardial layers contributed significantly to the overall improvement of the LV function. These results suggest that early thrombolysis may limit the transmural infarct progression and salvage the subepicardial layers.

In summary, myocardial MRI tagging offers the means to analyze noninvasively the myocardial deformation three-dimensionally independently of any external reference system.

Wall Velocity Mapping

The basic principles of myocardial tagging also define its main limitations. By applying tag lines or a grid pattern on the myocardium, the myocardial signal is voluntarily destroyed in a part of the image. To increase the sensitivity of the technique, multiple tag lines have to be defined. The more tag lines are used, the more signal is omitted, and because tag lines possess a certain thickness, information is lost and not every point of the myocardial wall can be tallied. Second, the lifespan of tag lines is unavoidably limited. As mentioned before, this poses certain limitations on this technique by inducing intensity variations in the images and sometimes yielding to lesser image quality. Third, notwithstanding considerable progress in automated analysis speed, delineation of data still remains a tedious labor, reducing its clinical capability.

Phase imaging has been proposed as an alternative to tagging for quantification of myocardial deformation and motion (124,125). Magnetic resonance imaging are normally reconstructed from the magnitude of the received signal, but images can alternatively also be calculated based on the phase of the spins in the imaging volume. It is possible to make these "phase images" sensible to speed, so that the intensity of the voxels in the image are not directly proportional to the signal magnitude, but rather to the velocity of the structure in that image point. This technique is routinely used for flow quantification in blood vessels and through the cardiac

valves (49,126,127). In a similar manner, the motion, speed, and direction of motion of solid organs such as the myocardium can be quantified (128). With its specific properties, it overcomes the main limitations of myocardial tagging by persisting throughout the cardiac cycle, accounting for every point within the myocardium, and maintains signal.

Nevertheless, this technique has not yet known a breakthrough in clinical cardiology, mainly because of its own major limitations. By giving up tag pulses, reference points within the myocardium are lost, the later being exactly the reason why tagging was created. Furthermore, velocity mapping measures wall speed. Assessing the position or displacement of a point in space with a reliable degree of accuracy requires multiplying the velocity of that point by its timecourse. This implies that the accuracy of the calculation of the displacement is directly proportional to the accuracy of the velocity measurements. Velocity mapping only measures changes in speed along one axis; namely, perpendicular to the imaging plane. Given the complex rotational and multiaxial motion of myocardial tissue, several acquisitions have to be performed, increasing the duration of the measurement.

Phase imaging must certainly be considered as a powerful and potentially useful diagnostic technique, but its laborious analysis and execution in measuring myocardial wall motion has extensively limited its clinical use. Its accuracy has nevertheless been effectively demonstrated in healthy subjects and in patients with cardiomyopathy.

Stress Imaging

Detection of Ischemic Heart Disease

Accurate noninvasive detection of coronary artery disease remains one of the great challenges in clinical cardiology. Myocardial ischemia leads to a series of clinical, metabolic, electrical, functional, and, later on, morphological changes. Within seconds, a depression of the ST-segment is visible on the EKG. Because myocardial ischemia is provoked by conditions with an increased myocardial oxygen demand, such as exercise, the latter is often clinically used to detect (exercise-induced) EKG changes. Though exercise-EKG has a fairly good specificity, however, this technique lacks sensitivity (129). Furthermore, there is a poor correlation between the extent of myocardial ischemia and the extent of ST-segment depression of a standard 12-lead EKG. Alternative methods, therefore, have been developed to detect myocardial ischemia.

As already mentioned, systolic dysfunction is another early indicator of ischemic heart disease. Stress-induced 2-D echocardiography has therefore been used to define LV dyssynergy, but several limitations compromise the accuracy of this technique (130,131). Main drawbacks are poor LV endocardial visualization and chest wall interference. By its ability to acquire reliable short- and long-axis images of the LV, its excellent contrast between the myocardial wall and the blood pool and its accurate visualization of endo- and epicardial borders, MRI offers a theoretical advantage in stress imaging of the myocardium.

Stress-induced systolic dysfunction can be obtained by exercise, although this approach is less practical to perform in a magnet (132). Another approach is pharmacological stress with vasodilators such as adenosine and dipyridamole or β-agonists such as dobutamine (133,134). Progressive β-agonist stimulation increases myocardial blood demand and is very effective in eliciting or worsening myocardial ischemic symptoms (135). Coronary vasodilators actually increase coronary flow to nonischemic areas and create flow redistribution abnormalities (136). The ideal dose of dobutamine that should be administered is not yet clearly defined, but the maximum dose should not exceed 20 μg/kg body weight. Ischemic regions will be visible on cine MRI as wall segments with an abnormal (i.e., hypo-, a-, or dyskinetic) wall motion, reduced wall thickening, or even wall thinning. For safety purposes concerning the patient, imaging is best performed under control of blood pressure and is generally discontinued in case of exaggerated chest pain, systolic blood pressure exceeding 200 mmHg, diastolic blood pressure exceeding 110 mmHg, dyspnea, and/or tachycardia.

Pennell and co-workers were the first to report on a comparative study using a blinded dobutamine-based qualitative cine MRI analysis (135). In a group of 25 patients with clinical suspicion of ischemic heart disease, dobutamine stress MRI was compared with thallium-201 dobutamine scintigraphy and coronary angiography. Twenty-two patients showed significantly diseased coronary vessels on angiography, and 21 patients of this group had evidence for reversible ischemia on thallium SPECT scanning. Twenty patients showed wall motion abnormalities on dobutamine stress MRI. Abnormal wall motion was induced in three patients with no evidence of coronary stenosis on coronarography.

In a study by Van Rugge and co-workers, the clinical value of dobutamine stress cine MRI in the detection of coronary artery disease was evaluated in a group of patients with coronary stenosis of 50% or greater (137). All underwent cine MRI at rest and at maximum dose dobutamine. Comparison was made with dobutamine echocardiography, angiography, and an exercise test. After independent analysis of the MRIs in a blinded experiment by two experienced readers, the sensitivity of detection for one-, two-, and three-vessel disease was found to be 75, 80, and 100%, respectively. This resulted

in a total sensitivity of 81% and a specificity of 100%. These results are similar to or even better than those obtained with exercise echocardiography (70% sensitivity and 63% specificity). In a follow-up study, these investigators used a more quantitative approach in detecting ischemic heart disease by calculating percentual wall thickening on short-axis cine MRIs (94). The tests were considered positive if the percentual regional wall thickening was less than 2 standard deviations from the values of a normal population. Global sensitivity and specificity of dobutamine cine MRI in the detection of coronary artery disease was 91 and 80%, respectively. The increased sensitivity in comparison to the qualitative approach in the first study is a strong argument for improved detection rate of the quantitative method. The lower specificity may be attributable to physiological variations in regional wall thickening in normal subjects.

The main limitation of current dobutamine stress MRI investigations is the rather long duration of the imaging series. If the LV is studied by contiguous short-axis slices, this may especially prove to be hazardous in a patient experiencing chest pain. By using the more recently developed faster cine MRI sequences, in which one slice can be obtained in a breathhold period with superior image quality, total imaging time can be efficiently reduced.

In summary, pharmacological stress cine MRI is a powerful tool to detect noninvasively ischemic regions in patients with coronary artery disease.

Differentiation between Dysfunctional but Viable and Infarcted Myocardial Tissue

The impact of a coronary artery occlusion on the myocardial viability is highly heterogeneous. It is strongly influenced by many factors (e.g., the rapidity and duration of the occlusion, the relation between myocardial oxygen consumption and supply) and the presence of collateral circulation. During the 1980s and 1990s several therapeutic strategies to salvage the myocardium distal to the occlusion have been developed. Therapeutic approaches (e.g., a mechanical or a pharmacological revascularization of the occluded artery and reduction of the myocardial oxygen consumption) are now routinely used clinically, whereas newer strategies (e.g., angiogenesis of collateral vessels by gene therapy) are still under investigation (138,139).

Prolonged ischemia will lead to an irreversible damage of the myocardium. Acute and extensive myocardial ischemia leads to apoptosis of myocytes (i.e., myocardial infarction) in the vascular territory distal to the coronary artery occlusion. Chronic myocardial ischemia, on the other hand, leads to a series of morphological (e.g., dedifferentiation of the myocytes, progressive loss of myocytes, and replacement fibrosis), functional (wall dyssynergia), and metabolic (increased glucose metabolism) changes (29). This condition is better known as hibernating myocardium and can be considered as a protective functional downloading of the myocardium (140). In other words, hibernating myocardium represents a "last defense mechanism" in response to profound and chronic ischemia; however, it does not occur in all patients with chronic myocardial ischemia. In some circumstances the myocardium might undergo ischemic necrosis instead of hibernation, with irreversible structural and functional damage. The mechanism leading to one or another response to chronic ischemia is unclear and might depend on the degree and duration of myocardial ischemia. Because the myocardium at least partially survives, some improvement of the myocardial function can be expected after revascularization (141). Thus, the detection of hibernating myocardium is clinically important because it constitutes a potentially salvageable myocardium.

Temporary occlusion of a coronary artery leads to a reversible postischemic contractile dysfunction after reperfusion has been achieved (i.e., stunned myocardium) (142). The length of the contractile dysfunction is out of proportion to the length of coronary artery occlusion, but the longer the ischemia time, the longer will be the contractile dysfunction. For instance, an occlusion of several minutes will cause a contractile dysfunction of several hours (143).

In a patient with single- or multivessel coronary artery disease presenting with angor or myocardial infarction, an important issue to solve is the differentiation between dysfunctional but viable myocardium and irreversible damaged myocardium because revascularization procedures will only improve the myocardial function in the first condition (144). Both hibernating and stunned myocardium possess a certain inotropic reserve (96,142,145). In hibernating myocardium the increase in contractile function is at the expense of metabolic recovery, whereas no metabolic deterioration occurs during inotropic stimulation in stunned myocardium. In contrast, infarcted myocardium has no inotropic reserve left and will not show any improvement under inotropic stimulation. This approach, therefore, may be helpful to identify viable, dysfunctional myocardium. Stunned and hibernating myocardium can be differentiated from each other by myocardial perfusion studies because the first has a normal myocardial perfusion by definition.

Several strategies have been proposed to assess the myocardial viability with MRI in patients with an acute previous myocardial infarction or a history of one (146). First, acute and subacute myocardial infarctions may be depicted by changes in signal intensity on spin-echo images, especially T2-weighted sequences (147). Second,

the use of paramagnetic contrast media (especially the use of infarct-avid contrast agents) may be appealing in the localization and quantification of infarcted myocardium (Fig. 30.14) (148,149). Third, measurement of metabolite concentrations within the infarct area using magnetic resonance spectroscopy is another approach to assess myocardial viability (150,151). Finally, viable but dysfunctional myocardial tissue can differentiate from infarcted myocardium by means of low-dose dobutamine infusion because wall thickening will improve in the viable but dysfunctional segments under inotropic stimulation, but remains unchanged or even gets worse in infarcted myocardium (145,152). In chronic infarcts, quantification of myocardial thickness and systolic wall thickening with and without positive inotropic stimulation can be applied to detect dysfunctional but viable myocardium (146). In myocardial infarcts older than 4 months the necrotic tissue has been transformed into scar tissue, and can be considered as "healed." Magnetic resonance imaging is ideally suited to detect and to characterize chronic myocardial scar and to distinguish it from viable but hibernating myocardium because it clearly depicts the regional wall thinning that is a typical feature of (transmural) infarcts. Viable myocardium in contrast is characterized by preserved end-diastolic wall thickness and a dobutamine-inducible contraction reserve (153).

To summarize, MRI is helpful for both accurate infarct localization and infarct quantitation and to differentiate between nonviable, infarcted, and viable but dysfunctional myocardial tissue in patients with coronary artery disease.

Conclusions

A comprehensive study of the heart in patients with ischemic heart disease requires detailed knowledge of the cardiac anatomy, global and regional ventricular function, the vascular supply during rest and stress conditions, myocardial viability, and metabolism. These parameters are now obtained through a multiplicity of separate methods, including echocardiography, coronary angiography, radionuclide imaging, and MRI. A single-step comprehensive examination of the heart within a reasonable time would both reduce the financial cost and benefit the cardiac patient. Cardiac MRI has the ability to quantify ventricular function accurately as well as to assess precisely the myocardial deformation three-dimensionally unmatched by any other existing methods. This, together with the ability accurately to quantify myocardial flow, perfusion, and cardiac anatomy at spatial and temporal resolutions, makes MRI a cost-effective, high diagnostic-value alternative in cardiac imaging.

A

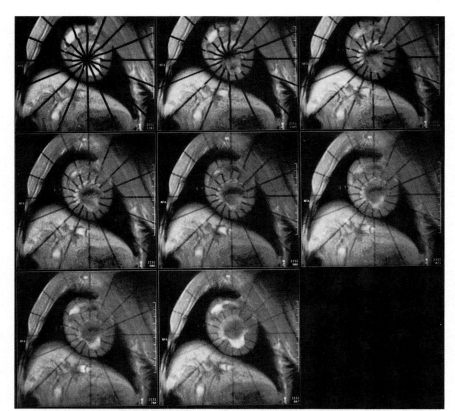

B

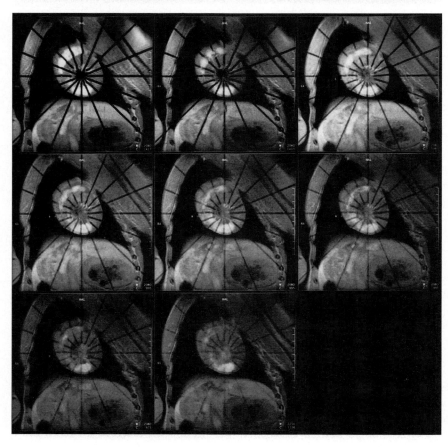

Figure 30.14. Combination of MRI tagging and administration of paramagnetic contrast agents in an animal model with a reperfused acute inferior myocardial infarction (courtesy of Prof. Dr. Ni and Prof. Dr. J. Bogaert). (A) MRI myocardial tagging in the cardiac short-axis plane before acute myocardial infarction. (B) MRI myocardial tagging in the cardiac short-axis plane 11 hours after the onset of acute myocardial infarction and seven hours after intravenous administration of paramagnetic contrast agent (Gadophrin-2). In this experimental animal model, a large infarct is clearly visible after administration of Gadophrin-2 in the inferior LV wall, which is edematously thickened. The area of enhancement corresponds very well with the infarcted (i.e., nonviable or necrotic) myocardium. MRI myocardial tagging reveals an absence of systolic wall thickening in the infarcted area. This combination provides a unique opportunity to assess the myocardial function in infarcted myocardium directly.

Acknowledgments. The authors would like to thank Frank E. Rademakers, MD, PhD, from the department of cardiology for his expertise and cooperation in the field of the myocardial MR tagging; Hilde Bosmans, PhD, our MR physicist for the application of the new cardiac MR techniques; Ycheng Ni for his experimental work on new MR contrast agents for myocardial infarction detection and quantification; and finally Guy Marchal, MD, PhD, chairman of the department of radiology.

References

1. Bloch F. Nuclear induction. Phys Rev 1946;70:460–74.

2. Purcell EM, Torrey HC, Pound RV. Resonance absorption by nuclear magnetic moments in a solid. Phys Rev 1946;69:37–38.

3. Lauterbur P. Image formation by induced local interactions: examples employing nuclear magnetic resonance. Nature 1973;242:190–91.

4. Higgins CB. New horizons in cardiac imaging? Radiology 1985;156:577–88.

5. Mousseaux E, Sapoval M, Gaux JC. [MRI in cardiology: clinical applications and perspectives]. Ann Radiol Paris 1995;38:55–68.

6. Streeter DD. Gross morphology and fiber geometry of the heart. *In*: Berne RM, Sperelakis N, eds. Handbook of Physiology. Section 2. The Cardiovascular System, Vol. 1. Baltimore: Williams & Wilkins, 1979:61–112.

7. Zerhouni EA, Parish DM, Rogers WJ, Yang A, Shapiro EP. Human heart: tagging with MR imaging—a new method for noninvasive assessment of myocardial motion. Radiology 1988;169:59–63.

8. Atkinson DJ, Edelman RR. Cineangiography of the heart in a single breath hold with a segmented turboflash sequence. Radiology 1991;178:357–60.

9. Stehling MK, Turner R, Mansfield P. Echo-planar imaging: magnetic resonance imaging in a fraction of a second. Science 1991;254:43–50.

10. Matthaei D, Haase A, Henrich D, Dühmke E. Cardiac and vascular imaging with an MR snapshot technique. Radiology 1990;177:527–32.

11. Wendland MF, Saeed M, Masui T, Derugin N, Moseley ME, Higgins CB. Echo-planar MR imaging of normal and ischemic myocardium with gadodiamide injection. Radiology 1993;186:535–42.

12. Guilfoyle DN, Gibbs P, Ordidge RJ, Mansfield P. Real-time flow measurements using echo-planar imaging. Magn Reson Med 1991;18:1–8.

13. Griswold MA, Sodickson DK, Jakob PM, Chen Q, Goldfarb JW, Edelman RR. Resolution enhancement and artifact reduction in single shot MR imaging using simultaneous acquisition of spatial harmonics (SMASH). Radiology 1997;205:387.

14. Unterweger M, Debatin JF, Leung DA, Wildermuth S, McKinnon GC, von Schulthness GK. Cardiac volumetry: comparison of echoplanar and conventional cine magnetic resonance data acquisition strategies. Invest Radiol 1994;29:994–1000.

15. Mancini GB, De Boe SF, Anselmo E, Simon SB, Le Free MT, Vogel RA. Quantitative regional curvature analysis: an application of shape determination for the assessment of segmental left ventricular function in man. Am Heart J 1987;113:326–34.

16. Nguyen TN, Glantz SA. Floating axis does not reduce motion artifacts in a model of left ventricular wall motion in dogs. Am J Physiol 1993;264:h631–638.

17. Assmann PE, Slager CJ, Van Der Borden SG, Sutherland GR, Roelandt JR. Reference systems in echocardiographic quantitative wall motion analysis with registration of respiration. J Am Soc Echocardiogr 1991;4:224–234.

18. Calenda P, Jain P, Smith LG. Utilization of echocardiography by internists and cardiologists: a comparative study. Am J Med 1996;101:584–591.

19. Waggoner AD, Harris KM, Braverman AC, Barzilai B, Geltman EM. The role of transthoracic echocardiography in the management of patients seen in an outpatient cardiology clinic. J Am Soc Echocardiogr 1996;9:761–68.

20. Pattynama PM, Doornbos J, Hermans J, van der Wall EE, de Roos A. Magnetic resonance evaluation of regional left ventricular function. Effect of through-plane motion. Invest Radiol 1992;27:681–85.

21. Rogers WJ, Shapiro EP, Weiss JL, Buchalter MB, Rademakers FE, Weisfeldt ML, et al. Quantification of and correction for left ventricular systolic long-axis shortening by magnetic resonance tissue tagging and slice isolation. Circulation 1991;84:721–31.

22. Waltman TJ, Dittrich HC. What's new in transesophageal echocardiography? Curr Opin Cardiol 1994;9:709–20.

23. Milner M. Transesophageal echocardiography. Md Med J 1994;43:791–93.

24. Liu N, Darmon PL, Saada M, Catoire P, Rosso J, Berger G, et al. Comparison between radionuclide ejection fraction and fractional area changes derived from transesophageal echocardiography using automated border detection. Anesthesiology 1996;85:468–74.

25. Antunes ML, Tresgallo ME, Seldin DW, Bhatia K, Johnson LL. Effect of infarct size measured from antimyosin single-photon emission computed tomographic scans on left ventricular remodeling. J Am Coll Cardiol 1991;18:1263–270.

26. Mochizuki T, Murase K, Fujiwara Y, Tanada S, Hamamoto K, Tauxe WN. Assessment of systolic thickening with thallium-201 ECG-gated single-photon emission computed tomography: a parameter for local left ventricular function. J Nucl Med 1991;32:1496–500.

27. Maes A, Van de Werf F, Nuyts J, Bormans G, Desmet W, Mortelmans L. Impaired myocardial tissue perfusion early after successful thrombolysis. Impact on myocardial flow, metabolism, and function at the late follow-up. Circulation 1995;92:2072–78.

28. Maes A, Mortelmans L, Nuyts J, Bormans G, Herregods MC, Bijnens B, et al. Importance of flow/metabolism studies in predicting late recovery of function following reperfusion in patients with acute myocardial infarction. Eur Heart J 1997;18:954–62.

29. Maes A, Flameng W, Nuyts J, Borgers M, Shivalkar B, Ausma J, et al. Histological alterations in chronically hypoperfused myocardium: correlation with PET findings. Circulation 1994;90:735–45.

30. Miron SD, Finkelhor R, Penuel JH, Bahler R, Bellon EM.

A geometric method of measuring the left ventricular ejection fraction on gated Tc-99m sestamibi myocardial imaging. Clin Nucl Med 1996;21:439–44.

31. Williams KA, Taillon LA. Left ventricular function in patients with coronary artery disease assessed by gated tomographic myocardial perfusion images: comparison with assessment by contrast ventriculography and first-pass radionuclide angiography. J Am Coll Cardiol 1996; 27:173–81.

32. Itchhaporia D, Cerqueira MD. New agents and new techniques in nuclear cardiology. Curr Opin Cardiol 1995; 10:650–55.

33. Sandler MP, Patton JA. Fluorine 18-labeled fluorodeoxyglucose myocardial single-photon emission computed tomography: an alternative for determining myocardial viability. J Nucl Cardiol 1996;3:342–49.

34. Bodemheimer MM, Banka VS, Helfant RH. Nuclear cardiology. I. radionuclide angiographic assessment of left ventricular contraction: uses, limitations and future directions. Am J Cardiol 1980;45:661–73.

35. Santinga JT, Kirsh MM, Brady TJ, Thrall J, Pitt B. Left ventricular function in patients with ventricular arrhythmias and aortic valve disease. Ann Thoracic Surg 1983;35:152–55.

36. Feiring AJ, Rumberger JA, Reiter SJ, Skorton DJ, Collins SM, Lipton MJ, et al. Determination of left ventricular mass in dogs with rapid-acquisition cardiac computed tomographic scanning. Circulation 1985;72:1355–64.

37. Hamada S, Naito H, Takamiya M. Evaluation of myocardium in ischemic heart disease by ultrafast computed tomography. Jpn Circ J 1992;56:627–31.

38. Gould RG. Perfusion quantitation by ultrafast computed tomography. Invest Radiol 1992;27:S18–21.

39. Coulden R, Lipton MJ. Noninvasive imaging for the diagnosis and management of myocardial ischemia. Adv Card Surg 1993;4:173–205.

40. Baumgartner F, Brundage B, Bleiweis M, Lee J, Ferrario T, Georgiou D, et al. Feasibility of ultrafast computed tomography in the early evaluation of coronary bypass patency. Am J Card Imag 1996;10:170–74.

41. Wolfkiel CJ, Brundage BH. Measurement of myocardial blood flow by UFCT: towards clinical applicability. Int J Card Imag 1991;7:89–100.

42. Yamaoka O, Yabe T, Okada M, Endoh S, Nakamura Y, Mitsunami K, et al. Evaluation of left ventricular mass: comparison of ultrafast computed tomography, magnetic resonance imaging, and contrast left ventriculography. Am Heart J 1993;126:1372–79.

43. Yamaoka O, Fujioka H, Haque T, Nakamura Y, Mitsunami K, Kinoshita M, et al. Low-dose dobutamine stress test for the evaluation of cardiac function using ultrafast computed tomography. Clin Cardiol 1993;16: 473–79.

44. Yamaoka O, Kinoshita M. Role of collateral flow in a pharmacological stress test (a combination of low-dose dobutamine and a vasodilator) as a predictor of wall motion reversibility. Jpn Circ J 1995;59:673–84.

45. Kosling S, Hoffmann U, Lieberenz S, Rother T, Weber P, Heywang KS, et al. First experiences with electron beam computed tomography of the heart: comparison with heart catheterization and echocardiographic findings.

Rofo Fortschr Geb Rontgenstr Neuen Bildgeb Verfahr 1995;163:111–18.

46. Higgins CB, Byrd BF II, McNamara MT, Lanzer P, Lipton MJ, Botvinick E, et al. Magnetic resonance imaging of the heart: a review of the experience in 172 subjects. Radiology 1985;155:671–79.

47. von Schulthess GK, Fisher M, Crooks LE, Higgins CB. Gated MR imaging of the heart: intracardiac signals in patients and healthy subjects. Radiology 1985;156:125–32.

48. Mayo JR. Thoracic magnetic resonance imaging: physics and pulse sequences. J Thorac Imag 1993;8:1–11.

49. Higgins CB, Caputo G, Wendland MF, Saeed M. Measurement of blood flow and perfusion in the cardiovascular system. Invest Radiol 1992;2:66–71.

50. von Schulthess G, Fisher MR, Higgins CB. Pathologic blood flow in pulmonary vascular disease as shown by gated magnetic resonance imaging. Ann Intern Med 1985;103:317–23.

51. Wagner S, Buser P, Auffermann W, Holt WW, Wolfe CL, Higgins CB. Cine magnetic resonance imaging: tomographic analysis of left ventricular function. Cardiol Clin 1989;7:651–59.

52. Matsumura K, Nakase E, Haiyama T, Takeo K, Shimizu K, Yamasaki K, et al. Determination of cardiac ejection fraction and left ventricular volume: contrast-enhanced ultrafast cine MR imaging vs IV digital subtraction ventriculography. Am J Roentgenol 1993;160:979–85.

53. Doherty NEI, Seelos KC, Suzuki J, Caputo GR, O'Sullivan M, Sobol SM, et al. Application of cine nuclear magnetic resonance imaging for sequential evaluation of response to angiotensin-converting enzyme inhibitor therapy in dilated cardiomyopathy. J Am Coll Cardiol 1992;19:1294–302.

54. Reichek N. Patterns of left ventricular response in essential hypertension. J Am Coll Cardiol 1992;7:1559–60.

55. Allison JD, Flickinger FW, Wright JC, Falls D III, Prisant LM, Von Dohlen TW, et al. Measurement of left ventricular mass in hypertrophic cardiomyopathy using MRI: comparison with echocardiography. Magn Reson Imag 1993;11:329–34.

56. Debatin JF, Nadel SN, Paolini JF, Sostman HD, Coleman RE, Evans AJ, et al. Cardiac ejection fraction: phantom study comparing cine MRI, radionuclide angiography and contrast ventriculography. J Magn Reson Imag 1992; 2:135–42.

57. Rehr RB, Malloy CR, Filipchuk NG, Peshock RM. Left ventricular volumes measured by MR imaging. Radiology 1985;156:717–19.

58. Soldo SJ, Norris SL, Gober JR, Haywood LJ, Colletti PM, Terk M. MRI-derived ventricular volume curves for the assessment of left ventricular function. Magn Reson Imag 1994;12:711–17.

59. Mogelvang J, Thomsen C, Mehlsen J, Bräckle G, Stubgaard M, Henriksen O. Evaluation of left ventricular volumes measured by magnetic resonance imaging. Eur Heart J 1987;1986:1016–21.

60. van Rossum AC, Visser FC, Sprenger M, Van Eenige MJ, Valk J, Roos JP. Evaluation of magnetic resonance imaging for determination of left ventricular ejection fraction and comparison with angiography. Am J Cardiol 1988; 1988:628–33.

61. Bogaert JG, Bosmans H, Rademakers F, Bellon E, Herregods MC, Verschakelen J. Left ventricular quantification with breath-hold MR imaging: comparison with echocardiography. MagMa 1995;3:5–12.

62. Longmore DB, Underwood SR, Hounsfield GN, Bland C, Poole-Wilson PA, Denison D, et al. Dimensional accuracy of magnetic resonance in studies of the heart. Lancet 1985;1:1360–62.

63. van Rossum AC, Visser FC, van Eenige MJ, Valk J, Roos JP. Magnetic resonance imaging of the heart for determination of ejection fraction. Int J Cardiol 1988;18:53–63.

64. Aurigemma G, Davidoff A, Silver K, Boehmer J. Left ventricular mass quantitation using single-phase cardiac magnetic resonance imaging. Am J Cardiol 1992;70: 259–62.

65. Debatin JF, Nadel SN, Sostman HD, Spritzer CE, Evans AJ, Grist TM. Magnetic resonance imaging-cardiac ejection fraction measurements: phantom study comparing four different methods. Invest Radiol 1992;27:198–204.

66. Caputo GR, Suzuki JI, Kondo C, Cho H, Quaife RA, Higgins CB, et al. Determination of left ventricular volume and mass with use of biphasic spin-echo MR imaging: comparison with cine MR. Radiology 1990;177:773–77.

67. Hunter GJ, Hamberg LM, Weisskoff RM, Halpern EF, Brady TJ. Measurement of stroke volume and cardiac output within a single breath hold with echo-planar MR imaging. J Magn Reson Imag 1994;4:51–58.

68. McDonald KM, Parrish T, Wennberg P, Stillman AE, Francis GS, Cohn JN, et al. Rapid, accurate and simultaneous noninvasive assessment of right and left ventricular mass with nuclear magnetic resonance imaging using the snapshot gradient method. J Am Coll Cardiol 1992; 19:1601–7.

69. Pattynama PM, Lamb HJ, van der Velde EA, van der Wall EE, de Roos A. Left ventricular measurements with cine and spin-echo MR imaging: a study of reproducibility with variance component analysis. Radiology 1993;187: 261–68.

70. Semelka RC, Tomei E, Wagner S, Mayo J, Caputo G, O'Sullivan M, et al. Interstudy reproducibility of dimensional and functional measurements between cine magnetic resonance studies in the morphologically abnormal left ventricle. Am Heart J 1990;119:1367–73.

71. Semelka RC, Tomei E, Wagner S, Mayo J, Kondo C, Suzuki JI, et al. Normal left ventricular dimensions and function: interstudy reproducibility of measurements with cine MR imaging. Radiology 1990;174:763–768.

72. Higgins CB. Which standard has the gold? J Am Coll Cardiol 1992;19:1608–9.

73. Markiewicz W, Sechtem U, Higgins CB. Evaluation of the right ventricle by magnetic resonance imaging. Am Heart J 1987;113:8–15.

74. Markiewicz W, Sechtem U, Kirby R, Derugin N, Caputo GC, Higgins CB. Measurement of ventricular volumes in the dog by nuclear magnetic resonance imaging. J Am Coll Cardiol 1987;10:170–77.

75. Pattynama PM, Lamb HJ, Van der Velde EA, Van der Geest RJ, Van der Wall EE, De Roos A. Reproducibility of MRI-derived measurements of right ventricular volumes and myocardial mass. Magn Reson Imag 1995;13:53–63.

76. Culham J, Vince DJ. Cardiac output by MR imaging: an experimental study comparing right ventricle and left ventricle with thermodilution. J Can Assoc Radiol 1988; 39:247–249.

77. Kondo C, Caputo GR, Semelka R, Foster E, Shimakawa A, Higgins CB. Right and left ventricular stroke volume measurements with velocity-encoded cine MR imaging: in vitro and in vivo validation. Am J Roentgenol 1991; 157:9–16.

78. Sechtem U, Pflugfelder PW, White RD, Gould RG, Holt W, Lipton MJ, et al. Cine MR imaging: Potential for the evaluation of cardiovascular function. Am J Roentgenol 1987;148:239–46.

79. Sechtem U, Sommerhoff BA, Markiewicz W, White RD, Cheitlin MD, Higgins CB. Regional left ventricular wall thickening by magnetic resonance imaging: evaluation in normal persons and patients with global and regional dysfunction. Am J Cardiol 1987;59:145–51.

80. Sechtem U, Plugfelder P, Higgins CB. Quantification of cardiac function by conventional and cine magnetic resonance imaging. Cardiovasc Intervent Radiol 1987;10; 365–73.

81. Herregods M, De Paep G, Bijnens B, Bogaert JG, Rademakers FE, Bosmans HT, et al. Determination of left ventricular volume by two-dimensional echocardiography: comparison with magnetic resonance imaging. Eur Heart J 1994;15:1070–73.

82. Buser PT, Auffermann W, Holt WW, Wagner S, Kircher B, Wolfe C, et al. Noninvasive evaluation of global left ventricular function with use of cine nuclear magnetic resonance. J Am Coll Cardiol 1989;13:1294–300.

83. Greenbaum RA, Ho SY, Gibson DG, Becker AE, Anderson RH. Left ventricular fibre architecture in man. Br Heart J 1981;45:248–63.

84. Rademakers FE. Three-dimensional strain analysis of the left ventricle. Proefschrift tot het behalen van de graad van geaggregeerde voor het hoger onderwijs (Universitaire instelling Antwerpen, 1991).

85. Bogaert J. Three-dimensional strain analysis of the human left ventricle. Doctoral Dissertation, Catholic University, Leuven, Belgium, 1997.

86. Fisher MR, Von Schulthess GK, Higgins CB. Multiphasic cardiac magnetic resonance imaging: normal regional left ventricular wall thickening. Am J Roentgenol 1985;145: 27–30.

87. White RD, Cassidy MM, Cheitlin MD, Emilson B, Ports TA, Lim AD, et al. Segmental evaluation of left ventricular wall motion after myocardial infarction: magnetic resonance imaging versus echocardiography. Am Heart J 1988;115:166–75.

88. White RD, Caputo GR, Mark AS, Modin GW, Higgins CB. Coronary artery bypass graft patency: noninvasive evaluation with MR imaging. Radiology 1987;164:681–86.

89. Buda AJ, Zotz RJ, Pace DP, Krause LC. Comparison of two-dimensional echocardiographic wall motion and wall thickening abnormalities in relation to the myocardium at risk. Am Heart J 1986;111:587–92.

90. Lieberman AN, Weiss JL, Jugdutt BI, Becker LC, Bulkley BH, Garrison JG, et al. Two-dimensional echocardiography and infarct size: relationship of regional wall motion and thickening to the extent of myocardial infarction in the dog. Circulation 1981;63:739–46.

91. Rademakers FE, Rogers WJ, Guier WH, Hutchins GM, Siu CO, Weisfeldt ML, et al. Relation of regional cross-fiber shortening to wall thickening in the intact heart: three-dimensional strain analysis by NMR tagging. Circulation 1994;89:1174–82.

92. Gallagher KP, Kumada T, Koziol JA, McKnown MD, Kemper WS, Ross JJ. Significance of regional wall thickening abnormalities relative to transmural myocardial perfusion in anesthetized dogs. Circulation 1980;62:1266–74.

93. Gallagher KP, Osakada G, Matsuzaki M, Miller M, Kemper WS, Ross JJ. Nonuniformity of inner and outer systolic wall thickening in conscious dogs. Am J Physiol 1985;249:H241–48.

94. van Rugge FP, van der Wall EE, Spanjersberg SJ, de Roos A, Matheijssen NA, Zwinderman AH, et al. Magnetic resonance imaging during dobutamine stress for detection and localization of coronary artery disease. Quantitative wall motion analysis using a modification of the centerline method. Circulation 1994;90:127–38.

95. Lima JAC, Jeremy R, Guier W, Bouton SA, Zerhouni EA, McVeigh E, et al. Accurate systolic wall thickening by nuclear magnetic resonance imaging with tissue ragging: correlation with sonomicrometers in normal and ischemic myocardium. J Am Coll Cardiol 1993;21:1741–51.

96. Cigarroa CB, de Filippi C, Brickner ME, Alvarez LG, Wait MA, Grayburn PA. Dobutamine stress echocardiography identifies hibernating myocardium and predicts recovery of left ventricular function after coronary revascularization. Circulation 1993;88:430–36.

97. Waldman LK, Fung YC, Covell JW. Transmural myocardial deformation in the canine left ventricle. Normal in vivo three-dimensional finite strains. Circ Res 1985;57:152–63.

98. Hansen DE, Daughters G, Alderman EL, Ingels NJ, Miller DC. Torsional deformation of the left ventricular midwall in human hearts with intramyocardial markers: regional heterogeneity and sensitivity to the inotropic effects of abrupt rate changes. Circ Res 1988;62:941–52.

99. Ingels NBJ, Daughters GTI, Davies SR. Stereo photogrammetic studies on the dynamic geometry of the canine left ventricular epicardium. J Biomech 1971;4:541–50.

100. Ingels NBJ, Daughters GT, Stinson EB, Alderman EL. Measurement of midwall myocardial dynamics in intact man by radiography of surgically implanter markers. Circulation 1975;52:859–67.

101. Zerhouni EA. Myocardial tagging by magnetic resonance imaging. Cor Art Dis 1993;4:334–39.

102. Bosmans H, Bogaert J, Rademakers FE, Marchal G, Laub G, Verschakelen J, et al. Left ventricular radial tagging acquisition using gradient-recalled-echo techniques: sequence optimization. MagMa 1996;4:123–33.

103. Azhari H, Weiss JL, Rogers WJ, Siu CO, Zerhouni EA, Shapiro EP. Noninvasive quantification of principal strains in normal canine hearts using tagged MRI images in 3-D. Am J Physiol Heart Circ Physiol 1993;264:33–41.

104. Pipe JG, Boes JL, Chenevert TL. Method for measuring three-dimensional motion with tagged MR imaging. Radiology 1991;181:591–95.

105. Axel L, Dougherty L. Heart wall motion: improved method for spatial modulation of magnetization for MR imaging. Radiology 1989;172:349–50.

106. Axel L, Dougherty L. MR imaging of motion with spatial modulation of magnetization. Radiology 1989;171:841–45.

107. McVeigh ER, Atalar E. Cardiac tagging with breath-hold cine MRI. Magn Reson Med 1992;28:318–27.

108. Moore CC, O'Dell WG, McVeigh ER, Zerhouni EA. Calculation of three-dimensional left ventricular strains from biplanar tagged MR images. J Magn Reson Imag 1992;2:165–75.

109. Rademakers FE, Buchalter MB, Rogers WJ, Zerhouni EA, Weisfeldt ML, Weiss JL, et al. Dissociation between left ventricular untwisting and filling: accentuation by catecholamines. Circulation 1992;85:1572–81.

110. Buchalter MB, Weiss JL, Rogers WJ, Zerhouni EA, Weisfeldt ML, Beyar R, et al. Noninvasive quantification of left ventricular rotational deformation in normal humans using magnetic resonance imaging myocardial tagging. Circulation 1990;81:1236–44.

111. Buchalter MB, Rademakers FE, Weiss JL, Rogers WJ, Weisfeldt ML, Shapiro EP. Rotational deformation of the canine left ventricle measured by magnetic resonance tagging: effects of catecholamines, ischaemia, and pacing. Cardiovasc Res 1994;28:629–35.

112. Young AA, Axel L, Dougherty L, Bogen DK, Parenteau CS. Validation of tagging with MR imaging to estimate material deformation. Radiology 1993;188:101–8.

113. Dong SJ, MacGregor JH, Crawley AP, McVeigh E, Belenkie I, Smith ER, et al. Left ventricular wall thickness and regional systolic function in patients with hypertrophic cardiomyopathy. Circulation 1994;90:1200–9.

114. Kramer CM, Reichek N, Ferrari VA, Theobald T, Dawson J, Axel L. Regional heterogeneity of function in hypertropic cardiomyopathy. Circulation 1994;90:186–94.

115. Maier SE, Fischer SE, McKinnon GC, Hess OM, Kraeyenbuehl HP, Boesiger P. Evaluation of left ventricular segmental wall motion in hypertrophic cardiomyopathy with myocardial tagging. Circulation 1992;86:1919–28.

116. Young AA, Kramer CM, Ferrari VA, Axel L, Reichek N. Three-dimensional left ventricular deformation in hypertrophic cardiomyopathy. Circulation 1994;90:854–67.

117. Dong SJ, Crawley AP, MacGregor JH, Petrank YF, Bergman DW, Belenkie I, et al. Regional left ventricular systolic function in relation to the cavity geometry in patients with chronic right ventricular pressure overload: a three-dimensional tagged magnetic resonance study. Circulation 1995;91:2359–70.

118. Bolster BJ, McVeigh ER, Zerhouni EA. Myocardial tagging in polar coordinates with use of striped tags. Radiology 1990;177:769–72.

119. McVeigh ER, Zerhouni EA. Noninvasive measurement of transmural gradients in myocardial strain with MR imaging. Radiology 1991;180:677–83.

120. Kramer CM, Lima JA, Reichek N, Ferrari VA, Llaneras MR, Palmon LC, et al. Regional differences in function within noninfarcted myocardium during left ventricular remodeling. Circulation 1993;88:1279–88.

121. Kramer CM, Rogers WJ, Theobald TM, Power TP,

Petruolo S, Reichek N. Remote noninfarcted region dysfunction soon after first anterior myocardial infarction: a magnetic resonance tagging study. Circulation 1996;94:660–66.

122. Bogaert J, Bosmans H, Herregods MC, Marchal G, De Geest H, Baert AL, et al. Early effects of acute anterior infarction on regional 3-dimensional left ventricular function using MRI tagging. Circulation 1995;92:I–669.

123. Bogaert J, Maes A, Van de Werf F, Desmet W, Mortelmans L, Marchal G, et al. Improvement of left ventricular function due to subepicardial recovery after acute Q-wave anterior myocardial infarction. Circulation 1996;94:I–244.

124. Wedeen VJ. Magnetic resonance imaging of myocardial kinematics: technique to detect, localize, and quantify the strain rates of the active human myocardium. Magn Reson Med 1992;27:52–67.

125. Wedeen VJ, Weisskoff RM, Reese TG, Beache GM, Poncelet BP, Rosen BR, et al. Motionless movies of myocardial strain-rates using stimulated echoes [published erratum appears in Magn Reson Med 1995;33(5):743]. Magn Reson Med 1995;33:401–8.

126. Firmin DN, Klipstein RH, Hounsfield GL, Paley MP, Longmore DB. Echo-planar high-resolution flow velocity mapping. Magn Reson Med 1989;12:316–27.

127. Kilner PJ, Firmin DN, Rees RSO, Martinez J, Pennell DJ, Mohiaddin RH. Valve and great vessel stenosis: assessment with MR jet velocity mapping. Radiology 1991;178:229–35.

128. Constable RT, Rath KM, Sinusas AJ, Gore JC. Development and evaluation of tracking algorithms for cardiac wall motion analysis using phase velocity MR imaging. Magn Reson Med 1994;32:33–42.

129. Detrano R, Gianrossi R, Mulvihill D, Lehmann KK, Dubach P, Colombo A, et al. Exercise induced ST segment depression in the diagnosis of multivessel coronary disease: a meta analysis. J Am Coll Cardiol 1998;14:1501–8.

130. Bartunek J, Marwick TH, Rodrigues AC, Vincent M, Van Schuerbeeck E, Sys SU, et al. Dobutamine-induced wall motion abnormalities: correlations with myocardial fractional wall reserve and quantitative coronary angiography. J Am Coll Cardiol 1996;27:1429–36.

131. Lanzer P, Garrett J, Lipton MJ, Gould R, Sievers R, O'Connell W. Quantification of regional myocardial function by cine computed tomography: pharmacologic changes in wall thickness. J Am Coll Cardiol 1986;8:682–92.

132. Schaefer S, Peshock RM, Parkey RW, Willerson JT. A new device for exercise MR imaging. Am J Roentgenol 1986;147:1289–90.

133. Baer FM, Theissen P, Smolarz K, Voth E, Sechtem U, Schicha H, et al. Dobutamine versus dipyridamole-magnetic resonance imaging: safety and sensitivity for the diagnosis of coronary artery stenoses. Z Kardiol 1993;82:494–503.

134. Pennell DJ. Magnetic resonance imaging during pharmacologic stress. Cor Art Dis 1993;4:345–53.

135. Pennell DJ, Underwood SR, Manzara CC, Howard SR, Malcolm WJ, Ell PJ. Magnetic resonance imaging during dobutamine stress in coronary artery disease. Am J Cardiol 1992;70:34–40.

136. Pennell DJ, Underwood SR, Longmore DB. Detection of coronary artery disease using MR imaging with dipyridamole infusion. JCAT 1990;14:167–70.

137. van Rugge FP, van der Wall EE, de Roos A, Bruschke AV. Dobutamine stress magnetic resonance imaging for detection of coronary artery disease. J Am Coll Cardiol 1993;22:431–39.

138. The TIMI study group. The thrombolysis in myocardial infarction (TIMI) trial: phase I findings. N Engl J Med 1985;312:932–36.

139. Takahashi JC, Saiki M, Miyatake S, Tani S, Kubo H, Goto K. Adenovirus-mediated gene transfer of basic fibroblast growth factor induces in vitro angiogenesis. Atherosclerosis 1997;132:199–205.

140. Rahimtoola SH. The hibernating myocardium in ischaemia and congestive heart failure. Eur Heart J 1993;14:22–26.

141. Braunwald E, Rutherford JD. Reversible ischemic left ventricular dysfunction: evidence for the "hibernating myocardium." J Am Coll Cardiol 1986;8:1467–70.

142. Trevi GP, Sheiban I. Chronic ischemic ("hibernating") and postischaemic ("stunned") dysfunctional but viable myocardium. Eur Heart J 1991;12:20–26.

143. Lawrence WE, Maughan WL, Kass DA. Mechanism of global functional recovery despite sustained postischemic regional stunning. Circulation 1992;85:816–27.

144. Galli M, Marcassa C, Bolli R, Giannuzzi P, Temporelli PL, Imparato A, et al. Spontaneous delayed recovery of perfusion and contraction after the first 5 weeks after anterior infarction. Evidence for the presence of hibernating myocardium in the infarcted area. Circulation 1994;90:1386–97.

145. Watada H, Ito H, Oh H, Masuyama T, Aburaya M, Hori M, et al. Dobutamine stress echocardiography predicts reversible dysfunction and quantitates the extent of irreversibly damaged myocardium after reperfusion of anterior myocardial infarction. J Am Coll Cardiol 1994;24:624–30.

146. Baer FM, Theissen P, Schneider CA, Voth E, Schicha H, Sechtem U. Magnetic resonance imaging techniques for the assessment of residual myocardial viability. Herz 1994;19:51–64.

147. Caputo GR, Sechtem U, Tscholakoff D, Higgins CB. Measurement of myocardial infarct size at early and late time intervals using MR imaging: an experimental study in dogs. Am J Roentgenol 1987;149:237–44.

148. De Roos A, Van Rossum AC, Van Der Wall E, Postema S, Doornbos J, Matheijssen N, et al. Reperfused and non-reperfused myocardial infarction: diagnostic potential of Gd-DTPA-enhanced MR imaging. Radiology 1989;172:717–20.

149. Marchal G, Ni Y, Herijgers P, Flameng W, Petré C, Bosmans H, et al. Paramagnetic metalloporphyrins: infarct avid contrast agents for diagnosis of acute myocardial infarction by MRI. Eur Radiol 1996;6:2–8.

150. Weiss RG, Bottomley PA, Hardy CJ, Gerstenblith G. Regional myocardial metabolism of high-energy phosphates during isometric exercise in patients with coronary artery disease. New Engl J Med 1990;323:1593–600.

151. Neubauer S, Krahe T, Schindler R, Hillenbrand H,

Entzeroth C, Horn M, et al. Direct measurement of spin-lattice relaxation times of phosphorus metabolites in human myocardium. Magn Reson Med 1992;26:300–7.

152. Piérard LA, De Landsheere CM, Berthe C, Rigo P, Kulbertus HE. Identification of viable myocardium by echocardiography during dobutamine infusion in patients with myocardial infarction after thrombolytic therapy: comparison with positron emission tomography. J Am Coll Cardiol 1990;15:1021–31.

153. Baer FM, Voth E, LaRosee K, Schneider CA, Theissen P, Deutsch HJ. Comparison of dobutamine transesophageal echocardiography and dobutamine magnetic resonance imaging for detection of residual myocardial viability. Am J Cardiol 1996;78:415–19.

31
MR Stress Ventriculography

Dudley Pennell

Introduction

Current Practice and Limitations of Stress Testing in Clinical Practice

Ever since the introduction of the concept of stress testing (ST) with exercise in 1929 (1), various techniques have been used to assess the response of the heart to challenge. This was initially the electrocardiogram, but more sophisticated techniques have become available as the limitations of using surrogate measures (e.g., ST-segment response) have become clear (2), including the poor correlation of the site of ST-segment changes with the underlying site of arterial disease (3), the poor sensitivity because electrocardiographic changes occur late in the cascade of physiological changes associated with ischemia (4), the poor specificity because numerous conditions exist where exercise ST-segment depression occurs for other reasons (5), and problems with exercise as the stress method as it is limited by physical or psychological problems rather than cardiovascular endpoints, which in one study occurred in one third of patients (6).

It is more common today for cardiologists to use myocardial perfusion imaging, radionuclide ventriculography, or stress echocardiography, but none of these techniques is ideal. Myocardial perfusion imaging (MPI) and radionuclide ventriculography (RNV) are radiotracer-based techniques that carry a small radiation burden, have low spatial resolution, and a long overall imaging duration for the patient of up to 6 hours. MPI, however, is widely used because it is the only currently available noninvasive technique that shows perfusion directly. In addition, it is extremely robust in clinical practice with very few imaging failures. Stress echocardiography has become more popular and shows good results in expert hands in the early days of its honeymoon period. In reality, it can often be suboptimal because of acoustic window limitation associated in particular with obesity or lung disease, and confidence in the results in these cases is limited. Even though transoesophageal approaches might be helpful, they render the test invasive. There is space, therefore, for the development of a high-resolution, noninvasive, rapid, non–X-ray-based technique that is clinically robust. This is the niche that magnetic resonance (MR) stress ventriculography might find. The approaches that allow both regional and global functional assessment during stress MR, and the new methods of quantification that are a significant problem for more established approaches, are of interest.

Stress Testing in Relation to Angiography

It is important to bear in mind that even though coronary angiography by traditional X-ray contrast methods, or possibly MR in the near future, gives important anatomical and localizing information on coronary artery disease, it does not provide all the information necessary for clinical management decisions in all cases. Important prognostic information is contained within the size and severity of ischemic defects during stress (7), and this has been shown to be equal or incremental in quantitative comparisons with angiography (8). This may preclude the use of the angiogram if prognosis can be defined as very good (9), even if coronary disease is known to be present (10). Viability is also not well assessed by angiography, but yields to an analysis of preserved muscle and its cellular integrity by other imaging techniques (11). Finally, newer indications (e.g., transmyocardial laser revascularization in areas of the myocardium that cannot be revascularized) need to be proven ischemic prior to undertaking the anaesthesia and the operative risk. This can again only be established with functional techniques (12), as can the improvement in perfusion and function with follow up (13).

Which Type of Stress in the Magnet?

Dynamic Exercise

There are no published reports of the use of dynamic exercise with magnetic resonance imaging (MRI) for the diagnosis of coronary artery disease. Exercise devices for fitting to the rear of the magnet have been described that are made from nonferromagnetic materials (14,15), but imaging during exercise has not been widely pursued. Low-level prone exercise during magnetic resonance spectroscopy has been reported (16). The main problems are that significant exercise in the magnet is awkward, particularly as the workload increases, and this leads to movement artifact exacerbated by hyperventilation. In addition, the sensation of exercising in a confined environment is unpleasant, and sustaining peak exercise for the duration of scanning is difficult. Faster imaging techniques have now begun to deal with some of these problems. Using spiral flow velocity mapping (17) in normals, Mohiaddin et al. imaged flow in the aorta throughout systole from a single heartbeat (15). Significant increases were documented in mean and peak aortic flow, whereas the time to peak flow fell. In a study of 10 young males at 1.5 T, Scheidegger et al. used an echo planar readout during a 10-heartbeat breathhold (5–10 seconds) to examine wall motion with tagging, as well as flow measurements in the aorta (18). For multi-heartbeat acquisitions, movement artifact became excessive above an exercise level of 65 W, but it was possible to stress up to 130 W with single heartbeat acquisitions. Oshinski et al. examined five normals and five patients with coronary artery disease using exercise in the magnet (19). Restraints across the hips and shoulder supports were used to restrict motion. A target heart rate of 65% of maximum predicted for age was achieved in all subjects, and fast gradient echo acquisitions were used to obtain six short-axis slices at rest and three during stress to estimate the ejection fraction. The stress images were acquired during a 6–8-second breathhold during temporary suspension of exercise. The ejection fraction rose from 55 to 62% in normals, but remained at 44% in patients with coronary artery disease; however, scan quality was not sufficient to allow regional wall motion analysis. These ejection fraction response differences are compatible with the findings long established in the nuclear cardiology literature (20). These results are encouraging, and suggest that there may be a happy marriage between exercise and ultrafast imaging; however, improvements in image resolution are necessary and direct comparisons need to be made with the pharmacological techniques in the induction of ischemia.

Alternatives to Dynamic Exercise

A number of stress techniques other than exercise have been used for the diagnosis of coronary artery disease, and these might be considered for stress in the magnet. Isometric exercise using the hand dynamometer is pos-

sible; however, the results of its use are unimpressive and muscle fatigue rapidly occurs. Atrial pacing is useful for invasive stress studies, but intracardiac electrodes are unsuitable for MRI. Transoesophageal pacing during MRI in animals has been developed (21), but very little has been attempted in humans (22). Cold pressor stress is impractical because of the difficulties of using iced water in the scanner and the capricious results with its use. Mental stress requires considerable patient cooperation and, together with the small changes observed, it, too, does not appear suitable. The most suitable alternative to exercise, therefore, is the use of pharmacological stress.

The vasodilator dipyridamole has been widely studied. Its mechanism of action in raising interstitial levels of adenosine is shown in Table 31.1. It is simple to administer in a 4-minute infusion of 0.56 mg/kg, and causes an increase in human coronary flow of up to six times baseline (23), with a half life of 30 minutes (24). In the presence of significant coronary stenoses, myocardial flow heterogeneity that can be detected by perfusion techniques occurs. Reduction in perfusion pressure distal to a stenosis, reduction in collateral flow, and redistribution of flow from subendocardium to subepicardium can cause ischemia and wall motion abnormalities (25), which can be detected by MRI. Adenosine at 140 μg/kg/min may also be given for a direct effect and it causes similar changes in coronary flow (26). Its side effects are shorter lived because of its half life of only 4 seconds, but it may be less effective in producing wall motion abnormalities (27,28). It is very useful for perfusion studies, and its mode of action is shown in Figure 31.2.

The β agonists may be used for cardiac imaging, but of those presently available only dobutamine produces hemodynamic effects similar to exercise, with a low arrhythmogenicity and good tolerance to peripheral vein infusion that makes it the most suitable for human use (other unsuitable agents for humans, such as isoproterenol, have been used in combination with MRI in animals for stress testing) (29). Dobutamine may be used for perfusion (30,31) and wall motion imaging (32) in doses up to 40 μg/kg/min. It has been shown to increase myocardial oxygen demand and, in the setting of acute ischemia, to increase oxygen demand above availability (33). It also dilates the distal coronary vessels which leads to an increase in coronary flow (34,35) and a fall in perfusion pressure distal to coronary stenoses. Flow therefore becomes heterogeneous (36) and may be redirected to the subepicardium (37). Dobutamine may also increase flow resistance at the site of a stenosis (37).

Both dipyridamole and dobutamine have been used for stress wall motion imaging by MRI. Dobutamine, however, has a number of advantages in the magnet, including operator controlled level of stress, a short half life of 120 seconds, physiological effects mimicking exercise more closely than dipyridamole, and stress-induced tachycardia which considerably shortens the stress imaging period when conventional MRI techniques are used.

Table 31.1. The alternatives to dynamic exercise for cardiac stress. Only the pharmacological techniques are presently suitable for clinical use in the magnet.

Form	Type	Comment
Isometric exercise		Useful in the magnet but causes rapid fatigue
Atrial pacing		Mainly confined to animal experiments
Cold pressor		Unwieldy for use in the magnet, and unreliable
Mental stress		Possible cardiac application, but more likely to be used for functional brain studies
Pharmacological	*Vasodilator*	
	Dipyridamole	Long acting
	Adenosine	Short acting
	Vasoconstrictor	
	Ergonovine	Research and invasive applications only
	Beta agonists	
	Dobutamine	Good tolerance makes this ideal for clinical inotropic stress

Pharmacological Stress in the Magnet

Dipyridamole MR Wall Motion Imaging

The first report of stress-induced regional wall motion abnormality in coronary artery disease detected by MRI was by Pennell et al. using dipyridamole at a dose of 0.56 mg/kg with a 10-mg bolus after 10 minutes (38). Gradient-echo cine imaging with velocity compensation at 0.5 T was used in the vertical and horizontal long axes and two short axis planes, with TE 14 msec, flip angle 45 degrees, 16 frames per cycle, and two averages. A follow-up study of this technique was subsequently performed in 40 patients. Despite the fact that 23 of the patients had previous infarction, the authors found only a sensitivity of 67% in the comparison of new wall motion abnormality in addition to any found at rest with areas of reversible ischemia assessed by thallium tomography (Fig. 31.2) (39). The sensitivity for detection of significant coronary artery disease was 62%. The poor sensitivity of detection of disease occurred because of the inability to detect smaller areas of ischemia (Fig. 31.3). The procedure was well tolerated, but side effects from the dipyridamole, both cardiac and noncardiac, were common. Imaging time before and after dipyridamole was 30 and 15–20 minutes, respectively.

In addition to the wall motion changes, a small fall in signal from areas of ischemic myocardium was shown (4% $p < 0.05$). This was visually appreciable in 38% of ischemic segments, but no clear changes were visualized in the majority. The signal changes were not explicable by changes in relaxation times with ischemia because these occur over a longer time frame, nor was it related to hypokinesis that would be expected to increase the myocardial signal. The likeliest explanation was thought to be a reduction in myocardial blood content, and this was supported by the finding of signal loss predominantly in the subendocardium where the most severe ischemia would be expected from the action of dipyridamole.

Further studies using dipyridamole have confirmed that regional wall abnormalities can be induced, although the sensitivity of detection showed some variability. Casolo et al. studied 10 patients at 0.5 T, seven of whom had had previous infarction, and infused 0.7

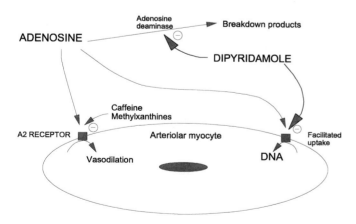

Figure 31.1. Dipyridamole raises interstitial adenosine by blocking its breakdown and facilitating its cellular uptake. The adenosine acts on the A2 receptor to cause vasodilatation. This binding is competitively antagonized by caffeine and aminophylline. Adenosine binds to A2 receptors and is greatly potentiated by oral dipyridamole treatment. The electrophysiological effects of adenosine are mediated by the A1 receptor and include slowed atrioventricular conduction and hyperpolarization of atrial cells.

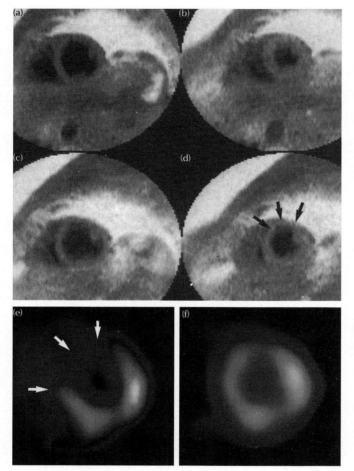

Figure 31.2. (A) Dipyridamole MRI in a patient with LAD artery disease. In the top row are images before dipyridamole with post-dipyridamole images below. End-diastole is on the left and end-systole on the right. Left ventricular contraction is normal prior to vasodilatation, but reduced in the anteroseptal region after dipyridamole. (B) The MRI abnormality is closely matched by the perfusion defect (left) seen during dipyridamole thallium myocardial perfusion tomography, which shows (right) full reversibility. (*From:* Pennell et al., British Heart Journal 1990;64:362–369, with permission from the BMJ Publishing Group.)

mg/kg dipyridamole over 5 minutes with comparison of wall motion changes with Tc^{99m}-MIBI perfusion tomography and angiography (40). Cine gradient-echo imaging with a temporal resolution of 50 msec was used, with a single midventricular short-axis slice. The sensitivity of detection of disease compared to both MIBI scanning and angiography was 100%. Baer et al. have published two studies using dipyridamole wall motion imaging. In the first, a homogeneous group of 23 patients with no resting wall motion abnormality at 1.5 T was studied (41), which allowed a more confident estimation of sensitivity of detection of ischemia in individual arterial territories. Again, cine gradient-echo imaging was used with TE 12 msec, flip angle 30 degrees, and a temporal resolution of 28 msec. Two midventricular short-axis slices were imaged using four repetitions to improve image quality. A dose of 0.75

mg/kg over 10 minutes was used and the overall detection rate of coronary artery disease was 78% compared with angiography. The sensitivity for one- and two-vessel disease was 69% and 90%, respectively. The sensitivity and specificity for each arterial territory are shown in Fig. 31.4. The higher sensitivity of the results compared with Pennell et al. might be explained by the higher dose of dipyridamole used. The side effects from the high dose dipyridamole, however, proved to be problematic. This may have been exacerbated by the mild sedation with valium that was used (U Sechtem, personal communication), which can potentiate the action of dipyridamole (42). In the second study of 33 patients (43), a similar protocol was used with a sensitivity of 84% for detection of coronary artery disease, with agreement between MIBI SPECT and MRI of 90% between segments for abnormality. It is interesting that the specificity dipyridamole MRI was marginally better than MIBI SPECT in the inferior wall abnormalities associated with right coronary artery (RCA) stenosis, (89% vs. 80%), which might reflect the known problems with inferior attenuation in nuclear techniques (44).

A comparison between MRI and transoesophageal echo (TEE) has been performed in 35 patients, of whom 29 had coronary artery disease (45). All patients had been shown to have poor echo windows for transthoracic echocardiography and a nondiagnostic exercise EKG. The sensitivity for detection of disease was 90% for TEE and 83% for MRI (p = NS) with specificity of 100% for both techniques. There was significant correlation between the techniques in a quantitative analysis for wall thickening, but there were a significantly higher number of abnormal chords by MRI than TEE. In addition, 75%

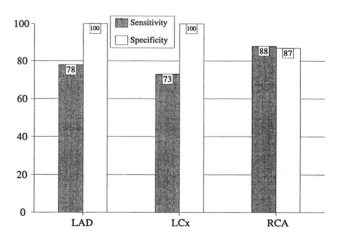

Figure 31.3. Sensitivity and specificity of dipyridamole MRI of wall motion in the detection of coronary artery disease in patients without resting wall motion abnormality. LAD, left anterior descending artery; LCx, left circumflex artery; RCA, right coronary artery. (Reprinted from American Journal of Cardiology, Volume 69, Baer et al., "Feasibility of high dose dipyridamole magnetic resonance imaging for detection of coronary artery disease and comparison with coronary angiography," pages 51–56, copyright 1992, with permission from Excerpta Media, Inc.)

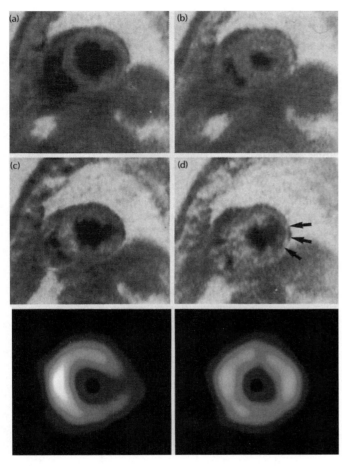

Figure 31.4. (A) Dobutamine MRI of a patient with LC artery disease. The format is the same as in Figure 31.3. Resting contraction is normal, but it is abnormal during dobutamine contraction in the lateral wall, which matches (B) the reversible perfusion defect seen during dobutamine thallium myocardial perfusion tomography. (Reprinted from American Journal of Cardiology, volume number 10, Pennell et al., "Magnetic resonance imaging during dobutamine stress in coronary artery disease," pages 34–40, copyright 1992, with permission from Excerpta Media, Inc.)

of patients indicated that they preferred the MRI to the TEE. Fedele et al. concluded that their results suggested benefit from the higher spatial resolution of MRI combined with its greater patient acceptability.

Finally, attempts to quantify dipyridamole-induced wall motion changes imaged using a breathhold cine technique have been examined (46). Using receiver operating characteristic (ROC) curve analysis, Croisille et al. showed superior results for the quantitative analysis using percent wall thickening as the test parameter. Comparison with thallium myocardial perfusion imaging showed equivalent results that were insensitive but specific (thallium 38%/90% and MRI 40%/91%).

Dobutamine MR Wall Motion Imaging

The first report of the diagnostic use of dobutamine MRI from Pennell et al. showed a considerable improvement

in sensitivity (47) when compared with the results from the same center with dipyridamole in similar patients (39). In 25 patients with coronary artery disease, gradient-echo cine imaging with velocity compensation was used at 0.5 T, with a TE of 14 msec, flip angle 45 degrees at rest, 35 degrees during stress, and 12 frames per cardiac cycle. Cines were once again acquired in the vertical and horizontal long axes and two short-axis planes. Dobutamine was infused up to 20 μg/kg/min, increasing the systolic blood pressure and heart rate, which had the advantage of shortening the imaging time during stress to 10–15 minutes. Of the patients with reversible ischemia identified by dobutamine thallium tomography, 95% had reversible myocardial wall motion abnormalities (Fig. 31.5). This represented a sensitivity for detection of significant coronary artery disease of 91%. There was a close concordance in site and extent of the perfusion and wall motion abnormalities, with 96% agreement at rest, 90% during stress, and 91% for the assessment of reversible ischemia. There were no significant differences between MRI and thallium in the detection or location of coronary stenoses (Fig. 31.6), but determination of specificity was hampered by small patient numbers. In common with the findings with dipyridamole, a small (9.2%) reduction in signal was found in the ischemic segments. Areas of signal reduction were seen in half of the patients with a new wall motion abnormality, but occasional areas of reduced signal were seen in nonischemic segments; therefore, the specificity of signal reduction for ischemia was reduced. The dobutamine was well tolerated overall in the magnet, but cardiac and noncardiac side effects were common; however, imaging proved to contain more artifacts as the heart rate increased. Intraventricular turbulence during ejection occurred, causing intense signal loss in the

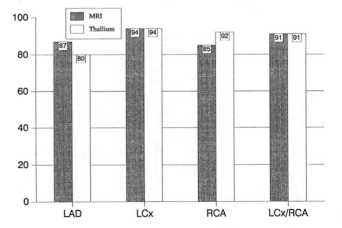

Figure 31.5. Comparison of sensitivity of detection of coronary artery disease by thallium tomography with MRI of wall motion during dobutamine stress. Abbreviations as in Figure 31.5 and LCx/RCA, combined left circumflex and right coronary artery territories. (Reprinted from American Journal of Cardiology, volume number 10, Pennell et al., "Magnetic resonance imaging during dobutamine stress in coronary artery disease," pages 34–40, copyright 1992, with permission from Excerpta Media, Inc.)

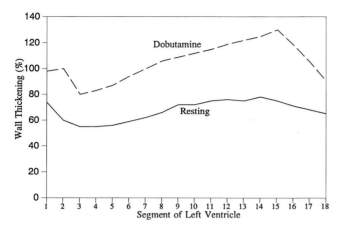

Figure 31.6. Normal wall thickening around the left ventricle at midpapillary muscle level, at rest and during dobutamine infusion measured by MRI. Such graphs may define limits of normality for quantitative analysis of stress wall contraction. Wall thickening was defined as (end-systolic-end-diastolic thickness)/ end-diastolic thickness. (Adapted from van Rugge et al., (48).)

dose of 15 μg/kg/min (48). Imaging was performed at 1.5 T using the cine gradient echo technique with TE 13 msec, flip angle 30 degrees, repetition time 30 msec, and eight short axis slices covering the left ventricle from base to apex. Normal ranges were established using a quantitative analysis for global ventricular function and regional wall thickening during rest and stress in the true short-axis plane. Heterogeneous values for resting wall thickening were found, as has been described using echocardiography, and significant increases in thickening occurred during stress. At rest, greatest thickening occurred at the apex with a decline in wall thickening in slices toward the base; however, the change in wall thickening from baseline with dobutamine stress was greatest at the base, with nonsignificant changes occurring in the apical portion of the left ventricle and the apex. By recording wall thickening in 20 segments around each short-axis slice, the thickening could be displayed graphically to show regional variation, with comparison of rest and dobutamine stress (Fig. 31.7). van Rugge et al. then reported their experience with dobutamine stress wall motion imaging in patients with coronary artery disease, with qualitative (49) and quantitative (50) analyses.

In the qualitative study, the authors examined short-axis cines only, using six slices to cover from base to apex. The imaging parameters were otherwise the same as discussed earlier. Of 45 patients studied, 37 had coronary artery disease and 30 (81%) showed wall motion abnormality with dobutamine stress. The specificity in this series was 100%. The results were better than exercise electrocardiography (70/63%) or dobutamine electrocardiography (51/63%). Single-, double-, and triple-

myocardium, and obliteration of the cavity in the apical short-axis view occurred. A lower echo time was helpful, but some of the stress cines were of low quality.

The results of dobutamine wall motion MRI in patients with coronary artery disease have also been reported by two other European groups. van Rugge et al. have reported their findings in normals and subsequently in patients with coronary artery disease. In 23 normal subjects, dobutamine was given to a maximum

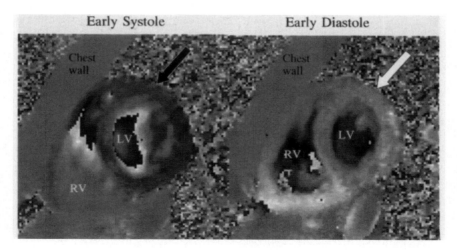

Figure 31.7. Short-axis myocardial velocity maps in early systole (left) and early diastole (right). Midgray represents stationary velocity. The myocardium is relatively thin in early systole and in dark shade (black arrow) representing increased velocities toward the apex. In early diastole the myocardium is thicker with white shading of the myocardium (white arrow), showing recoil toward the base. Aliazing of the ventricular blood velocities occurs be- cause the velocity window is set very low for the myocardium. Regional variations in velocity may be determined from segments around the myocardial circumference. (*From*: Noninvasive assessment of regional left ventricular long axis motion using magnetic resonance velocity mapping in normal subjects. Karwatowski et al., *J Magn Reson Imag*, copyright 1994. Reprinted with permission of Wiley-Liss, Inc., a subsidiary of John Wiley & Sons, Inc.)

vessel disease was detected with 75%, 80%, and 100% sensitivity, respectively. In the quantitative study, 39 patients without rest wall motion abnormality and 10 normal volunteers were stressed with dobutamine to 20 μg/kg/min. A short-axis stress cine that was judged to show wall motion abnormality was analyzed with a modified centerline method. In these preselected cuts, stress wall motion was considered abnormal if four or more adjacent chords (100 encompassed the ventricle) showed systolic wall thickening below 2 SD of that obtained from the normals. This resulted in a 91% sensitivity and a 80% specificity for detection of disease. Single-, double-, and triple-vessel disease was detected with 88%, 91%, and 100% sensitivity, respectively, whereas the sensitivity of detection of individual coronary artery stenosis was 75%, 87%, and 63% for the left anterior descending (LAD), RCA, and left circumflex (LCx) arteries, respectively. No direct comparison of the quantitative and qualitative methods was given to determine if the time-consuming task of endo- and epicardial tracing yielded a significant diagnostic improvement in the same patients; however, the advantages of a quantitative analysis in the reduction of observer variability are clear and the approach is laudible. Further questions needing to be answered concerning this approach include whether the quantification is significantly disturbed by the presence of resting wall motion abnormalities.

Baer et al. have also studied the role of dobutamine MRI of wall motion. In one study of 28 patients with coronary artery disease, but without previous infarction (51), imaging was performed at 1.5 T, with a gradient echo sequence with an echo-time (TE) of 12 msec and a flip angle of 30 degrees and a peak dobutamine dose of 20 μg/kg/min. Although the peak rate pressure product was lower during dobutamine MRI than exercise electrocardiography, the relative sensitivities were 85% and 77%. Single and multivessel disease was detected with 73% and 100% sensitivity, respectively. The sensitivity and specificity for detection of disease in the individual arteries was 87/100% in the LAD, 78/88% for the RCA, and 62/93% for the LCx arteries. In another study of 35 consecutive patients with coronary artery disease, comparison was made between dobutamine MRI and MIBI SPECT (52). The sensitivity of MRI and SPECT was 84% and 87%, respectively, for the detection of disease. Comparison of the detection of individual artery ischemia was very similar between the techniques, clearly indicating that MRI could be successfully used in the assessment of disease in comparison with a well-established clinical standard.

All three groups who have studied wall motion during dobutamine stress now report good results with excellent patient tolerance. The main problem with the current studies has been that they last too long and they need to be repeated using breathhold fast MRI. Comparison with thallium imaging and stress electrocardiography shows excellent correlation with the former, and significant improvement over the latter. In addition, the combination of perfusion and wall motion in the same dobutamine stress MR study has also been evaluated with good results (53).

Dobutamine MR Myocardial Velocity Imaging

The steady-state hemodynamics generated by infusion of dobutamine allows imaging of other aspects of cardiac function during stress using conventional imaging techniques with longer image acquisition times. Karwatowski et al. have studied ventricular long-axis motion before and after dobutamine stress in normal subjects (54) and in patients with coronary artery disease (55). Long-axis motion of the left ventricle is thought to be a particularly sensitive indicator of contractile dysfunction because the myocardial fibres in the subendocardium are aligned longitudinally and the subendocardium is the first portion of the myocardium to be affected by reduced perfusion (56). The technique uses velocity mapping of the myocardium in the short-axis plane just below the mitral annulus, with through-plane velocity sensitization (0.3–0.5 m/second) to measure the long axis velocities (Fig. 31.8). Karwatowski et al. defined normal long-axis dynamics in 31 normal subjects (54). The peak velocity of long-axis motion always occurred in early diastole, and significant heterogeneity occurred around the ventricular wall with greatest ve-

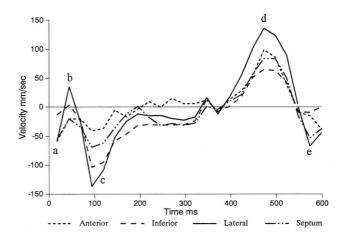

Figure 31.8. Regional myocardial velocity can be represented in graphical form to illustrate quantitative and regional abnormalities. Point (a) represents displacement of the heart with shape change, (b) isovolumic contraction prior to the descent of the base toward the apex in systole, (c) peak systolic long-axis velocity followed by rapid motion of the base away from the apex, (d) peak early diastolic velocity, and (e) brief period of movement back toward the base. Measurements of peak diastolic timing of velocity are made at point (d). (*From:* Noninvasive assessment of regional left ventricular long axis motion using magnetic resonance velocity mapping in normal subjects. Karwatowski et al., *J Magn Reson Imag,* copyright 1994. Reprinted with permission of Wiley-Liss, Inc., a subsidiary of John Wiley & Sons, Inc.)

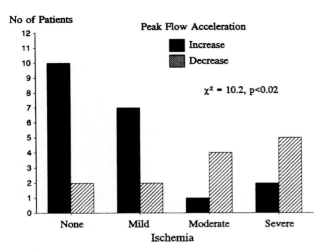

Figure 31.9. Peak flow acceleration usually increases during dobutamine stress. This may occur even in patients with mild ischemia, but there is an increasing likelihood that peak flow acceleration falls as ischemia becomes more severe, which is a significant finding of global contraction depression.

locities in the lateral wall. A mean figure for long-axis velocity was generated by considering the myocardial slice as a whole, and regional velocities were calculated by dividing the slice into 16 segments. These can be displayed graphically as shown in Figure 31.9.

Following this study of normals, Karwatowski et al. also studied nine normal subjects and 25 patients with coronary artery disease before and during dobutamine stress (55). The study concentrated on diastolic function because highest long-axis velocities occur at this time, and abnormalities of left ventricular function during ischemia may occur first in diastole (57). Diastolic function was assessed by measuring the time to peak early diastolic velocity, as well as the mean velocity of the myocardium, and the maximum and minimum regional segment velocity at this time point. The time to peak diastolic velocity decreased in both normals and patients from baseline to low-dose dobutamine (5–7.5 μg/kg/min), and from low- to high-dose dobutamine (10–15 μg/kg/min). The mean long axis velocity increased in the normals with low-dose dobutamine and remained elevated with the high dose. In the patients with reversible ischemia, however, 62% developed a reduced mean long-axis velocity. Those with previous infarction but no reversible ischemia behaved similarly to normals. Regional changes in long-axis velocity were also examined. In the normals, regional long-axis velocity increased with low-dose dobutamine, but some reduction was seen with high-dose, particularly in the inferoseptal wall. In patients with reversible ischemia, 62% developed abnormal regional velocities with dobutamine. Overall, 67% of patients with reversible ischemia had an abnormal global or regional response to stress. The

patients with anterior ischemia were more likely to develop abnormal velocity values during stress because of the greater contribution to mean myocardial long-axis velocity from these segments; therefore, there was a lower sensitivity for uncovering inferior ischemia.

Technical advances have now introduced new methods for the acquisition of myocardial velocity data that might prove useful. Segmented phase–contrast gradient-echo imaging permits acquisition of myocardial velocities within a period of a breathhold with high resolution. This improves image quality and significantly reduces velocity artifacts from respiratory motion (58). In addition, some interesting work from Arai et al. has been presented where components of velocity accounting for rigid body movement of the heart (translation and rotation) are calculated from short-axis myocardial velocity maps and then subtracted to yield velocity maps showing pure radial velocity in systole and diastole (59). These uncontaminated myocardial velocity maps might be useful for stress imaging in the quantification of myocardial mechanics. Using myocardial velocities has been suggested as an alternative to myocardial tagging (60,61), and, in addition, strain rate can be derived from the myocardial velocity data (62). There are no reports of stress studies to date.

Dobutamine MR Assessment of Global Ventricular Function

Dobutamine infusion also allows the measurement of aortic flow during stress by MRI velocity mapping. Absolute flow is measured from simultaneous area and velocity measurements of the ascending aorta yield. By also measuring the heart rate and blood pressure during stress, the stroke volume, cardiac output, aortic acceleration, cardiac power output, and flow wave velocity may be calculated. Pennell et al. have studied normal subjects and patients with coronary artery disease (63) to determine which parameters were predictive of the extent of reversible myocardial ischemia.

In normals, an increase in all parameters was seen with dobutamine stress, except for the stroke volume that rose and then fell, and the diastolic blood pressure that remained unchanged. In patients with coronary artery disease, the qualitative pattern of change in parameters was similar, except that a fall in peak flow acceleration at peak stress was found to occur significantly more frequently in patients with moderate and severe ischemia than in patients with mild or no ischemia (Fig. 31.10). The quantitative change from baseline to peak stress in five parameters was significantly related to the extent of myocardial ischemia (i.e., peak flow acceleration, peak flow, cardiac power output, maximum dobutamine dose tolerated, and systolic blood pressure). Using multivariate analysis, the peak flow acceleration was

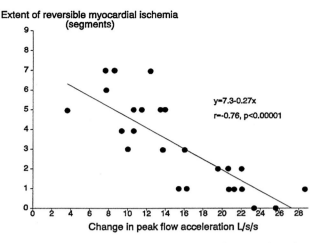

Figure 31.10. The change in peak flow acceleration from baseline to peak stress is inversely related to the extent of reversible myocardial ischemia (maximum number of segments was nine); therefore, it can be used as an assessment of global burden of ischemia on ventricular function during stress.

found to be the most predictive variable ($p < 0.00001$), and alone explained 58.4% of the variation in the observed myocardial ischemia. Only the cardiac power output retained predictive significance after allowing for the peak flow acceleration, but its contribution to the predictive accuracy of the model was small (4.2%). Attempts to reproduce this type of study using exercise have now been reported (15,64).

This study showed that an assessment of global ventricular function by MRI could be performed during dobutamine stress. There have been very few other attempts to study stress global function, which is surprising bearing in mind that it is standard practice with radionuclide ventriculography; however, the aortic flow MRI technique is unable to measure the ejection fraction. The ejection fraction, however, has been reported in stress wall motion studies. With dipyridamole, Pennell et al. found a nonsignificant difference between ischemic and nonischemic patients (+1% vs. +3%) (39). Pennell et al. also showed a significant reduction in ejection fraction during ischemia using dobutamine in patients only (−6.1%), accompanied by reductions in ventricular volumes and stroke volumes (47). Dobutamine has also been shown to increase ejection fraction in normals (48). Further work in this area would be useful.

Dobutamine Myocardial Viability Assessment

Although viability is not normally considered in the confines of stress imaging, the use of dobutamine or other inotropes to increase regional contraction in hibernating myocardium transiently is diagnostic (65), and of clinical value using echocardiography (66). The technique can also be performed using stress MRI (67),

and more reports are surfacing of its value, bearing in mind the common problem with echocardiography of poor image quality that makes the interpretation of the stress tests difficult with poor reproducibility (68). The most significant work was performed by Baer et al. (67), in which dobutamine MRI was compared with fluorodeoxyglucose (FDG) PET. The authors showed that the end-diastolic wall thickness predicted FDG uptake in chronic infarction, and that the addition of dobutamine added further sensitivity. Dendale studied patients with acute myocardial infarction in comparison with stress echocardiography (69), and showed an 81% concordance between the techniques and correctly predicted the evolution of wall motion with revascularization.

There have been reports of the use of myocardial tagging for the definition of viability. This is important because it allows a quantified approach to the assessment of ischemia. Sayad et al. used tagging to examine wall thickening and showed that a dobutamine contractile reserve was present in 89% of hibernating segments, but also in only 7% of nonhibernating segments (70). Using tagging to evaluate percent segmental shortening, Cubukcu et al. showed that postrevascularization improvement in wall motion was present in 79% of arterial territories in which dobutamine elicited an improvement (mean change 9.5–14.7% with stress) (71). This was also shown by Kramer et al., who used a threshold for a positive response to dobutamine of more than 3% in circumferential shortening. The responders increased shortening from 8 to 16% ($p < 0.001$) 8 weeks after acute MI, whereas the nonresponder had no significant increase (9–11%, $p = NS$) (72). Comparison of dobutamine tagging MR and echocardiography in preliminary studies has suggested that the quantitative MR approach is more sensitive [78% vs. 67% from Shigeru (73), and 73% vs. 53% from Isao (74)].

Choice of Pharmacological Agent

It is likely that the role of pharmacological vasodilatation and stress in the magnet will grow for the functional assessment of heart disease. This will require familiarity of the strengths of each technique and the important contraindications (75,76). The vasodilators should not be administered to asthmatics because of the risk of provocation of severe bronchospasm (77,78). Adenosine infusion in sinoatrial disease may lead to sinus arrest, and should also be avoided (79). Caffeine is a competitive antagonist of adenosine and should be avoided for at least 12 hours prior to scanning or attenuated vasodilatation will occur. The contraindications to dobutamine are the same as for dynamic exercise. Dobutamine is competitively antagonized by β-blockers. The longer-acting of these should be stopped 48 hours prior to imaging. This may occasionally lead to withdrawal angina and the patients need to be warned of this possibility. Some studies of wall motion suggest that cessation of β blockade may be unnecessary (32), but there is no consensus on this issue (80,81), with others showing that additional atropine is important in maintaining sensitivity when the heart rate response is attenuated (82). The vasodilators remain first-choice agents for studies of myocardial perfusion and coronary flow because dobutamine causes less coronary hyperemia (25), and the induced tachycardia causes problems with temporal resolution. Dobutamine is better suited to wall motion and global ventricular studies (25) whereas myocardial ischemia is more reliably provoked by increased myocardial oxygen demand.

Conclusions

There are a number of MRI stress techniques being developed that will be direct competitors with scintigraphic techniques for the evaluation of reversible myocardial ischemia. The most well developed is wall motion imaging that has been performed in a number of centers using both dipyridamole and dobutamine. This technique is analogous to stress echocardiography, but MRI has the inherent advantage of better resolution, and true long- and short-axis imaging with contiguous parallel slices. The results in comparison with myocardial perfusion imaging are reasonable, especially with dobutamine, but all the studies reported to date have been conducted in patients with a very high pretest likelihood of disease and much more intense scrutiny in patient populations with intermediate and low pretest risk are necessary before a confident and clinically robust investigation can be envisaged. A simple and rapid technique for quantification of wall motion would greatly help clinical use. The other techniques described earlier are more experimental at present. Long-axis velocity imaging and aortic flow imaging during dobutamine stress have only been performed in one center and their overall sensitivity needs further evaluation. They therefore remain speculative. Myocardial perfusion imaging by MRI is very attractive because of the lack of ionizing radiation, despite the need for intravenous cannulae (probably in a central vein or right atrium for quantitative work) and a contrast agent injection. Although FLASH imaging has been used by most investigators to date, coverage of the entire ventricle is difficult with this technique and multislice echo-planar imaging may be necessary in the clinical arena (83). Exercise stress in the magnet remains difficult despite some modest success, and many patients fail to exercise fully because of physical or psychological reasons, and therefore there is every likelihood that pharmacological stress will continue to be the technique of choice for stress MRI in the long term.

References

1. Master AM, Oppenheimer ET. A simple exercise tolerance test for circulatory efficiency with standard tables for normal individuals. Am J Med Sci 1929;177:223–42.
2. Gianrossi R, Detrano R, Mulvihill D, et al. Exercise induced ST depression in the diagnosis of coronary artery disease: a meta-analysis. Circulation 1989;80:87–98.
3. Abouantoun A, Ahnve S, Savvides M, Witztum K, Jensen D, Froelicher V. Can areas of myocardial ischemia be localised by the exercise electrocardiogram? a correlative study with thallium-201 scintigraphy. Am Heart J 1984;108:933–41.
4. Nesto RW, Kowalchuk GJ. The ischemic cascade: temporal sequence of hemodynamic, electrocardiographic and symptomatic expressions of ischemia. Am J Cardiol 1987;57:23C–30C.
5. Pennell DJ, Prvulovich E. Nuclear cardiology: clinician's guide. London: British Nuclear Medicine Society, 1995.
6. Zoghbi WA. Use of adenosine echocardiography for diagnosis of coronary artery disease. Am Heart J 1991;122:285–92.
7. Ladenheim ML, Pollock BH, Rozanski A, et al. Extent and severity of myocardial hypoperfusion as predictors of prognosis in patients with suspected coronary artery disease. J Am Coll Cardiol 1986;7:464–71.
8. Iskandrian AS, Chae SC, Heo J, Stanberry CD, Wasserleben V, Cave V. Independent and incremental prognostic value of exercise single photon emission computed tomography (SPECT) thallium imaging in coronary artery disease. J Am Coll Cardiol 1993;22:665–70.
9. Brown KA. Prognostic value of thallium-201 myocardial perfusion imaging. A diagnostic tool comes of age. Circulation 1991;83:363–81.
10. Fattah AA, Kamal AM, Pancholy S, Ghods M, Russel J, Cassel D, et al. Prognostic implications of normal exercise tomographic thallium images in patients with angiographic evidence of significant coronary artery disease. Am J Cardiol 1994;74:769–71.
11. Baer FM, Voth E, Schneider CA, Theissen P, Schicha H, Sechtem U. Comparison of low dose dobutamine gradient echo magnetic resonance imaging and positron emission tomography with fluorodeoxyglucose in patients with chronic coronary artery disease. A functional and morphological approach to the detection of residual myocardial viability. Circulation 1995;91:1006–15.
12. Frazier OH, Cooley DA, Kadipasaoglu KA, Pehlivanoglu S, Lindenmeir M, Barasch E, et al. Myocardial revascularisation with laser: preliminary findings. Circulation 1995;92(Suppl. II): 58–65.
13. Cayton M, Wang Y, Klassen C, Unress M, Campson C, Wann SL, Mirhoseni M. Transmyocardial laser revascularisation protects ischemic tissue: quantitative treatment monitoring with MRI (abstr.). Proc Int Soc Magn Reson Med 1996.
14. Schaefer S, Peshock RM, Parkey RW, Willerson JT. A new device for exercise MR imaging. Am J Roentgenol 1986;147:1289–90.

15. Mohiaddin RH, Gatehouse PD, Firmin DN. Exercise related changes in aortic flow measured by magnetic resonance spiral echo-planar phase-shift velocity mapping. J Magn Reson Imag 1994; (in press).

16. Conway MA, Bristow JD, Blackledge MJ, Rajagopalan B, Radda GK. Cardiac metabolism during exercise in healthy volunteers measured by ^{31}P magnetic resonance spectroscopy. Br Heart J 1991;65:25–30.

17. Gatehouse PD, Firmin DN, Collins S, Longmore DB. Real time blood flow imaging by spiral scan phase velocity mapping. Magn Reson Med 1994;31:504–12.

18. Scheidegger MB, Stuber M, Pederson EM, Koxerke S, Boesiger P. Methodological and technical aspects of physiological (ergometer) stress for cardiovascular examinations in MR scanners (abstract). Proc Int Soc Magn Reson Med 1997;899.

19. Oshinski JN, Ferichs F, Doyle JA, Dixon WT, de Boer R, Pettigrew RI. Exercise stress measurements of cardiac performance using an MR compatible cycle ergometer (abstr.). Proc Int Soc Magn Reson Med 1997;900.

20. Udelson JE, Leppo JA. Single photon myocardial perfusion imaging and exercise radionuclide angiography in the detection of coronary artery disease. In: Murray IPC, Ell PJ, eds. Nuclear medicine in clinical diagnosis and management. Churchill Livingstone, 1994, 1129–56.

21. Hofman MBM, de Cock C, van der Linden JC, van Rossum AC, Visser FC, Sprenger M. Transesophageal cardiac pacing during magnetic resonance imaging: feasibility and safety considerations. Magn Reson Med 1996;35:413–22.

22. Jadvar H, Gober J, Schaefer S, Schwartz G, Weiner M, Massie GB. Esophageal pacing: Potential utility of esophageal pacing during cardiac magnetic resonance studies. Med Electron 1989;10:134–36.

23. Wilson RF, Laughlin DE, Ackell PH, Chilian WM, Holida MD, Hartley CJ, et al. Transluminal, subselective measurement of coronary artery blood flow velocity and vasodilator reserve in man. Circulation 1985;72:82–92.

24. Brown G, Josephson MA, Petersen RD, Pierce CD, Wong M, Hecht HS et al. Intravenous dipyridamole combined with isometric handgrip for near maximal coronary flow in patients with coronary artery disease. Am J Cardiol 1981;48:1077–85.

25. Fung AY, Gallagher KP, Buda AJ. The physiological basis of dobutamine as compared with dipyridamole stress interventions in the assessment of critical coronary stenosis. Circulation 1987;76:943–51.

26. Wilson RF, Wyche K, Christensen BV, Zimmer S, Laxson DD. Effects of adenosine on human coronary arterial circulation. Circulation 1990; 82:1595–606.

27. Zoghbi WA, Cheirif J, Kleiman NS, Verani MS, Trakhtenbroit A. Diagnosis of ischemic heart disease with adenosine echocardiography. J Am Coll Cardiol 1991;18:1271–79.

28. Nguyen T, Heo J, Ogilby D, Iskandrian AS. Single photon emission computed tomography with thallium-201 during adenosine induced coronary hyperaemia: correlation with coronary arteriography, exercise thallium imaging and two-dimensional echocardiography. J Am Coll Cardiol 1990;16:1375–83.

29. Pettigrew RI, Martin S, Eisner R, Oh D, Leyendecker J, Schmarkey S, et al. Detection of partial coronary artery stenosis with isoproterenol stress cine MRI in dogs: Vali-

dation by on-line ultrasonic crystals and flow probes (abstr.). Proc Soc Magn Reson Med 1991;243.

30. Pennell DJ, Underwood SR, Swanton RH, Walker JM, Ell PJ. Dobutamine thallium myocardial perfusion tomography. J Am Coll Cardiol 1991;18:1471–79.

31. Pennell DJ, Underwood SR, Ell PJ. Safety of dobutamine stress for thallium myocardial perfusion tomography in patients with asthma. Am J Cardiol 1993;71:1346–50.

32. Sawada SG, Segar DS, Ryan T, Brown SE, Dohan AM, Williams R, et al. Echocardiographic detection of coronary artery disease during dobutamine infusion. Circulation 1991;83:1605–14.

33. Willerson JT, Hutton I, Watson JT, Platt MR, Templeton GH. Influence of dobutamine on regional myocardial blood flow and ventricular performance during acute and chronic myocardial ischemia in dogs. Circulation 1976;53: 828–33.

34. Vasu MA, O'Keefe DD, Kapellakis GZ, Vezeridis MP, Jacobs ML, Daggett WM, et al. Myocardial oxygen consumption: effects of epinephrine, isoproterenol, dopamine, norepinephrine and dobutamine. Am J Physiol 1978;235: 237–41.

35. Fowler MB, Alderman EL, Oesterle SN, Derby G, Daughters GT, Stinson EB, et al. Dobutamine and dopamine after cardiac surgery: greater augmentation of myocardial blood flow with dobutamine. Circulation 1984;70(Suppl. I):103–11.

36. Meyer SL, Curry GC, Donsky MS, Twieg DB, Parkey RW, Willerson JT. Influence of dobutamine on hemodynamics and coronary blood flow in patients with and without coronary artery disease. Am J Cardiol 1976;38:103–8.

37. Warltier DC, Zyvlowski M, Gross GJ, Hardman HF, Brooks HL. Redistribution of myocardial blood flow distal to a dynamic coronary arterial stenosis by sympathomimetic amines: comparison of dopamine, dobutamine and isoproterenol. Am J Cardiol 1981;48:269–79.

38. Pennell DJ, Underwood SR, Longmore DB. The detection of coronary artery disease by magnetic resonance imaging using intravenous dipyridamole. JCAT 1990;14:167–70.

39. Pennell DJ, Underwood SR, Ell PJ, Swanton RH, Walker JM, Longmore DB. Dipyridamole magnetic resonance imaging: a comparison with thallium-201 emission tomography. Br Heart J 1990;64:362–69.

40. Casolo GC, Bonechi F, Taddei T, Fortini A, Dabizzi RP, Bisi, et al. Alterations in dipyridamole induced LV wall motion during myocardial ischemia studied by NMR imaging: comparison with Tc-99m-MIBI myocardial scintigraphy. G Ital Cardiol 1991;21:609–17.

41. Baer FM, Smolarz K, Jungehulsing M, Theissen P, Sechtem U, Schicha H, et al. Feasibility of high dose dipyridamole magnetic resonance imaging for detection of coronary artery disease and comparison with coronary angiography. Am J Cardiol 1992;69:51–56.

42. Kanekin TP. The potentiation of cardiac responses to adenosine by benzodiazepines. J Pharmacol Exp Ther 1982;222:752–58.

43. Baer FM, Smolarz K, Theissen P, et al. Identification of haemodynamically significant coronary stenoses by dipyridamole magnetic resonance imaging and 99mTc methoxyisobutyl-isonitrile SPECT. Int J Card Imag 1993;9: 133–45.

44. Perault C, Loboguerrero A, Liehn JC, Wampach H, Gibold C, Ouzan J. Quantitative comparison of prone and supine myocardial SPECT MIBI images. Clin Nucl Med 1995;20: 678–84.

45. Fedele F, Rosaanio S, Tocchi M, di Renzi P, Trambaiolo P, Cacciotti L, et al. Comparison of cine magnetic resonance imaging and multiplane transesophageal echocardiography during dipyridamole stress for detecting coronary artery disease: qualitative and quantitative analysis (abstr.). Circulation 1996;94:I–180.

46. Croisille P, Zhao S, Janier M, Roux JP, Plana A, Revel D. Dipyridamole stress breath-hold cine MRI in patients with severe coronary artery stenosis: comparison between qualitative and quantitative wall motion analyses (abstr.). Proc Int Soc Magn Reson Med 1997;389.

47. Pennell DJ, Underwood SR, Manzara CC, Ell PJ, Swanton RH, Walker JM, et al. Magnetic resonance imaging during dobutamine stress in coronary artery disease. Am J Cardiol 1992;70;34–40.

48. van Rugge FP, Holman ER, van der Wall EE, de Roos A, van der Laarse A, Bruschke AVG. Quantitation of global and regional left ventricular function by cine magnetic resonance imaging during dobutamine stress in normal human subjects. Eur Heart J 1993;14:456–63.

49. van Rugge P, van der Wall EE, de Roos A, Bruschke AVG. Dobutamine stress magnetic resonance imaging for detection of coronary artery disease. J Am Coll Cardiol 1993; 22:431–39.

50. van Rugge FP, van der wall EE, Spanjersberg SJ, et al. Magnetic resonance imaging during dobutamine stress for detection and localisation of coronary artery disease: quantitative wall motion analysis using a modification of the centerline method. Circulation 1994;90:127–38.

51. Baer FM, Voth E, Theissen P, Schicha H, Sechtem U. Gradient echo magnetic resonance imaging during incremental dobutamine infusion for the localisation of coronary artery stenosis. Eur Heart J 1994;15:218–25.

52. Baer FM, Voth E, Theissen P, Schneider CA, Schicha H, Sechtem U. Coronary artery disease: findings with GRE MR imaging and Tc-99m-methoxyisobutyl-isonitrile SPECT during simultaneous dobutamine stress. Radiology 1994; 193:203–9.

53. Hartnell G, Cerel A, Kamalesh M, et al. Detection of myocardial ischemia: value of combined myocardial perfusion and cineangiographic MR imaging. Am J Roentgenol 1994; 163:1061–67.

54. Karwatowski SP, Mohiaddin RH, Yang GZ, et al. Noninvasive assessment of regional left ventricular long axis motion using magnetic resonance velocity mapping in normal subjects. J Magn Reson Imag 1994;4:151–55.

55. Karwatowski SP, Forbat SM, Mohiaddin RH, Cronos NA, Yang GZ, Firmin DN, et al. Regional left ventricular long axis function in controls and patients with ischaemic heart disease pre and post angioplasty (abstr.) Circulation 1993;88(Suppl): I–83.

56. Jones CJH, Raposo L, Gibson DG. Functional importance of the long axis dynamics of the left ventricle. Br Heart J 1990;63:215–20.

57. Reduto LA, Wickermeyer WJ, Young JB, et al. Left ventricular diastolic performance at rest and during exercise in patients with coronary artery disease: assessment with first pass radionuclide ventriculography. Circulation 1981; 63:1228–37.

58. Hennig J, Markl M, Peschl S, Schmialek A, Schneider B, Krause T, et al. Measurement of myocardial wall motion with segmented breath-hold phase contrast gradient echo imaging (abstr.). Proc Int Soc Magn Reson Med 1997;390.

59. Arai AE, Gaither CC, Epstein FH, Balaban RS, Wolff SD. Velocity gradient of phase contrast MRI to quantify regional contractile abnormalities with myocardial infarction (abstr.). Proc Int Soc Magn Reson Med 1997;384.

60. Ligamenei A, Hardy PA, Powell KA, Pelc NJ, White RD. Validation of cine phase contrast MR imaging for motion analysis. J Magn Reson Imag 1995;5:331–38.

61. Pelc NJ, Drangova M, Pelc LR, Zhu Y, Noll DC, Bowman BS. Tracking of cyclic motion with phase contrast cine MR velocity data. J Magn Reson Imag 1995;5:339–45.

62. Wedeed VJ. Magnetic resonance imaging of myocardial kinematics: techniques to detect, localise and quantify the strain rates of active human myocardium. Magn Reson Med 1992;27:52–67.

63. Pennell DJ, Underwood SR, Manzara CC, Mohiaddin RH, Firmin DN, Poole-Wilson PA. The assessment of aortic flow and acceleration during dobutamine stress by magnetic resonance imaging (abstr.). Eur Heart J (Suppl.) 1990;11a:26.

64. Niezen RA, Doornbos J, de Boer RW, van der Wall EE, de Roos A. Great vessel flow studies with MRI at rest and during physical exercise (abstr.). Proc Int Soc Magn Reson Med 1997;867.

65. Schulz R, Guth BD, Pieper K, Martin C, Heuisch G. Recruitment of an inotropic reserve in moderately ischemic myocardium at the expense of metabolic recovery. A model of short term hibernation. Circ Res 1992;70:1282–95.

66. Alfridi I, Kleiman NS, Raizner AE, Zoghbi WA. Dobutamine echocardiography in myocardial hibernation. Optimal dose and accuracy in predicting recovery of ventricular function after coronary angioplasty. Circulation 1995;91:663–70.

67. Baer FM, Voth E, Schneider CA, Theissen P, Schicha H, Sechtem U. Comparison of low dose dobutamine gradient echo magnetic resonance imaging and positron emission tomography with fluorodeoxyglucose in patients with chronic coronary artery disease. A functional and morphological approach to the detection of residual myocardial viability. Circulation 1995;91:1006–15.

68. Hoffman R, Lethen H, Marwick T, Arnese M, Fioretti P, Pingitore A, et al. Analysis of interinstitutional observer agreement in interpretation of dobutamine stress echocardiograms. J Am Coll Cardiol 1996;27:330–36.

69. Dendale PAC, Franken PR, Waldman GJ, Demoor DGE, Tombeur DAM, Block PFC, et al. Low-dosage dobutamine magnetic resonance imaging as an alternative to echocardiography in the detection of viable myocardium after acute infarction. Am Heart J 1995;130:134–40.

70. Sahad DE, Willett DL, Hundley WG, Grayburn PA, Peshock RM. Dobutamine magnetic resonance imaging with myocardial tagging predicts quantitative improvement in regional function after revascularisation (abstr.). Circulation 1995;92(Suppl.):I–507.

71. Cubukcu AA, Ridgway JP, Sivanathan UM, Cooke A, Nair UR, Tan LB. Detection of contractile reserve by tagged MRI during low dose dobutamine infusion (abstr.). Circulation 1995;92(Suppl.):I–508.

72. Kramer CM, Geskin G, Rogers WJ, Theobald TM, Hu YL, Reichek N. Assessment of myocardial viability after reperfused first infarction by low dose dobutamine MR tagging (abstr.). Proc Int Soc Magn Reson Med 1997;387.

73. Shigeru W, Isao S, Miharu U, et al. Detection of viable myocardium by tagging with magnetic resonance imaging during dobutamine infusion in patients with acute myocardial infarction (abstr.). Circulation 1996;94(Suppl.): I-540.

74. Isao S, Shigeru W, Yoshiaki M. Detection of hibernation myocardium by tagging with dobutamine stress MRI by automatic trace method (abstr.). Proc Int Soc Magn Reson Med 1997;897.

75. Pennell DJ. Cardiac stress in nuclear medicine. *In:* Nuclear medicine in clinical diagnosis and management. Murray IPC, Ell PJ, eds. London: Churchill Livingstone, 1994.

76. Pennell DJ. Pharmacological cardiac stress: when and how? Nuc Med Commun 1994;15:578–85.

77. Homma S, Gilliland Y, Guiney TE, Strauss H, Boucher CA. Safety of intravenous dipyridamole for stress testing with thallium imaging. Am J Cardiol 1987;59:152–54.

78. Taviot B, Pavheco Y, Coppere B, Pirollet B, Rebaudet P, Perrin-Fayolle M. Bronchospasm induced in an asthmatic by the injection of adenosine. Presse Med 1986;15:1103.

79. Pennell DJ, Mahmood S, Ell PJ, Underwood SR. Bradycardia progressing to cardiac arrest during adenosine thallium myocardial perfusion imaging in covert sino-atrial disease. Eur J Nucl Med 1994;21:170–72.

80. Weissman NJ, Levangie MW, Newell JB, Guerrero JL, Weyman AE, Picard MH. Effect of beta-adrenergic receptor blockade on the physiologic response to dobutamine stress echocardiography. Am Heart J 1995;130;248–53.

81. Weissman NJ, Levangie MW, Guerrero JL, Weyman AE, Picard MH. Effect of beta-blockade on dobutamine stress echocardiography. Am Heart J 1996;131:698–703.

82. Fioretti P, Poldermans D, Salustri A, et al. Atropine increases the accuracy of dobutamine stress echocardiography in patients taking beta blockers. Eur Heart J 1994;15: 355–60.

83. Edelman RR, Li W. Contrast enhanced echo planar MR imaging of myocardial perfusion: preliminary study in humans. Radiology 1994;190:771–77.

32
Conclusions

André J. Duerinckx

Many questions about the future technical developments in coronary magnetic resonance angiography (MRA) are still unanswered (1,2). In 1996 the questions were as follows (1): Will the best coronary MRA technique require a two-dimensional (2-D), a three-dimensional (3-D), a projectional, or a HYBRID approach? Will an echoplanar approach (which allows almost real-time imaging) or spiral approach really make a difference? Will MR contrast agents be needed to better visualize certain lesions? Given that coronary MRA is not as good as the existing "gold standard," are there specific clinical problems where it would be good enough to be able to replace or complement conventional coronary angiography?

Several of these questions have since been answered. The first- and second-generation techniques have now reached a level of stability and commercial implementation such that most MR users can use them. The distinction between 2-D and 3-D techniques may no longer be so great because both approaches can benefit from second- and third-generation technical improvements (hybrid with navigator echoes and breathhold acquisi-

tions of thin-3-D slab). Magnetic resonance contrast agents do appear to have a major future role. The new targeted breathhold 3-D thin-slab techniques show great promise. Changes in technique development have been and continue to be so fast that there has been no time or interest for in-depth large-scale clinical testing of any of the coronary MRA techniques. The work by Meyer et al. (3) and others demonstrates in vivo visualization of the coronary artery vessel wall by magnetic resonance imaging (MRI), as shown in Figure 32.1.

Both the second- and third-generation improvements to coronary MRA techniques are still evolving (4–7). This and the use of contrast agents (8–10) may make coronary MRA an important component of a comprehensive MR-based noninvasive evaluation of patients with ischemic heart disease. Coronary flow reserve assessment by MRI can be added to the evaluation of anatomy. Such a combined noninvasive MR study of anatomy and flow may become the ultimate cost-effective coronary screening tool. Despite their current limitations, first- and second-generation MRA techniques can help in many clinical applications (e.g., in the identification of congenital coronary anatomy variants), and in the noninvasive follow up of patients who have undergone coronary angioplasty, coronary stent placement, or bypass grafting.

In the year 2000, cardiac-gated multislice computed tomography (CT) has emerged as a very serious competitor for both coronary electron-beam computed tomography (EB-CT) and coronary MRI/MRA. The jury is still out as to which imaging modality will ultimately prevail. This topic continues to be hotly debated at many cardiac imaging meetings (11,12).

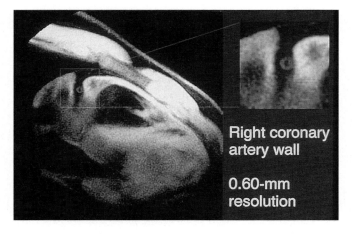

Figure 32.1. High-resolution imaging of the vessel wall of the right coronary artery using spiral coronary MRA. (From Craig-Meyers et al., Stanford University, 1998; with permission.)

References

1. Duerinckx AJ. Coronary MR angiography. *In*: Cardiac MR Imaging, Boxt LM, guest ed. MRI Clin North Am 1996;4(2): 361–418.
2. Duerinckx AJ. (Clinics) Coronary magnetic resonance angiography. Radiol Clin North Am 1999;37:273–318.
3. Meyer CH, Hu BS, Macovski A, Nishimura DG. Coronary vessel wall imaging (abstr.). *In*: Proceedings of the Sixth

Scientific Meeting of the International Society for Magnetic Resonance in Medicine (ISMRM), April 18–24, 1998 (paper #15). Sydney, Australia, 1998; 1: 15.

4. Wielopolski PA, van Geuns RJ, de Feyter PJ, Oudkerk M. Coronary arteries. Eur Radiol 1998;8(6):873–85.

5. Wielopolski P, vanGeuns RJ, deFeyter PJ, Oudkerk M. Breath-hold coronary MR angiography with volume targeted imaging. Radiology 1998;209:209–20.

6. Hardy CJ. Real-time cardiovascular MR imaging. *In*: Reiber JHC, vanderWall EE, eds. What's New in Cardio-Vascular Imaging? Dordrecht: Kluwer Academic Publishers, 1998:207–19.

7. Danias PG, Edelman RR, Manning WJ. Coronary MR angiography. Cardiol Clin 1998;16(2):207–25.

8. Li D, Dolan RP, Walovitch RC, Lauffer RB. Three-dimensional MRI of coronary arteries using an intravascular contrast agent. Magn Reson Med 1998;39(6):1014–18.

9. Johansson LO, Nolan NM, Taniuchi M, Fischer SE, Wick-line SA, Lorenz CH. High resolution magnetic resonance coronary angiography of the entire heart using a new blood-pool agent NC100150 injection: comparison with invasive x-ray angiography in pigs. J Cardiovasc Magn Reson 1999;2(1):139–44.

10. Goldfarb JW, Edelman RR. Coronary arteries: breath-hold, gadolinium-enhanced, three-dimensional MR angiography. Radiology 1998;206(3):830–34.

11. Book of Abstracts of the First International Workshop on Coronary MR & CT Angiography. Lyon, France, Oct 1–3, 2000. Organized and published by the North American Society for Cardiac Imaging. Reprinted in: Inter J Card Imag 2000;16:3:185–224.

12. Book of Abstracts of the Second International Workshop on Coronary MR & CT Angiography. Chicago, IL, Sept 29–Oct 2, 2001. Organized and published by the North American Society for Cardiac Imaging. Reprinted in: Inter J Card Imag 2001;17:5 (in press).

Index